PHYSICAL AGENTS IN REHABILITATION
From Research to Practice

evolve

To access your Instructor Resources, visit:

http://evolve.elsevier.com/Cameron/Physical

Evolve® Student Resources for **Cameron: Physical Agents in Rehabilitation,
3th Edition**, offers the following features:

- *Electrical Stimulation, Ultrasound, and Laser Light Handbook*
- **Application Techniques**
- **Glossary activities**
- **Figure-labeling exercises**
- **Interactive test questions**
- **Links to Medline**
- **Additional resource links**

PHYSICAL AGENTS IN REHABILITATION

From Research to Practice

Third Edition

Michelle Cameron, MD, PT, OCS
Oregon Health & Science University
Portland, Oregon

SAUNDERS

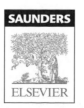

ELSEVIER

SAUNDERS
ELSEVIER

11830 Westline Industrial Drive
St. Louis, Missouri 63146

PHYSICAL AGENTS IN REHABILITATION: FROM   ISBN-13: 978-1-4160-3257-1
RESEARCH TO PRACTICE   ISBN-10:   1-4160-3257–1

Notice

Knowledge and best practice in this field are constantly changing. As new research and experience broaden our knowledge, changes in practice, treatment and drug therapy may become necessary or appropriate. Readers are advised to check the most current information provided (i) on procedures featured or (ii) by the manufacturer of each product to be administered, to verify the recommended dose or formula, the method and duration of administration, and contraindications. It is the responsibility of the practitioner, relying on their own experience and knowledge of the patient, to make diagnoses, to determine dosages and the best treatment for each individual patient, and to take all appropriate safety precautions. To the fullest extent of the law, neither the Publisher nor the [Editors/Authors] assumes any liability for any injury and/or damage to persons or property arising out or related to any use of the material contained in this book.

The Publisher

Library of Congress Control Number: 2007939521

ISBN-13: 978-1-4160-3257-1
ISBN-10: 1-4160-3257-1

Publisher: Linda Duncan
Senior Editor: Kathy Falk
Developmental Editor: Megan Fennell
Publishing Services Manager: Julie Eddy
Senior Project Manager: Celeste Clingan
Design Direction: Kim Denando

Printed in China

Last digit is the print number: 9 8 7 6 5 4 3 2

DEDICATION

*This book is dedicated to my friends, and especially my partner
Roland Brady, whose support, encouragement, and patience kept me going
through the ups and downs of this endeavor.*

BIOGRAPHY

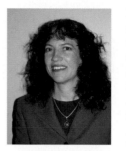 Michelle H. Cameron, MD, PT, OCS, is the owner of Health Potentials, a health education and consulting company. She is a physical therapist and physician, a teacher, researcher, and author and the primary author of this book, *Physical Agents in Rehabilitation: From Research to Practice*. Michelle also recently co-edited a new text, *Physical Rehabilitation: Physical Rehabilitation: Evidence-Based Examination, Evaluation, and Intervention*. In addition, her research on phonophoresis is published in Physical Therapy, the Journal of the American Physical Therapy Association, and in Clinical Management magazine, and earned her the California APTA Clinician Research Award. Michelle has written and edited many articles on electrical stimulation, ultrasound and phonophoresis, laser light therapy and wound management, and wrote the section on ultrasound in Saunders' *Manual for Physical Therapy Practice*. Michelle's discussions of physical agents bring together current research and practice to provide the decision-making and hands-on tools to support optimal care within today's health care environment.

ACKNOWLEDGMENTS

First and foremost, I want to thank the readers and purchasers of the previous editions of this book. Without you, this book would not exist. In particular, I would like to thank those readers who took the time to contact me with their comments, thoughts, and suggestions about what worked for them and what could be improved.

I would also like to give special thanks to: Amy Sutkus, Research Assistant, for her help with updating this edition of the book, and particularly for her attention to detail, organization, reliability and insight; Megan Fennell, Associate Developmental Editor at Elsevier, for her consistent support throughout this project; Diane Allen, Linda Monroe, Sara Shapiro and Gail Widener, contributing authors to this and previous editions, who updated their respective chapters thoroughly and promptly; Stephen Campbell for his comments and help with updating Chapter 2; David Sibell for his comments and help with updating Chapter 3; Naomi Kall for her comments on the paraffin bath section of Chapter 6; Michelle Pinard for her comments and help with updating Chapter 8; Chris Durall, Ginny Gibson, Rose Hamm, Kevin Helgeson, Lori Quinn, Vince Lepak and Diane Allen who reviewed this book in its entirety at the beginning of this process and offered comments.

Thank you also to those who provided photos and pictures for illustrations, space and equipment for photos to be taken, and helped smooth the way through the myriad of details that add up to a book.

Thank you all,
Michelle H. Cameron

CONTRIBUTORS

Diane D. Allen, PhD, PT
Adjunct Assistant Professor
Samuel Merritt College
Oakland, California
Physical Therapist
Interim Health Care
San Jose, California

Linda G. Monroe, MPT, OCS
Physical Therapist
Lafayette, California

Julie A. Pryde, MS, PA-C, PT, OCS, SCS, ATC, CSCS
Adjunct Assistant Professor
Samuel Merritt College
Oakland, California
Physician Assistant
Muir Orthopaedic Specialists
Walnut Creek, California

Sara Shapiro, MPH, PT
Assistant Clinical Professor
University of California San Francisco
San Francisco, California
Owner
Apex Wellness & Physical Therapy
San Francisco, California

Gail L. Widener, PhD, PT
Associate Professor
Samuel Merritt College
Oakland, California

REVIEWERS

Diane D. Allen, PhD, PT
Adjunct Assistant Professor
Samuel Merritt College
Oakland, California
Physical Therapist
Interim Health Care
San Jose, California

Stephen Campbell, MD
Salem Hospital
West Linn, Oregon

Christopher J. Durall, DPT, PT, MS, SCS, LAT, CSCS
Senior Clinical Physical Therapist
Student Health Center
University of Wisconsin—LaCrosse
LaCrosse, Wisconsin

Ginny Gibson, MS, OTR/L, CHT
Assistant Professor
Department of Occupational Therapy
Samuel Merritt College
Oakland, California

Rose Little Hamm, DPT, PT, CWS, FCCWS
Assistant Professor of Clinical Physical
  Therapy
Department of Biokinesiology and Physical
  Therapy
University of Southern California
Los Angeles, California

Kevin Helgeson, DHSc, PT, SCS
Assistant Professor
Department of Physical and Occupational
  Therapy
Idaho State University
Pocatello, Idaho

Naomi Kall
Marketing Manager
The Hygenic Corporation
Akron, Ohio

Michelle Pinard
VQ Orthocare
Irvine, California

Lori Quinn, EdD, PT
Clinical Faculty Associate
Program in Physical Therapy
New York Medical College
Valhalla, New York

Dave Sibell, MD
Associate Professor
Department of Anesthesiology &
  Perioperative Medicine
Oregon Health & Science University
Portland, Oregon

PREFACE

In writing the first edition of this book I tried to meet a need that I believed existed—the need for a book on the use of physical agents in rehabilitation that covered the breadth and depth of this material in a readily accessible and easy to understand manner. I put together a text that leads the reader from the basic scientific and physiological principles underlying the application of physical agents to the research evaluating their clinical use and then to the practical details of selecting and applying each specific physical agent to optimize patient outcome. The enthusiasm with which the first and second editions of this book were received—including complimentary comments, adoption by many educational programs, and purchase by many clinicians—shows that the need was there and was met.

In this new edition I have done my best to keep the best of previous editions while bringing the reader new and updated information and further clarifying the presented material. This book has always provided easy-to-follow guidelines for safe application of all physical agents. It has also provided the essential scientific rationale and evidence-base to select and apply interventions with physical agents safely and effectively. As the quantity of research has increased, along with the quality, this text has become even more important for making clinical decisions. To keep up with the pace of research and new developments in the field of rehabilitation, I have added a number of new features to this edition.

In previous editions, the topic of laser and light therapy was covered briefly within a chapter on electromagnetic agents. In this edition, a complete chapter on laser and light therapy was added because, since the initial FDA clearance of a laser therapy device in 2002, laser and light therapy has grown in popularity and become an essential tool for many clinicians. This edition now includes a full discussion of the principles underlying laser and light therapy, the indications and contraindications for this intervention, clinical application guidelines, and clinical case studies.

The second biggest change in this new edition is the addition of color. The art from the previous edition is now presented in full-color to enhance the quality of the figures and the overall design. **Clinical Pearls** were added to all chapters to emphasize important clinical points. The **Case Studies** were enhanced to include an ICF model evaluation at the level of body structure and function, activity, and participation. The Case Studies also include sections on documentation with a sample progress note in SOAP note format.

In response to reviewers' and readers' requests, a **Glossary** of useful terms and concepts is now included in every chapter. The terms are in bold within the text and the Glossary appears at the end of the chapter. To enhance learning, vocabulary-building activities based on these glossaries are also included on the updated Evolve website (http://evolve.elsevier.com/Cameron/physical).

The **Evolve** site also underwent other major changes. There are boards-style practice test questions, figure-labeling activities, links to Medline from the textbook reference lists, and additional resource links. For instructors, the Evolve site has all of the student resources as well as lab activities for all the physical agent chapters based on chapter content (including competency checklists) and an electronic image collection that includes all figures from the textbook ready for use in PowerPoint presentations. Also, PDF versions of the glossaries, case studies, application techniques, and the **Electrical Stimulation, Ultrasound, and Laser Light Handbook** are available on Evolve for readers to create and print custom study or clinical quick-reference guides.

CONTENTS

Chapter 1

Introduction to Physical Agents and How They Are Used

This book is intended primarily as a course text for those learning to use **physical agents** in **rehabilitation**. It was written to meet the needs of students learning about the theory and practice of applying physical agents and to assist practicing rehabilitation professionals in reviewing and updating their knowledge about the use of physical agents. This book describes the effects of physical agents, gives guidelines on when and how physical agents can be most effectively and safely applied, and describes the outcomes that can be expected from integrating physical agents within a program of rehabilitation. The book covers the theory underlying the application of each agent and the research concerning its effects, providing a rationale for the treatment recommendations. There is also information on the physiological processes influenced by physical agents. After reading this book, the reader will be able to integrate the ideal physical agent(s) and intervention parameters within a complete rehabilitation program to promote optimal patient outcome.

This book's recommendations regarding the clinical use of physical agents integrate concepts from a variety of sources. Specific recommendations are derived from the best available research-based evidence on the physiologic effects and clinical outcomes of applying physical agents to patients. The World Health Organization's (WHO) International Classification for Functioning, Disability, and Health (ICF) model is used to consider and describe the impact of physical agent interventions on patient outcomes. This model was developed in 2001, as an approach to describing functional abilities and differences and has been adopted globally, particularly among rehabilitation professionals.[1] Additionally, the American Physical Therapy Association's Guide to Physical Therapist Practice, 2nd edition (the Guide) is widely used by physical therapists to categorize patients according to preferred practice patterns.[2] These patterns include typical findings and descriptive norms of types and ranges of interventions for conditions in each pattern.

After this introductory chapter, the book is divided into two sections. The first section discusses typical musculoskeletal and neuromuscular problems that may be addressed by the use of physical agents. The second section describes the physical properties, physiologic effects, and application techniques for the types of physical agents currently available.

An appendix added to this edition includes a full-color version of the Electrical Stimulation, Ultrasound, and Laser Light Handbook. The handbook is now also available on the accompanying Evolve site along with boards-style examination questions, figure exercises, links to Medline for all the cited journal references, glossary activities, and links to additional resources. PDF versions of the chapter glossaries, case studies, application techniques, and the handbook are also available for use as custom quick-reference or study guides. The instructor's site includes structured lab activities and downloadable copies of all the figures in the book for use in power-point presentations.

WHAT ARE PHYSICAL AGENTS?

Physical agents are energy and materials applied to patients to assist in rehabilitation. Physical agents include heat, cold, water, pressure, sound, electromagnetic radiation, and electrical currents. The term physical agent can be used to describe the general type of energy, such as electromagnetic radiation or sound; a specific range within the general type, such as **ultraviolet (UV) radiation** or **ultrasound**; and the actual means of applying the energy, such as an UV lamp or an ultrasound transducer. The terms **physical modality**, physical agent modality, and **modality** are also frequently used in place of the term physical agent and are used interchangeably in this book.

CATEGORIES OF PHYSICAL AGENTS

Physical agents can be categorized as thermal, mechanical, or electromagnetic (Table 1-1). **Thermal agents** include deep-heating agents, superficial heating agents, and superficial cooling agents. **Mechanical agents** include **traction**, **compression**, water, and sound. **Electromagnetic agents** include electromagnetic fields and electrical currents. Some physical agents fall into more than one category. Water and ultrasound, for example, can have mechanical and thermal effects.

THERMAL AGENTS

Thermal agents transfer energy to a patient to produce an increase or decrease in tissue temperature. Examples of thermal agents include hot packs, ice packs, ultrasound, whirlpool, and **diathermy**. **Cryotherapy** is the therapeutic application of cold, whereas **thermotherapy** is the therapeutic application of heat. Depending on the thermal agent and the body part to which it is applied, temperature changes may be superficial or deep and may affect one type of tissue more than another. For example, a hot pack produces the greatest temperature increase in superficial tissues with high thermal conductivity in the area directly below it. In contrast, ultrasound produces heat in deeper tissues and produces the most heat in tissues with high ultrasound absorption coefficients such as tendon and bone. Diathermy, which involves the application of shortwave or microwave electromagnetic energy, heats deep tissues with high electrical conductivity.

Thermotherapy is used to increase circulation, metabolic rate, and soft tissue extensibility or to decrease **pain**. Cryotherapy is applied to decrease circulation, metabolic

rate, or pain. A full discussion of the principles underlying the processes of heat transfer, the methods of heat transfer used in rehabilitation, and the effects, **indications**, and **contraindications** for applying superficial heating and cooling agents is provided in Chapter 6. The principles and practice of applying deep heating agents are discussed in Chapter 7 in the section on thermal applications of ultrasound and in Chapter 14 in the section on diathermy.

Ultrasound is a physical agent that has both thermal and nonthermal effects. Ultrasound is defined as sound with a frequency of greater than 20,000 cycles/second. It cannot be heard by humans because of its high frequency. Ultrasound is a mechanical form of energy composed of alternating waves of compression and rarefaction. Thermal effects, including increased deep and superficial tissue temperature, are produced by continuous ultrasound waves of a sufficient intensity, and nonthermal effects are produced by both continuous and **pulsed ultrasound**. Continuous ultrasound is used to heat deep tissues to increase circulation, metabolic rate, and soft tissue extensibility and decrease pain. Pulsed ultrasound is used to facilitate tissue healing or promote transdermal drug penetration by nonthermal mechanisms. Further information on the theory and practice of applying ultrasound can be found in Chapter 7.

MECHANICAL AGENTS

Mechanical agents apply force to increase or decrease pressure on the body. Examples of mechanical agents include water, traction, compression, and sound. Water can provide resistance, hydrostatic pressure, and buoyancy for exercise or apply pressure to clean open wounds. Traction decreases the pressure between structures, and compression increases the pressure on and between structures. Ultrasound is discussed in the previous section.

The therapeutic use of water is called **hydrotherapy**. Water can be applied with or without immersion. Immersion in water increases the pressure around the immersed area, provides buoyancy, and if there is a difference in temperature between the area and the water, transfers heat to or from the area. Movement of the water produces local pressure that can be used as resistance for exercise when an area is immersed and for cleansing or debriding open wounds with or without immersion. Further information on the theory and practice of hydrotherapy is provided in Chapter 9.

Traction is most commonly used to alleviate pressure on structures such as nerves or joints that produce pain or other sensory changes or that become inflamed when compressed. Traction can normalize sensation and prevent or reduce damage or **inflammation** of compressed structures. The pressure-relieving effects of traction may be temporary or permanent, depending on the nature of the underlying **pathology** and the force, duration, and means of traction application used. Further information on the theory and practice of applying traction is provided in Chapter 10.

Compression is used to counteract fluid pressure and control or reverse edema. The force, duration, and means of applying compression can be varied to control the mag-

TABLE 1-1	Categories of Physical Agents	
Category	**Types**	**Clinical Examples**
Thermal	Deep heating agents	Ultrasound, diathermy
	Superficial heating agents	Hot pack
	Cooling agents	Ice pack
Mechanical	Traction	Mechanical traction
	Compression	Elastic bandage, stockings
	Water	Whirlpool
	Sound	Ultrasound
Electromagnetic	Electromagnetic fields	Ultraviolet, laser
	Electric currents	TENS

TENS, Transelectrical nerve stimulation.

nitude of the effect and to accommodate different patient needs. Further information on the theory and practice of applying compression is provided in Chapter 11.

ELECTROMAGNETIC AGENTS

Electromagnetic agents apply energy in the form of electromagnetic radiation or an electrical current. Examples of electromagnetic agents include UV radiation, **infrared (IR) radiation**, **laser**, diathermy, and electrical current. Variation of the frequency and intensity of electromagnetic radiation changes its effects and depth of penetration. For example, UV radiation, which has a frequency of 7.5×10^{14} to 10^{15} cycles/second, produces erythema and tanning of the skin but does not produce heat, whereas IR radiation, which has a frequency of 10^{11} to 10^{14} cycles/second, produces heat only in superficial tissues. Lasers output monochromatic, coherent, directional electromagnetic radiation that is generally in the frequency range of visible light or IR radiation. Continuous shortwave diathermy, which has a frequency of 10^5 to 10^6 cycles/second, produces heat in both superficial and deep tissues. When shortwave diathermy is pulsed (**pulsed shortwave diathermy** [PSWD]) to provide a low average intensity of energy, it does not produce heat; however, the electromagnetic energy is thought to modify cell membrane permeability and cell function by nonthermal mechanisms and may thus control pain and edema. These agents are thought to facilitate healing via biostimulative effects on cells. Further information on the theory and practice of applying electromagnetic radiation and on lasers and other forms of light is provided in Chapter 12. UV radiation and diathermy are discussed in Chapters 13 and 14 respectively.

Electrical stimulation (ES) is the use of electrical current to induce muscle contraction (motor-level ES) and changes in sensation (sensory-level ES), reduce edema, or accelerate tissue healing. The effects and clinical applications of electrical currents vary according to the waveform, intensity, duration, and direction of the current flow and according to the type of tissue to which the current is applied. Electrical currents of sufficient intensity and duration can depolarize nerves, causing sensory or motor responses that may be used to control pain or increase muscle strength and control. Electrical currents with an appropriate direction of flow can also attract or repel charged particles and alter cell membrane permeability to control the formation of edema, promote tissue healing, and facilitate transdermal drug penetration. Further information on the theory and practice of electrical current application is provided in Chapter 8.

HISTORY OF PHYSICAL AGENTS IN MEDICINE AND REHABILITATION

Physical agents have been a component of medical and rehabilitation treatment for many centuries and are used across a wide variety of cultures. Ancient Romans and Greeks used heat and water to maintain health and to treat various musculoskeletal and respiratory problems, as evidenced by the remains of ancient bath houses with steam rooms and pools of hot and cold water still present in many major Roman and Greek cities.[3] The health benefits of soaking and exercising in hot water regained popularity centuries later with the advent of health spas in Europe in the late 19th century in areas of natural hot springs. Today, the practices of soaking and exercising in water continue to be popular throughout the world because water provides resistance and buoyancy, allowing the development of strength and endurance while reducing weight bearing on compression-sensitive joints.

Other historic applications of physical agents include the use of electrical torpedo fish in approximately 400 BCE to treat headaches and arthritis by applying electrical shocks to the head and feet. Amber was used in the 17th century to generate static electricity for the treatment of skin diseases, inflammation, and hemorrhage.[4] There are also reports from the 17th century of charged gold leaf being used to prevent scarring from smallpox lesions.[5]

Before the widespread availability of antibiotics and effective analgesic and antiinflammatory drugs, physical agents were commonly used to treat infection, pain, and inflammation. Sunlight was used for the treatment of tuberculosis, bone and joint diseases, as well as dermatological disorders and infections. Warm Epsom salt baths were used for the treatment of sore or swollen limbs.

Although physical agents have been used for their therapeutic benefits throughout history, over time, new uses, applications, and agents have been developed and certain agents and applications have fallen out of favor. New uses of physical agents have developed as a result of increased understanding of the biological processes underlying disease, dysfunction, and recovery and in response to the availability of advanced technology. For example, the use of **transcutaneous electrical nerve stimulation** (TENS) for the treatment of pain was developed based on the **gate control theory of pain modulation**, as proposed by Melzack and Wall.[6] The gate control theory states that that nonpainful stimuli can inhibit the transmission of pain at the spinal cord level. The various modes of TENS application now available are primarily the result of the recent development of electrical current generators that allow fine control of the applied electrical current.

Physical agents usually fall out of favor because the intervention is ineffective or because more effective interventions are developed. For example, IR lamps were commonly used to treat open wounds because the superficial heat they provide can dry out the wound bed; however, these lamps are no longer used for this application because we now know that wounds heal more rapidly when kept moist.[7,8] During the early years of the 20th century, sunlight was used to treat tuberculosis; however, since the advent of antibiotics, which are generally effective in eliminating bacterial infections, physical agents are now rarely used to treat tuberculosis or other infectious diseases.

A number of physical agents have waned in popularity because they are cumbersome, have excessive associated risks, or interfere with other aspects of treatment. For example, the use of diathermy as a deep-heating agent was very popular 20 to 30 years ago, but because the machines are large and awkward to move around, can easily burn patients if not used appropriately, and can interfere with

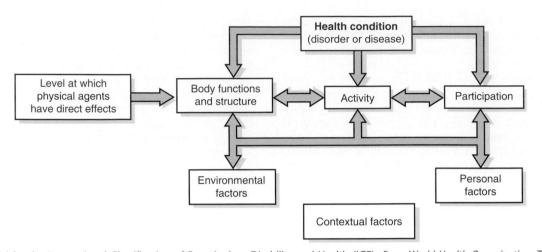

FIG 1-1 Model for the International Classification of Functioning, Disability and Health (ICF). *From World Health Organization*: Towards a Common Language for Functioning, Disability, and Health: International Classification of Functioning, Disability and Health (ICF), *Geneva, 2002, WHO.*

the functioning of computer-controlled equipment nearby, diathermy is not commonly used today in the United States (US). However, diathermy is covered is this book because it is used in some practices and falls within the scope of physical therapist practice.

This book focuses on the physical agents most commonly used in the US today. Physical agents that are not commonly used in the US but were popular in the recent past and those that are popular abroad or expected to come back into favor as new delivery systems and applications are developed are covered more briefly. The popularity of particular physical agents is based on their history of clinical use and in most cases, research data supporting their efficacy; however, in some cases, their clinical application has continued despite lacking or limited supporting evidence. More research is needed to clarify which interventions and patient characteristics provide optimal results. Further study is also needed to determine precisely what outcomes should be expected from the application of physical agents in rehabilitation.

APPROACHES TO REHABILITATION

Rehabilitation is a goal-oriented intervention designed to maximize independence in individuals who have compromised function. Function is usually compromised by some underlying pathology and secondary **impairments** and is affected by environmental and personal factors. Compromised function may lead to **disability**. Rehabilitation generally addresses the sequelae of pathology to maximize a patient's function and ability to participate in usual activities, rather than being directed at resolving the pathology itself, and should take into consideration the environmental and personal factors affecting each patient's individual activity and participation limitations and goals.

A number of classification schemes exist to categorize the sequelae of pathology. In 1980, WHO published the first classification scheme for the consequences of diseases, known as the International Classification of Impairments, Disabilities and Handicaps (ICIDH).[9] This scheme, based

primarily on the work of Wood, is based on a linear model in which the sequelae of pathology or disease are impairments that lead to disabilities and handicaps.[10,11] Impairment is characterized as an abnormality of structure or function of body or organ, including mental function. Disability is characterized as a restriction of activities resulting from an impairment, and handicap is the social level of the consequences of diseases characterized as the individual's disadvantage resulting from impairment or disability. Shortly after the **ICIDH model** was published, Nagi developed a similar model that classified the sequelae of pathology as impairments, **functional limitations**, and disabilities.[12] He defined impairments as alterations in anatomical, physiological, or psychological structures or functions that result from an underlying pathology. In the **Nagi model**, functional limitations were defined as restrictions in the ability to perform an activity in an efficient, typically expected, or competent manner and disabilities were defined as the inability to perform activities required for self-care, home, work, or community roles.

Over the years, the WHO has worked to update the ICIDH model to reflect and create changes in perceptions of people with disabilities and to meet the needs of different groups of individuals. In 2001 the WHO published the ICIDH-2, also known as the International Classification of Functioning, Disability and Health (ICF) (Fig. 1-1).[1] In contrast to the earlier linear model, the **ICF model** views functioning and disability as a complex dynamic interaction between the health condition of the individual and the contextual factors of the environment, as well as personal factors. It is applicable to all people, whatever their health condition. The language of the ICF is neutral to etiology, placing the emphasis on function rather than condition or disease. It is also designed to be relevant across cultures, as well as age groups and genders, making it appropriate for heterogeneous populations.

The original models were intended to differentiate disease and pathology from the limitations they produced. These models were developed primarily for use by rehabilitation professionals. The new model has a more positive perspective on the changes associated with pathology and disease and is intended for use by a wide range of people, including community, national, and global institutions that create policy and allocate resources for persons with disabilities. Specifically, the ICF has tried to change the perspective of disability from the negative focus of "consequences of disease" used in the ICIDH to a more positive focus on "components of health." Thus the ICIDH used categories of impairments, disabilities, and handicaps to describe sequelae of pathology, whereas the ICF uses categories of health conditions, body functions, activities, and participation to focus on abilities rather than limitations.

This book uses the terminology and framework of the ICF model to evaluate clinical findings and determine a plan of care for the individuals described in the case studies. The ICF model reflects the interaction between health conditions and contextual factors as they affect disability and functioning. Health conditions include diseases, disorders, and injuries. Contextual factors include environmental and personal factors. Social attitudes and structures, legal structures, terrain, and climate are examples of environmental factors. Personal factors are those things that influence how disability is experienced by a person, such as gender, age, education, experience, and character. The ICF model is designed to be used in conjunction with the International Classification of Diseases (ICD), a classification used throughout the US health care system to document and code medical diagnoses.

The ICF model is structured around three levels of functioning: the body or a part of the body, the whole person, and the whole person in a social context.

> #### ◎ Clinical Pearl
>
> The ICF model considers the body, the whole person, and the person in society.

Dysfunction at any of these levels is called a disability and results in impairments (at the body level), activity limitations (at the whole person level), and participation restrictions (at the social level). For example, a person who suffers a stroke may be weak on one side of the body (an impairment). This impairment may cause difficulty with activities of daily living (activity limitation). The person may also be unable to attend social gatherings he or she once enjoyed (participation restriction).

The ICF resulted from combining medical and social models of disability. In the medical model, disability is the result of an underlying pathology, and to treat the disability one must treat the pathology. In the social model, disability is the result of the social environment, and to treat the disability, one must change the social environment to make it more accommodating.

Thus medical treatment is generally directed at the underlying pathology or disease, whereas rehabilitation focuses primarily on reversing or minimizing impair-

ments, activity limitations, and participation restrictions. Rehabilitation professionals must assess and set goals not only at the level of impairment, such as pain, decreased range of motion, or **hypertonicity** (increased **muscle tone**), but also at the level of activity and participation. These goals should include the patient's goals, such as being able to get out of bed, ride a bicycle, work, or compete in a marathon.

THE ROLE OF PHYSICAL AGENTS IN REHABILITATION

Physical agents are tools to be used when appropriate as components of rehabilitation. The American Physical Therapy Association's (APTA) position statement concerning the exclusive use of physical agents, published in 1995 and reiterated in 2005, states that "Without documentation which justifies the necessity of the exclusive use of physical agents/modalities, the use of physical agents/modalities, in the absence of other skilled therapeutic or educational interventions should not be considered physical therapy."[13] In other words, the APTA believes that the use of physical agents alone does not generally constitute physical therapy and that in most cases, physical agents should be applied in conjunction with other interventions.

> #### ◎ Clinical Pearl
>
> Physical agents are usually used with other interventions and not as the sole intervention.

The use of physical agents as a component of physical therapy involves the integration of appropriate interventions. This integration may include applying a physical agent or educating the patient in its application as part of a complete program to help patients achieve their activity and participation goals. However, since the aim of this text is to give clinicians a better understanding of the theory and appropriate application of physical agents, it focuses on the use of physical agents and describes other components of the rehabilitation program in less detail.

Physical agents have direct effects primarily at the level of impairment. These effects can promote improvements in activity and participation. For example, for a patient with pain that impairs motion, electrical currents can be used to stimulate sensory nerves to control pain and allow the patient to increase their motion and thus increase their activity, such as lifting objects, and their participation, such as returning to work. Physical agents can also increase the effectiveness of other interventions. They are used in conjunction with or in preparation for therapeutic exercise, functional training, and manual mobilization. For example, a hot pack may be applied before stretching to increase the extensibility of the superficial soft tissues and promote a more effective and safe increase in soft tissue length when the stretching force is applied.

EVALUATION AND PLANNING FOR THE USE OF PHYSICAL AGENTS

When considering the application of a physical agent, one should first check the physician's referral, if one is required, for a medical diagnosis of the patient's condition and any necessary **precautions**. Precautions are conditions under which a particular treatment should be applied with special care or limitations. The therapist's examination should include but not be limited to the patient's history, which would include information about the history of the current complaint, relevant medical history, and information about current and expected level of activity and participation; a review of systems; and specific tests and measures. The examination findings are then evaluated to establish a diagnosis, prognosis, and plan of care, including anticipated goals. Given an understanding of the effects of different physical agents, the clinician can assess whether intervention using a physical agent may help the patient progress toward the anticipated goals. The clinician can then determine the treatment plan, including the ideal physical agent(s) and intervention parameters if indicated. The plan may be modified as indicated through ongoing reexamination and reevaluation. The sequence of examination, evaluation, and intervention is followed in the case studies described in Part II of this book.

DOCUMENTATION

Documentation involves putting information into a patient's medical record, whether handwritten, dictated, or typed into a computer. The purposes of documentation include communicating the examination findings, evaluations, interventions, and plans to other health care professionals; serving as a long-term record; and supporting reimbursement for services provided.

Documentation of a patient encounter may follow any format but is usually done in the traditional SOAP note format to include the four components of subjective (S), objective (O), assessment (A), and plan (P).

◎ Clinical Pearl

Documentation generally follows the SOAP note format.

Within each component of the SOAP note, details vary depending on the patient's condition, patient assessment, and the interventions applied. In general, when documenting the use of a physical agent, information should be included on the physical agent used; the area of the body treated; and intervention duration, parameters, and outcomes, including progress toward goals; and regressions or complications arising from the application of the physical agent.

The following is an example of a SOAP note written after applying a hot pack to the lower back:

S: Pt reports low back pain and decreased sitting tolerance.
O: Pretreatment: Pain level 7/10. Forward and sidebending ROM restricted due to pain.

Intervention: Hot pack to low back, 20 minutes, pt prone, six layers of towels.
Posttreatment: Pain level 4/10. Sitting tolerance increased from 30 to 60 minutes.
A: Pain decreased, sitting tolerance increased, no side effects.
P: Continue use of hot pack as above before stretching. Continue exercise program.

Specific recommendations for SOAP note documentation and examples are given for all physical agents discussed in this book.

PRACTITIONERS USING PHYSICAL AGENTS

Physical therapists, physical therapy assistants, occupational therapists, occupational therapy assistants, athletic trainers, physiatrists, and patients all apply physical agents. Physical therapists commonly use physical agents and supervise physical therapy assistants in their use. As mentioned earlier, the APTA has made it clear that physical therapists use physical agents as part of a complete rehabilitation program. Training in physical agents is a required part of physical therapist and physical therapist assistant education and licensure.

Occupational therapists, especially those involved in hand therapy, also commonly use physical agents. In a position statement published in 2003, the American Occupational Therapy Association (AOTA) stated that "physical agent modalities may be used by occupational therapists and occupational therapy assistants as an adjunct to or in preparation for intervention that ultimately enhances engagement in occupation."[14] Physical therapy students receive training in physical agents as a required part of an academic physical therapy program, although occupational therapists do not always receive this training. The AOTA states that occupational therapists must be able to demonstrate competence to use physical agents in practice but provide no explicit guidelines for how this competence should be demonstrated. As a result, several states have instituted guidelines, licensing laws, specific educational requirements, and restrictions regarding physical agent use by occupational therapists and occupational therapist assistants. Occupational therapists and occupational therapist assistants must adhere to the regulations of the state(s) in which they practice.

The National Athletic Trainers' Association (NATA) states that training in therapeutic modalities is a required part of the curriculum to become a certified athletic trainer at accredited programs[15] and continuing education in physical modalities is required to maintain athletic trainer certification.[16]

Patients can learn about and apply physical agents to themselves, in addition to having them applied by these professionals. For example, agents, such as heat, cold, compression, and TENS, can be safely applied at home after the patient demonstrates proper use of the agent. Patient education has several advantages, including the option for more prolonged and frequent application, as well as decreased cost and increased convenience for the patient. Most importantly, it allows a patient to be an active participant in achieving therapeutic goals.

GENERAL CONTRAINDICATIONS AND PRECAUTIONS FOR PHYSICAL AGENT USE

Restrictions on the use of particular treatment interventions are categorized as contraindications or precautions. Contraindications are conditions under which a particular treatment should not be applied, and precautions are conditions under which a particular form of treatment should be applied with special care or limitations.[8] The terms absolute contraindications and relative contraindications can be used in place of contraindications and precautions, respectively.

Although the contraindications and precautions for the application of specific physical agents vary, a number of conditions are contraindications or precautions for the use of most physical agents. Therefore caution should be used when considering application of a physical agent to a patient with any of these conditions. In patients with such conditions, the nature of the restriction, the nature and distribution of the physiological effects of the physical agent, and the distribution of the energy produced by the physical agent must be considered.

CONTRAINDICATIONS

for Application of a Physical Agent

- Pregnancy
- Malignancy
- Pacemaker or other implanted electronic device
- Impaired sensation
- Impaired mentation

PREGNANCY

Pregnancy is generally a contraindication or precaution for the application of a physical agent if the energy produced by the agent or the physiological effects of the agent may reach the fetus. These restrictions apply because the influences of these types of energy on fetal development are usually not known and because fetal development is adversely affected by many influences, some of which are subtle.

MALIGNANCY

Malignancy is a contraindication or precaution for the application of physical agents if the energy produced by the agent or the physiological effects of the agent may reach malignant tissue or alter the circulation to such tissue. Some physical agents are known to accelerate the growth, or metastasis, of malignant tissue. These effects are thought to result from increased circulation or altered cellular function. Care must also be taken when considering treating any area of the body that currently has or previously had cancer cells because malignant tissue can metastasize and may therefore be present in areas where it has not yet been detected.

PACEMAKER OR OTHER IMPLANTED ELECTRONIC DEVICE

The use of physical agents is generally contraindicated when the energy of the agent can reach a pacemaker or any other implanted electronic device (e.g., deep brain stimulator, spinal cord stimulator) because the energy produced by some of these agents may alter the functioning of the device and thus adversely affect the patient.

IMPAIRED SENSATION AND MENTATION

Impaired sensation and mentation are contraindications or precautions for the use of many physical agents because the end limit for the application of these agents is the patient's report of how the intervention feels. For example, for most thermal agents, the patient's report of the sensation of heat as comfortable or painful is used as a guide to limit the intensity of the treatment. If the patient cannot feel heat or pain because of impaired sensation or cannot report this sensation accurately and consistently because of impaired mentation or other factors affecting the ability to communicate, the application of the treatment would not be safe and is therefore contraindicated.

Although these conditions indicate the need for caution with the use of most physical agents, the specific contraindications and precautions for the agent being considered and the patient situation must be evaluated before an intervention may be used or should be rejected. For example, although the application of ultrasound to a pregnant patient is contraindicated in any area where the ultrasound may reach the fetus, this physical agent may be applied to the distal extremities of a pregnant patient because ultrasound penetration is limited to the area close to the applicator. In contrast, it is recommended that diathermy not be applied to any part of a pregnant patient because the electromagnetic radiation produced by this type of agent reaches areas distant from the applicator. Specific contraindications and precautions, including questions to ask the patient and features to assess before the application of each physical agent, are provided in Part II of this book.

CHOOSING A PHYSICAL AGENT

Physical agents generally assist in rehabilitation by affecting inflammation and tissue healing, pain, muscle tone, or motion restrictions. Guidelines for intervention selection based on the direct effects of physical agents are presented here in narrative form and are summarized in Tables 1-2 to 1-5. If the patient presents with more than one problem and has numerous goals for treatment, a limited number of the goals may need to be addressed at any one time. It is generally recommended that the primary problems and those most likely to respond to the available interventions be addressed first; however, the ideal intervention will facilitate progress in a number of areas (Fig. 1-2). For example, if a patient has knee pain caused by acute joint inflammation, treatment should first be directed at resolving the inflammation; however, the ideal intervention would also help to relieve pain. When the primary underlying problem, such as arthritis, cannot benefit directly from an intervention with a physical agent, treatment with physical agents may still be used to help alleviate the sequelae of these problems, such as pain or swelling.

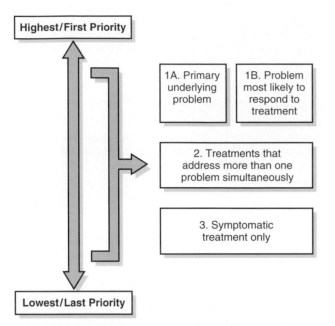

FIG 1-2 Prioritizing goals and effects of treatment.

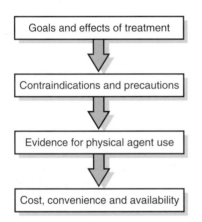

FIG 1-3 Attributes to be considered in the selection of physical agents.

ATTRIBUTES TO CONSIDER IN THE SELECTION OF PHYSICAL AGENTS

Given the variety of available physical agents and the unique characteristics of each patient, it is helpful to have a systematic approach to the selection of physical agents so that the ideal physical agent is applied in each situation (Fig. 1-3). The first consideration should be the goals of the intervention and the physiological effects required to reach these goals. If the patient has inflammation, pain, motion restrictions, or problems with muscle tone, the use of a physical agent may be appropriate. Looking at the effects of a particular physical agent on these conditions is the next step. Having determined which physical agents can promote progress toward the determined goals, the clinician should then decide which of the potentially effective interventions would be most appropriate for the particular patient and his or her current clinical presentation. Attending to the rule of "do no harm," all contrain-

dicated interventions should be rejected and all precautions should be adhered to. If a number of methods would be effective and could be applied safely, the evidence on the intervention, the ease and cost of application, and the availability of resources should also be considered. Having selected the physical agent(s), the clinician must then select the ideal treatment parameters and means of application and appropriately integrate the chosen physical agent(s) into a complete rehabilitation program.

Because physical agents have differing levels of associated risk, when all other factors are equal, those with a lower level of risk should be selected. Physical agents with a low level of associated risk have a potentially harmful dose that is difficult to achieve or is much greater than the effective therapeutic dose and have contraindications that are easy to detect. In contrast, physical agents with a high level of associated risk have an effective therapeutic dose that is close to the potentially harmful dose and have contraindications that are difficult to detect. For example, hot packs that are heated in hot water and used with sufficient insulation have a low associated risk because although they can heat superficial tissues to a therapeutic level in 15 to 20 minutes, they are unlikely to cause a burn if applied for a longer period because they start to cool as soon as they are removed from the hot water. In contrast, UV radiation has a high associated risk because a slight increase in the treatment duration, for example, from 5 to 10 minutes, or using the same treatment duration for patients with different skin sensitivity may change the effect of the treatment from a therapeutic level to a severe burn. Diathermy also has a high associated risk because it preferentially heats metal, which may have been previously undetected, and can burn tissue that is near any metal object(s) in the treatment field. It is generally recommended that agents with higher associated risk be used only if those with lower risks would not be as effective and that special care be taken to minimize these risks when these agents are used.

EFFECTS OF PHYSICAL AGENTS

The application of physical agents primarily results in modification of tissue inflammation and healing, relief of pain, alteration of **collagen** extensibility, or modification of muscle tone. A brief review of these processes follows; more complete discussions of these processes are provided in Chapters 2 through 5. A brief discussion of physical agents that modify each of these conditions is included here, and the chapters in Part II of this book cover each physical agent in detail.

INFLAMMATION AND HEALING

When tissue is damaged, it usually responds predictably. Inflammation is the first phase of recovery, followed by the proliferation and maturation phases. Modifying this healing process can accelerate rehabilitation and reduce adverse effects, such as prolonged inflammation, pain, and disuse. This in turn leads to improved patient function and more rapid achievement of therapeutic goals.

Thermal agents modify inflammation and healing by changing the rates of circulation and chemical reactions. Mechanical agents control motion and alter fluid flow,

TABLE 1-2	Physical Agents for Promoting Tissue Healing		
Stage of Tissue Healing	**Goals of Treatment**	**Effective Agents**	**Contraindicated Agents**
Initial injury	Prevent further injury or bleeding	Static compression, cryotherapy	Exercise Intermittent traction Motor-level ES Thermotherapy
	Clean open wound	Hydrotherapy (immersion or nonimmersion)	
Chronic inflammation	Prevent/decrease joint stiffness	Thermotherapy Motor ES Whirlpool Fluidotherapy	Cryotherapy
	Control pain	Thermotherapy ES Laser	Cryotherapy
	Increase circulation	Thermotherapy ES Compression Hydrotherapy (immersion or exercise)	
	Progress to proliferation stage	Pulsed ultrasound ES PSWD	
Remodeling	Regain or maintain strength	Motor ES Water exercise	Immobilization
	Regain or maintain flexibility	Thermotherapy	Immobilization
	Control scar tissue formation	Brief ice massage Compression	

ES, Electrical stimulation; *PSWD,* pulsed shortwave diathermy.

and electromagnetic agents alter cell function, particularly membrane permeability and transport. Many physical agents affect inflammation and healing and, when appropriately applied, can accelerate progress, limit adverse consequences of the healing process, and optimize the final patient outcome (see Table 1-2). However, when poorly selected or misapplied, physical agents may impair or potentially prevent complete healing.

During the inflammation phase of healing, which generally lasts for 1 to 6 days, the cells that remove debris and limit bleeding enter the traumatized area. The **inflammatory phase** is characterized by heat, swelling, pain, redness, and loss of function. The more quickly this phase is completed and resolved, the more quickly healing can proceed and the lower the probability of joint destruction, excessive pain, swelling, weakness, immobilization, and loss of function. Physical agents generally assist during the inflammation phase by reducing circulation, reducing pain, reducing enzyme activity rate, controlling motion, and promoting progression to the **proliferative phase** of healing.

During the proliferation phase, which generally starts within the first 3 days after injury and lasts for approximately 20 days, collagen is deposited in the damaged area to replace tissue that was destroyed by the trauma. In addition, if necessary, myofibroblasts contract to accelerate closure, and epithelial cells migrate to resurface the wound. Physical agents generally assist during the proliferation phase of healing by increasing circulation and enzyme activity rate and promoting collagen deposition and progression to the remodeling phase of healing.

During the **maturation phase**, which usually starts approximately 9 days after the initial injury and can last

for up to 2 years, both deposition and resorption of collagen occur. The new tissue remodels itself to resemble the original tissue as closely as possible to best serve its original function. During this phase, the healing tissue changes both in shape and structure to allow for optimal functional recovery. The shape conforms more closely to the original tissue, often decreasing in size from the proliferation phase, and the structure becomes more organized. Thus greater strength is achieved with no change in tissue mass. Physical agents generally assist during the remodeling phase of healing by altering the balance of collagen deposition and resorption and improving the alignment of the new collagen fibers.

Physical Agents for Tissue Healing

The stage of tissue healing determines the goals of intervention and the physical agents to be used. The following discussion is summarized in Table 1-2.

Initial Injury. Immediately after an injury or trauma, the goals of intervention are to prevent further injury or bleeding and to clean away wound contaminants if the skin has been broken. Immobilization and support of the injured area with a static compression device, such as an elastic wrap, a cast, or a brace, or reduction of stress on the area by use of assistive devices, such as crutches, can limit further injury and bleeding. Motion of the injured area, whether active, electrically stimulated, or passive, is contraindicated at this stage because this can lead to further tissue damage and bleeding. Cryotherapy will contribute to the control of bleeding by limiting blood flow to the injured area through vasoconstriction and increased blood viscosity.[17,18] Thermotherapy is contraindicated at this early stage because it can increase bleeding at the site of injury by increasing blood flow or reopening vascular lesions because of vasodilation.[19-21] Hydrotherapy, involving immersion or nonimmersion techniques, can be used to cleanse the injured area if the skin has been broken and the wound has become contaminated; however, because thermotherapy is contraindicated, only neutral warmth or cooler water should be used.[22]

Acute Inflammation. During the acute inflammatory stage of healing, the goals of intervention are to control pain, edema, bleeding, and the release and activity of inflammatory mediators and to facilitate progression to the proliferation stage. A number of physical agents, including cryotherapy, hydrotherapy, ES, and PSWD, can be used to control pain; however, the use of thermotherapy, intermittent traction, and motor-level ES is not appropriate.[23-27] Thermotherapy is not recommended because it causes vasodilation, which may aggravate edema, and it increases the metabolic rate, which may increase the inflammatory response. Intermittent traction and motor-level ES should be used with caution because the movement produced by these physical agents may cause further tissue irritation and thereby aggravate the inflammatory response. A number of physical agents, including cryotherapy, compression, sensory-level ES, PSWD, and **contrast bath**, may be used to control or reduce edema.[28-31] Cryotherapy and compression can also help to control bleeding; furthermore, cryotherapy will inhibit the activity and release of inflammatory mediators. If healing is delayed because of the inhibition of inflammation, which may occur in the patient who is on high-dose catabolic corticosteroids, cryotherapy should not be used because it may further impair the process of inflammation and thus potentially delay tissue healing. There is some evidence to indicate that pulsed ultrasound, laser light, and PSWD may promote progression from the inflammation stage of healing to the proliferation stage.[32-34]

Chronic Inflammation. If the inflammatory response persists and become chronic, the goals and thus the selection of interventions will change. During this stage of healing, the goals of treatment are to prevent or decrease joint stiffness, control pain, increase circulation, and promote progression to the proliferation stage. The most effective interventions for reducing joint stiffness are thermotherapy and motion.[35,36] Superficial structures, such as the skin and subcutaneous fascia, may be heated by superficial heating agents, for example, hot packs or **paraffin**, which is a waxy substance that can be warmed and used to coat the extremities for thermotherapy. However, to heat deeper structures, such as the shoulder or hip joint capsules, deep-heating agents, such as ultrasound or diathermy, must be used.[37-39] Motion may be produced by active exercise or ES, and motion can be combined with heat by having the patient exercise in warm water or **fluidotherapy**. Thermotherapy and ES can be used to relieve pain during the chronic inflammatory stage;

however, cryotherapy is generally not recommended during this stage because it can increase the joint stiffness frequently associated with chronic inflammation. Selection between thermotherapy and ES will generally depend on the need for the additional benefits of each modality and the other selection factors discussed later. Circulation may be increased by the use of thermotherapy, ES, compression, water immersion or exercise, and possibly by the use of contrast baths.[19,40-44] A final goal of treatment at the chronic inflammatory phase of tissue healing is to promote progression to the proliferation phase. Some studies indicate that pulsed ultrasound, electrical currents, and electromagnetic fields may promote this transition.

Proliferation. Once the injured tissue moves beyond the inflammation stage to the proliferation stage of healing, the primary goals of intervention become controlling scar tissue formation, ensuring adequate circulation, maintaining strength and flexibility, and promoting progression to the remodeling stage. Static compression garments can control superficial scar tissue formation, promoting enhanced cosmesis and reducing the severity and incidence of contractures.[45-47] Adequate circulation is required to provide oxygen and nutrients to the newly forming tissue. Circulation may be enhanced by the use of thermotherapy, electrotherapy, compression, water immersion or exercise, and possibly by the use of contrast baths. Although active exercise can increase or maintain strength and flexibility during the proliferation stage of healing, the addition of motor-level ES or water exercise may accelerate recovery and provide additional benefits. The water environment reduces loading and thus the potential for trauma to weight-bearing structures and may thereby decrease the risk of regression to the inflammatory stage.[48] The support provided by the water may also assist motion should the muscles be very weak, and water-based exercise and thermotherapy may promote circulation and help to maintain or increase flexibility.[49,50]

Maturation. During the final stage of tissue healing, maturation, the goals of intervention are to regain or maintain strength and flexibility and to control scar tissue formation. At this point in the healing process, the injured tissues are approaching their final form. The focus of treatment should therefore be on reversing any adverse effects of the earlier stages of healing, such as weakening of muscles or loss of flexibility. Strengthening and stretching exercises most effectively address these problems. Strengthening may be more effective with the addition of motor-level ES or water exercise, whereas stretching may be more effective with the prior application of thermotherapy or brief ice massage.[35,51] If the injury be is the type particularly prone to excessive scar formation, such as a burn, control of scar formation with compression garments should be continued throughout the remodeling stage.

PAIN

Pain is an unpleasant sensory and emotional experience associated with actual or threatened tissue damage. Pain usually protects individuals by preventing them from performing activities that would cause tissue damage; however, it may also interfere with normal activities and cause functional limitation and disability. For example, pain can interfere with sleep, work, or exercise. Relieving pain can allow patients to participate more fully in normal activities of daily living and may accelerate the initiation of an active rehabilitation program, thereby limiting the adverse consequences of disuse and allowing more rapid progress toward the patient's functional goals.

Pain may be the result of an underlying pathology, such as joint inflammation or pressure on a nerve, that is in the process of resolution or by a pathology, such as a malignancy, that is not expected to fully resolve. In either circumstance, relieving pain may improve the patient's level of activity and participation. The use of pain-relieving interventions, including physical agents, may be continued as long as pain persists and should be discontinued when the pain resolves.

Physical agents can control pain by modifying pain transmission or perception or by changing the underlying process causing the sensation. Physical agents may act by modulating transmission at the spinal cord level, changing the rate of nerve conduction, or altering the central or peripheral release of neurotransmitters. Physical agents can change the processes that cause pain by modifying tissue inflammation and healing, altering collagen extensibility, or modifying muscle tone. The processes of pain perception and pain control are explained in greater detail in Chapter 3.

Physical Agents for Pain Modulation

The choice of a physical agent for treating pain depends on the type and etiology of the pain. Physical agents used for pain are summarized in Table 1-3.

Acute Pain. When treating acute pain, the goals of intervention are to control the pain and any associated inflammation and to prevent aggravation of the pain or its cause. Many physical agents, including sensory-level ES, cryotherapy, and laser light, can relieve or reduce the severity of acute pain.[23,24] Thermotherapy may reduce the severity of acute pain; however, because acute pain is frequently associated with acute inflammation, which is aggravated by thermotherapy, thermotherapy is generally not recommended for the treatment of acute pain.[52] Cryotherapy is thought to control acute pain by modulating transmission at the spinal cord, by slowing or blocking nerve conduction, and by controlling inflammation and its associated signs and symptoms.[23] Sensory-level ES also relieves acute pain by modulating transmission at the spinal cord or by stimulating the release of endorphins. Briefly limiting motion of a painful area with the aid of a static compression device, an assistive device, or bed rest can prevent aggravation of the symptom or cause of acute pain. Very low-load, prolonged static traction may be used for a number of hours or even a few days to immobilize a symptomatic spinal area temporarily, thereby relieving the spinal pain and inflammation that would be aggravated by lumbar spine motion.[53,54] Excessive movement or muscle contraction in the area of acute pain is generally contraindicated, thus exercise or motor-level ES of this area should be avoided or restricted to a level that does not exacerbate pain. As acute pain starts to resolve, controlled reactivation of the patient may accelerate pain resolution. The water environment may be used to facilitate such activity.

Chronic Pain. Pain that does not resolve in the normal recovery time expected for an injury or disease is known as chronic pain.[55] The goals of intervention for chronic pain shift from resolution of the underlying pathology and control of symptoms to promotion of function, enhancement of strength, and improvement of coping skills. Although psychological interventions are the mainstay of improving coping skills in patients with chronic pain, exercise should be used to regain strength and function. The water environment may be used to promote the development of the functional abilities and the capacity of certain patients with chronic pain, and both motor-level ES and water exercise may be used to increase muscle strength in weak or deconditioned patients. Bed rest, which can result in weakness and further reduce function, should be discouraged in this patient population, and because passive physical agent treatments provided by a clinician can encourage dependence on the clinician rather than improving the patient's own coping skills, such interventions are generally not recommended for the treatment of chronic pain. The judicious use of pain-controlling physical agents by patients themselves may be

TABLE 1-3	Physical Agents for the Treatment of Pain		
Type of Pain	**Goals of Treatment**	**Effective Agents**	**Contraindicated**
Acute	Control pain	Sensory ES, cryotherapy	
	Control inflammation	Cryotherapy	Thermotherapy
	Prevent aggravation of pain	Immobilization	Local exercise, motor ES
		Low-load static traction	
Referred	Control pain	ES, cryotherapy, thermotherapy	
Spinal radicular	Decrease nerve root inflammation	Traction	
	Decrease nerve root compression		
Pain caused by malignancy	Control pain	ES, cryotherapy, superficial thermotherapy	

ES, Electrical stimulation.

indicated when this helps to improve the patient's ability to cope with pain on a long-term basis; however, it is important that such interventions do not excessively disrupt the patient's functional activities. For example, TENS applied by a patient to relieve or reduce his chronic back pain may promote function by allowing him to participate in work-related activities; however, a hot pack applied by the patient for 20 minutes every few hours would interfere with his ability to perform normal functional activities and would therefore not be recommended.

Referred Pain. If the patient's pain is referred to a musculoskeletal area from an internal organ or from another musculoskeletal area, physical agents may be used to control it; however, the source of the pain should also be treated if possible. Pain-relieving physical agents, such as thermotherapy, cryotherapy, or ES, may control referred pain and may be particularly beneficial if complete resolution of the problem is prolonged or cannot be achieved. For example, although surgery may be needed to fully relieve pain caused by endometriosis, if the disease does not place the patient at risk, pain-controlling interventions, such as physical or pharmacological agents, may be used to control the associated pain.

Radicular pain in the extremities caused by spinal nerve root dysfunction may be effectively treated by the application of spinal traction or by the use of physical agents that cause sensory stimulation of the involved dermatome, such as thermotherapy, cryotherapy, or ES.[56,57] Spinal traction is effective in such circumstances because it can reduce nerve root compression, addressing the source of the pain, whereas sensory stimulation may modulate the transmission of pain at the spinal cord level.[58]

Pain Caused by Malignancy. The treatment of pain caused by malignancy may differ from the treatment of pain of other etiologies because particular care must be taken to avoid using agents that can promote the growth or metastasis of malignant tissue. Because the growth of some malignancies can be accelerated by increasing local circulation, agents, such as ultrasound and diathermy, which are known to increase deep tissue temperature and circulation, should generally not be used in an area of malignancy.[59,60] However, in patients with end-stage malignancies, pain-relieving interventions that can improve the patient's quality of life but may adversely affect disease progression may be used with the patient's informed consent.

Complex Regional Pain Syndrome. Complex regional pain syndrome (CRPS) is pain believed to involve overactivation of the sympathetic nervous system. Physical agents can be used to control the pain of CRPS with sympathetic nervous system involvement. In general, low-level sensory stimulation of the involved area, as can be provided by neutral warmth, mild cold, water immersion, or gentle agitation of fluidotherapy, may be effective,

whereas more aggressive stimulation, as can be provided by very hot water, ice, or aggressive agitation of water or fluidotherapy, will probably not be tolerated and may aggravate this type of pain.

COLLAGEN EXTENSIBILITY AND MOTION RESTRICTIONS

Collagen is the main supportive protein of skin, tendon, bone cartilage, and connective tissue.[61] Tissues that contain collagen can become shortened as a result of being immobilized in a shortened position or being moved only through a limited range of motion (ROM). Immobilization may result from disuse caused by debilitation or neural injury or may be caused by the application of an external device such as a cast, brace, or external fixator. Movement may be limited by internal derangement, pain, weakness, poor posture, or an external device. Shortening of muscles, tendons, or joint capsules may cause restricted joint ROM.

To return soft tissue to its normal functional length and thereby allow full motion without damaging other structures, the collagen must be stretched. Collagen can be stretched most effectively and safely when it is most extensible. Because the extensibility of collagen increases in response to increased temperature, thermal agents are frequently applied before soft tissue stretching to optimize the stretching process (Fig. 1-4).[62-65] The processes underlying the development and treatment of motion restrictions are discussed in detail in Chapter 5.

Physical Agents for the Treatment of Motion Restrictions

Physical agents can be effective adjuncts to the treatment of motion restrictions caused by muscle weakness, pain, soft tissue shortening, or a bony block; however, the appropriate interventions for these different sources of motion restriction vary (Table 1-4). When active motion is restricted by muscle weakness, the treatment should be aimed at increasing muscle strength. This can be achieved by repeated overload muscle contraction through active

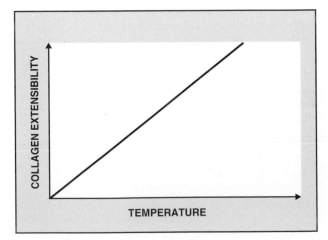

FIG 1-4 Changes in collagen extensibility in response to changes in temperature.

TABLE 1-4	Physical Agents for the Treatment of Motion Restrictions		
Source of Motion Restriction	**Goals of Treatment**	**Effective Agents**	**Contraindicated**
Muscle weakness	Increase muscle strength	Water exercise, motor ES	Immobilization
Pain			
At rest and with motion	Control pain	ES, cryotherapy, thermotherapy, PSWD, spinal traction	Exercise
With motion only	Control pain Promote tissue healing	ES, cryotherapy, thermotherapy, PSWD	Exercise into pain
Soft tissue shortening	Increase tissue extensibility Increase tissue length	Thermotherapy Thermotherapy or brief ice massage and stretch	Prolonged cryotherapy
Bony block	Remove block Compensate	None Exercise Thermotherapy or brief ice massage and stretch	Stretching blocked joint

ES, Electrical stimulation; *PSWD*, pulsed shortwave diathermy.

exercise and may be enhanced by exercise in water or motor-level ES. Water can provide support to allow weaker muscles to move joints through greater range and can provide resistance for stronger muscles to work against. Motor-level ES can provide preferential training of larger muscle fibers, isolation of specific muscle contraction, and precise control of the timing and number of muscle contractions. When ROM is limited by muscle weakness alone, rest and immobilization of the area are contraindicated because restricting the active use of weakened muscles will further reduce their strength and thus exacerbate the existing motion restriction.

When motion is restricted by pain, treatment selection will depend on whether the pain occurs at rest and with all motion or if it occurs in response to active or passive motion only. When motion is restricted by pain that is present at rest and with all motion, the first goal of treatment is to reduce the severity of the pain. This can be achieved, as previously described, with the use of ES, cryotherapy, thermotherapy, or PSWD. If the pain and motion restriction are related to a compressive spinal dysfunction, spinal traction may also be used to alleviate the pain and promote increased motion. When pain restricts motion with active motion only, this indicates an injury of contractile tissue, such as muscle or tendon, without complete rupture.[66] When active and passive motion are both restricted by pain, noncontractile tissue, such as ligament or meniscus, is involved. Physical agents may help restore motion after an injury to contractile or noncontractile tissue by promoting tissue healing or by controlling pain, as described previously.

When active and passive motion are restricted by soft tissue shortening or a bony block, the restriction is generally not accompanied by pain. Soft tissue shortening may be reversed by stretching, and thermal agents may be used before or in conjunction with stretching to increase soft tissue extensibility and thus promote a safer, more effective stretch.[49,50,67] The ideal thermal agent depends on the depth, size, and contouring of the tissue to be treated. Deep-heating agents, such as ultrasound or diathermy, should be used when motion is restricted by shortening of deep tissues, such as the shoulder joint capsule, whereas superficial heating agents, such as hot packs, paraffin,

warm whirlpools, or IR lamps, should be used when motion is restricted by shortening of superficial tissues such as the skin or subcutaneous fascia. Ultrasound should be used for treating small areas of deep tissue, whereas diathermy is more appropriate for larger areas. Hot packs can be used to treat large or small areas of superficial tissue with little or moderate contouring. Paraffin or a whirlpool is more appropriate for treating small areas with greater contouring. IR lamps can be used to heat large or small areas, but they provide consistent heating only to relatively flat surfaces. Because increasing tissue extensibility alone will not decrease soft tissue shortening, thermal agents must be used in conjunction with stretching techniques to increase soft tissue length and reverse motion restrictions caused by soft tissue shortening. Brief forms of cryotherapy, such as brief ice massage or vapocoolant sprays, may also be used before stretching to facilitate greater increases in muscle length by reducing the discomfort of stretching; however, prolonged cryotherapy should not be used before stretching because cooling soft tissue decreases its extensibility.[68,69]

When a bony block restricts motion, the goals of intervention are to remove the block or to compensate for the loss of motion. Physical agents cannot remove a bony block, but they may help with compensation for the loss of motion by facilitating increased motion at other joints. Motion may be increased at other joints by the judicious use of thermotherapy or brief cryotherapy with stretching, as described previously. Such treatment should be applied with caution to avoid causing injury, hypermobility, or other dysfunctions in previously normal joints. Applying a stretching force to a joint that is blocked by a bony obstruction is not recommended because this force will not increase ROM at that joint and may cause inflammation by traumatizing the intraarticular structures.

MUSCLE TONE

Muscle tone is the underlying tension that serves as a background for contraction in a muscle.[70] Muscle tone is affected by neural and biomechanical factors and can vary in response to a pathology, expected demand, pain, and position.[71] Abnormal muscle tone is usually the direct result of nerve pathology or is a secondary sequela of pain that results from injury of other tissues.[72]

Central nervous system injury, as may occur with head trauma or a stroke, can result in increased or decreased muscle tone in the affected area, whereas peripheral motor nerve injury, as may occur with nerve compression, traction, or sectioning, can decrease muscle tone in the affected area. For example, a patient who has had a stroke may have increased tone in the flexor muscles of the upper extremity and the extensor muscles of the lower extremity on the same side, whereas a patient who has had a compression injury to the radial nerve as it passes through the radial groove in the arm may have decreased tone in the wrist and finger extensors.

Pain may cause an increase or decrease in muscle tone. Muscle tone may be increased in the muscles surrounding a painful injured area in order to splint the area and limit motion, or tone in a painful area may be decreased as a result of inhibition. Although protective splinting may prevent further injury from excessive activity, if prolonged, it can also impair circulation, retarding or preventing healing. Decreased muscle tone as a result of pain—as occurs, for example, with the reflexive **hypotonicity** (decreased muscle tone) of the knee extensors that causes buckling of the knee, when knee extension is painful—can limit activity.

Physical agents can alter muscle tone either directly, by altering nerve conduction, nerve sensitivity, or the biomechanical properties of muscle, or indirectly, by reducing pain or the underlying cause of the pain. Normalizing muscle tone will generally reduce functional limitations and disability, allowing the individual to improve the performance of functional and therapeutic activities. Attempting to normalize muscle tone may also promote better outcomes from passive treatment techniques such as passive mobilization or positioning. The processes underlying changes in muscle tone are discussed fully in Chapter 4.

Physical Agents for Tone Abnormalities

Physical agents can temporarily modify muscle hypertonicity, hypotonicity, or fluctuating tone (Table 1-5). Hypertonicity may be reduced directly by the application of neutral warmth or prolonged cryotherapy to the hypertonic muscles, or it may be reduced indirectly by stimulation of antagonist muscle contraction with motor-level ES or quick icing. Stimulation of antagonist muscles indirectly reduces hypertonicity because the stimulated activity in these muscles causes reflex relaxation and tone reduction in opposing muscles.[4] In the past, stimulation of hypertonic muscles with motor-level ES or quick icing

was generally not recommended because of concern that this would further increase muscle tone; however, reports indicate that ES of hypertonic muscles improves patient function by increasing the strength and voluntary control of these muscles.[73,74]

In patients with muscle hypotonicity, in which the goal of intervention is to increase tone, quick icing or motor-level ES of the hypotonic muscle(s) may be beneficial. In contrast, the application of heat to these muscles should generally be avoided because this may further reduce muscle tone. In patients with fluctuating tone, where the goal of treatment is to normalize tone, functional ES may be applied to cause a muscle or muscles to contract at the appropriate time during functional activities. For example, if a patient cannot maintain a functional grasp because he cannot contract the wrist extensors while contracting the finger flexors, contraction of the wrist extensors could be produced by ES at the appropriate time during active grasping.

EVIDENCE-BASED PRACTICE

If several agents may promote progress toward the goals of treatment, are not contraindicated, and can be applied with the appropriate precautions, selection should be based on evidence for or against the intervention. **Evidence-based practice** (EBP) is "the conscientious, explicit, and judicious use of current best evidence in making decisions about the care of individual patients."[75,76] EBP is based on the application of the scientific method to clinical practice. EBP requires that clinical practice decisions be guided by the best available relevant clinical research data in conjunction with the clinician's experience and also takes into account what is known about the pathophysiology of the patient's condition, the individual patient's values and preferences, and what is available in the clinical practice setting.

The goal of EBP is to provide the best possible patient care by assessing available research and applying it to each individual patient. Research studies vary in quality, from the case report (an individual description of a particular patient) to the randomized controlled trial (the gold standard of EBP in which bias is minimized through blinded, randomized application of interventions and assessment of outcomes). To use EBP, the clinician needs to understand the differences between different types of research studies and the advantages and disadvantages of each. The evidence used in EBP can be classified by factors such as study design, types of subjects, nature of controls, outcome measures, and type of statistical analysis.

Using EBP to guide the selection and application of physical agents as part of rehabilitation is often challeng-

TABLE 1-5	Physical Agents for the Treatment of Tone Abnormalities		
Tone Abnormality	**Goals of Treatment**	**Effective Agents**	**Contraindicated**
Hypertonicity	Decrease tone	Neutral warmth or prolonged cryotherapy to hypertonic muscles Motor ES or quick ice of antagonists	Quick ice of agonist
Hypotonicity	Increase tone	Quick ice or motor ES of agonists	Thermotherapy
Fluctuating tone	Normalize tone	Functional ES	

ES, Electrical stimulation.

ing. It is often difficult to find studies of the highest quality because blinding patients and clinicians to treatment may not be possible, outcomes may be hard to assess, subject numbers are often small, and there may be many studies of varying quality in a given area. A good initial approach to evaluating the quality of an individual study is to examine the quality of the question being asked. All well-built questions should have four readily identifiable components—the patients, the intervention, the comparison intervention, and the outcome. These components can be readily remembered by the mnemonic PICO.

P: Patient or Population—The question should apply to a specific population (e.g., adults with low back pain, children with lower extremity spasticity caused by spinal dysraphism).

I: Intervention—The intervention should be specific (e.g., specified exercises applied for a specified period of time at a specified frequency).

C: Comparison intervention/measure—The intervention (or measure) should be compared to some current commonly used treatment (or gold standard measure) or to no intervention if no intervention is usually provided.

O: Outcome—The outcome should be defined as precisely as possible, ideally using a clinically relevant, reliable, and validated measure (e.g., walking speed, level of independence with activities of daily living [ADLs]).

When there are many studies in an area, published **systematic reviews**, **metaanalyses**, and **clinical practice guidelines** may be helpful. These types of publications use systematic methods to find and evaluate the quality of studies and to derive composite conclusions and recommendations from high-quality studies that address a particular question. This may help the clinician keep abreast of current evidence and is easier than searching for and evaluating individual studies.

Systematic reviews answer clearly formulated questions by systematically searching for, assessing, and evaluating literature from multiple sources. Systematic reviews are not all equal, and it is important to be aware of the quality of the literature included and the methods used to evaluate the literature. Metaanalyses are systematic reviews that use statistical analysis to integrate data from a number of independent studies.[77] The specialized databases of systematic reviews and metaanalyses of medical and rehabilitation-related research are the Cochrane Database of Systematic Reviews, the Database of Abstracts of Reviews of Effects (DARE), and Patient-Oriented Evidence that Matters (POEMS) (Box 1-1). For clinical questions not included in these databases, individual studies may be found in online libraries of medical and rehabilitation-oriented publications (Box 1-2), such as Medline, the Cumulative Index of Nursing and Allied Health Literature (CINAHL), and PEDro (the Physiotherapy Evidence Database).

Clinical practice guidelines are systematically developed statements that attempt to interpret current research to provide evidence-based guidelines to guide practitioner and patient decisions about appropriate health care for

---

BOX 1-1	**Databases of Systematic Reviews and Metaanalyses**

- Cochrane Database of Systematic Reviews
- Database of Abstracts of Reviews of Effects (DARE)
- Patient-Oriented Evidence that Matters (POEMS)

BOX 1-2	**Sources of Studies Answering Specific Clinical Questions**

- Medline
- Cumulative Index of Nursing and Allied Health Literature (CINAHL)
- PEDro (the Physiotherapy Evidence Database)

BOX 1-3	**Sources of Clinical Practice Guidelines**

- National Guideline Clearinghouse (NCG)
- Journal of the American Physical Therapy Association

---

specific clinical circumstances.[78] Clinical practice guidelines give recommendations for diagnostic and prognostic measures and for preventive or therapeutic interventions. For any of these, the specific types of patients or problems, the nature of the intervention or test, the alternatives to the intervention being evaluated, and the outcomes of the intervention for which these guidelines apply will be stated. For example, there are guidelines for the treatment of acute low back pain and for the treatment of pressure ulcers that include evidence-based recommendations for tests and measures, interventions, prevention, and prognosis. Often, such recommendations are classified according to the strength of the evidence supporting them. General clinical practice guidelines can be found at the National Guideline Clearinghouse (NCG) web site, and clinical practice guidelines for the use of physical agents can be found at the Journal of the American Physical Therapy Association web site (Box 1-3).

EBP is becoming accepted practice and should be incorporated into every patient's plan of care. However, it is important to remember that every study does not apply to every patient, and research-supported interventions should not be applied without considering each patient's situation. EBP requires the careful combination of patient preference, clinical circumstances, clinician's expertise, and research findings.

USING PHYSICAL AGENTS IN COMBINATION WITH EACH OTHER OR WITH OTHER INTERVENTIONS

To promote progress toward the goals of intervention, a number of physical agents may be used simultaneously and sequentially, and generally, physical agents are applied in conjunction with or during the same treatment session as other interventions. Interventions are generally combined when they have similar effects or when they address different aspects of a common array of symptoms. For example, splinting, ice, pulsed ultrasound, laser light, PSWD, and **phonophoresis** or **iontophoresis** may be used during the acute inflammatory phase of healing. Splinting can limit further injury; ice may control pain and limit circulation; pulsed ultrasound, laser light, and PSWD may promote progress to the proliferation stage of healing; and phonophoresis and iontophoresis may limit the inflammatory response. During the proliferation stage of healing, heat, motor-level ES, and exercise may all be used, and ice or other inflammation-controlling interventions may continue to be applied after activity to reduce the risk of recurring inflammation.

Rest, ice, compression, and elevation (RICE) are frequently combined for the treatment of inflammation and edema because these interventions can control inflammation and edema. Rest limits and prevents further injury, ice reduces circulation and inflammation, compression elevates hydrostatic pressure outside the blood vessels, and elevation reduces hydrostatic pressure within the blood vessels of the elevated area to decrease capillary filtration pressure at the arterial end and facilitate venous and lymphatic outflow from the limb.[79-82] ES may also be added to this combination to further control inflammation and the formation of edema by repelling negatively charged blood cells and ions associated with inflammation.

When the goal of intervention is to control pain, a number of physical agents may be used to impact different mechanisms of pain control. For example, cryotherapy or thermotherapy may be used to modulate pain transmission at the spinal cord, whereas motor-level ES may be used to modulate pain through stimulation of endorphin release. These physical agents may be combined with other pain-controlling interventions, such as medications, and may also be used in conjunction with treatments such as joint mobilization and dynamic stabilization exercise, which are intended to address the underlying impairment causing the pain.

When the goal of intervention is to alter muscle tone, a number of tone-modifying physical agents or other interventions may be applied during or before activity to promote more normal movement and increase the efficacy of other aspects of treatment. For example, ice may be applied for 30 to 40 minutes to the leg of a patient with hypertonicity of the ankle plantar flexors caused by a stroke to control the hypertonicity of these muscles temporarily and thereby promote a more normal gait pattern during gait training. Because practicing normal movement is thought to facilitate the recovery of more normal movement patterns, such treatment may promote a superior outcome.

When the goal of intervention is to reverse soft tissue shortening, the application of thermal agents before or during stretching or mobilization is recommended to promote relaxation and increase soft tissue extensibility, thereby increasing the efficacy and safety of the treatment. For example, hot packs are often applied in conjunction with mechanical traction to promote relaxation of the paraspinal muscles and increase the extensibility of the

superficial soft tissues in the area to which the traction is being applied.

Physical agents are generally used more extensively during the initial rehabilitation sessions when inflammation and pain control are a priority, with progression over time to more active or aggressive interventions, such as exercise or passive mobilization. Progression from one physical agent to another or from the use of a physical agent to another intervention should be based on the progression of the patient's problem. For example, hydrotherapy may be applied to cleanse and débride an open wound during the initial treatment sessions; however, once the wound is clean, this treatment should be stopped, whereas the use of ES may be initiated to promote collagen deposition.

USING PHYSICAL AGENTS WITHIN DIFFERENT HEALTH CARE DELIVERY SYSTEMS

Clinicians may be called on to treat patients within different health care delivery systems in the US and abroad. These systems may vary in both the quantity and nature of available health care resources. Some systems provide high levels of resources, in the forms of skilled clinicians and costly equipment, and others do not. At the present time, the health care delivery system in the US is undergoing change because of the need and desire to contain the growing costs of medical care. Utilizing available resources of both personnel and equipment in the most cost-effective manner is being emphasized, resulting in new systems of reimbursement and increased monitoring of intervention outcomes.

To improve the efficiency and efficacy of health care as it relates to patient function, both health care providers and those paying for treatment are attempting to assess functional outcome in response to different interventions. These changes in reimbursement and outcome assessment are pressuring both service providers and third-party payers to find the most cost-efficient means to provide rehabilitation services and to demonstrate the efficacy of their interventions in improving patient function and reducing disability.

Some payers are attempting to improve the cost-effectiveness of care by denying or reducing reimbursement for certain physical agent treatments or by including the cost of physical agent treatments in the reimbursement for other services. For example, before January 1995, many third-party payers provided a higher level of reimbursement for treatments involving physical agents than for other interventions; however, since that time, reimbursement for these services has been reduced to reflect the lower perceived level of skill required to apply these agents. In January 1997, Medicare changed its reimbursement schedule, bundling the payment for hot pack and cold pack treatments into the payment for all other services rather than reimbursing separately for these treatments.[83] This is because "hot and cold packs are easily self-administered . . . hot and cold packs, by their nature, do not require the level of professional involvement as do the other physical medicine and rehabilitation modalities. . . . Although . . . professional judgment is involved in the use of hot and cold packs, much less judgment is demanded for them than for other modalities." Nonetheless, this intervention may be indicated, and patients may benefit from instruction in applying these agents themselves at home.

Although there is a growing emphasis on the cost-effectiveness of care, the goals of intervention continue to be, as they always have been, to obtain the best outcome for the patient within the constraints of the health care delivery system. Although it has been suggested that the need for cost efficiency may eliminate the use of physical agents, this is not so. Rather, this requirement pushes the clinician to find and use the most efficient ways to provide those interventions that can be expected to help the patient progress toward the goals of treatment. To use physical agents in this manner, the clinician must be able to assess the presenting problem and know when physical agents can be an effective component of treatment. The clinician must also know when and how to use physical agents most effectively and know which ones can be used by patients to treat themselves (Box 1-4). To achieve the most cost-effective treatment, the clinician should optimize the use of the varied skill levels of different practitioners and the use of home programs when appropriate. In many cases, the licensed therapist may not need to apply the physical agent but instead may assess and analyze the presenting clinical findings, determine the intervention plan, provide those aspects of care requiring the skills of the licensed therapist, and then train the patient or supervised unlicensed personnel to apply those interventions requiring a lower level of skill. The therapist can then reassess the patient regularly to determine the effectiveness of the interventions provided and the patient's progress toward his or her goals, and adjust the plan of care accordingly.

Cost efficiency may also be increased by providing intervention to groups of patients, such as group water exercise programs for patients recovering from total joint arthroplasty or for those with osteoarthritis. Such programs may be designed to facilitate the transition to a community-based exercise program when the patient reaches the appropriate level of function and recovery. Used in this manner, physical agents can provide cost-effective care and involve the patient in promoting recovery and achieving the goals of treatment.

CHAPTER REVIEW

1. Physical agents are materials or energy applied to patients to assist in rehabilitation. Physical agents include heat, cold, water, pressure, sound, electromagnetic radiation, and electrical currents. These agents can be categorized as thermal (e.g., hot packs, cold packs), mechanical (e.g., compression, traction), or electromagnetic (e.g., lasers, ES, UV radiation). Some physical agents fall into more than one category. Water and ultrasound, for example, are both thermal and mechanical agents.
2. Physical agents are components of a complete rehabilitation program. They should not be used as the sole intervention for a patient.
3. The ICF model assesses the impact of a disease or condition on a patient's function. It considers the effects of a patient's health condition, environment, and personal circumstances on his or her impairments, activity limitations, and participation restrictions. The ICF model looks at the patient on three levels: body, whole person, and social. Physical agents primarily affect the patient at the body, or impairment, level. A complete rehabilitation program should affect the patient at all levels of functioning, disability, and health.
4. Selection of a physical agent is based on integrating findings from the patient examination and evaluation with the evidence regarding the effects (positive and negative) of the available agent(s).
5. Physical agents primarily affect inflammation and healing, pain, motion restrictions, and tone abnormalities. Knowledge of normal and abnormal physiology in each of these areas can help in selection of a physical agent for a patient. These are discussed in Chapters 2 through 5. The specific effects of particular physical agents are discussed in Chapters 6 through 14.
6. Contraindications are circumstances in which a physical agent should not be used. Precautions are circumstances in which a physical agent should be used with caution. There are general contraindications and precautions, such as pregnancy, malignancy, pacemaker, and impaired sensation and mentation, to the application of physical agents. Specific contraindications and precautions for each physical agent are discussed in Chapters 6 through 14.
7. EBP is the incorporation of research-based evidence into a patient's rehabilitation plan. EBP integrates the clinician's experience and judgment with the patient's preferences, the clinical situation, and the available evidence. Although EBP is ideally a rigorous approach to patient care, many studies have not yet been done in the area of physical agents, partly because of the difficulty in blinding patients and clinicians to the intervention being used. This book attempts to include the most current and best-quality evidence available.

| **BOX 1-4** | **Requirements for Cost-Effective Use of Physical Agents** |

- Assess and analyze the presenting problem.
- Know when physical agents can be an effective component of treatment.
- Know when and how to use physical agents most effectively.
- Know the skill level required for the application of different physical agents.
- Optimize the use of the skill levels of different practitioners.
- Use home programs when appropriate.
- Treat in groups when appropriate.
- Reassess patients regularly to determine the efficacy of the treatments provided.
- Adjust the plan of care according to the findings of reassessments.

8. Physical agents are commonly used in conjunction with each other and with other interventions. They are used in the clinic, at home, and in various health care delivery systems. Depending on the system, the selection and application of physical agents may vary. Reimbursement for applying physical agents is constantly in flux, and the potential for conflict between minimizing cost and maximizing benefit can make intervention selection difficult.

ADDITIONAL RESOURCES evolve

Web Sites

American Occupation Therapy Association (AOTA): US national professional society. The web site has a link to evidence-based practice resources which is available only to members. www.aota.org.

American Physical Therapy Association (APTA): US national professional organization. The web site includes current research, physical therapy news, consumer information, career advice, and access to back issues of *Physical Therapy*, the journal of the APTA. www.apta.org.

Centre for Evidence-Based Medicine (CEBM): The CEBM web site includes information for health care professionals on learning, practicing, and teaching EBM, as well as definitions of terminology and calculators. www.cebm.net.

CINAHL: A database of studies from the nursing allied health literature since 1982. www.cinahl.com

Cochrane Collaboration: International not-for-profit organization that provides up-to-date information about the effects of health care via systematic reviews and metaanalyses. www.cochrane.org.

Database of Abstracts of Reviews of Effects (DARE): The DARE web site contains summaries of systematic reviews that have met strict quality criteria. Included reviews have to be about the effects of interventions. Each summary also provides a critical commentary on the quality of the review. The database covers a broad range of health and social care topics and can be used for answering questions about the effects of interventions, as well as for developing guidelines and policy making. www.york.ac.uk/inst/crd/index.htm.

Hooked on Evidence web site: An APTA database that provides abstracts and summarizes articles related to specific physical therapy–related problems. www.apta.org/hookedonevidence/index/cfm.

Medline: An online database of 11 million citations and abstracts from health and medical journals and other news sources. www.ncbi.nlm.nih.gov/sites/entrez

National Athletic Trainers' Association (NATA): The NATA professional membership association web site for certified athletic trainers and others who support the athletic training profession. The website allows members access to the *Journal of Athletic Training*. www.nata.org.

National Guideline Clearinghouse (NCG): The NCG is a public resource for evidence-based clinical practice guidelines and is an initiative of the Agency for Healthcare Research and Quality (AHRQ), US Department of Health and Human Services. The NGC was originally created by the AHRQ in partnership with the American Medical Association and the American Association of Health Plans (now America's Health Insurance Plans [AHIP]). The web site allows searches by keyword, disease, intervention, measures, or organization. www.guideline.gov.

PEDro (the Physiotherapy Evidence Database): PEDro is an Australian website that was developed to give rapid access to bibliographical details and abstracts of randomized controlled trials, systematic reviews, and evidence-based clinical practice guidelines in physiotherapy. Most trials on the database have been rated for quality to help the reader quickly discriminate between trials that are likely to be valid and interpretable and those that are not. www.pedro.fhs.usyd.edu.au/.

World Health Organization (WHO): The WHO web site contains information on the ICF model including an interactive section on the classifications. http://www.who.int/en/.

GLOSSARY evolve

Clinical practice guidelines: Systematically developed statements that attempt to interpret current research to provide evidence-based guidelines to guide practitioner and patient decisions about appropriate health care for specific clinical circumstances.

Collagen: A glycoprotein that provides the extracellular framework for all multicellular organisms.

Complex regional pain syndrome (CRPS): Pain believed to involve sympathetic nervous system overactivation; previously called reflex sympathetic dystrophy and sympathetically maintained pain.

Compression: The application of a mechanical force that increases external pressure on a body part to reduce swelling, improve circulation, or modify scar tissue formation.

Contraindications: Conditions in which a particular treatment should not be applied; also called absolute contraindications.

Contrast bath: Alternating immersion in hot and cold water.

Cryotherapy: The therapeutic use of cold.

Diathermy: The application of shortwave or microwave electromagnetic energy to produce heat within tissues, particularly deep tissues.

Disability: The inability to perform activities required for self-care, home, work, or community roles.

Electrical stimulation (ES): The use of electrical current to induce muscle contraction (motor level) or changes in sensation (sensory level).

Electromagnetic agents: Physical agents that apply energy to the patient in the form of electromagnetic radiation or electrical current.

Evidence-based practice (EBP): The conscientious, explicit, and judicious use of current best evidence in making decisions about the care of individual patients.

Fluidotherapy: A dry heating agent that transfers heat by convection. It consists of a cabinet containing finely ground particles of cellulose through which heated air is circulated.

Functional limitations: Restrictions in the ability to perform an activity in an efficient, typically expected, or competent manner.

Gate control theory of pain modulation: A theory of pain control and modulation that states that pain is modulated at the spinal cord level by inhibitory effects of nonnoxious afferent input.

Guide to Physical Therapist Practice (the Guide): A book used by physical therapists to categorize patients according to preferred practice patterns that include typical findings and descriptive norms of types and ranges of interventions for patients in each pattern.

Hydrotherapy: The therapeutic use of water.

Hypertonicity: High tone or increased resistance to stretch compared with normal muscles.

Hypotonicity: Low tone or decreased resistance to stretch compared with normal muscles.

ICF model: International Classification of Functioning, Disability and Health (ICF) model of disability and health created by the WHO that views functioning and disability as a complex interaction between the health condition of the individual and contextual factors, including environmental and personal factors. ICF uses categories of health conditions, body functions, activities, and participation to focus on abilities rather than limitations.

ICIDH model: International Classification of Impairments, Disabilities and Handicaps (ICIDH) model of disability created by the WHO that was a precursor to the ICF model and focused on disability rather than ability.

Impairments: Alterations in anatomical, physiological, or psychological structures or functions as the result of an underlying pathology.

Indications: Conditions under which a particular treatment should be applied.

Inflammation: The body's first response to tissue damage, characterized by heat, redness, swelling, pain, and often loss of function.

Inflammatory phase: The first phase of healing after tissue damage.

Infrared (IR) radiation: Electromagnetic radiation in the IR range (wavelength range approximately 750 to 1300 nm) that can be absorbed by matter and, if of sufficient intensity, can cause an increase in temperature.

Iontophoresis: The transcutaneous delivery of ions into the body for therapeutic purpose using an electrical current.

Laser: The acronym for light amplification by stimulated emission of radiation is LASER; laser light is monochromatic, coherent, and directional.

Maturation phase: The final phase of healing after tissue damage. During this phase scar tissue is modified into its mature form.

Mechanical agents: Physical agents that apply force to increase or decrease pressure on the body.

Metaanalyses: Systematic reviews that use statistical analysis to integrate data from a number of independent studies.

Modality/physical modality: Other terms for physical agent.

Muscle tone: The underlying tension in a muscle that serves as a background for contraction.

Nagi model: A linear model of disability in which a pathology causes impairments, leading to functional limitations that lead to disabilities. A precursor to the ICF model.

Pain: An unpleasant sensory and emotional experience associated with actual or threatened tissue damage.

Paraffin: A waxy substance that can be warmed and used to coat the extremities for thermotherapy.

Pathology: Alteration of anatomy or physiology as a result of disease or injury.

Phonophoresis: The application of ultrasound with a topical drug to facilitate transdermal drug delivery.

Physical agents: Energy and materials applied to patients to assist in rehabilitation.

Precautions: Conditions in which a particular treatment should be applied with special care or limitations; also called relative contraindications.

Proliferative phase: The second phase of healing after tissue damage in which damaged structures are rebuilt and the wound is strengthened.

Pulsed shortwave diathermy (PSWD): The therapeutic use of intermittent shortwave radiation in which heat is not the mechanism of action.

Pulsed ultrasound: Intermittent delivery of ultrasound during the treatment period.

Rehabilitation: Goal-oriented intervention designed to maximize independence in individuals who have compromised function.

Systematic reviews: Reviews of studies that answer clearly formulated questions by systematically searching for, assessing, and evaluating literature from multiple sources.

Thermal agents: Physical agents that cause an increase or decrease in tissue temperature.

Thermotherapy: The therapeutic application of heat.

Traction: The application of a mechanical force to the body in a way that separates, or attempts to separate, the joint surfaces and elongates the surrounding soft tissues.

Transcutaneous electrical nerve stimulation (TENS): The application of electrical current through the skin to modulate pain.

Ultrasound: Sound with a frequency greater than 20,000 cycles per second that is used as a physical agent to produce thermal and nonthermal effects.

Ultraviolet (UV) radiation: Electromagnetic radiation in the ultraviolet range (wavelength < 290 to 400 nm) that lies between x-ray and visible light and has nonthermal effects when absorbed through the skin.

REFERENCES

1. World Health Organization: *Towards a common language for functioning, disability and health: International Classification of Functioning, Disability and Health (ICF)*, Geneva, 2002, WHO.
2. American Physical Therapy Association: *Guide to physical therapist practice*, ed 2, Alexandria, VA, 2001, The Association.
3. Johnson EW: Back to water (or hydrotherapy), *J Back Musculoskel Med* 4(4):ix, 1994.
4. Baker LL, McNeal DR, Benton LA, et al: *Neuromuscular electrical stimulation: a practical guide*, ed 3, Downey, CA, 1993, Los Amigos Research & Education Institute.
5. Roberson WS: Digby's receipts, *Ann Med Hist* 7(3):216, 1925.
6. Melzack JD, Wall PD: Pain mechanisms: a new theory, *Science* 150:971-979, 1965.

7. Hyland DB, Kirkland VJ: Infrared therapy for skin ulcers, *Am J Nurs* 80(10):1800-1801, 1980.

8. Cummings J: Role of light in wound healing. In Kloth L, McCulloch JM, Feedar JA, eds: *Wound healing: alternatives in management,* Philadelphia, 1990, FA Davis.

9. World Health Organization: *International Classification of Impairments, Disabilities and Handicaps* (ICIDH), Geneva, 1980, WHO.

10. Wood PHN: The language of disablement: a glossary relating to disease and its consequences, *Int Rehab Med* 2:86-92, 1980.

11. Wagstaff S: The use of the International Classification of Impairments, Disabilities and Handicaps in rehabilitation, *Physiotherapy* 68:548-553, 1982.

12. Nagi S: Disability concepts revisited. In Pope AM, Tarlov AR, eds: *Disability in America: toward a national agenda for prevention,* Washington, DC, 1991, National Academy Press,

13. American Physical Therapy Association: *Position on exclusive use of physical agents modalities,* Alexandria, VA, House of Delegates Reference Committee, P06-95-29-18, 2005.

14. American Occupational Therapy Association: Physical agent modalities: a position paper, *Am J Occup Ther* 57:650-651, 2003.

15. Education section of National Association of Athletic Trainers: http://www.nata.org/student/education.htm. Accessed June 28, 2006.

16. Draper D: Are certified athletic trainers qualified to use therapeutic modalities? *J Ath Train* 37(1):11-12, 2002.

17. Weston M, Taber C, Casgranda L, et al: Changes in local blood volume during cold gel pack application to traumatized ankles, *J Orthop Sport Phys Ther* 19(4):197-199, 1994.

18. Wolf SL: Contralateral upper extremity cooling from a specific cold stimulus, *Phys Ther* 51:158-165, 1971.

19. Bickford RH, Duff RS: Influence of ultrasonic irradiation on temperature and blood flow in human skeletal muscle, *Circ Res* 1:534-538, 1953.

20. Fox HH, Hilton SM: Bradykinin formation in human skin as a factor in heat vasodilation, *J Physiol* 142:219, 1958.

21. Schmidt KL: Heat, cold, and inflammation, *Rheumatology* 38:391-404, 1979.

22. McCulloch J: Physical modalities in wound management: ultrasound, vasopneumatic devices and hydrotherapy, *Ostomy Wound Manage* 41(5):30-32, 35-37, 1995.

23. Ernst E, Fialka V: Ice freezes pain? A review of the clinical effectiveness of analgesic cold therapy, *J Pain Symptom Manage* 9(1):56-59, 1994.

24. Benson TB, Copp EP: The effects of therapeutic forms of heat and ice on the pain threshold of the normal shoulder, *Rheumatol Rehabil* 13:101-104, 1974.

25. Wilson DH: Treatment of soft tissue injuries by pulsed electrical energy, *Br Med J* 2:269-270, 1972.

26. Pennington GM, Danley DL, Sumko MH: Pulsed, nonthermal, high frequency electromagnetic field (Diapulse) in the treatment of Grade I and Grade II ankle sprains, *Milit Med* 153:101-104, 1993.

27. Kaplan EG, Weinstock RE: Clinical evaluation of Diapulse as adjunctive therapy following foot surgery, *J Am Podiatr Assoc* 58(5):218-221, 1968.

28. Cote DJ, Prentice WE, Hooker DN, et al: Comparison of three treatment procedures for minimizing ankle sprain swelling, *Phys Ther* 68(7):1072-1076, 1988.

29. Wilkerson GB: Treatment of inversion ankle sprain through synchronous application of focal compression and cold, *J Athl Train* 26:220-237, 1991.

30. Quillen WS, Roullier LH: Initial management of acute ankle sprains with rapid pulsed pneumatic compression and cold, *J Orthop Sports Phys Ther* 4:39-43, 1982.

31. Pilla AA, Martin DE, Schuett AM, et al: Effect of PRF therapy on edema from grades I and II ankle sprains: a placebo controlled randomized, multi-site, double-blind clinical study, *J Athl Train* 31:S53, 1996.

32. Grossman N, Schneid N, Reuveni H, et al: 780 nm low power diode laser irradiation stimulates proliferation of keratinocyte cultures: involvement of reactive oxygen species, *Lasers Surg Med* 22(4):212-218, 1998.

33. Young SR, Dyson M: Macrophage responsiveness to therapeutic ultrasound, *Ultrasound Med Biol* 16(8):809-816, 1990.

34. Bansal PS, Sobti VK, Roy KS: Histomorphochemical effects of shortwave diathermy on healing of experimental muscular injury in dogs, *Ind J Exper Biol* 28(8):766-770, 1990.

35. Lehmann J, Masock A, Warren C, et al: Effect of therapeutic temperatures on tendon extensibility, *Arch Phys Med Rehabil* 51:481-487, 1970.

36. Lehmann JF, DeLateur BJ: Application of heat and cold in the clinical setting. In Lehmann JF, DeLateur BJ, eds: *Therapeutic heat and cold,* ed 4, Baltimore, 1990, Williams & Wilkins.

37. Lehmann JF, DeLateur BJ: *Therapeutic heat and cold,* ed 4, Baltimore, 1990, Williams & Wilkins.

38. Lehmann JF, DeLateur BJ, Stonebridge JB, et al: Therapeutic temperature distribution produced by ultrasound as modified by dosage and volume of tissue exposed, *Arch Phys Med Rehabil* 48:662-666, 1967.

39. Lehmann JF, DeLateur BJ, Warren G, et al: Bone and soft tissue heating produced by ultrasound, *Arch Phys Med Rehabil* 48:397-401, 1967.

40. Kamm RD: Bioengineering studies of periodic external compression as prophylaxis against deep venous thrombosis: Part I: Numerical studies, *J Biomech Eng* 104:87-95, 1982.

41. Olson DA, Kamm RD, Shapiro AH: Bioengineering studies of periodic external compression as prophylaxis against deep venous thrombosis. Part II: experimental studies on a simulated leg, *J Biomech Eng* 104:96-104, 1982.

42. Risch WD, Koubenec HJ, Beckmann U, et al: The effect of graded immersion on heart volume, central venous pressure, pulmonary blood distribution and heart rate in man, *Pfluegers Arch* 374:117, 1978.

43. Haffor AA, Mohler JG, Harrison AAC: Effects of water immersion on cardiac output of lean and fat male subjects at rest and during exercise, *Aviat Space Environ Med* 62:125, 1991.

44. Balldin UI, Lundgren CEG, Lundvall, J et al: Changes in the elimination of 133 Xenon from the anterior tibial muscle in man induced by immersion in water and by shifts in body position, *Aerospace Med* 42(5):489, 1971.

45. Ward RS: Pressure therapy for the control of hypertrophic scar formation after burn injury: a history and review, *J Burn Care Rehabil* 12:257-262, 1991.

46. Larson DL, Abston S, Evans EB, et al: Techniques for decreasing scar formation and contractures in the burned patient, *J Trauma* 11:807-823, 1971.

47. Kircher CW, Shetlar MR, Shetlar CL: Alteration of hypertrophic scars induced by mechanical pressure, *Arch Dermatol* 111:60-64, 1975.

48. Wade J: Sports splash, *Rehabil Manage* 10(4):64-70, 1997.

49. Warren C, Lehmann J, Koblanski J: Elongation of rat tail tendon: effect of load and temperature, *Arch Phys Med Rehabil* 52:465-474, 484, 1971.

50. Warren C, Lehmann J, Koblanski J: Heat and stretch procedures: an evaluation using rat tail tendon, *Arch Phys Med Rehabil* 57:122-126, 1976.

51. Gersten JW: Effect of ultrasound on tendon extensibility, *Am J Phys Med* 34:362-369, 1955.

52. Lehmann JF, Brunner GD, Stow RW: Pain threshold measurements after therapeutic application of ultrasound, microwaves and infrared, *Arch Phys Med Rehabil* 39:560-565, 1958.

53. Judovich B: Lumbar traction therapy, *JAMA* 159:549, 1955.

54. Cheatle MD, Esterhai JL: Pelvic traction as treatment for acute back pain, *Spine* 16:1379-1381, 1991.

55. Bonica JJ: *The Management of pain,* ed 2, Philadelphia, 1990, Lea & Febiger.

56. Hood LB, Chrisman D: Intermittent pelvic traction in the treatment of the ruptured intervertebral disc, *Phys Ther* 48:21-30, 1968.

57. Mathews JA, Mills SB, Jenkins VM, et al: Back pain and sciatica: controlled trials of manipulation, traction, sclerosant, and epidural injections, *Br J Rheumatol* 26:416-423, 1987.

58. Lidstrom A, Zachrisson M: Physical therapy on low back pain and sciatica: an attempt at evaluation, *Scand J Rehabil Med* 2:37-42, 1970.

59. Sicard-Rosenbaum L, Lord D, Danoff JV, et al: Effects of continuous therapeutic ultrasound on growth and metastasis of subcutaneous murine tumors, *Phys Ther* 75(1):3-11, 1995.

60. Burr B: *Heat as a therapeutic modality against cancer. Report 16,* Bethesda, MD, 1974, US National Cancer Institute.

61. *Dorland's Illustrated medical dictionary,* ed 29, Philadelphia, 2000, WB Saunders.
62. Lentell G, Hetherington T, Eagan J, et al: The use of thermal agents to influence the effectiveness of low load prolonged stretch, *J Orthop Sport Phys Ther* 16(5):200-207, 1992.
63. Warren C, Lehmann J, Koblanski J: Elongation of rat tail tendon: Effect of load and temperature, *Arch Phys Med Rehabil* 52:465-474, 484, 1971.
64. Warren C, Lehmann J, Koblanski J: Heat and stretch procedures: An evaluation using rat tail tendon, *Arch Phys Med Rehabil* 57:122-126, 1976.
65. Gersten JW: Effect of ultrasound on tendon extensibility, *Am J Phys Med* 34:362-369, 1955.
66. Cyriax J: Diagnosis of soft tissue lesions. In *Textbook of orthopedic medicine,* vol I, London, 1982, Bailliere Tindall.
67. Lentell G, Hetherington T, Eagan J, et al: The use of thermal agents to influence the effectiveness of low load prolonged stretch, *J Orthop Sport Phys Ther* 16(5):200-207, 1992.
68. Travell JG, Simons DG: *Myofascial pain and dysfunction: the trigger point manual,* Baltimore, 1983, Williams & Wilkins.
69. Simons DG, Travell JG: Myofascial origins of low back pain. 1. Principles of diagnosis and treatment, *Postgrad Med* 73(2):70-77, 1983.
70. Lehmann J, Masock A, Warren C, et al: Effect of therapeutic temperatures on tendon extensibility, *Arch Phys Med Rehabil* 51:481-487, 1970.
71. Keshner EA: Reevaluating the theoretical model underlying the neurodevelopmental theory: A literature review, *Phys Ther* 61:1035-1040, 1981.
72. Brooks VB: Motor control: how posture and movements are governed, *Phys Ther* 63:664-673, 1983.
73. Carmick J: Clinical use of neuromuscular electrical stimulation for children with cerebral palsy, *Phys Ther* 73:505-513, 1993.
74. Carmick J: Use of neuromuscular electrical stimulation and a dorsal wrist splint to improve hand function of a child with spastic hemiparesis, *Phys Ther* 77(6):661-671, 1997.
75. Sackett DL, Rosenberg WMC, Gray JAM, et al: Evidence based medicine: what it is and what it isn't, *BMJ* 312:71-72, 1996.
76. Sackett DL, Straus SE, Richardson WS, et al: *Evidence based medicine: How to practice and teach EBM,* ed 2, Edinburgh, 2000, Churchill Livingstone.
77. *Dorland's illustrated medical dictionary,* ed 30, Philadelphia, 2003, WB Saunders.
78. Field MJ, Lohr KN: *Clinical practice guidelines: directions of a new program,* Washington, DC, 1990, National Academy Press.
79. Abramson DI: Physiological basis for the use of physical agents in peripheral vascular disorders, *Arch Phys Med Rehabil* 46:216-244, 1965.
80. Stillwell GK: Physiatric management of postmastectomy lymphedema, *Med Clin North Am* 46:1051-1063, 1962.
81. Rucinski TJ, Hooker D, Prentice W: The effects of intermittent compression on edema in post acute ankle sprains, *J Orthop Sport Phys Ther* 14(2):65-69, 1991.
82. Sims D: Effects of positioning on ankle edema, *J Orthop Sport Phys Ther* 8:30-35, 1986.
83. *PT Bulletin:* 12/20/1997, p 11.

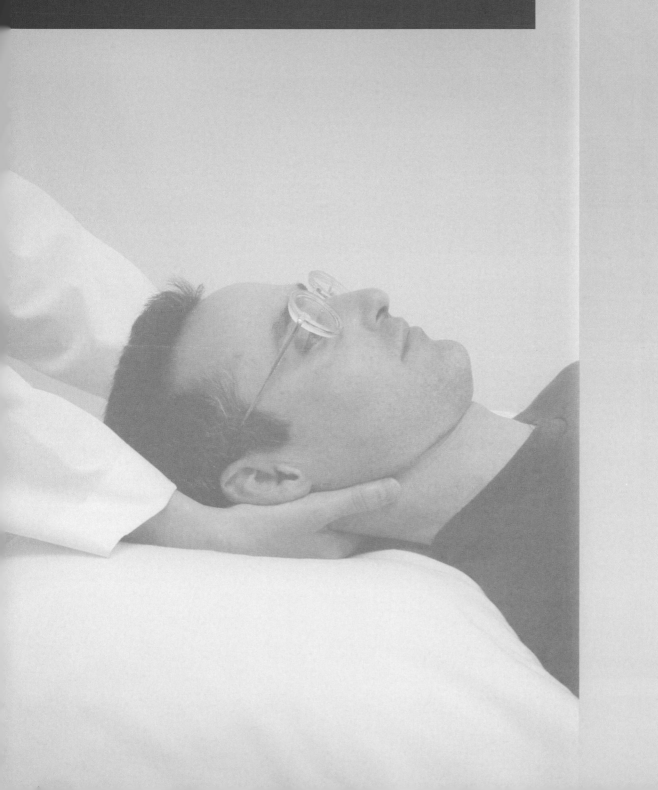

PART I

Pathology and Patient Problems

Chapter 2

Inflammation and Tissue Repair

Julie A. Pryde

Injury to vascularized tissue results in a coordinated, complex, and dynamic series of events collectively referred to as **inflammation** and repair. Although there are variations between the responses of different tissue types, overall the processes are remarkably similar. The sequelae depend on the source and site of injury, the state of local homeostasis, and whether the injury is acute or chronic. The ultimate goal of inflammation and repair is to restore function by eliminating the pathological or physical insult, replacing the damaged or destroyed tissue, and promoting regeneration of normal tissue structure.

Rehabilitation professionals treat a variety of inflammatory conditions resulting from trauma, surgical procedures, or problematic healing. The clinician who is called on to manage such injuries needs to understand the physiology of inflammation and healing and how it can be modified. The clinician can enhance healing by the appropriate application of various physical agents, therapeutic exercises, or manual techniques. The foundation for a successful rehabilitation program requires an understanding of biomechanics, the phases of tissue healing, and the effects of immobilization and therapeutic interventions on the healing process.

THE PHASES OF INFLAMMATION AND HEALING

This chapter will provide readers with information on the processes involved in inflammation and tissue repair so they can understand how physical agents may be used to modify these processes and improve patient outcome.

The process of inflammation and repair consists of three phases: inflammation, proliferation, and maturation. The **inflammation phase** prepares the wound for healing; the **proliferation phase** rebuilds the damaged structures and strengthens the wound; and the **maturation phase** modifies the scar tissue into its mature form (Fig. 2-1). The duration of each phase varies to some degree, and the phases generally overlap. Thus the timetables for the various phases of healing provided in this chapter are only general guidelines not precise definitions (Fig. 2-2).

INFLAMMATION PHASE (DAYS 1-6)

Inflammation, from the Latin *inflamer*, meaning "to set on fire," begins when the normal physiology of tissue is altered by disease or trauma.[1] This immediate protective response attempts to destroy, dilute, or isolate the cells or agents that may be at fault. It is a normal and necessary prerequisite to healing. If there is no inflammation, healing cannot occur. Inflammation can also be harmful, particularly when it is directed at the wrong tissue or is overly exuberant. For example, inappropriately directed inflammatory reactions that underlie autoimmune diseases, such as rheumatoid arthritis, can cause excessive scarring, which can damage and destroy joints. Although the inflammatory process follows the same sequence regardless of the cause of injury, some causes result in exaggeration or prolongation of certain events.

Cornelius Celsus first described the inflammatory phase nearly 2000 years ago as being characterized by the four cardinal signs of *calor, rubor, tumor,* and *dolor* (Latin terms for heat, redness, swelling, and pain). *Functio laesa* (loss of function) was later added to this list by Virchow, bringing the number of cardinal signs of inflammation to five (Table 2-1).

An increase in blood in a given area, known as **hyperemia**, accounts primarily for the increased temperature and redness in the area of **acute inflammation**. The onset of hyperemia at the beginning of the inflammatory

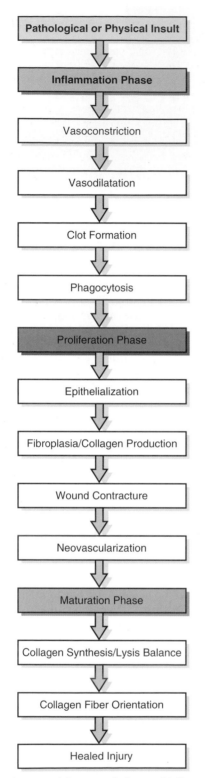

FIG 2-1 Flow diagram of the normal phases of inflammation and repair.

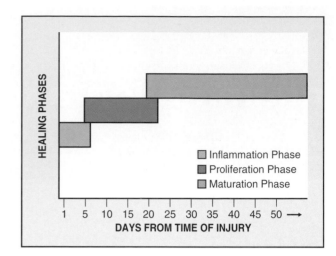

FIG 2-2 Timeline of the phases of inflammation and repair.

TABLE 2-1	Cardinal Signs of Inflammation	
Sign (English)	Sign (Latin)	Cause
Heat	Calor	Increased vascularity
Redness	Rubor	Increased vascularity
Swelling	Tumor	Blockage of lymphatic drainage
Pain	Dolor	Physical pressure or chemical irritation of pain-sensitive structures
Loss of function	Functio laesa	Pain and swelling

response is controlled by neurogenic and chemical mediators.[2] Local swelling results from increased permeability and vasodilation of the local blood vessels and infiltration of fluid into the interstitial spaces of the injured area. Pain results from the pressure of the swelling and from irritation of pain-sensitive structures by chemicals released from damaged cells.[2] Both pain and swelling may result in loss of function.

There is some disagreement in the literature about the duration of the inflammation phase. Some investigators state that it is relatively short, lasting for less than 4 days,[3,4] and others believe it may last for up to 6 days.[5,6] This discrepancy may be the result of individual and injury-specific variation or the overlapping nature of phases of inflammation and tissue healing.

The inflammatory phase involves a complex sequence of interactive and overlapping events including vascular, cellular, hemostatic, and immune processes. **Humoral** and **neural mediators** act to control the inflammatory phase. There is evidence that immediately after injury, **platelets** and **neutrophils** predominate and release a number of factors that amplify the platelet aggregation response, initiate a coagulation cascade, or act as chemoattractants for cells involved in the inflammatory phase.[7] Neutrophil infiltration ceases after a few days, and neutrophils are replaced by **macrophages** starting 2 days after injury.[8] This shift in cell type at the site of injury correlates with a shift from the inflammation to the proliferation phase of healing.

Vascular Response

Alterations in the anatomy and function of the microvasculature, including the capillaries, postcapillary venules, and lymphatic vessels, are among the earliest responses in the inflammatory phase.[9] Trauma, such as a laceration, sprain, or contusion, physically disrupts these structures and may produce bleeding, fluid loss, cell injury, and exposure of tissues to foreign material, including bacteria. The damaged vessels respond rapidly with transient constriction in an attempt to minimize blood loss. This response, which is mediated by norepinephrine, generally lasts for 5 to 10 minutes but can be prolonged in the small vessels by serotonin released from mast cells and platelets.

After the transient vasoconstriction of injured vessels, the noninjured vessels near the injured area dilate. Capillary permeability is also increased by injury of the capillary walls and in response to chemicals released from injured tissues (Fig. 2-3). The vasodilation and increase in

capillary permeability are initiated by histamine, Hageman factor, bradykinin, prostaglandins, and complement fractions. Vasodilation and increased capillary permeability last for up to 1 hour after tissue damage.

Histamine is released primarily by mast cells, as well as by platelets and basophils at the injury site.[10] Histamine causes vasodilation and increased vascular permeability in venules, which contributes to local **edema** (swelling). Histamine also attracts **leukocytes** (white blood cells) to the damaged tissue area.[11] The ability of a chemical to attract cells is known as **chemotaxis**. Histamine is one of the first inflammatory mediators released after tissue injury and is active for approximately 1 hour after injury (Fig. 2-4).[12]

Hageman factor (also known as clotting factor XII), an enzyme found in the blood, is activated by contact with the negatively charged surfaces of the endothelial lining of vessels that are exposed when vessels are damaged. The role of Hageman factor is twofold. First, it activates the coagulation system to stop local bleeding. Second, it causes vasoconstriction and increased vascular permeability by activating other **plasma** proteins. It converts plasminogen to plasmin and prekallikrein to kallikrein, and it activates the alternative complement pathway (Fig. 2-5).[13]

Plasmin augments vascular permeability in both the skin and lungs by inducing breakdown of fibrin and by cleaving components of the **complement system**. Plasmin also activates Hageman factor, which initiates the cascade that generates bradykinin.

Plasma kallikrein attracts neutrophils and cleaves kininogen to generate several kinins such as bradykinin. Kinins are biologically active peptides that are potent inflammatory substances derived from plasma. Kinins, particularly bradykinin, function similarly to histamine, causing a marked increase in permeability of the microcirculation. They are most prevalent in the early phases of

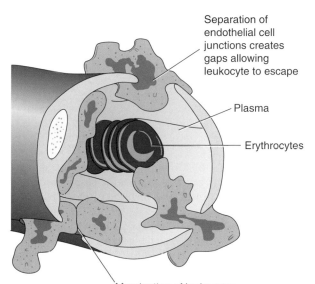

Separation of endothelial cell junctions creates gaps allowing leukocyte to escape

Plasma

Erythrocytes

Margination of leukocytes on endothelial surface

FIG 2-3 Vascular response to wound healing.

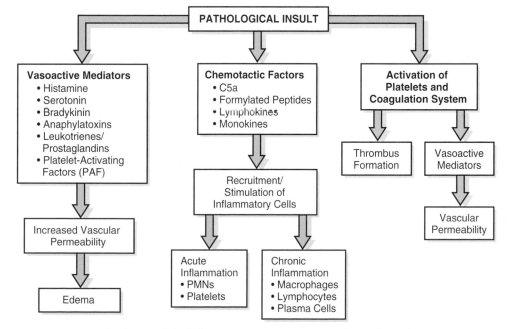

FIG 2-4 Mediators of the inflammatory response. *PMN*, Polymorphonucleocytes.

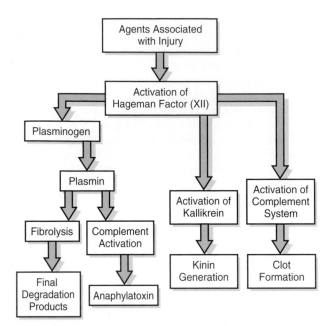

FIG 2-5 Hageman factor activation and inflammatory mediator production.

TABLE 2-2	Mediators of the Inflammatory Response
Response	**Mediators**
Vasodilation	Histamine Prostaglandins Serotonin
Increased vascular permeability	Bradykinin C3a, C5a PAF Histamine Serotonin Prostaglandins
Chemotaxis	Histamine C5a Monokines Kallikrein Lymphokines
Fever	Prostaglandins
Pain	Prostaglandins Hageman factor Bradykinin

PAF, Platelet-activating factor.

inflammation, after which they are rapidly destroyed by tissue proteases or kininases.[14]

Prostaglandins are produced by nearly all cells in the body and are released in response to any damage to the cell membrane. Two prostaglandins affect the inflammatory phase: prostaglandin E_1 (PGE_1) and prostaglandin E_2 (PGE_2). PGE_1 increases vascular permeability by antagonizing vasoconstriction, and PGE_2 attracts leukocytes and synergizes the effects of other inflammatory mediators such as bradykinin. Proinflammatory prostaglandins are also thought to be responsible for sensitizing pain receptors. In the early stages of the healing response, prostaglandins may regulate the repair process; they are also responsible for the later stages of inflammation.[15] Nonsteroidal antiinflammatory drugs (NSAIDs) specifically work by inhibiting prostaglandin synthesis, whereas **corticosteroids** inhibit inflammation by this and other mechanisms. Because prostaglandins are responsible for febrile states, these medications are also effective in reducing fever.

The anaphylatoxins C3a, C4a, and C5a are important products of the complement system. These complement fractions cause increased vascular permeability and induce mast cell and basophil degranulation, causing a further release of histamine and further increasing vascular permeability.

Aside from the chemically mediated vascular changes (Table 2-2), changes in physical attraction between blood vessel walls also alter blood flow. During the initial vasoconstriction, the opposing walls of the small vessels become approximated, causing the lining of the blood vessels to stick together. Under normal physiological conditions, the cell membranes of the inflammatory cells and the basement membranes have mutually repulsive negative charges; however, after injury, this repulsion decreases and the polarity may actually be reversed. This results in

a decrease in the repulsion between the circulating inflammatory cells and the vessel walls and contributes to the adherence of inflammatory cells to the blood vessel linings.

As vasoconstriction of the postcapillary venules and increased permeability of the microvasculature causes blood flow to slow, an increase in the cellular concentration occurs in the vessels, resulting in increased viscosity. In the normal physiological state, the cellular components of blood within the microvasculature are confined to a central axial column and the blood in contact with the vessel wall is relatively cell-free plasma.

Early in the inflammatory response, neutrophils, a type of leukocyte, in the circulating blood begin migrating to the injured area. Within a few hours of injury, the bulk of neutrophils in the wound transmigrate across the capillary endothelial cell walls. The sequence of events in the journey of these cells from inside the blood vessel to the tissue outside the blood vessel is known as **extravasation**. The neutrophils break away from the central cellular column of blood and start to roll along the blood vessel lining (the endothelium) and adhere. They line the walls of the vessels in a process known as **margination**. Within 1 hour, the endothelial lining of the vessels can be completely covered with neutrophils. As these cells accumulate, they lay down in layers in a process known as **pavementing**. Certain mediators control the adherence of leukocytes to the endothelium, either enhancing or inhibiting this process. For example, fibronectin, a glycoprotein present in plasma and basement membranes, has an important role in the modulation of cellular adherence to vessel walls. After injury to the vessels, increased amounts of fibronectin are deposited at the injury site. The adherence of the leukocytes to the endothelium or vascular basement membrane is critical for their recruitment to the site of the injury.

After margination, neutrophils begin to squeeze through the vessel walls in a process known as **diapedesis**. Endothelial P- and E-selectin and intercellular adhesion molecule-1 (ICAM-1) and ICAM-2 are adhesion molecules crucial to the process of diapedesis. These adhesion molecules interact with integrins on the surface of neutrophils as they insert their pseudopods into the junctions between the endothelial cells, crawl through the widened junctions, and assume a position between the endothelium and the basement membrane. Then, attracted by chemotactic agents, they escape to reach the interstitium. This process of leukocyte migration from the blood vessels into the perivascular tissues is known as **emigration** (Fig. 2-6). The receptors on white blood cells and endothelial cells that allow rolling, margination, and diapedesis have now been identified, and drugs affecting these functions have been developed. In the future, these drugs may play an important role in treating severe inappropriate inflammation.[16,17]

Edema is an accumulation of fluid within the extravascular space and interstitial tissues. Edema is the result of increased capillary hydrostatic pressure, increased interstitial osmotic pressure, increased venule permeability, and an overwhelmed lymphatic system that is unable to accommodate this substantial increase in fluid and plasma proteins. Edema formation and control are discussed in detail in Chapter 11. The clinical manifestation of edema is swelling.

> **◎ Clinical Pearl**
>
> Edema is swelling caused by fluid accumulation outside the vessels.

The fluid that first forms edema during inflammation has very few cells and very little protein. This fluid is known as **transudate**. Transudate is made up of predominantly dissolved electrolytes and water and has a specific gravity of less than 1.0. As the permeability of the vessels increases, more cells and lower molecular weight plasma proteins cross the vessel wall, making the extravascular fluid more viscous and cloudy. This cloudy fluid, known as **exudate**, has a specific gravity greater than 1.0. It is also characterized by a high content of lipids and cellular debris. Exudate is often observed early in the acute

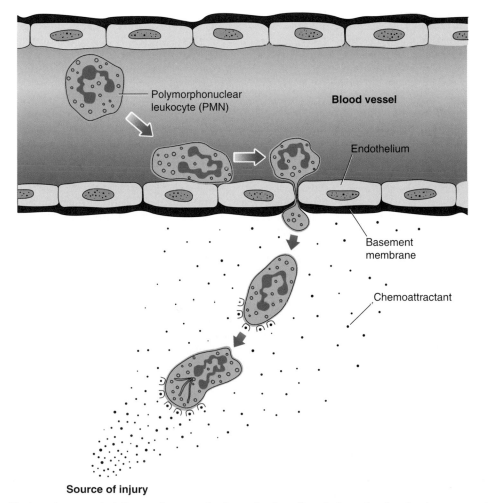

Source of injury

FIG 2-6 Illustration of leukocytic events in inflammation: margination, adhesion, diapedesis, and emigration in response to a chemoattractant emanating from the source of the injury.

inflammatory process and forms in response to such minor injuries as blisters and sunburns.

The loss of protein-rich fluid from the plasma reduces the osmotic pressure within the vessels and increases the osmotic pressure of the interstitial fluids, which in turn increases the outflow of fluid from the vessels, resulting in an accumulation of more fluid in the interstitial tissue. When the exudate concentration of leukocytes increases, it is known as **pus** or suppurative exudate. Pus consists of neutrophils, liquefied digestion products of underlying tissue, fluid exudate, and often bacteria if an infection is present. When localized suppurative exudate occurs within a solid tissue, it results in an abscess, which is a localized collection of pus buried in a tissue, organ, or confined space. Pyogenic bacteria produce abscesses.

Four mechanisms are responsible for the increased vascular permeability seen in inflammation. The first mechanism is endothelial cell contraction, which leads to a widening of the intercellular junctions or gaps. This mechanism affects venules while sparing capillaries and arterioles. It is controlled by chemical mediators and is relatively short-lived, lasting for only 15 to 30 minutes.[18] The second mechanism is a result of direct endothelial injury and is an immediate, sustained response potentially affecting all levels of the microcirculation. This effect is often seen in severe burns or lytic bacterial infections and is often associated with platelet adhesion and thrombosis or clot formation. Leukocyte-dependent endothelial injury is the third mechanism. Leukocytes bind to the area of injury and release various chemicals and enzymes that damage the endothelium and thus increase permeability. The final mechanism is leakage by regenerating capillaries that lack a differentiated endothelium and therefore do not have tight gaps. This may account for the edema characteristic of later healing inflammation (Fig. 2-7).

Hemostatic Response

The hemostatic response to injury controls the blood loss when vessels are damaged or ruptured. Immediately after injury, platelets enter the area and bind to the exposed **collagen**, releasing fibrin to stimulate clotting. Platelets also release a regulatory protein known as **platelet-derived growth factor** (PDGF), which is chemotactic and mitogenic to **fibroblasts** and may also be chemotactic to macrophages, **monocytes**, and neutrophils.[19] Thus platelets play a role not only in hemostasis but also contribute to the control of fibrin deposition, fibroblast proliferation, and angiogenesis.

When fibrin and fibronectin enter the injured area, they form cross-links with the collagen to create a fibrin lattice. This tenuous structure provides a temporary plug in the blood and lymph vessels, limiting local bleeding and fluid drainage. The lattice seals off damaged vessels and confines the inflammatory reaction to the area immediately surrounding the injury. The damaged, plugged vessels do not reopen until later in the healing process. The fibrin lattice serves as the wound's only source of tensile strength during the inflammatory phase of healing.[20]

Cellular Response

Circulating blood is composed of specialized cells suspended in a fluid known as plasma. These cells include erythrocytes (red blood cells), leukocytes (white blood cells), and platelets. Red blood cells play a minor role in the inflammatory process, although they may migrate into the tissue spaces if the inflammatory reaction is intense. The primary role of the red blood cells, oxygen transport, is carried out within the confines of the vessels. An inflammatory exudate that contains blood usually indicates severe injury to the microvasculature. The accumulation of blood in a tissue or organ is referred to as a **hematoma**; bloody fluid that is present in a joint is called a **hemarthrosis**. Hematomas in muscle can cause pain and limit motion or function; they can also increase scar tissue formation.

> ### Clinical Pearl
>
> Muscle hematomas can cause pain, limit motion, and increase scar tissue formation.

A critical function of inflammation is to deliver leukocytes to the area of injury via the circulatory system. Leukocytes are classified according to their structure into **polymorphonucleocytes** (PMNs) and mononuclear cells (Fig. 2-8). PMNs have nuclei with several lobes and contain cytoplasmic granules. They are further categorized as neutrophils, basophils, and eosinophils by their preference for specific histological stains. Monocytes are larger than PMNs and have a single nucleus. In the inflammatory process, leukocytes play the important role of clearing the injured site of debris and microorganisms to set the stage for tissue repair.

Migration of leukocytes into the area of injury occurs within hours of the injury. Each leukocyte is specialized and has a specific purpose. Some leukocytes are more prominent in early inflammation, whereas others become more important during the later stages. Initially the number of leukocytes at the injury site is proportional to their concentration in the circulating blood.

Because neutrophils have the highest concentration in the blood, they predominate in the early phases of inflammation. Chemotactic agents released by other cells, such as mast cells and platelets, attract leukocytes at the time of injury. Neutrophils rid the injury site of bacteria and debris by **phagocytosis**. When lysed, the lysosomes of the neutrophils release proteolytic enzymes (proteases) and collagenolytic enzymes (**collagenases**), which begin the débridement process. Neutrophils remain at the site of the injury for only 24 hours, after which time they disintegrate. However, they help to perpetuate the inflammatory response by releasing chemotactic agents to attract other leukocytes into the area.

Basophils release histamine after injury and contribute to early increased vascular permeability. Eosinophils may be involved in phagocytosis to some degree.

For 24 to 48 hours after an acute injury, monocytes predominate. Monocytes make up between 4% and 8% of

MECHANISMS OF LEAKAGE
AND DISTRIBUTION

Endothelial cell contraction
• venules

Direct endothelial injury
• all microvessels

NORMAL

Leukocyte-dependent
endothelial injury
• mostly venules
• lung capillaries

INFLAMED

Regenerating capillary
endothelium
• capillaries
• other vessels

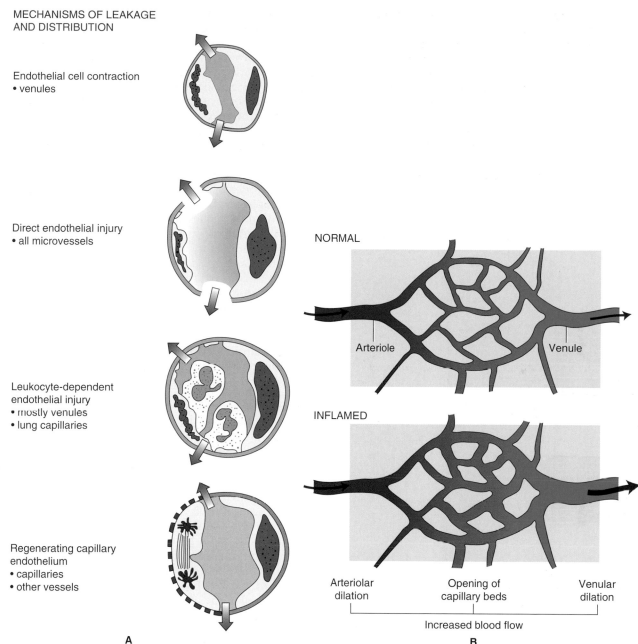

Arteriole   Venule

Arteriolar
dilation

Opening of
capillary beds

Venular
dilation

Increased blood flow

A   **B**

FIG 2-7 **A,** Illustration of four mechanisms of increased vascular permeability in inflammation. **B,** Vascular changes associated with acute inflammation.

the total white blood cell count. The predominance of these cells at this stage of inflammation is thought to result in part from their longer lifespan. Lymphocytes supply antibodies to mediate the body's immune response. They are prevalent in chronic inflammatory conditions.

Monocytes are converted into macrophages when they migrate from the capillaries into the tissue spaces. The macrophage is considered the most important cell in the inflammatory phase and is essential for wound healing. Macrophages are important because they produce a wide range of chemicals (Box 2-1). They play a major role in phagocytosis by producing enzymes such as collagenase (Fig. 2-9). These enzymes facilitate the removal of necrotic

BOX 2-1	Macrophage Products

- Proteases
- Elastase
- Collagenase
- Plasminogen activator
- Chemotactic factors for other leukocytes
- Complement components of the alternative and classical pathways
- Coagulation factors
- Growth-promoting factors for fibroblasts and blood vessels
- Cytokines
- Arachidonic acid metabolites

tissue and bacteria. Macrophages also produce factors that are chemotactic for other leukocytes and growth factors that promote cell proliferation and the synthesis of extracellular matrix molecules by resident skin cells.[21]

Macrophages also probably play a role in localizing the inflammatory process and attracting fibroblasts to the injured area by releasing chemotactic factors such as fibronectin. Macrophages chemically influence the number of fibroblastic repair cells activated; therefore, in the absence of macrophages, fewer, less mature fibroblasts migrate to the injured site. PDGF released by platelets during clotting is also released by macrophages and can activate fibroblasts. In the later stages of **fibroplasia**, macrophages

may also enhance collagen deposition by causing fibroblasts to adhere to fibrin.

As macrophages phagocytose organisms, they release a variety of substances, such as hydrogen peroxide, ascorbic acid, and lactic acid, that enhance killing of microorganisms.[22] Hydrogen peroxide inhibits anaerobic microbial growth. The other two products signal the extent of the damage in the area, and their concentration is interpreted by the body as a need for more macrophages in the area.[23] This interpretation in turn causes increased production of these substances, which then results in an increased macrophage population and a more intense and prolonged inflammatory response.

Macrophages are most effective when oxygen is present in the injured tissues. However, they can tolerate low oxygen conditions, as is apparent by their presence in chronic inflammatory states. Adequate oxygen tension in the injured area is also necessary to minimize the risk of infection. Tissue oxygen tension depends on the concentration of atmospheric oxygen available for breathing, the amount of oxygen absorbed by the respiratory and circulatory systems, and the volume of blood available for transportation, as well as the state of the tissues. Local topical application of oxygen to an injured area does not influence tissue oxygen tension as much as the level of oxygen brought to the injured area by the circulating blood.[24-26]

Immune Response

The immune response is mediated by cellular and humoral factors. On a cellular level, macrophages present foreign antigens to T lymphocytes to activate them. Activated T lymphocytes elaborate a host of inflammatory mediators and activate B cells, causing them to evolve into plasma cells, which make antibodies that specifically bind foreign antigens. These antibodies can coat bacteria and viruses, inhibiting their function and opsonizing them so that they are more readily ingested and cleared from the system by phagocytic cells. Antibodies bound to antigens, bacteria, and viruses also activate the complement system, an important source of vasoactive mediators. The complement system is one of the most important plasma protein systems of inflammation because its components participate in virtually every inflammatory response.

The complement system is a series of enzymatic plasma proteins that is activated by two different pathways, the classical and the alternative.[27] Activation of the first com-

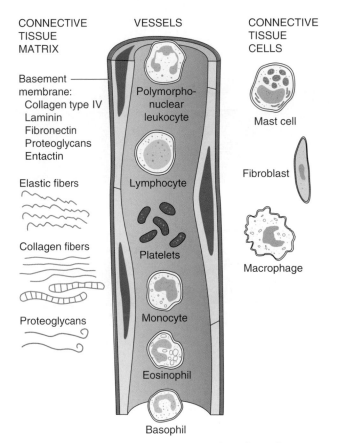

FIG 2-8 Connective tissue matrix, intravascular cells, and connective tissue cells involved in the inflammatory response.

CONNECTIVE TISSUE MATRIX

Basement membrane:
  Collagen type IV
  Laminin
  Fibronectin
  Proteoglycans
  Entactin

Elastic fibers

Collagen fibers

Proteoglycans

VESSELS

Polymorpho-nuclear leukocyte

Lymphocyte

Platelets

Monocyte

Eosinophil

Basophil

CONNECTIVE TISSUE CELLS

Mast cell

Fibroblast

Macrophage

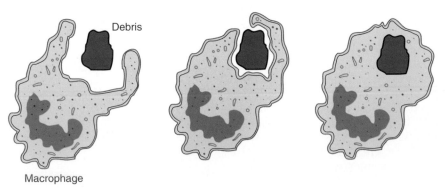

Debris

Macrophage

FIG 2-9 Diagrammatic representation of the process of phagocytosis.

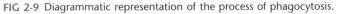

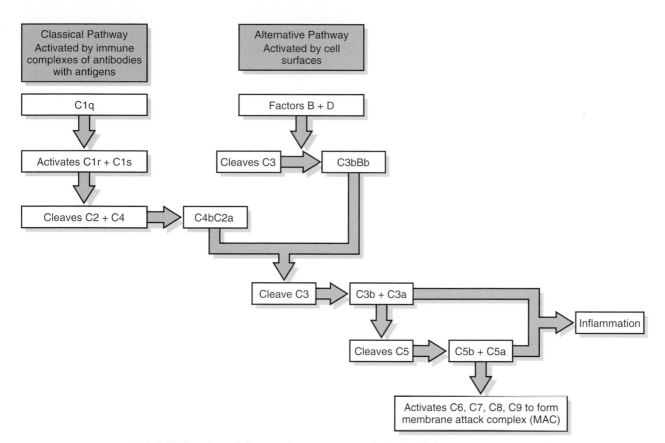

FIG 2-10 Overview of the complement system—classical and alternative activation pathways.

ponent of either pathway of the cascade results in the sequential enzymatic activation of the downstream components of the cascade (Fig. 2-10). The classical pathway is activated by an antibody-antigen association, and the alternative pathway is activated by cellular or microbial substances. The end product of the cascade, by either pathway, is a complex of C6, C7, C8, and C9, which form the membrane attack complex (MAC). The MAC creates pores in plasma membranes, thereby allowing water and ions into the cell, leading to cell lysis and death.

The subcomponents generated earlier in the cascade also have important functions. Activation of components C1 to C5 produces subunits that enhance inflammation by making bacteria more susceptible to phagocytosis (known as **opsonization**), attracting leukocytes by chemotaxis and acting as anaphylatoxins. Anaphylatoxins induce mast cell and basophil degranulation, causing the release of histamine, platelet-activating factor, and leukotrienes. These further promote increased vascular permeability.

In summary, there are three major consequences of the inflammatory phase. First, fibrin, fibronectin, and collagen cross-link to form a fibrin lattice that limits blood loss and provides the wound with some initial strength. Then neutrophils followed by macrophages begin to remove damaged tissue. Finally, endothelial cells and fibroblasts are recruited and stimulated to divide. This sets the stage for the proliferation phase of healing. Table 2-3 summarizes the events of the inflammatory phase of healing.

TABLE 2-3	Summary of Events of the Inflammatory Phase
Response	**Changes in the Injured Area**
Vascular	Vasodilation followed by vasoconstriction at the capillaries, postcapillary venules, and lymphatics.
	Vasodilation mediated by chemical mediators—histamine, Hageman factor, bradykinin, prostaglandins, complement fractions.
	Slowing of blood flow.
	Margination, pavementing, and ultimately emigration of leukocytes.
	Accumulation of fluid in the interstitial tissues resulting in edema.
Hemostatic	Retraction and sealing off of blood vessels.
	Platelets form clots and assist in building of fibrin lattice, which serves as the wound's source of tensile strength in the inflammatory phase.
Cellular	Delivery of leukocytes to the area of injury to rid the area of bacteria and debris by phagocytosis.
	Monocytes, the precursors of macrophages, are considered the most important cell in the inflammatory phase.
	Macrophages produce a number of products essential to the healing process.
Immune	Mediated by both cellular and humoral factors.
	Activation of the complement system via the alternative and classical pathways resulting in components that increase vascular permeability, stimulate phagocytosis, and act as chemotactic stimuli for leukocytes.

PROLIFERATION PHASE (DAYS 3-20)

The second phase of tissue healing is known as the proliferation phase. This phase generally lasts for up to 20 days and involves both **epithelial cells** and **connective tissues**.[20] Its purpose is to cover the wound and impart strength to the injury site.

◎ Clinical Pearl

During the proliferation phase of healing, the wound is covered, and the injury site starts to regain some of its initial strength.

Epithelial cells form the covering of mucous and serous membranes and the epidermis of the skin. Connective tissue consists of fibroblasts, ground substance, and fibrous strands and provides the structure for other tissues. The structure, strength, and elasticity of connective tissue varies, depending on the type of tissue it comprises. Four processes occur simultaneously in the proliferation phase to achieve coalescence and closure of the injured area: **epithelialization**, collagen production, **wound contraction**, and **neovascularization**.

Epithelialization

Epithelialization, the reestablishment of the epidermis, is initiated early in proliferation when a wound is superficial, often within a few hours of injury.[28] When a wound is deep, epithelialization occurs later, after collagen production and neovascularization. Epithelialization provides a protective barrier to prevent fluid and electrolyte loss and to decrease the risk of infection. Healing of the wound surface by epithelialization alone does not provide adequate strength to meet the mechanical demands placed on most tissues. Such strength is provided by the collagen produced during fibroplasia.

During epithelialization, uninjured epithelial cells from the margins of the injured area reproduce and migrate over the injured area, covering the surface of the wound and closing the defect. It is hypothesized that the stimulus for this activity is the loss of contact inhibition that occurs when epithelial cells are normally in contact with one another. The migrating epithelial cells stay connected to their parent cells, thereby pulling the intact epidermis over the wound edge. When epithelial cells from one edge meet migrating cells from the other edge, they stop moving because of contact inhibition (Fig. 2-11). Although clean, approximated wounds can be clinically resurfaced within 48 hours; larger open wounds take longer to resurface.[29] It then takes several weeks for this thin layer to become multilayered and to differentiate into the various strata of normal epidermis.

Collagen Production

Fibroblasts make collagen. Fibroblast growth, known as fibroplasia, takes place in connective tissue. Fibroblasts

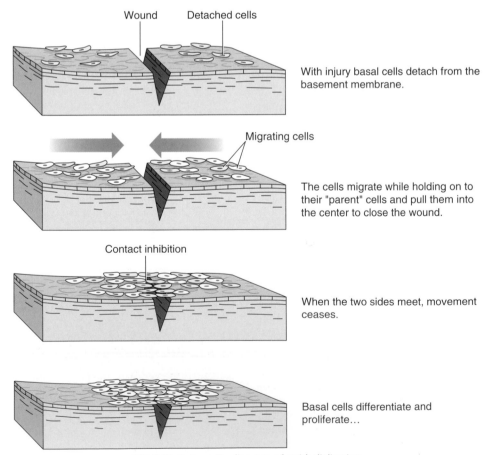

Wound   Detached cells

With injury basal cells detach from the basement membrane.

Migrating cells

The cells migrate while holding on to their "parent" cells and pull them into the center to close the wound.

Contact inhibition

When the two sides meet, movement ceases.

Basal cells differentiate and proliferate...

FIG 2-11 Schematic diagram of epithelialization.

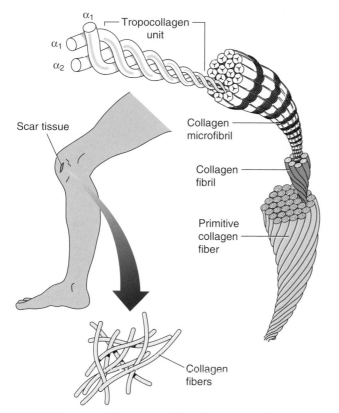

FIG 2-12 Diagrammatic representation of one tropocollagen unit joining with others to form collagen filaments and, ultimately, collagen fibers.

develop from undifferentiated mesenchymal cells located around blood vessels and in fat. They migrate to the injured area along fibrin strands, in response to chemotactic influences, and are present throughout the injured area.[30] Adequate supplies of oxygen, ascorbic acid, and other cofactors, such as zinc, iron, manganese, and copper, are necessary for fibroplasia to occur.[31] As the number of fibroblasts increases, they begin to align themselves perpendicular to the capillaries.

Fibroblasts synthesize procollagen, which is composed of three polypeptide chains coiled and held together by weak electrostatic bonds into a triple helix. These chains undergo cleavage by collagenase to form tropocollagen. Multiple tropocollagen chains then coil together to form collagen microfibrils, which then make up collagen fibrils and ultimately combine to form collagen fibers (Fig. 2-12). Cross-linking between collagen molecules provides further tensile strength to the injured area. Collagen serves a dual purpose in wound healing, providing increased strength and facilitating the movement of other cells, such as endothelial cells and macrophages, while they participate in wound healing.[32,33]

Tissue containing the newly formed capillaries, fibroblasts, and **myofibroblasts** is referred to as **granulation tissue**. As the amount of granulation tissue increases, there is a concurrent reduction in the size of the fibrin clot, allowing for the formation of a more permanent support structure. These events are mediated by chemotactic factors that stimulate increased fibroblastic activity and by fibronectin that enhances migration and adhesion of the fibroblasts. The fibroblasts initially produce a thin, weak-structured collagen with no consistent organization known as **type III collagen**. This period is the most tenuous time during the healing process because of the limited tensile strength of the tissue. During the proliferation phase, an injured area has the greatest amount of collagen, yet its tensile strength can be as low as 15% of the tensile strength of normal tissue.[34]

> ### ◉ Clinical Pearl
> During the proliferation phase, an injured area has the greatest amount of collagen, yet its tensile strength can be as low as 15% of the tensile strength of normal tissue.

Fibroblasts also produce hyaluronic acid, a glycosaminoglycan (GAG), which draws water into the area, increases the amount of intracellular matrix, and facilitates cellular migration. It is postulated that the composition of this substance is related to the number and location of the cross-bridges, thereby implying that the relationship between GAG and collagen dictates the scar architecture.[22,35]

The formation of cross-links allows the newly formed tissue to tolerate early, controlled movement without disruption. However, infection, edema, or excessive stress on the healing area may result in further inflammation and additional deposition of collagen. Excessive collagen deposition will result in excessive scarring that may limit the functional outcome.

By the seventh day after injury there is a significant increase in the amount of collagen, causing the tensile strength of the injured area to increase steadily. By day 12, the initial immature type III collagen starts to be replaced by **type I collagen**, a more mature and stronger form.[20,36,37] The ratio of type I to type III collagen increases steadily from this point on. Production of collagen is maximal at day 21 of healing, but the wound strength at this time is only approximately 20% of the normal dermis. By about 6 weeks after injury, when a wound is healing well, it has about 80% of its long-term strength.[38]

Wound Contraction

Wound contraction is the final mechanism for repairing an injured area. In contrast to epithelialization, which covers the wound surface, contraction pulls the edges of the injured site together, in effect shrinking the defect. Successful contraction results in a smaller area to be repaired by scar formation. Contraction of the wound begins approximately 5 days after injury and peaks after about 2 weeks.[39] Myofibroblasts are the primary cells responsible for wound contraction. Myofibroblasts, identified by Gabbiani et al in 1971, are derived from the same mesenchymal cells as fibroblasts.[40] Myofibroblasts are similar to fibroblasts except that they also possess the contractile properties of smooth muscle. Myofibroblasts

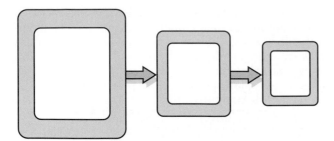

FIG 2-13 Illustration of the picture-frame theory of wound contraction.

attach to the margins of the intact skin and pull the entire epithelial layer inward. The rate of contraction is proportional to the number of myofibroblasts at and under the cell margins and is inversely proportional to the lattice collagen structure.

According to the "picture-frame" theory, the wound margin beneath the epidermis is the location of myofibroblast action.[41] A ring of myofibroblasts moves inward from the wound margin. Although contractile forces are initially equal, the shape of the picture frame predicts the resultant speed of closure (Fig. 2-13). Linear wounds with one narrow dimension contract rapidly; square or rectangular wounds, with no close edges, progress at a moderate pace; and circular wounds contract most slowly.[42]

If wound contraction is uncontrolled, it can result in the formation of **contractures**. Contractures are conditions of fixed high resistance to passive stretch that may result from fibrosis of tissues surrounding a joint.[43] Contractures may also result from adhesions, muscle shortening, or tissue damage. Contractures are discussed in greater depth in Chapter 5.

When the initial injury causes minimal tissue loss and minimal bacterial contamination, the wound can be closed with sutures and can thus heal without wound contraction. This is known as **healing by primary intention** (also known as primary union) (Fig. 2-14). When the initial injury causes significant loss of tissue or bacterial contamination, the wound must first undergo the process of wound contraction to close the wound; this is known as **healing by secondary intention** (also known as indirect union) (see Fig. 2-14).[44] Later approximation of a wound's edges with sutures or the application of skin grafts can reduce wound contraction and is known as **healing by delayed primary intention**.[45,46] To minimize contraction, grafts must be applied early in the inflammatory phase, before the process of contraction begins.[47]

As scar tissue matures, it develops pressure and tension-sensitive nerve endings to protect the immature vascular system, which is weak and can bleed easily with any insult. During the proliferation phase, the scar is red and swollen from the increase in vascularity and fluid, the innervation of the healing site, and the relative immaturity of the tissue. The tissue can easily be damaged and is tender to tension or pressure.

Neovascularization

Neovascularization, the development of a new blood supply to the injured area, occurs as a result of **angiogenesis**, the growth of new blood vessels. Healing cannot occur without angiogenesis. These new vessels are needed to supply oxygen and nutrients to the injured and healing tissue. It is thought that macrophages signal the initiation of neovascularization through the release of growth factors.[38] Angiogenesis can occur by three different mechanisms: generation of a new vascular network, anastomosis to preexisting vessels, or coupling of the vessels in the injured area.[48]

Vessels in the wound periphery develop small buds that grow into the wound area. These outgrowths eventually come in contact with and join other arterial or venular buds to form a capillary loop. These vessels fill the injured area, giving it a pinkish to bright red hue. As the wound heals, many of these capillary loops cease to function and retract, giving the mature scar a more whitish appearance than the adjacent tissues. Initially the walls of these capillaries are thin, making them prone to injury. Therefore immobilization at this stage may help to protect these vessels and permit further regrowth, whereas excessive early motion can cause microhemorrhaging and increase the likelihood of infection.

MATURATION PHASE (DAY 9 ON)

As the transition from the proliferation to the maturation stage of healing is made, changes occur in the size, form, and strength of the scar tissue. The maturation phase is the longest phase in the healing process. It can persist for over a year after the initial insult. During this time, the number of fibroblasts, macrophages, myofibroblasts, and capillaries decrease and the water content of the tissue declines. The scar becomes whiter in appearance as the collagen matures and the vascularity decreases. The ultimate goal of this phase is restoration of the prior function of the injured tissue.

Several factors determine the rate of maturation and the final physical characteristics of the scar. These include fiber orientation and the balance of collagen synthesis and lysis.

Throughout the maturation phase, synthesis and lysis of collagen occur in a balanced fashion. Hormonal stimulation that results from inflammation causes increased collagen destruction by the enzyme collagenase. Collagenase is derived from polymorphogranular leukocytes, the migrating epithelium, and the granulation bed. Collagenase is able to break the strong cross-linking bonds of the tropocollagen molecule, causing it to become soluble. It is then excreted as a waste by-product. Although collagenase is most active in the actual area of the injury, its effects can also be noticed to a lesser extent in areas adjacent to the injury site. Thus remodeling occurs through a process of collagen turnover.

Collagen, a glycoprotein, provides the extracellular framework for all multicellular organisms. Although more than 27 types of collagen have been identified, the following discussion is limited to types I, II, and III (Table 2-4).[49] All collagen molecules are made up of three separate polypeptide chains wrapped tightly together in a triple left-

HEALING BY PRIMARY INTENTION   HEALING BY SECONDARY INTENTION

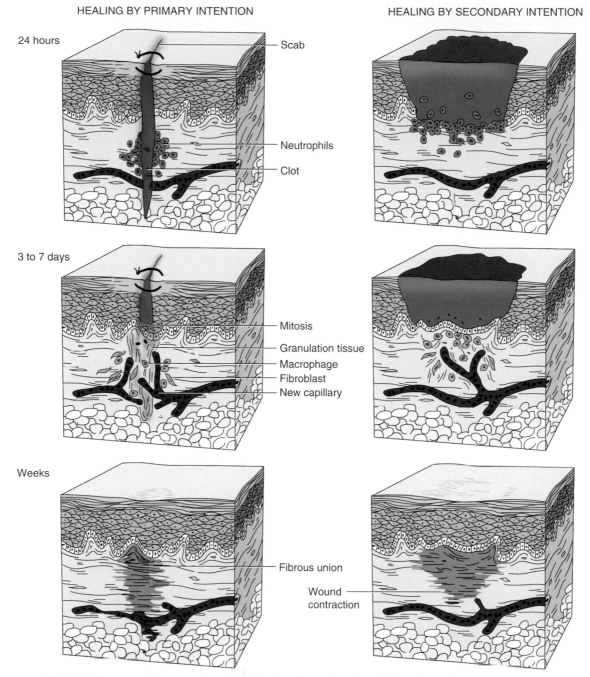

FIG 2-14 Diagrammatic comparison of healing by primary intention (*left*) and secondary intention (*right*).

handed helix. Type I collagen is the primary collagen found in bone, skin, and **tendon** and is the predominant collagen in mature scars. **Type II collagen** is the predominant collagen in **cartilage**. Type III collagen is found in the gastrointestinal tract, uterus, and blood vessels in adults. It is also the first type of collagen to be deposited during the healing process.

During the maturation phase, the collagen synthesized and deposited is predominantly type I. The balance between synthesis and lysis generally slightly favors synthesis. Because type I collagen is stronger than the type III collagen deposited in the proliferation phase, tensile strength increases faster than mass. If the rate of collagen production is much greater than the rate of lysis, a keloid or hypertrophic scar can result. Both keloids and hypertrophic scars are the result of excessive collagen deposition as a result of inhibition of lysis. It is believed that this inhibition of lysis is caused by a genetic defect. Keloids extend beyond the original boundaries of an injury and invade the surrounding tissue, whereas hypertrophic scars, although raised, remain within the margins of the original wound. The treatment of keloid scars through surgery, medications, pressure, and irradiation has only limited success.[50-52]

TABLE 2-4	Collagen Types
Type	**Distribution**
I	Most abundant form of collagen: skin, bone, tendons, and most organs
II	Major cartilage collagen, vitreous humor
III	Abundant in blood vessels, uterus, skin
IV	All basement membranes
V	Minor component of most interstitial tissues
VI	Abundant in most interstitial tissues
VII	Dermal-epidermal junction
VIII	Endothelium
IX	Cartilage
X	Cartilage

Collagen synthesis is oxygen dependent, whereas collagen lysis is not.[53] Thus, when oxygen levels are low, the process of maturation is weighted toward lysis, resulting in a softer, less bulky scar. Hypertrophic scars can be managed clinically with prolonged pressure, which causes a decrease in oxygen, resulting in decreased overall collagen synthesis while maintaining the level of collagen lysis.[45] This is one of the bases for the use of pressure garments in the treatment of patients suffering from burns and for the use of elastomer in the management of scars in hand therapy. Eventually, balance is achieved when the scar bulk is flattened to approximate normal tissue.

Collagen synthesis and lysis may last for up to 12 to 24 months after an injury. The high rate of collagen turnover during this period can be viewed as both detrimental and beneficial. As long as the scar tissue appears redder than the surrounding tissue, remodeling is still occurring. Although a joint or tissue structure can lose mobility quickly during this stage, such a loss can still be reversed through appropriate intervention.

The physical structure of the collagen fibers is largely responsible for the final function of the injured area. Collagen in scar tissue is always less organized than collagen in the surrounding tissue. Scars are inelastic because elastin, a normal skin component, is not present in scars,[38] so redundant folds are necessary to permit mobility of the structures to which they are attached. To understand this concept better, one may consider a spring, which, although made of an inelastic material, has a spiraled form (like the redundant folds of a scar) that allows it to expand and contract. If short, dense adhesions are formed, these will restrict motion because they cannot elongate.

Two theories have been proposed to explain the orientation of the collagen fibers in scar tissue: the induction theory and the tension theory. According to the induction theory, the scar attempts to mimic the characteristics of the tissue it is healing.[54] Thus a dense tissue induces a dense, highly cross-linked scar, whereas a more pliable tissue results in a loose, less cross-linked scar. Dense tissue types have a preferential status when multiple tissue types are in close proximity. Based on this theory, surgeons attempt to design repair fields that separate dense and soft tissues. If this is not possible, as in the case of repaired tendon left immobile over bone fractures, adhesions and

poorly gliding tendons can result. In such cases, early controlled movement may be beneficial.

According to the tension theory, the internal and external stresses placed on the injured area during the maturation phase determine the final tissue structure.[48] Muscle tension, joint movement, soft tissue loading and unloading, fascial gliding, temperature changes, and mobilization are all forces that are thought to affect collagen structure. Thus the length and mobility of the injured area may be modified by the application of stress during the appropriate phases of healing. This theory has been supported by the work of Arem and Madden, which has shown that the two most important variables responsible for successful remodeling are the phases of the repair process in which mechanical forces were introduced and the nature of the applied forces.[55] Scars need low-load, long-duration stretch during the appropriate phase for permanent changes to occur.

Studies have shown that the application of tension during healing causes an increase in tensile strength, and immobilization and stress deprivation reduce tensile strength and collagen structure. The recovery curves for tissue experimentally immobilized for between 2 and 4 weeks reveal that these processes can take months to reverse, and reversal is often never complete.

Each phase of the healing response is necessary and essential to the subsequent phase. In the optimal scenario, inflammation is a necessary aspect of the healing response and the first step toward recovery, setting the stage for the other phases of healing. If repeated insults or injury occur, however, a chronic inflammatory response may develop that can adversely affect the outcome of the healing process.

Acute inflammatory processes can have one of four outcomes. First and most beneficial is the complete resolution and replacement of the injured tissue with like tissue. Second and most common is healing by scar formation. The third is the formation of an abscess. Fourth is the possibility of progression to **chronic inflammation**.[12]

CHRONIC INFLAMMATION

Chronic inflammation is the simultaneous progression of active inflammation, tissue destruction, and healing. Chronic inflammation can arise in one of two ways. The first follows acute inflammation and can be a result of the persistence of the injurious agent (such as a cumulative trauma) or some other interference with the normal healing process. The second is the result of an immune response to either an altered host tissue or a foreign material (such as an implant or a suture) or the result of an autoimmune disease (such as rheumatoid arthritis).

The normal acute inflammatory process lasts for no more than 2 weeks. If it continues for more than 4 weeks, it is known as **subacute inflammation**.[3] Chronic inflammation is inflammation that lasts for months or years.

The primary cells present during chronic inflammation are mononuclear cells, including lymphocytes, macrophages, and monocytes (Fig. 2-15). Occasionally, eosinophils are also present.[13] The progression of the inflammatory response to a chronic state is a result of both immunologi-

Leukocyte	Characteristics/Functions

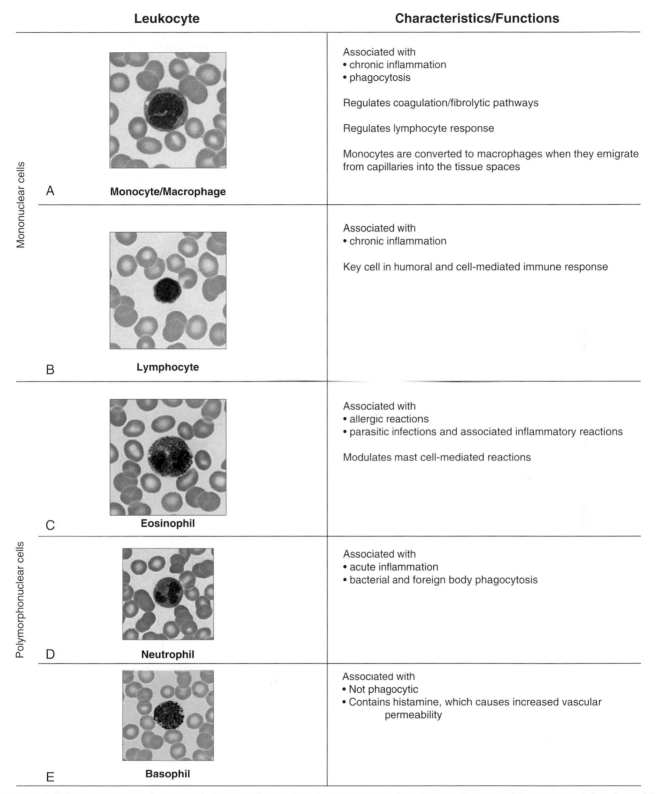

Mononuclear cells

A — Monocyte/Macrophage

Associated with
• chronic inflammation
• phagocytosis

Regulates coagulation/fibrolytic pathways

Regulates lymphocyte response

Monocytes are converted to macrophages when they emigrate from capillaries into the tissue spaces

B — Lymphocyte

Associated with
• chronic inflammation

Key cell in humoral and cell-mediated immune response

Polymorphonuclear cells

C — Eosinophil

Associated with
• allergic reactions
• parasitic infections and associated inflammatory reactions

Modulates mast cell-mediated reactions

D — Neutrophil

Associated with
• acute inflammation
• bacterial and foreign body phagocytosis

E — Basophil

Associated with
• Not phagocytic
• Contains histamine, which causes increased vascular permeability

FIG 2-15 Cellular components of acute and chronic inflammation. **A,** Monocyte; **B,** lymphocyte; **C,** eosinophil; **D,** neutrophil; **E,** basophil. *Adapted from McPherson & Pincus:* Henry's clinical diagnosis and management by laboratory methods, *ed 21, Philadelphia, 2006, Saunders.*

BOX 2-2 Factors Influencing Healing

Local
- Type, size, and location of injury
- Infection
- Vascular supply
- Movement/excessive pressure
- Temperature deviation
- Topical medications
- Electromagnetic energy
- Retained foreign body

Systemic
- Age
- Infection or disease
- Metabolic status
- Nutrition
- Hormones
- Medication
- Fever
- Oxygen

---

cal and nonimmunological factors. The macrophage is an important source of inflammatory and immunological mediators and is an important component in the regulation of their actions. The role of eosinophils is much less clear, although they are often present in chronic inflammatory conditions that are caused by allergic reactions or parasitic infection.[13]

Chronic inflammation also results in increased fibroblast proliferation, which in turn increases collagen production and ultimately increases scar tissue and adhesion formation. This may lead to a loss of function as the delicate balance between optimal tensile strength and mobility of the involved tissues is lost.

FACTORS AFFECTING THE HEALING PROCESS

A number of factors, either local or systemic, can impact or modify the processes of inflammation and repair (Box 2-2). Local factors that can affect wound healing include the type, size, and location of the injury; infection; blood supply; and external physical forces.

LOCAL FACTORS

Type, Size, and Location of the Injury

Injuries located in well-vascularized tissue, such as the scalp, heal faster than those in poorly vascularized areas.[20] Injuries in areas of ischemia, such as those that may be caused by arterial obstruction or excessive pressure, heal more slowly.[20]

Smaller wounds heal faster than larger wounds, and surgical incisions heal faster than wounds caused by blunt trauma.[20] Soft tissue injuries over bones tend to adhere to the bony surfaces, preventing contraction and adequate opposition of the edges and delaying healing.[20]

Infection

Infection in an injured area is the most problematic local factor that can affect healing. Among the complications of wound healing, 50% are the result of local infection.[13] Infections affect collagen metabolism, reducing collagen production and increasing lysis.[56] Infection often prevents or delays healing and encourages excessive granulation tissue formation.[20]

Vascular Supply

The healing of injuries largely depends on the availability of a sufficient vascular supply. Nutrition, oxygen tension, and the inflammatory response all depend on the microcirculatory system to deliver their components.[57] Decreased oxygen tension resulting from a compromised blood supply can result in the inhibition of fibroblast migration and collagen synthesis, leading to decreased tensile strength of the injured area and increased susceptibility to infection.[25]

External Forces

The application of physical agents, including thermal agents, electromagnetic energy, and mechanical forces, may also influence inflammation and healing. Cryotherapy (cold therapy), thermotherapy (heat), therapeutic ultrasound, electromagnetic radiation, light, electrical currents, and mechanical pressure have all been used by rehabilitation professionals in an attempt to modify the healing process.

Clinical Pearl

Physical agents used to modify the healing process include cryotherapy, thermotherapy, ultrasound, electromagnetic radiation, light, electrical currents, and compression.

The impact of these physical agents on tissue healing is discussed in Part II of this book which describes each type of physical agent, its effects, and its clinical applications.

Movement

Early movement of a newly injured area may delay healing. Therefore immobilization may be used to aid early healing and repair. However, because immobility can result in adhesions and stiffness by altering collagen cross-linking and elasticity, continuous passive motion (CPM) with strictly controlled parameters is often used to remobilize and restore function safely.[58] The use of CPM in conjunction with short-term immobilization, compared to immobilization alone, has been shown to achieve a better functional outcome in some studies; however, other studies have found differences only in early range of motion (ROM).[59,60] It has also been reported that patients utilizing CPM during the inflammatory phase of soft tissue healing after anterior cruciate ligament reconstruction use significantly less pain-relieving narcotics than patients not using CPM,[61] and CPM in conjunction with physical therapy after total knee arthroplasty resulted in improved knee ROM and decreased analgesic medication use.[62]

SYSTEMIC FACTORS

Age

Age should be considered because of variations in healing between the pediatric, adult, and geriatric populations. In childhood, wound closure occurs more rapidly than in adulthood because the physiological changes and cumulative sun exposure that occur with aging can reduce the healing rate.[63] A decrease in the density and cross-linking of collagen, which results in reduced tensile strength, decreased numbers of mast cells and fibroblasts, and a lower rate of epithelialization, occurs in the elderly.[64,65] The poor organization of cutaneous vessels in older people also adversely affects wound healing.

Disease

A number of diseases can affect wound healing either directly or indirectly. For example, poorly controlled diabetes mellitus impairs collagen synthesis, increases the risk of infection as a result of a dampened immune response, and decreases phagocytosis as a result of alterations in leukocyte function.[57,66] Peripheral vascular compromise is also prevalent in this population, leading to a decrease in local blood flow. Neuropathies, which are also common, can increase the potential for trauma and decrease the ability of soft tissue lesions to heal.

Patients who are immunocompromised, such as those with acquired immune deficiency syndrome (AIDS) or those taking immunosuppressive drugs after organ transplantation, are more prone to wound infections because they have an inadequate inflammatory response. AIDS also affects many other facets of the healing process through its impairment of phagocytosis, fibroblast function, and collagen synthesis.[67]

Problems involving the circulatory system, including atherosclerosis, sickle cell disease, and hypertension, can also have an adverse effect on wound healing because inflammation and healing depend on the cardiovascular system for the delivery of components to the local area of injury. Decreased oxygen tension resulting from a reduced blood supply can result in an inhibition of fibroblast migration and a decreased collagen synthesis, resulting in decreased tensile strength and making the injured area more susceptible to reinjury. Wounds with a decreased blood supply are also more susceptible to infection.[25,68]

Medications

Patients with injuries or wounds often take medications with systemic effects that alter tissue healing. For example, antibiotics can prevent or fight off infection, which can help speed healing, but they may also have toxic effects that inhibit healing. Corticosteroids, such as prednisone and dexamethasone, block the inflammatory cascade at a variety of levels, inhibiting many of the pathways involved in inflammation. At this time, it is thought that glucocorticoids act mainly by affecting gene transcription inside cells to inhibit the formation of inflammatory molecules, including cytokines, enzymes, receptors, and adhesion molecules.[69] They are also thought to stimulate the production of antiinflammatory molecules. Corticosteroids decrease the margination, migration, and accumulation of monocytes at the site of inflammation.[70] They also induce antiinflammatory actions by monocytes, such as phagocytosis of other inflammatory molecules, while repressing adhesion, apoptosis, and oxidative burst.[71] They severely inhibit wound contracture, decrease the rate of epithelialization, and decrease the tensile strength of closed, healed wounds.[72-75] Corticosteroids administered at the time of injury have a greater impact because decreasing the inflammatory response at this early stage delays subsequent phases of healing and increases the incidence of infection.

In comparison to corticosteroids, NSAIDs, such as ibuprofen, are less likely to impair healing. They interrupt the production of prostaglandins from arachidonic acid but are not thought to adversely affect the function of fibroblasts or tissue macrophages.[76] NSAIDs can cause vasoconstriction and suppress the inflammatory response,[14] however, and some NSAIDs have been found to inhibit cell proliferation and migration during tendon healing.[77,78]

Nutrition

Nutrition can have a profound effect on healing tissues. Deficiency of any of a number of important amino acids, vitamins, minerals, or water, as well as insufficient caloric intake, can result in delayed or impaired healing. This is because physiological stress from the injury induces a hypermetabolic state. Thus if insufficient "fuel" is available for the process of inflammation and repair, healing is slowed.

In most cases, healing abnormalities are associated with general protein-calorie malnutrition rather than depletion of a single nutrient.[79] Such is the case with patients with extensive burns who are in a prolonged hypermetabolic state. A protein deficiency can result in decreased fibroblastic proliferation, reduced proteoglycan and collagen synthesis, decreased angiogenesis, and disrupted collagen remodeling.[80] Protein deficiency can also adversely affect phagocytosis, which may lead to an increased risk of infection.[68]

Studies have shown that a deficiency of specific nutrients may also affect healing. Vitamin A deficiency can retard epithelialization, the rate of collagen synthesis, and cross-linking.[81] Thiamine (vitamin B1) deficiency decreases collagen formation, and vitamin B5 deficiency decreases the tensile strength of healed tissue and reduces the fibroblast number.[82,83] Vitamin C deficiency impairs collagen synthesis by fibroblasts, increases the capillary rupture potential, and increases the susceptibility of wounds to infection.[84]

Many minerals also play an important role in healing. Insufficient zinc can decrease the rate of epithelialization, reduce collagen synthesis, and decrease tensile strength.[85,86] Magnesium deficiency may also cause decreased collagen synthesis, and copper insufficiency may alter cross-linking, leading to a reduction in tensile strength.[84]

HEALING OF SPECIFIC MUSCULOSKELETAL TISSUES

The primary determinants of the outcome of any injury are the type and extent of the injury, the regenerative capacity of the tissues involved, the vascular supply of the injured site, and the extent of damage to the extracellular framework. The basic principles of inflammation and healing apply to all tissues; however, there is some tissue specificity to the healing response. For example, the liver can regenerate even when over half of it is removed, whereas even a thin fracture line in cartilage is unlikely to heal.

CARTILAGE

Cartilage has a limited ability to heal because it lacks lymphatics, blood vessels, and nerves.[87] However, cartilage reacts differently when injured alone than when injured in conjunction with the subchondral bone to which it is attached. Injuries confined to the cartilage do not form a clot or recruit neutrophils or macrophages, and the cells adjacent to the injury show a limited capacity to induce healing. This limited response generally fails to heal the defect, and these lesions seldom resolve.[88]

In injuries that involve both articular cartilage and subchondral bone, the vascularization of the subchondral bone allows for the formation of fibrin-fibronectin gel, giving access to the inflammatory cells and permitting the formation of granulation tissue. Differentiation of granulation tissue into chondrocytes can begin within 2 weeks. Normal-appearing cartilage can be seen within 2 months after the injury. However, this cartilage has a low proteoglycan content and is therefore predisposed to degeneration and erosive changes.[89] Recent research has explored the use of stem cells for cartilage repair.

TENDONS AND LIGAMENTS

Tendons and **ligaments** pass through similar stages of healing. Inflammation occurs in the first 72 hours, and collagen synthesis occurs within the first week. Fibroplasia occurs from intrinsic sources, such as adjacent cells, and from extrinsic sources, such as those brought in via the circulatory system.

The repair potential of tendon is somewhat controversial. Both intrinsic cells, such as epitendinous and endotendinous cells, and extrinsic peritendinous cells participate in tendon repair. The exact role of these cells and the final outcome depend on several factors, including the type of tendon, the extent of damage to the tendon sheath, the vascular supply, and the duration of immobilization. The first two stages of tendon healing, inflammation and proliferation, are similar to the healing phases of other tissues. The third phase, scar maturation, is unique to tendons in that this tissue can achieve a state of repair close to regeneration.

During the first 4 days after an injury, the inflammatory phase progresses with an infiltration of both extrinsic and intrinsic cells. Many of these cells develop phagocytic capabilities, while others become fibroblastic. Collagen synthesis becomes evident by days 7 to 8, with fibroblasts predominating at around day 14. Early in this stage, both cells and collagen are oriented perpendicular to the tendon's long axis.[90] This orientation changes at day 10, when new collagen fibers begin to align themselves parallel to the old longitudinal axis of the tendon stumps.[91] For the next 2 months, there is a gradual transition of alignment, through remodeling and reorientation, parallel to the long axis. Ultimate maturation of the tissue depends on sufficient physiological loading.

If the synovial sheath is absent or uninjured, the relative contributions of the intrinsic and extrinsic cells are balanced and adhesions are minimal. If the synovial sheath is injured, the contributions of the extrinsic cells overwhelm the capacities of the intrinsic cells, and adhesions are common.

Factors affecting the repair of tendons are different from those associated with the repair of ligaments.[92] Studies have shown that mobilization of tendons by controlled forces accelerates and enhances strengthening of tendon repair, but mobilization by active contraction of the attached muscle less than 3 weeks after repair generally results in a poor outcome. The poor outcome may be a result of the fact that high tension can lead to ischemia and tendon rupture. Studies have found no significant difference in tendon strength when tendons are exposed to controlled low or high levels of passive force after repair.[93,94] It appears that mechanical stress is needed to promote appropriate orientation of the collagen fibrils and remodeling of collagen into its mature form and to optimize strength, but the amount of tension necessary to promote the optimal clinical response is not certain.[95,96]

Many variables influence the healing of ligamentous tissue, the most important of which are the type of ligament, the size of the defect, and the amount of loading applied. For example, injuries to capsular and extracapsular ligaments generally stimulate an adequate repair response, whereas injuries to intracapsular ligaments often do not. In the knee, the medial collateral ligament often heals without surgical intervention, whereas the anterior cruciate ligament does not. These differences in healing may be a result of the synovial environment, the limited neovascularization, or the fibroblast migration from surrounding tissues. Treatments that stabilize the injury site and maintain the apposition of the torn ligament can help the ligament heal in its optimal length and minimize scarring. However, mature ligamentous repair tissue is still 30% to 50% weaker than uninjured ligament.[97] This weakness does not usually significantly impair joint function because the repaired tissue is usually larger than the uninjured ligament. Early, controlled loading of healing ligaments can also promote healing, although excessive loading may delay or disrupt the healing process.[98,99]

SKELETAL MUSCLE

Muscles may be injured by blunt trauma causing a contusion, by violent contraction or excessive stretch causing a strain, or by muscle-wasting diseases. Although skeletal muscle cells cannot proliferate, stem or reserve cells, known as satellite cells, can proliferate and differentiate in some circumstances to form new skeletal muscle cells after the death of adult muscle fibers.[89] Skeletal muscle regeneration has been documented in muscle biopsy specimens from patients with diseases, such as muscular dystrophy and polymyositis; however, skeletal muscle regeneration in humans after trauma has not been documented. After a severe contusion, a calcified hematoma, known as *myositis ossificans*, may develop. Myositis ossificans is rare after surgery if hemostasis is controlled.

BONE

Bone is a specialized tissue that is able to heal itself with like tissue. Bone can heal by two mechanisms: primary or secondary healing. Primary healing occurs with rigid internal fixation of the bone, whereas secondary healing occurs in the absence of such fixation.

Bone goes through a series of four histologically distinct stages in the healing process: inflammation, soft callus, hard callus, and bone remodeling. Some investigators also include the stages of **impaction** and **induction** before inflammation in this scheme.

Impaction is the dissipation of the energy from an insult. The impact of an insult is proportional to the energy applied to the bone and is inversely proportional to the volume of the bone. Thus a fracture is more likely to occur if the force is great or the bone is small. Energy dissipated by a bone is inversely proportional to its modulus of elasticity. Therefore the bone of a person suffering from osteoporosis, which has low elasticity, will sustain a fracture more easily. Young children have a more elastic bone structure that allows their bones to bend, accounting for the greenstick-type fractures seen in this population (Box 2-3).

Induction is the stage when cells that possess osteogenic capabilities are activated. Induction is the least understood stage of bone healing. It is thought that the cells may be activated by oxygen gradients, forces, bone morphogenic proteins, or noncollagenous proteins. Although the timing of this process is not known exactly, it is thought to be initiated after the moment of impact. The duration of this stage is also not known, although the influence of the induction forces seems to lessen with time. Therefore optimizing the early conditions for healing to minimize the potential for delayed union or nonunion is imperative.

Inflammation begins shortly after impact and lasts until some fibrous union at the fracture site occurs. At the time of the fracture, there is disruption of the blood supply and formation of a fracture hematoma, as well as a decrease in oxygen tension and pH. This environment favors the growth of the early fibrous or cartilaginous callus. This callus forms more easily than bone and helps to stabilize the fracture site, decrease pain, and lessen the likelihood of a fat embolism. It also rapidly and efficiently provides a scaffold for further circulation and for cartilage and endosteal bone production. The amount of movement at the fracture site influences the amount and quality of the callus. Small amounts of movement stimulate callus formation, whereas excessive movement can disrupt callus formation and inhibit bony union.

The soft callus stage begins when the pain and swelling subside and lasts until the bony fragments are united by fibrous or cartilaginous tissue. This period is marked by a great increase in vascularity, growth of capillaries into the fracture callus, and increased cell proliferation. The tissue oxygen tension remains low, but the pH returns to normal. The hematoma becomes organized with fibrous tissue cartilage and bone formation; however, no callus is visible radiographically. The callus is electronegative relative to the rest of the bone during this period. Osteoclasts remove the dead bone fragments.

The hard callus stage begins when a sticky, hard callus covers the ends of the fracture and ends when new bone unites with the fragments. This period corresponds to the period of clinical and radiological fracture healing. The duration of this period depends on the fracture location and the patient's age and can range from 3 weeks to 4 months.

The remodeling stage begins when the fracture is both clinically and radiologically healed. It ends when the bone has returned to its normal state and the patency of the medullary canal is restored. The fibrous bone is converted to lamellar bone, and the medullary canal is revised. This process can take several months to several years to complete.[100]

BOX 2-3   **Stages of Fracture Healing**
1. Impaction 2. Induction 3. Inflammation 4. Soft callus 5. Hard callus 6. Remodeling

CLINICAL CASE STUDY

The following case study summarizes the concepts of inflammation and repair discussed in this chapter. Based on the scenario presented, an evaluation of the clinical findings and goals of treatment are proposed.

CASE STUDY 2-1

Inflammation and Repair
Examination
History

JP is a 16-year-old high school student. She injured her right ankle 1 week ago playing soccer and was treated conservatively with crutches; rest, ice, compression, and elevation (RICE); and NSAIDs. She reports some improvement, although she is unable to play soccer because of continued complaints of right lateral ankle pain. Her x-ray films showed no fracture, and her family physician diagnosed the injury as a grade II lateral ankle sprain. She comes to your clinic with an order to "evaluate and treat."

JP sustained this injury during a cutting motion while dribbling a soccer ball. She noted an audible pop, immediate pain and swelling, and an inability to bear weight. She reports that her pain has decreased in intensity from 8/10 to 6/10, but the pain increases with weight bearing and with certain demonstrated movements.

Tests and Measures

The objective examination reveals moderate warmth of the skin of the anterolateral aspect of the right ankle. Moderate ecchymosis and swelling are also noted, with a girth measurement of 34 cm on the right ankle compared with 30 cm on the left. Her ROM is restricted to 0 degrees dorsiflexion, 30 degrees plantarflexion, 10 degrees inversion, and 5 degrees eversion, with pain noted especially with plantarflexion and inversion. She exhibits a decreased stance phase on the right lower extremity. Pain and weakness occur on strength tests of the peroneals, gastrocnemius, and soleus muscles. JP also exhibits a marked decrease in proprioception, as evidenced by the single-leg balance test. Her anterior drawer test is positive, and her talar tilt is negative.

What stage of healing is this patient in? What kind of injury does she have? What physical agents could be useful for this patient?

Evaluation, Diagnosis, Prognosis, and Goals
Evaluation and Goals

ICF Level	Current Status	Goals
Body structure and function	Right ankle: Pain Loss of subtalar and talocrural motion Increased girth Decreased strength of evertors and plantarflexors Decreased proprioception	Reduce inflammation, thereby reducing pain and edema and increasing ROM
Activity	Difficulty ambulating	Increase ability to walk
Participation	Unable to play soccer	Return to playing soccer in next 2 to 3 months

Diagnosis

Preferred practice pattern 4D: Impaired joint mobility, motor function, muscle performance, and ROM associated with connective tissue dysfunction.

Prognosis/Plan of Care

This patient has had a recent injury and is in the inflammatory phase of tissue healing, as evidenced by her signs of pain, edema, bruising, and warmth at the injured site. She is likely also at the beginning of the proliferative phase of healing. Given her positive anterior drawer test, it is likely that she has injured her anterior talofibular ligament. The expected time of healing with a grade II ankle sprain and partial tear of the talofibular ligament is 2 to 3 months. At this stage of healing, the plan is to minimize the effects of inflammation and accelerate the healing process so that she can move on to the proliferative and maturation phases and regain normal function.

Intervention

Physical agents that may be used to help accelerate the acute inflammatory phase of healing include cryotherapy and compression. She should avoid applying heat. The patient should continue the RICE regimen accompanied by NSAIDs as needed for pain. Physical agents should be used as part of a rehabilitation program in which the patient slowly resumes passive motion followed by active motion and motion with weight bearing. Hydrotherapy may be used to facilitate non–weight-bearing movement.

CHAPTER REVIEW

1. The processes of inflammation and tissue repair involve a complex and dynamic series of events, the ultimate goal of which is the restoration of normal function. In these events the involved tissue progresses through three sequential but overlapping stages: inflammation, proliferation, and maturation. This series of events follows a timely and predictable course.

2. The inflammation phase involves interaction of hemostatic, vascular, cellular, and immune responses mediated by a number of neural and chemical factors. Characteristics of the inflammation phase include heat, redness, swelling, pain, and loss of function in the injured area.

3. The proliferation phase is characterized by epithelialization, fibroplasia, wound contraction, and neovascularization. During this phase, the wound appears red and swelling decreases, but the wound is still weak and therefore easily susceptible to damage from excessive pressure and tension.

4. The maturation phase involves balanced collagen synthesis and lysis to ultimately remodel the injured area. The optimal outcome of the maturation phase is to new tissue that resembles the previously uninjured tissue. More frequently, scar tissue forms that is slightly weaker than the original tissue. Over time, the scar lightens in color.

5. If the normal healing process is disturbed, healing may be delayed or chronic inflammation may result. Drugs, such as corticosteroids, NSAIDs, and antibiotics, are used to limit inflammation, but they can also hinder healing.

6. Physical agents may influence the progression of inflammation and tissue repair. Physical agents used at various stages of the healing process include thermotherapy, cryotherapy, electromagnetic radiation, light, electrical stimulation, ultrasound, and compression. The rehabilitation specialist must assess the stage of inflammation and repair to determine the appropriate agent to incorporate into the treatment plan for an optimal outcome.

8. The reader is referred to the Evolve web site for study questions pertinent to this chapter.

ADDITIONAL RESOURCES *evolve*

Textbooks

Kumar V, Abbas AK, Fausto N, et al: *Robbins basic pathology,* ed 8, Philadelphia, 2007, Elsevier.

Sussman C, Bates-Jensen B: *Wound care: a collaborative practice manual for health professionals,* ed 3, Philadelphia, 2007 Lippincott Williams & Wilkins.

GLOSSARY *evolve*

Acute inflammation: Inflammation that occurs immediately after tissue damage.

Angiogenesis: The growth of new blood vessels.

Cartilage: A fibrous connective tissue that lines the ends of the bones in joints providing the weight-bearing surface of joints and that helps form the flexible portions of the nose and ears.

Chemotaxis: The movement of cells toward or away from chemicals.

Chronic inflammation: The simultaneous progression of active inflammation, tissue destruction, and healing. Chronic inflammation may last for months or years.

Collagen: The protein of the fibers of skin, tendon, bone, cartilage, and all other connective tissue. Collagen is made up of individual polypeptide molecules combined together in triplets to form helical tropocollagen molecules that then associate to form collagen fibrils.

Collagenases: Enzyme that destroy collagen.

Complement system: A system of enzymatic plasma proteins activated by antigen-antibody complexes, bacteria, and foreign material that participates in the inflammatory response through cell lysis, opsonization, and the attraction of leukocytes by chemotaxis.

Connective tissues: Tissues consisting of fibroblasts, ground substance, and fibrous strands that provides the structure for other tissues.

Contractures: Permanent shortening of muscle or scar tissue that produces deformity or distortion.

Corticosteroids: Drugs that decrease the inflammatory response by many mechanisms involving many cell types.

Diapedesis: The process by which leukocytes squeeze through the intact blood vessel walls; a part of the process of extravasation.

Edema: Swelling that results from accumulation of fluid in the interstitial space.

Emigration: The process by which leukocytes migrate from blood vessels into perivascular tissues; a part of the process of extravasation.

Epithelial cells: Cells that form the epidermis of the skin and the covering of mucous and serous membranes.

Epithelialization: Healing by growth of epithelium over a denuded surface, thus reestablishing the epidermis.

Erythrocytes: Red blood cells.

Extravasation: The movement of leukocytes from inside a blood vessel to the tissue outside the blood vessel.

Exudate: Wound fluid composed of serum with a high content of protein and white blood cells or solid materials from cells.

Fibroblasts: Cells in many tissues and particularly wounds that are the primary producers of collagen.

Fibroplasia: Fibroblast growth.

Granulation tissue: Tissue composed of new blood vessels, connective tissue, fibroblasts, and inflammatory cells that fills an open wound when it starts to heal; typically appears deep pink or red with an irregular, berrylike surface.

Healing by delayed primary intention: Healing in which wound contraction is reduced by delayed approximation of a wound's edges with sutures or the application of skin grafts.

Healing by primary intention: Healing without wound contraction that occurs when wounds are rapidly closed with sutures with minimal loss of tissue and minimal bacterial contamination.

Healing by secondary intention: Healing with wound contraction that occurs when there is significant loss of tissue or bacterial contamination and the wound edges are not approximated.

Hemarthrosis: Bloody fluid present in a joint.

Hematoma: The accumulation of blood in a tissue or organ.

Humoral mediators: Antibodies, hormones, cytokines, and a variety of other soluble proteins and chemicals that contribute to the inflammatory process.

Hyperemia: An excess of blood in a given area that causes redness and temperature increase in the area.

Impaction: The dissipation of the energy from an insult to bone.

Induction: The stage of bone healing when cells with osteogenic capabilities are activated.

Inflammation: The body's first response to tissue damage, characterized by heat, redness, swelling, pain, and often loss of function.

Inflammation phase: The first phase of healing after tissue damage.

Leukocytes: White blood cells.

Ligaments: Bands of fibrous tissue that connect bone to bone or cartilage to bone, supporting or strengthening a joint at the extremes of motion.

Macrophages: Phagocytic cells that are derived from monocytes and important for attracting other immune cells to a site of inflammation.

Margination: A part of the process of extravasation in which leukocytes line the walls of blood vessels.

Maturation phase: The final phase of tissue healing in which scar tissue is modified into its mature form.

Monocytes: Leukocytes that are larger than PMNs, have a single nucleus, and become macrophages when in connective tissue and outside the bloodstream.

Myofibroblasts: Cells similar to fibroblasts that also have the contractile properties of smooth muscles and are responsible for wound contraction.

Neovascularization: The development of a new blood supply to an injured area.

Neural mediators: Nerve-related contributions to the inflammatory process.

Neutrophils: White blood cells present early in inflammation that have the properties of chemotaxis and phagocytosis.

Opsonization: The coating of bacteria with protein that makes them more susceptible to phagocytosis.

Pavementing: A part of the process of extravasation in which leukocytes lay down in layers inside the blood vessel.

Phagocytosis: Ingestion and digestion of bacteria and particles by a cell.

Plasma: The acellular, fluid portion of blood.

Platelet-derived growth factor: A protein produced by platelets that stimulates cell growth and division and is involved in normal wound healing.

Platelets: Small, anuclear cells in the blood that assist in clotting.

Polymorphonucleocytes (PMNs): Leukocytes whose nuclei have several lobes and contain cytoplasmic granules and that include neutrophils, basophils, and eosinophils.

Proliferation phase: The second phase of tissue healing during which damaged structures are rebuilt and the wound is strengthened.

Pus: Opaque wound fluid that is thicker than exudate and contains white blood cells, tissue debris, and microorganisms Also called suppurative exudate.

Subacute inflammation: An inflammatory process that has continued for more than 4 weeks.

Tendon: Fibrous band of tissue that connects muscle with bone.

Transudate: Thin, clear wound fluid composed primarily of serum.

Type I collagen: The most abundant form of collagen found in skin, bone, tendons, and most organs.

Type II collagen: the predominant collagen in cartilage.

Type III collagen: A thin, weak-structured collagen with no consistent organization, initially produced by fibroblasts after tissue damage.

Wound contraction: The pulling together of the edges of an injured site to accelerate repair.

REFERENCES evolve

1. *Stedman's medical dictionary*, ed 25, Baltimore, 1990, Williams & Wilkins.
2. Price SA, Wilson LM: *Pathophysiology: Clinical concepts of disease processes*, ed 2, New York, 1982, McGraw Hill.
3. Kellett J: Acute soft tissue injuries—a review of the literature, *Med Sci Sports Exerc* 18:489-500, 1986.
4. Garrett WE Jr, Lohnes J: Cellular and matrix responses to mechanical injury at the myotendinous junction. In Leadbetter WB, Buckwalter JA, Gordon SL, eds: *Sports-induced inflammation*, Park Ridge, IL, 1990, American Academy of Orthopaedic Surgeons.
5. Andriacchi T, Sabiston P, DeHaven K, et al: Ligament: Injury and repair. In Woo SL-Y, Buckwalter JA, eds: *Injury and repair of the musculoskeletal soft tissues*, Park Ridge, IL, 1988, American Academy of Orthopaedic Surgeons.
6. Garrett WE Jr: Muscle strain injuries: Clinical and basic aspects, *Med Sci Sports Exerc* 22:436-443, 1990.
7. Szpaderska A, Egozi E, Gamelli RL, et al: The effect of thrombocytopenia on dermal wound healing, *J Invest Dermatol* 120:1130-1137, 2003.
8. Eming SA. Krieg T. Davidson JM: Inflammation in wound repair: molecular and cellular mechanisms, *J Invest Dermatol* 127(3):514-525, 2007.
9. Fantone JC, Ward PA: Inflammation. In Rubin E, Farber JL, eds: *Pathology*, Philadelphia, 1988, JB Lippincott.
10. Wilkerson GB: Inflammation in connective tissue: etiology and management, *Athl Training* 20:298-301, 1985.
11. Christie AL: The tissue injury cycle and new advances toward its management in open wounds, *Athl Training* 26:274-277, 1991.
12. Cotran RS, Kumar V, Collins T: *Robbins pathologic basis of disease*, ed 6, Philadelphia, 1999, WB Saunders.
13. Fantone JC: Basic concepts in inflammation. In Leadbetter WB, Buckwalter JA, Gordon SL, eds: *Sports-induced inflammation*, Park Ridge, IL, 1990, American Academy of Orthopaedic Surgeons.
14. Peacock EE: *Wound repair*, ed 3, Philadelphia, 1984, WB Saunders.
15. Salter RB, Simmons DF, Malcolm BW, et al: The biological effects of continuous passive motion on the healing of full thickness defects in articular cartilage, *J Bone Joint Surg* 62A:1232-1251, 1980.
16. Egan BM, Chen G, Kelly CJ, et al: Taurine attenuates LPS-induced rolling and adhesion in rat microcirculation, *J Surg Res* 95(2):85-91, 2001.

17. Xia G, Martin AE, Besner GE: Heparin-binding EGF-like growth factor downregulates expression of adhesion molecules and infiltration of inflammatory cells after intestinal ischemia/reperfusion injury, *J Pediatr Surg* 38(3):434-439, 2003.
18. Majno G, Palade GE: Studies on inflammation. I. The effect of histamine and serotonin on vascular permeability: an electron microscopic study, *J Biophys Biochem Cytol* 11:571, 1961.
19. Pierce GF, Mustoe TA, Senia RM, et al: In vivo incisional wound healing augmented by PDGF and recombinant c-sis gene homodimeric proteins, *J Exp Med* 167:975-987,1988.
20. Martinez-Hernandez A, Amenta PS: Basic concepts in wound healing. In Leadbetter WB, Buckwalter JA, Gordon SL, eds: *Sports-induced inflammation*, Park Ridge, IL, 1990, American Academy of Orthopaedic Surgeons.
21. DiPietro LA, Polverini PJ: Role of the macrophage n the positive and negative regulation of wound neovascularization, *Am J Pathol* 143:678-784, 1993.
22. Hardy M: The biology of scar formation, *Phys Ther* 69:1014-1024, 1989.
23. Rutherford R, Ross R: Platelet factors stimulate fibroblasts and smooth muscle cells quiescent in plasma serum to proliferate, *J Cell Biol* 69:196-203, 1976.
24. Mathes S: Roundtable discussion: problem wounds, *Perspect Plastic Surg* 2:89-120, 1988.
25. Whitney JD, Heiner S, Mygrant BI, et al: Tissue and wound healing effects of short duration postoperative oxygen therapy, *Biol Res Nurs* 2(3):206-215, 2001.
26. Davidson JD, Mustoe TA: Oxygen in wound healing: more than a nutrient, *Wound Repair Regen* 9(3):175-177, 2001.
27. Bellanti JA, ed: *Immunology III*, ed 3, Philadelphia, 1985, WB Saunders.
28. Werb A, Gordon S: Elastase secretion by stimulated macrophages, *J Exp Med* 142:361-377, 1975.
29. Madden JW: Wound healing: biologic and clinical features. In Sabiston DC, ed: *Davis-Christopher textbook of surgery*, ed 11, Philadelphia, 1997, WB Saunders.
30. Clark RAF: Overview and general considerations of wound repair. In Clark RAF, Henson PM, eds: *The molecular and cellular biology of wound repair*, New York, 1988, Plenum Press.
31. Stotts NA, Wipke-Tevis D: Co-factors in impaired wound healing, *Ostomy* 42(2):44-56, 1996.
32. Monaco JL, Lawrence WT: Acute wound healing: an overview, *Clin Plast Surg* 30:1-12, 2003.
33. Lawrence WT: Physiology of the acute wound, *Clin Plast Surg* 25:321-340, 1998.
34. Levenson S: Practical applications of experimental studies in the care of primary closed wounds, *Am J Surg* 104:273-282, 1962.
35. Nemeth-Csoka M, Kovacsay A: The effect of glycosaminoglycans (GAG) on the intramolecular bindings of collagen, *Acta Biol* 30(4):303-308, 1979.
36. Lachman SM: *Soft tissue injuries in sports*, St. Louis, 1988, Mosby.
37. Hunt TK, Van Winkle W Jr: Wound healing. In Heppenstall RB, ed: *Fracture treatment and healing*, Philadelphia, 1980, WB Saunders.
38. Baum CL, Arpey CJ: Normal cutaneous wound healing: clinical correlation with cellular and molecular events, *Dermatol Surg* 31(6):674-686; discussion 686, 2005.
39. Daly T: The repair phase of wound healing: re-epithelialization and contraction. In Kloth L, McCulloch J, Feeder J, eds: *Wound healing: alternatives in management*, Philadelphia, 1990, FA Davis.
40. Gabbiani G, Ryan G, Majeno G: Presence of modified fibroblasts in granulation tissue and their possible role in wound contraction, *Experientia* 27:549-550, 1971.
41. Watts GT, Grillo HC, Gross J: Studies in wound healing. II. The role of granulation tissue in contraction, *Ann Surg* 148:153-160, 1958.
42. McGrath MH, Simon RH: Wound geometry and the kinetics of the wound contraction, *Plast Reconstr Surg* 72:66-73, 1983.
43. *Taber's cyclopedic medical dictionary*, ed 15, Philadelphia, 1985, FA Davis.
44. Billingham RE, Russell PS: Studies on wound healing, with special reference to the phenomena of contracture in experimental wounds in rabbit skin, *Ann Surg* 144:961, 1956.
45. Sawhney CP, Monga HL: Wound contracture in rabbits and the effectiveness of skin grafts in preventing it, *Br J Plast Surg* 23:318-321, 1970.
46. Stone PA, Madden JW: Biological factors affecting wound contraction, *Surg Forum* 26:547-548, 1975.
47. Rudolph R: Contraction and the control of contraction, *World J Surg* 4:279-287, 1980.
48. Alvarez OM: Wound healing. In Fitzpatrick T, ed: *Dermatology in general medicine*, ed 3, New York, 1986, McGraw-Hill.
49. Eyre DR: The collagens of musculoskeletal soft tissues. In Leadbetter WB, Buckwalter JA, Gordon SL, eds: *Sports-induced inflammation*, Park Ridge, IL, 1990, American Association of Orthopaedic Surgeons.
50. McPherson JM, Piez KA: Collagen in dermal wound repair. In Clark RAF, Henson PM, eds: *The molecular and cellular biology of wound repair*, New York, 1988, Plenum Press.
51. Kosaka M, Kamiishi H: New concept of balloon-compression wear for the treatment of keloids and hypertrophic scars, *Plast Reconstr Surg* 108(5):1454-1455, 2001.
52. Uppal RS, Khan U, Kakar S, et al: The effects of a single dose of 5-fluorouracil on keloid scars: a clinical trial of timed wound irrigation after extralesional excision, *Plast Reconstr Surg* 108(5):1218-1224, 2001.
53. Hunt TK, Van Winkle W: *Wound healing: normal repair—fundamentals of wound management in surgery*, South Plainfield, NJ, 1976, Chirurgecom, Inc.
54. Madden J: Wound healing: the biological basis of hand surgery, *Clin Plast Surg* 3:3-11, 1976.
55. Arem AJ, Madden JW: Effects of stress on healing wounds. I. Intermittent noncyclical tension, *J Surg Res* 20:93-102, 1976.
56. Irvin T: Collagen metabolism in infected colonic anastomoses, *Surg Gynecol Obstet* 143:220-224, 1976.
57. Carrico T, Mehrhof A, Cohen I: Biology of wound healing, *Surg Clin North Am* 64:721-733, 1984.
58. Woo SL, Gelberman RM, Cobb NG, et al: The importance of controlled passive mobilization on flexor tendon healing: a biochemical study, *Acta Orthop Scand* 52:615-622, 1981.
59. Gelberman RH, Woo SL, Lothringer K, et al: Effects of early intermittent passive immobilization on healing canine flexor tendons, *J Hand Surg* 7:170-175, 1982.
60. Lau SK, Chiu KY: Use of continuous passive motion after total knee arthroplasty, *J Arthroplasty* 16(3):336-339, 2001.
61. McCarthy MR, Yates CK, Anderson MA, et al: The effects of immediate continuous passive motion on pain during the inflammatory phase of soft tissue healing following anterior cruciate ligament reconstruction, *J Orthop Sport Phys Ther* 17(2):96-101, 1993.
62. Brosseau L, Milne S, Wells G, et al: Efficacy of continuous passive motion following total knee arthroplasty: a metaanalysis, *J Rheumatol* 31(11):2251-2264, 2004.
63. Thomas DR: Age-related changes in wound healing, *Drugs Aging* 18(8):607-620, 2001.
64. Holm-Peterson P, Viidik A: Tensile properties and morphology of healing wounds in young and old rats, *Scand J Plast Reconstr Surg* 6:24-35, 1972.
65. van de Kerkhoff PCM, van Bergen B, Spruijt K, et al: Age-related changes in wound healing, *Clin Exerc Dermatol* 19:369-374, 1994.
66. Goodson W, Hunt T: Studies of wound healing in experimental diabetes mellitus, *J Surg Res* 22:221-227, 1997.
67. Peterson M, Barbul A, Breslin R, et al: Significance of T-lymphocytes in wound healing, *Surgery* 2:300-305, 1987.
68. Gogia PP: The biology of wound healing, *Ostomy* 38(9):12-22, 1992.
69. Adcock IM, Ito K, Barnes PJ: Glucocorticoids: effects on gene transcription, *Proc Am Thorac Soc* 1(3):247-254, 2004.
70. Behrens TW, Goodwin JS: Oral corticosteroids. In Leadbetter WB, Buckwalter JA, Gordon SL, eds: *Sports-Induced Inflammation*, Park Ridge, IL, 1990, American Academy of Orthopaedic Surgeons.
71. Ehrchen J, Steinmuller L, Barczyk K, et al: Glucocorticoids induce differentiation of a specifically activated, anti-inflammatory subtype of human monocytes, *Blood* 109(3):1265-1274, 2007.

72. Ehlrich H, Hunt T: The effect of cortisone and anabolic steroids on the tensile strength of healing wounds, *Ann Surg* 170:203-206, 1969.

73. Baker B, Whitaker W: Interference with wound healing by the local action of adrenocortical steroids, *Endocrinology* 46:544-551, 1950.

74. Howes E, Plotz C, Blunt J, et al: Retardation of wound healing by cortisone, *Surgery* 28:177-181, 1950.

75. Stephens F, Dunphy J, Hunt T: The effect of delayed administration of corticosteroids on wound contracture, *Ann Surg* 173:214-218, 1971.

76. Abramson SB: Nonsteroidal anti-inflammatory drugs: mechanisms of action and therapeutic considerations. In Leadbetter WB, Buckwalter JA, Gordon SL, eds: *Sports-Induced Inflammation*, Park Ridge, IL, 1990, American Academy of Orthopaedic Surgeons.

77. Riley GP, Cox M, Harrall RL et al: Inhibition of tendon cell proliferation and matrix glycosaminoglycan synthesis by non-steroidal anti-inflammatory drugs in vitro, *J Hand Surg* 26(3)B:224-228, 2001.

78. Tsai WC, Hsu CC, Chou SW: Effects of celecoxib on migration, proliferation and collagen expression of tendon cells, *Connect Tissue Res* 48(1):46-51, 2007.

79. Albina JE: Nutrition in wound healing, *J Parenter Enteral Nutr* 18(4):367-376, 1994.

80. Pollack S: Wound healing: a review. III. Nutritional factors affecting wound healing, *J Dermatol Surg Oncol* 5:615-619, 1979.

81. Freiman M, Seifter E, Connerton C: Vitamin A deficiency and surgical stress, *Surg Forum* 21:81-82, 1970.

82. Alverez OM, Gilbreath RL: Thiamine influence on collagen during granulation of skin wounds, *J Surg Res* 32:24-31, 1982.

83. Grenier JF, Aprahamian M, Genot C, et al: Pantothenic acid (vitamin B5) efficiency on wound healing, *Acta Vitaminol Enzymol* 4:81-85, 1982.

84. Pollack S: Systemic drugs and nutritional aspects of wound healing, *Clin Dermatol* 2:68-80, 1984.

85. Sandstead HH, Henriksen LK, Grefer JL, et al: Zinc nutriture in the elderly in relation to taste acuity, immune response, and wound healing, *Am J Clin Nutr* 36(suppl 5):1046-1059, 1982.

86. Maitra AK, Dorani B: Role of zinc in post-injury wound healing, *Arch Emerg Med* Jun;9(2):122-124, 1992.

87. Athanasiou KA, Shah AR, Hernandez RJ, et al: Basic science of articular cartilage repair, *Clin Sports Med* Apr;20(2):223-247, 2001.

88. Gelberman R, Goldberg V, An K-N, et al: Tendon. In Woo SL-Y, Buckwalter JA, eds: *Injury and repair of musculoskeletal soft tissues*, Park Ridge, IL, 1988, American Academy of Orthopaedic Surgeons.

89. Caplan A, Carlson B, Faulkner J, et al: Skeletal muscle. In Woo SL-Y, Buckwalter JA, eds: *Injury and repair of musculoskeletal soft tissues*, Park Ridge, IL, 1988, American Academy of Orthopaedic Surgeons.

90. Strickland JW: Flexor tendon injuries, *Orthop Rev* 15(10):21, 1986.

91. Lindsay WK: Cellular biology of flexor tendon healing. In Hunter JM, Schneider LH, Mackin EJ, eds: *Tendon surgery of the hand*, St Louis, 1987, Mosby.

92. Akeson WH, Frank CB, Amiel D, et al: Ligament biology and biomechanics. In Finnerman G, ed: *American Academy of Orthopaedic Surgeon's symposium on sports medicine*, St Louis, 1985, Mosby.

93. Ketchum LD: Primary tendon healing: a review, *J Hand Surg* 2:428-435, 1977.

94. Goldfarb CA, Harwood F, Silva MJ, et al: The effect of variations in applied rehabilitation force on collagen concentration and maturation at the intrasynovial flexor tendon repair site, *J Hand Surg* 26(5)A:841-846, 2001.

95. Peacock EE Jr: Biological principles in the healing of long tendons, *Surg Clin North Am* 45:461-476, 1965.

96. Potenza AD: Tendon healing within the flexor digital sheath in the dog, *J Bone Joint Surg* 44A:49-64, 1962.

97. Frank C, Woo SL-Y, Amiel D, et al: Medial collateral ligament healing: a multidisciplinary assessment in rabbits, *Am J Sports Med* 11:379-389, 1983.

98. Fronek J, Frank C, Amiel D, et al: The effects of intermittent passive motion (IPM) in the healing of medial collateral ligaments, *Trans Orthop Res Soc* 8:31, 1983.

99. Long M, Frank C, Schachar N, et al: The effects of motion on normal and healing ligaments, *Trans Orthop Res Soc* 7:43, 1982.

100. McKibben B: The biology of fracture healing in long bones, *J Bone Joint Surg* 60B:150-162, 1978.

Pain

Pain is an experience based on a complex interaction of physical and psychological processes. It has been defined as an unpleasant sensory and emotional experience associated with actual or potential tissue damage or described in terms of such damage.[1-3] Pain usually acts as a warning to protect the body from damage and thus serves an essential function in survival.[4] It is important to realize that pain is not just the activation of receptors of noxious stimuli, known as **nociception**, but also the sensory experiences, suffering, and alterations in behavior associated with such activation.

Pain is the most common symptom prompting patients to seek medical attention and is a predominant symptom leading patients to receive rehabilitation.[5] Many patients with musculoskeletal or neurological impairments report pain, and most of these individuals consider pain control or relief to be the primary goal of treatment.[6] Pain may alter body structure and function, limiting participation in home, work, and recreational activities. Pain symptoms encountered by rehabilitation professionals are generally related to inflammation of musculoskeletal or neurological structures caused by injury, trauma, or degenerative disease. These structures can be sources of pain and can increase the responsiveness of peripheral pain receptors to other painful stimuli.[8-10]

The goals of pain management include resolving the underlying condition causing the pain, when possible; modifying the patient's perception of the discomfort; and maximizing function within the limitations imposed by the source of pain, whether the source of pain can or cannot be modified. Even when the source of pain is identified and can be modified, pain control during recovery is important. Limiting pain helps the patient fully participate in rehabilitation and reach goals of increased activity and participation. Examples include pain caused by structural malalignment from poor posture or imbalanced muscle length, or a self-limiting condition such as inflammation after an acute soft tissue injury. When the pain is caused by a condition that cannot be directly modified, such as phantom limb pain or rheumatoid arthritis, pain control may facilitate increased participation in a rehabilitation program and increased patient activity and participation.

TYPES OF PAIN

Pain can be categorized according to its duration or source as acute, chronic, or referred. **Acute pain** is generally defined as pain of less than 6 months' duration for which an underlying pathology can be identified.[11] Acute pain is felt in response to actual or potential tissue damage that resolves when tissue damage or the threat of damage passes. **Chronic pain** persists beyond the normal time for tissue healing.[10] Chronic pain conditions are usually the result of activation of dysfunctional neurological or psychological responses that cause the individual to continue to experience the sensation of pain even when no damaging or threatening stimulus is present. **Referred pain** is the experience of pain in one area when the actual or potential tissue damage is in another area. Knowing whether a patient's pain is acute, chronic, or referred will help the clinician determine the mechanisms and processes that may be contributing to the sensation and facilitate selection of the most appropriate intervention to control or relieve this symptom.

ACUTE PAIN

Acute pain is a complex combination of unpleasant sensory, perceptual, and emotional experiences with associated autonomic, psychological, emotional, and behavioral reactions that occur in response to a **noxious stimulus** provoked by acute injury or disease.[12,13] Acute pain is generally viewed as biologically meaningful, useful, and time-limited. Acute pain is mediated through rapidly conducting pathways and is associated with increases in muscle tone, heart rate, blood pressure, skin conductance, and other manifestations of increased **sympathetic nervous system** activity.[14] The intensity and location of the pain are usually related to the degree of tissue inflammation, damage, or destruction in the area in which the pain is felt. Acute pain is generally well-localized and defined, although its degree of localization varies to some extent with the type of tissue involved. Pain sensations from the skin are localized with great accuracy, whereas muscle pain is frequently more diffuse.[15,16] Acute pain lasts as long as the noxious stimulation persists. Acute pain serves a protective function after an injury by limiting activity to prevent further damage and promote tissue healing and recovery; however, it may also adversely affect an individual's quality of life and impair the ability to function. For example, when a patient sustains a rotator cuff injury while playing racquetball, he or she will feel acute pain in the shoulder. This pain will probably cause the patient to restrict shoulder motion and thereby avoid further injury. This acute pain will likely prevent the patient from playing raquetball for a number of days or weeks but will gradually resolve as the injured tissues heal allowing return to full activity.

Treatment of acute pain resulting from musculoskeletal injury generally attempts to resolve the underlying disorder, reduce inflammation, and modify the transmission of pain from the periphery to the central nervous system (CNS).

CHRONIC PAIN

Chronic pain may start as acute pain related to a chronic disease as with peripheral polyneuropathy, poststroke, or spinal cord injury pain syndrome, and fibromyalgia, or it may have no identifiable cause. Chronic pain is usually defined as pain that does not resolve in the usual time it takes for the disorder to heal or that continues beyond the duration of noxious stimulation.[17] Some authors and organizations use time-based definitions, defining chronic pain as any pain lasting longer than 3 months or 6 months.[18,19] Whatever its precise definition, chronic pain is an ongoing condition that is difficult to manage. It has been estimated that approximately one third of the United States (US) population has chronic pain, and 14% of the US population suffers from chronic pain related to the joints and the musculoskeletal system.[20,21] Other disease states, such as cancer, are also commonly associated with chronic pain. A study of pain in 13,625 elderly and minor-ity nursing home residents with cancer found that more than 25% reported daily pain.[22]

Chronic pain may be classified according to pathophysiology.[23-25] Nociceptive pain is caused by the stimulation of pain receptors by noxious mechanical, chemical, or thermal stimuli and associated with ongoing tissue damage. Conditions associated with chronic nociceptive pain include arthritis, ischemia, cancer, and chronic pancreatitis. Neuropathic pain is the result of peripheral or central nervous system dysfunction without ongoing tissue damage. Neuropathic pain is seen in diabetic neuropathy, postherpetic neuralgia, and phantom limb pain. Mixed pain syndromes are those with multiple or uncertain pathophysiology. Examples include recurrent headache and some vasculitic syndromes. Psychological pain syndromes are those in which psychological processes play a large role. This kind of pain may be seen in somataform disorders and conversion reactions. Although this classification of pain can be helpful for systematically approaching a patient with pain, the pathophysiology of chronic pain in an individual patient is often only partially understood. In addition, chronic pain may have more than one cause. The pain associated with arthritis, for example, may be caused by inflammation, joint distortion, strain on muscles and connective tissue, and microfracture from eroded cartilage or bone. This pain may also be magnified by psychological distress related to loss of function.[25]

Chronic pain may be the result of changes in sympathetic nervous system and adrenal activity, reduced production of endogenous opioids, or **sensitization** of primary afferent (**peripheral sensitization**) and spinal cord neurons. Decreased levels of **enkephalins** and increased numbers and sensitivity of **nociceptors** have been observed in individuals with chronic pain.[29] These individuals frequently have increased sensitivity to both noxious (**hyperalgesia**) and innocuous (**allodynia**) stimuli.[30] These changes in pain perception may in part be the result of a process known as wind-up, or **central sensitization**, in which the pathways that transmit pain continue to discharge after the discontinuation of intense or repeated stimulation. Then, even a small additional stimulus exceeds the threshold that is perceived as painful.[31-34] Thus, for an individual with a painful condition that is severe or long-lasting, the noxious stimulation may result in increased pain receptor activity and a consequent reduced tolerance for noxious or innocuous stimuli. Understanding of this sensitization mechanism has led to increased study and use of preemptive **analgesia** before procedures that are known to be painful in an attempt to reduce postprocedural pain and reduce recovery time.[35-37]

Although many patients with chronic pain have found ways to adapt and cope with their condition, there are some who catastrophize or perceive their symptoms to be debilitating. These patients are more likely to have difficulties with social function and employment. Some individuals, such as those with preexisting affective or anxiety disorders, or chemical dependence, are predisposed to becoming more dysfunctional in the face of chronic pain. Psychological and social factors associated with chronic pain include depression; catastrophizing; decreased function, quality of life, and ability to work; and increased dependence on others. In a study of 5,800 patients, 41% of those with depression reported disabling chronic pain compared with 10% of those without depression.[38] Patients with concurrent depression and disabling chronic pain had significantly poorer health-related quality of life, greater somatic symptom severity, and higher prevalence of panic disorder than other patients.[38] A study of 1,800 depressed older adults also found that patients with coexisting arthritis (56%) who were treated for depression not only had decreased depressive symptoms but also had reduced pain and improved function and quality of life.[39] Catastrophizing has been positively correlated with the reported severity of pain, affective distress, muscle and joint tenderness, pain-related disability, poor outcomes of pain treatment, and possibly inflammatory disease activity.[40] These associations exist even after controlling for depression. Proposed effects of catastrophizing range from maladaptive influences on the social environment to direct amplification of the processing of pain by the CNS.[40] Although most studies have found a correlation between chronic pain and psychological factors, no studies have confirmed this relationship, making this an area in need of further research.[41]

Chronic pain can decrease a person's participation in normal activities. A study in Europe found that more than half of a group of patients with chronic pain were less able or unable to work outside the home, 19% had lost their jobs and 13% had changed jobs because of their pain.[42] Chronic pain also impacts a person's relationship to others, particularly those in the caregiving role. In an enmeshed or solicitous relationship, the patient assumes a sick role that is unknowingly reinforced by the caregiver through "checking" behaviors and excessively supportive responses. It is important to note that although health care professionals may suspect that a patient is using chronic pain for secondary gain, to play the sick role, or to justify certain behaviors, this attitude may obstruct a patient's adjustment to chronic pain, prolong sick leave, and hinder rehabilitation.[43]

Ideally, the development of chronic pain should be prevented by early identification of individuals at risk. Patients with prolonged, severe, or disabling acute pain are at increased risk of developing chronic pain. To reduce this risk, pain-controlling interventions, such as physical agents or medications, should be applied during the acute stage of an injury and during the later recovery phases, when pain is still the result of pain receptor activation.[46] The prevention of chronic pain in patients who have had surgery should include avoiding nerve damage while in surgery and effective pain control immediately after surgery, because the intensity of acute postoperative pain correlates with the risk of developing chronic pain.[47]

If chronic pain develops, successful treatment usually requires that all components of the dysfunction be addressed. Multidisciplinary treatment programs based on a biopsychosocial model of pain have been specifically developed to address these problems.[4] These treatment programs are described in the section on pain management.

REFERRED PAIN

Referred pain is felt at a location distant from its source. Pain may be referred from one joint to another, from a peripheral nerve to a distal area of innervation, or from an internal organ to an area of musculoskeletal tissue (Fig. 3-1). For example, hip joint pathology occasionally refers pain to the knee, particularly in children, and compression of the spinal nerve roots at the L5 to S1 level as they exit through the spinal foramen may cause pain in the lateral leg because this is the area of sensory innervation.[48,49] Common referral patterns from internal organs to musculoskeletal tissue include the pain associated with myocardial infarction or angina caused by cardiac ischemia that is felt in the upper chest, left shoulder, jaw and arm, and pain originating from the central portion of the diaphragm that is frequently felt in the lateral tip of either shoulder. The gallbladder also frequently refers pain to the right shoulder or the inferior angle of the right scapula, and the spleen refers pain to the left shoulder.

It is proposed that pain is referred in one of three ways: from a nerve to its area of innervation, from one area to another derived from the same dermatome, or from one area to another derived from the same embryonic segment. The peripheral neural pathways from these different areas converge on the same or similar areas of the spinal cord and **synapse** with the same second-order neurons to ascend the spinal cord and reach the central cortex.[50] For example, pain is referred from the diaphragm to the tip of the shoulder because both of these areas initially develop in the neck region during embryonic development, causing them both to have efferent innervation from the phrenic nerve and afferent innervation to the second through fourth levels of the cervical spine. When pain that may be of either visceral or musculoskeletal origin converges on the same neuron in the spinal cord, it is usually interpreted to be of musculoskeletal origin. This may be because musculoskeletal injury and pain are so much more common that the brain "learns" that activity arriving along that pathway is associated with pain stimulus in a particular musculoskeletal area.

Clinicians who treat neuromusculoskeletal dysfunction must be aware of the potential for pain referral and be familiar with common pain referral patterns to determine the source of a patient's complaints and select appropriate treatment methods. Therefore, when a patient with pain in a musculoskeletal area seeks treatment, the clinician should first determine if the source of the pain is located in the area of this sensation. Pain of musculoskeletal origin generally varies with position or movement of the painful area, whereas pain caused by dysfunction in other systems generally varies with stress on those systems. For example, shoulder pain that is aggravated by raising the arm is likely to originate in the shoulder, whereas left shoulder pain that is aggravated by all forms of strenuous exercise may be caused by a cardiac condition. When assessing pain that is determined to be of musculoskeletal origin, it is also important to accurately determine the structure(s) at fault to provide the most effective treatment. This can be done by performing provocative tests to reproduce the patient's chief complaint. Physical agents may effectively relieve referred pain; however, they should not be used as

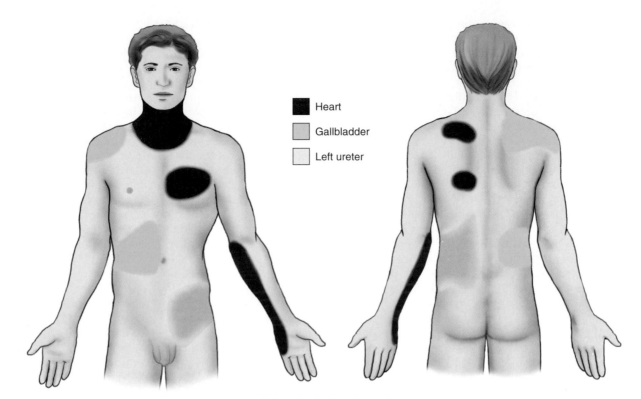

Heart

Gallbladder

Left ureter

FIG 3-1 Referred pain from internal organs.

a substitute for determining the true source of the pain or for treating its underlying cause. They may be used for pain relief while the source of the pain is being investigated, during the recovery process, and for controlling referred pain in which the underlying cause cannot be directly treated.

MECHANISMS OF PAIN RECEPTION AND TRANSMISSION

Pain is generally felt in response to stimulation of peripheral nociceptive structures. The stimulus is transmitted along peripheral nerves to the CNS, from where it can reach the cortex and consciousness. The sensation of pain and the individual's response to the sensation are influenced by a variety of factors, including the physiological mechanisms of the pain receptors, the anatomy of pain-transmitting structures, **neurotransmitter** levels, and the motivation, behavior, and physiological and emotional state of the individual. Variations in any of these factors can alter the individual's perception of pain severity, type, location, and duration.

SPECIFICITY AND PATTERN THEORIES

Over the years, various theories regarding the nature of peripheral pain reception and transmission have been proposed. The primary early theories were the specificity theory and the pattern theory. Current theories integrate components of both of these with more recent findings and observations. According to the specificity theory, as described by Von Frey and others, the sensation of pain depends on the stimulation of nerve endings that are

specialized for each type of sensation.[51-53] For example, a nerve fiber that responds to heat will always transmit the sensation of heat and not pain, no matter how intensely or frequently it is stimulated; similarly, pain fibers will only transmit a sensation of pain and never a sensation of heat. According to this theory, specific pain fibers are responsible for the transmission of the sensation of pain (Fig. 3-2, *A*). Von Frey supported this theory with his identification of free nerve endings widely distributed in the skin that caused a sensation of pain when stimulated. He proposed that these free nerve endings were specific pain receptors.[53] Although the specificity theory is consistent with Von Frey's findings, scientists have since learned that the sensation of pain involves more than the simple stimulation of a specific receptor. The specificity theory also fails to account for the fact that many types of stimuli are perceived as painful and that pain can be modulated by input from the spinal cord or brain. The limitations of the specificity theory led to the development of an alternative explanation of pain perception, the pattern theory.

According to the pattern theory, the sensation of pain results from an increase in the frequency or intensity of stimulation of receptors that also respond to nonnoxious stimuli such as touch, pressure, or temperature.[54] Neural impulses from the periphery are combined and modified to summate in CNS structures, where the pain is localized and interpreted. According to the pattern theory, summation of impulses along the pathways from the skin to the brain determines the individual's sensation of pain (Fig. 3-2, *B*). For example, a nerve may transmit the sensation of heat when stimulated lightly, but the same nerve may

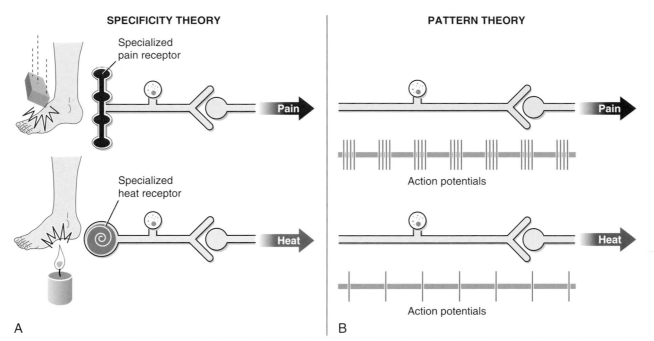

FIG 3-2 Specificity versus pattern theory of pain. **A,** Specific receptors for each type of sensation. **B,** Pattern of action potentials resulting in sensation of pain.

transmit pain when stimulated intensely. This theory accounts for the fact that a wide variety of stimuli cause the sensation of pain and also suggests central influence by pain summation; however, it fails to consider the role of specialized pain receptor structures and to account for central pain modulation.

Current theories integrate components of the specificity theory and the pattern theory with more recent findings regarding neural anatomy and the functions of endogenous neurotransmitters. Current findings indicate that specific nerve endings called nociceptors respond to all painful stimuli, and specific nerve types, small myelinated **A-delta fibers** and unmyelinated **C fibers**, transmit the sensation of pain from these nerve endings to the spinal cord and then, within specific tracts, to the brain. The quality of the pain depends on the type of tissue from which the stimulus originates and on which of the two nerve types transmits the pain; the intensity of the pain is related to the firing rate of the nerves. Pain from cutaneous noxious stimulation is usually perceived as sharp, pricking, or tingling and is easy to localize, whereas pain from musculoskeletal structures is usually dull, heavy, or aching and is harder to localize.[55] Visceral pain has an aching quality similar to that of musculoskeletal pain but tends to refer superficially rather than deeply.[15]

> **Ⓠ Clinical Pearl**
>
> Cutaneous pain is usually well-localized and sharp, pricking, or tingling. Musculoskeletal pain is usually poorly localized and is dull, heavy, or aching. Visceral pain refers superficially and has an aching quality.

Pain transmitted by C fibers is usually dull, long-lasting, and aching, whereas pain transmitted by A-delta fibers is generally sharp. The intensity of the pain and the responses to it are thought to be more severe when the intensity of nociceptive receptor stimulation is greater than that of nonnociceptive receptor stimulation, when levels of endogenous opioids are low, and with certain variations in the individual's psychological state.[56]

PAIN RECEPTORS

Nociceptors are free, noncorpuscular peripheral nerve endings consisting of a series of spindle-shaped, thick segments linked by thin segments to produce a "string-of-beads" appearance. The beads and end bulbs contain mitochondria, glycogen particles, vesicles, and bare areas of axolemma that are not covered by Schwann cell processes.[57] Nociceptors are present in almost all types of tissue. For example, low back pain is thought to be transmitted from free nerve endings that have been found in facet joints, discs, ligaments, nerve roots, and muscles.[58] In damaged discs, nerves also penetrate areas where they would normally not be present, such as the inner anulus fibrosis and the nucleus pulposus, thus contributing to discogenic pain.[59]

Nociceptors can be activated by intense thermal, mechanical, or chemical stimuli from exogenous or endogenous sources. For example, intense mechanical stimulation, such as that caused by a brick falling on someone's foot or a piece of broken bone compressing a nociceptor, will result in nociceptor activation. Chemical stimulation by exogenous substances, such as acid or bleach, or by endogenously produced substances, such as bradykinin, histamine, and arachidonic acid, which are released as

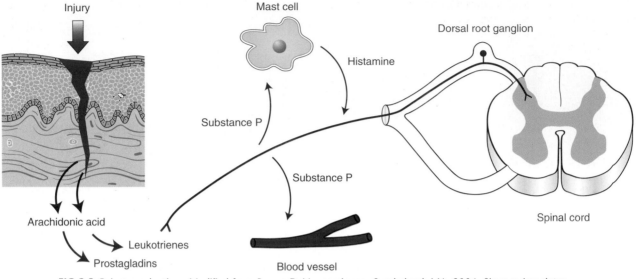

FIG 3-3 Pain transduction. *Modified from Purves D:* Neuroscience, *Sunderland, MA, 2004, Sinauer Associates.*

part of the inflammatory response to tissue damage, can also activate nociceptors. Because these chemical mediators remain after the initial physical stimulus has passed, they generally cause pain to persist beyond the duration of the initial noxious stimulation. It is important to note that chemical mediators of inflammation also sensitize nociceptors, reducing their activation threshold to other stimuli.[64,65] This is the reason that clinically many activities and stimuli to recently injured areas are perceived as painful even when they are not damaging.

When nociceptors are activated, they release a variety of neuropeptides from their peripheral terminals, including **substance P** and a number of breakdown products of arachidonic acid such as prostaglandins and leukotrienes.[29] Nociceptors also convert the initial stimulus into electrical activity, in the form of action potentials, by a process known as **transduction** (Fig. 3-3). It is thought that the released neuropeptides may initiate or participate in transduction because they sensitize nociceptors.[53] The action potentials resulting from the process of transduction propagate from the nociceptors along **afferent nerves** toward the spinal cord.

PERIPHERAL NERVE PATHWAYS

Nociceptors give rise to two types of first-order afferent nerve fibers, C fibers and A-delta fibers. The activity in both types of fibers increases in response to peripheral noxious stimulation, including that associated with acute inflammation or muscle ischemia.[54-69] Eighty percent of afferent pain-transmitting fibers are C fibers, and the remaining 20% are A-delta fibers.[70] Generally, about 50% of the sensory fibers in a cutaneous nerve have nociceptive functions.[56]

C fibers, also known as group IV afferents, are small, unmyelinated nerve fibers that transmit action potentials quite slowly, at the rate of 1.0 to 4.0 m/sec.[71] They respond to noxious levels of mechanical, thermal, and chemical stimulation, causing pain that is generally described as dull, throbbing, aching, or burning and may also be

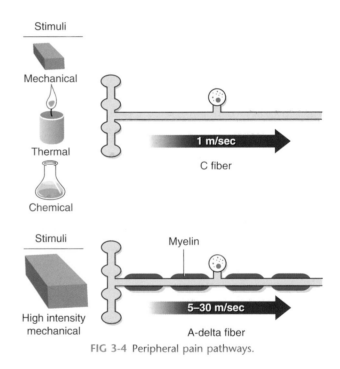

FIG 3-4 Peripheral pain pathways.

reported as tingling or tapping[72,73] (Fig. 3-4). The pain sensations transmitted by these fibers have a slow onset after the initial painful stimulus, are long-lasting, emotionally difficult for the individual to tolerate, and tend to be diffusely localized, particularly when the stimulus is intense.[74,75] They can be accompanied by autonomic responses such as sweating, increased heart rate and blood pressure, or nausea.[76] The pain associated with C-fiber activation can be reduced by opiates, and this pain relief is blocked by the opiate antagonist naloxone.[77]

A-delta fibers, also known as group III afferents, are also small-diameter fibers; however, they transmit more rapidly than C fibers, at a rate of about 30 m/sec, because they are myelinated.[71,78] They are most sensitive to high-intensity mechanical stimulation, although they can also respond to stimulation by heat or cold and are capable of transmitting innocuous information.[79] The sensations associated with A-delta fiber activity are generally described as sharp, stabbing, or pricking.[56] The pain sensations transmitted by these fibers have a quick onset after the painful stimulus, last only for a short time, are generally localized to the area from which the stimulus arose, and are not generally associated with emotional involvement. The pain associated with A-delta fiber activation is generally not blocked by opiates.[80]

Mechanical trauma usually activates both C and A-delta fibers. Take the example of a brick landing on someone's foot. Almost immediately the individual feels a sharp sensation of pain. The initial pain is followed by a deep ache that may last for several hours or days. The initial sharp pain is transmitted by the A-delta fibers and is produced in response to the high-intensity mechanical stimulation of the nociceptors as a result of the impact of the brick. The later, deep ache is transmitted by the C fibers and is produced in response to stimulation by chemical mediators of inflammation released by the tissue after the initial injury.

A-beta nerve fibers can also be involved in abnormal pain transmission and perception. **A-beta fibers**, or wide dynamic-range neurons, have relatively large myelinated axons that conduct impulses more quickly than A-delta and C fibers. Their receptors are located in the skin, bones, and joints. Normally, they transmit sensation related to vibration, stretching of skin, and mechanoreception and do not transmit pain. However, in states such as neuropathic pain and central sensitization, these neurons alter their transduction so that normal stimuli result in pain. There are three theories on how A-beta fibers contribute to pain.[81] The first theory states that firing of A-beta fibers activates spinal neurons that have undergone central sensitization. The second theory posits that A-beta fibers might sprout into spinal cord layers normally targeted by C-fibers and when activated, stimulate the wrong neurons.[82] A third theory states that intact A-beta nerve fibers near damaged nociceptive nerves begin firing abnormally.[83] This alteration in nerve function is key in prolonged pain.

CENTRAL PATHWAYS

The peripheral first-order C and A-delta afferents project from the periphery to the grey matter of the spinal cord. The C and A-delta fibers synapse, either directly or via interneurons, with second-order neurons in the superficial dorsal horn of the grey matter (the substantia gelatinosa).[71,84-87] Some A-delta fibers penetrate more deeply into the dorsal horn to terminate at the normal termination sites of A-beta afferents. The interneurons in the dorsal horn are also known as **transmission cells**, or T cells (Fig. 3-5).

T cells make local connections within the spinal cord, either with efferent neurons as part of spinal cord reflexes or with afferent neurons that project toward the cortex. Continued or repetitive C-fiber activation can sensitize the T cells, causing them to fire more rapidly and to increase their receptor field size, and input from other interneurons

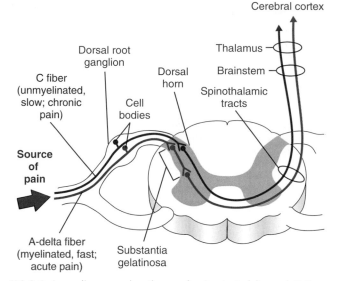

FIG 3-5 Ascending neural pathway of pain via A-delta and C fibers.

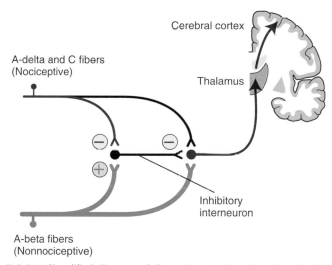

FIG 3-6 Simplified diagram of the gate control mechanism of pain modulation.

originating in the substantia gelatinosa of the spinal cord or from descending fibers originating in higher brain centers can inhibit T-cell activity.[88] Inhibitory interneurons in the substantia gelatinosa are activated by input from large-diameter, myelinated, low-threshold sensory neurons (primarily A-beta nerves) that respond to non-painful stimuli.[89,90] These inhibitory interneurons release various neurotransmitters, including norepinephrine, serotonin, and enkephalins, to modulate the flow of the afferent pain pathways.[91-93] Thus the transmission cells receive excitatory input from the C fibers and A-delta nociceptor afferents and inhibitory input from large-diameter, nonnociceptor sensory afferents and from descending fibers from higher brain centers[56] (Fig. 3-6).

The balance of these excitatory and inhibitory inputs influences whether the individual feels pain and how severe the pain sensation is.[89] The inhibition of pain by inputs from nonnociceptor afferents is known as **pain gating** and is discussed in greater detail in the section on pain modulation and control theories.

Transmission cell activation can increase muscle spasm via a spinal cord reflex in which the transmission cell synapses with anterior horn cells to cause muscle contractions. The ongoing muscle contractions can cause accumulation of fluid and tissue irritants. The contracting muscles may also initiate further nociceptive impulses by mechanically compressing the nociceptors. In this way the combination of ongoing chemical and mechanical stimuli can set up a self-sustaining cycle of pain causing muscle spasm, which then causes more pain. This is known as the **pain-spasm-pain cycle** (Fig. 3-7). Many interventions indirectly reduce pain, even after their direct analgesic effect has passed, because they reduce muscle spasms and thereby interfere with this self-perpetuating cycle.

Ascending second-order nerves carry stimuli within the spinal cord toward the higher brain centers (Fig. 3-8). The second-order pathways that carry pain stimuli are located primarily in the anterolateral aspect of the cord.[94] This area of the spinal cord also transmits information about temperature and touch. Most axons in the anterolateral system cross midline in the spinal cord to ascend contralaterally. Information regarding pain is transmitted within the anterolateral cord via both the lateral spinothalamic tract and the larger anterospinothalamic tract to project to the thalamus. The lateral spinothalamic tract projects directly to the medial area of the thalamus, whereas the anterospinothalamic tract separates from the lateral spinothalamic tract in the brain stem to synapse with neurons in the reticular formation and the hypothalamic and limbic systems to then project to lateral, ventral, and caudal areas of the thalamus. The anterospinothalamic tract also relays information to the periaqueductal grey matter, where there is a large concentration of opiate receptors and is thought to be associated with pain modulation. Impulses relayed via the lateral spinothalamic tract are involved in transmission of sharp pain and in localization of the painful stimulus, whereas those sent via the anterospinothalamic tract are involved in transmission of more prolonged, aching pain and are thought to have stronger association with the disturbing emotions that accompany the pain sensation. The second-order neurons synapse in the thalamus with third-order neurons to project to the cortex, from which the sensation of pain can reach consciousness.

SYMPATHETIC NERVOUS SYSTEM INFLUENCES

The sympathetic nervous system is a component of the **autonomic nervous system**. The autonomic nervous system consists of the sympathetic and parasympathetic systems and is concerned with the activities of smooth and cardiac muscles and with glandular secretion. This contrasts with most of the nervous system, which is concerned with voluntary activation of the skeletal muscles or with transmission of sensory impulses from the periphery[95,96] (Fig. 3-9). The sympathetic nervous system is considered to be primarily involved in producing effects that prepare the body for "fight or flight," such as increasing heart rate and blood pressure, constricting cutaneous blood vessels, and increasing sweating in the palms of the hands. Although it is normal for the sympathetic nervous system to be activated by acute pain or injury, stimulation of the sympathetic nervous system efferents does not usually cause pain.[97] However, abnormal sympathetic activation, caused by a hyperactive response of the sympathetic nervous system to an acute injury or by a failure of its response to subside, can increase pain severity and cause exaggerated signs and symptoms of sympathetic activity such as excessive vasomotor or sweating reactions. In patients with these signs and symptoms, pain relief can often be achieved by interrupting sympathetic nervous system activity by chemical or surgical means.[98-100] In addition, stimuli that evoke sympathetic discharges, such as the startle reflex or emotional events, frequently exacerbate pain. It has therefore been proposed that excessive sympathetic nervous system activation may increase or maintain pain.[96,95] Although anesthetic blockade of the

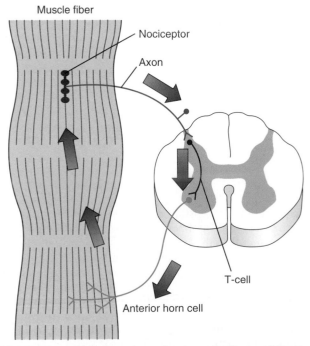

FIG 3-7 Pain-spasm-pain cycle: nociceptor activation resulting in T-cell activation stimulating an anterior horn cell to cause a muscle fiber to contract, resulting in accumulation of fluid and tissue irritants and mechanical compression of the nociceptor and increasing nociceptor activation.

Muscle fiber

Nociceptor

Axon

T-cell

Anterior horn cell

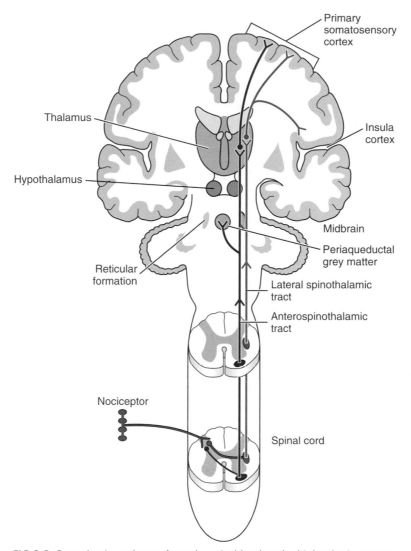

FIG 3-8 Central pain pathways from the spinal level to the higher brain centers.

sympathetic nervous system is widely used to reduce pain in complex regional pain syndrome, its effectiveness has not yet been proven.[101,102]

Pain that is believed to involve sympathetic nervous system overactivation has a variety of names, including causalgia, reflex sympathetic dystrophy (RSD), shoulder-hand syndrome, posttraumatic dystrophy, Sudeck's atrophy, and sympathetically maintained pain.[103] Currently, the International Association for the Study of Pain (IASP) recommends the use of the term **complex regional pain syndrome** (CRPS).[86] CRPS involving tissue damage without nerve damage is categorized as type I, and CRPS associated with nerve involvement is categorized as type II.[86] In addition, pain that reduces with sympathetic blockade may be called sympathetically maintained pain (SMP), whereas pain that does not respond to sympthetic blockade may be called sympathetically independent pain (SIP).[86]

CRPS generally includes the following signs and symptoms: severe pain that is out of proportion to the inciting injury or disease, hyperesthesia (excessive reaction to

painful stimuli), and allodynia (the sensation of pain in response to stimuli that are not usually painful). CRPS frequently also includes trophic changes such as skin atrophy and hyperhidrosis, edema, stiffness, increased sweating, and decreased hair growth.[86] These symptoms generally result in decreased function and if the syndrome is prolonged, spotty osteoporosis in the affected area.[105] Other sensory, vasomotor, and skeletal motor abnormalities have also been associated with this syndrome.[106] CRPS can occur in any area of the body but is most common in the hand and in such cases, is frequently associated with ipsilateral restriction of shoulder motion. CRPS may develop as a consequence of major or minor trauma, after visceral disease or CNS lesions, or without any known antecedent event.

The mechanism by which the sympathetic nervous system affects pain is not well understood; however, it may be the result of direct excitation of the nociceptors by the sympathetic efferent fibers or by the neurotransmitters released by the sympathetic nerves. The normal activation of sympathetic activity caused by pain may in some

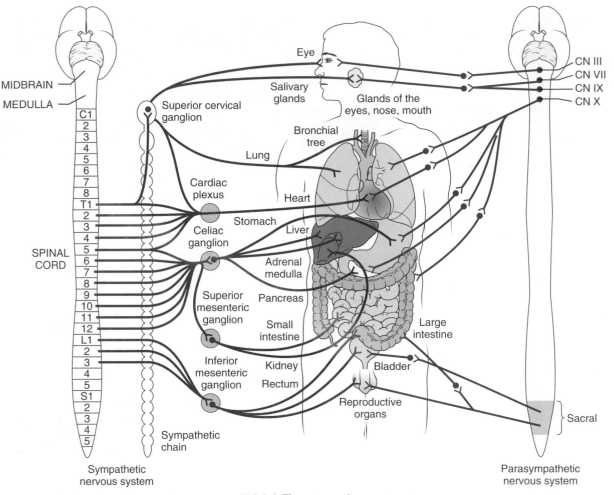

FIG 3-9 The autonomic nervous system.

cases activate the afferent C fibers, further increasing pain, which could then increase sympathetic activation, creating a self-sustaining vicious cycle. This cycle could amplify the sensation of pain and the signs of sympathetic activity, causing them to persist long after an injury or disease has resolved.[89] It has also been proposed that faulty sympathetic effector mechanisms that cause inappropriate vasoconstriction, vasodilation, increased capillary permeability, or smooth muscle tone may indirectly cause or exacerbate pain.[56]

THE ROLE OF SUBSTANCE P

Substance P is a neurotransmitter thought to be involved in the transmission of neuropathic and inflammatory pain. Substance P is present in both the central and peripheral nervous systems. In the CNS, it is found in approximately 20% of C fibers.[107] It is also released from peripheral nociceptors and has been detected in inflammatory exudate.[108-110] Substance P release can excite pain-transmitting neurons in the dorsal horn of the spinal cord and is involved in nociceptive processing at the spinal cord level.[93-113] Although less than 5% of the neurons in the dorsal horn express substance P receptors, the majority of pain-transmitting neurons express these receptors. Substance P levels in the spinal cord increase in response to

induction of joint inflammation and in response to movement of inflamed joints. Elevated levels of substance P in both the cerebrospinal fluid (CSF) and blood of fibromyalgia patients correlate with elevated inflammatory markers in the blood.[114] Substance P receptor activation appears to be involved in the sensitization of pain-transmitting neurons and in the development of hyperalgesia.[113-117] Substance P release and receptor activation is thought to be a response to tissue injury and stress.

A number of mechanisms have been proposed for the action of substance P on pain transmission. Substance P may facilitate excitation of afferent pain fibers by activating the neurokinin-1 receptors in the spinal cord.[118,119] Substance P may also contribute to localized inflammation by causing mast cells to release proinflammatory and neurosensitizing molecules.[114,120] When released into the periphery, substance P increases the production of the inflammatory mediator prostaglandin E_2 (PGE_2) and the release of cytokines from macrophages and neutrophils.[121] Both prostaglandins and cytokines sensitize primary afferent nociceptors.[122]

Treatments to control pain based on inhibiting substance P release or using substance P receptor antagonists seem promising but have shown poor results thus far. Although certain substances have been found to inhibit the release of substance P in rats,[123] it is uncertain if these substances would affect pain in humans. Substance P receptor antagonists have not been found to decrease pain in human subjects[124] or relieve depression, another condition associated with elevated levels of substance P.[125] Opiates may in part exert an analgesic effect by inhibiting the release of substance P from peripheral nerves, although substance P receptor–expressing neurons are not the major site of action of opiates.[115,126] One study found that opiates reduced the sensation of pain related to substance P by inhibiting its effects both presynaptically and postsynaptically.[127] By activating the mu opioid receptor, morphine may also impact the neurokinin-1 receptor and substance P, impacting immune responses in the CNS.[128] Noradrenalin may be the link between opiate-induced pain relief and substance P. In mice without noradrenalin, morphine was not effective and levels of substance P and pain were elevated; this effect was reversed with administration of noradrenalin or substance P receptor antagonists.[129] Substance P has also been linked to the paradoxical increased pain seen with high-dose opiates in animals.[130]

PAIN MODULATION AND CONTROL

Pain transmission and perception are subject to inhibition and modification. For example, rubbing or shaking an area that hurts can relieve pain in that area, and stress can cause pain not to be felt at the time an injury occurs. Several mechanisms have been proposed to explain pain control and modulation. These proposed mechanisms attempt to correlate what is known regarding the experience of pain with the structures and physiological processes thought to be involved in pain transmission. According to the gate control theory, pain is modulated at the spinal cord level by inhibitory effects of innocuous afferent input. According to the theory of endogenous opiates, pain is modulated at the peripheral, spinal cord, and cortical levels by endogenous neurotransmitters that have the same effects as opiates. Psychological central control mechanisms are also thought to affect pain perception and control.

Various physical, chemical, and psychological interventions have been developed based on the current understanding of the mechanisms underlying pain modulation. For example, transcutaneous electrical nerve stimulation (TENS) devices were developed based on the gate control theory of pain modulation. Also, the efficacy of a number of established treatment approaches is now better understood because the underlying mechanisms of pain control have become clearer. For example, it is now thought that thermal agents, which have been used to control pain for centuries, may be effective for this purpose because they gate pain transmission at the spinal cord.

GATE CONTROL THEORY

The **gate control theory of pain modulation** was first proposed by Melzack and Wall in 1965.[89] According to this theory, severity of the pain sensation is determined by the balance of excitatory and inhibitory inputs to the T cells in the spinal cord. These cells receive excitatory input from C and A-delta nociceptor afferents and inhibitory input via the substantia gelatinosa from large-diameter A-beta nonnociceptor sensory afferents. Increased activity of the nonnociceptor sensory afferents causes presynaptic inhibition of the T cells and thus effectively closes the spinal gate to the cerebral cortex and decreases the sensation of pain (see Fig. 3-6).

Many physical agents and interventions are thought to control pain in part by activating nonnociceptive sensory nerves, thereby inhibiting activation of pain transmission cells and closing the gate to the transmission of pain.[131,132] For example, electrical stimulation (ES), traction, compression, and massage can all activate low-threshold, large-diameter, nonnociceptive sensory nerves and therefore may inhibit pain transmission by closing the gate to pain transmission at the spinal cord level.

Although the gate control theory explains many observations regarding pain control and modulation, it fails to account for the finding that descending controls from higher brain centers, in addition to ascending input from sensory afferents, can affect pain perception.[133,134] Therefore the gate theory has been modified to include influences from descending neurons from the limbic system, the raphe nucleus, and the reticular systems, which affect pain perception, the emotional aspects of pain, and motor responses to pain.[135]

THE ENDOGENOUS OPIOID SYSTEM

Pain perception is also modulated by endogenous opiate-like peptides. These peptides are called **opiopeptins** (previously known as **endorphins**). Opiopeptins control pain by binding to specific opiate receptors in the nervous system.

An endogenous system of analgesia was first discovered by three independent groups of researchers who were investigating the mechanisms of morphine-induced analgesia. In 1973, they discovered specific opiate-binding sites in the CNS.[136-138] In 1975, two peptides, met-enkephalin (methionine-enkephalin) and leu-enkephalin (leucine-enkephalin), which were isolated from the CNS of a pig, were shown to produce physiological effects similar to those of morphine.[139] These peptides also bind specifically to the opiate receptors, and their action and binding are blocked by naloxone, an opiate antagonist.[140] These findings demonstrated that these endogenous peptides are similar to exogenous opiates such as morphine. Consequently, researchers identified and isolated other similar-acting endogenous peptides, such as beta-endorphin and dynorphin A and B.[141]

Opiopeptins and opiate receptors have been found in many peripheral nerve endings and in neurons in several regions of the nervous system.[142] Concentrations of opiopeptins and opiate receptors have been identified in various areas of the brain, including the periaqueductal grey matter (PAGM) and the raphe nucleus of the brain stem, which are structures that induce analgesia when electrically stimulated, and in various areas of the limbic system. Opiopeptins are also found in high concentrations in the superficial layers of the dorsal horn of the spinal cord (layers I and II) and in the enteric nervous system, as well as in the nerve endings of C fibers. It has been proposed that opiate receptors inhibit the release of substance P from C-fiber terminals because local opiate application to C-fiber terminals depresses pain transmission at the spinal cord level.[143]

Opioids and opiopeptins always have an inhibitory action. They cause presynaptic inhibition by suppressing the inward flux of calcium and cause postsynaptic inhibition by activating an outward potassium current. In addition, opiopeptins indirectly inhibit pain transmission by inhibiting the release of **gamma-aminobutyric acid** (GABA) in the PAGM and the raphe nucleus.[144] GABA inhibits the activity of various pain-controlling structures, including A-beta afferents, the PAGM, and the raphe nucleus, and can thus increase pain transmission in the spinal cord.

ES of areas with high levels of opiopeptins, such as the PAGM and the raphe nucleus, strongly inhibits the transmission of pain messages by some spinal dorsal horn neurons, thereby causing analgesia.[145,146] ES of these areas of the brain can also relieve intractable pain in humans and increase the amount of beta-endorphin in their CSF.[147] Because these effects are reversed by the administration of naloxone, they have been attributed to the release of opiopeptins.[148] The concentration of opiate receptors and opiopeptins in the limbic system, an area of the brain largely associated with emotional phenomena, also provides an explanation for the emotional responses to pain and for the euphoria and relief of emotional stress associated with the use of morphine and the release of opiopeptins.[149]

The release of opiopeptins is thought to play an important role in the modulation and control of pain during times of emotional stress. Levels of opiopeptins in the brain and CSF become elevated, and pain thresholds increase in both animals and humans when stress is induced experimentally by the anticipation of pain.[150,151] Experimentally, animals have been shown to experience a diffuse analgesia when placed under stress. Humans demonstrate a naloxone-sensitive increase in pain threshold and a parallel depression of the nociceptive flexion reflex when subjected to emotional stress.[151,152] These findings indicate that pain suppression by stress is most likely caused by increased opiopeptin levels at the spinal cord and higher CNS centers.

The **endogenous opiate theory** also provides an explanation for the paradoxical pain-relieving effects of painful stimulation and acupuncture. Bearable levels of painful stimulation, such as topical preparations that cause the sensation of burning or noxious TENS that causes the sensation of pricking or burning, have been shown to reduce the intensity of less bearable preexisting pain in the area of application and in other areas.[152] Painful stimuli have also been shown to reduce the nociceptive flexion reflex of the lower limb in animals.[153] Because these effects of painful stimulation are blocked by naloxone, they are thought to be mediated by opiopeptins.[151,152,154,155] Pain may be relieved because the applied painful stimulus causes neurons in the PAGM regions of the midbrain and thalamus to produce and release opiopeptins.[155]

Placebo analgesia is also thought to be mediated in part by opiopeptins. This claim is supported by the observation that the opiate antagonist naloxone can reverse placebo analgesia and that placebos can also produce respiratory depression, a typical side effect of opioids.[156,157]

MEASURING PAIN

To determine the most appropriate treatment for a patient's pain and to assess the efficacy of such treatment, it is helpful to assess the nature and severity of the patient's pain. Such an assessment should attempt to ascertain the causes and sources of pain, the intensity and duration of pain, and the degree to which the pain affects body function, activity, and participation.

Ⓠ Clinical Pearl

When evaluating a patient's pain, consider the pain's source, intensity, and duration and how it affects a person's function, activity, and participation.

Various methods and assessment tools have been developed to quantify and qualify both experimentally induced and clinical pain. These methods are based on patients rating their pain on a visual analog or numeric scale; comparing their present pain with that experienced in response to a predefined, quantifiable pain stimulus; or selecting words from a list to describe their present experience of pain. In cases where a person cannot express their pain by one of these methods, as with infants, observational scales are used. These tools provide different amounts and types of information and require varying amounts of time and cognitive ability to complete.

VISUAL ANALOG AND NUMERIC SCALES

Visual analog and numeric scales assess pain severity by asking the patient to indicate the present level of pain on a drawn line or to rate the pain numerically on a scale of 0 to 10 or 0 to 100.[158] With a visual analog scale, the patient marks a position on a horizontal or vertical line, where one end of the line represents no pain and the other end represents the most severe pain possible or the most severe pain the patient can imagine (Fig. 3-10). With a numeric rating scale, 0 is no pain and 10 or 100, depending on the scale used, is the most severe pain possible or the most severe pain the patient can imagine.

Scales similar to the visual analog or numeric scales have been developed for use with individuals who have difficulty using numeric or standard visual analog scales. For example, children who understand words or pictures but are too young to understand numeric representations of pain can use a scale with faces with different expressions to represent different experiences of pain, as shown in Fig. 3-11. This type of scale can also be used to assess pain in patients with limited comprehension because of language barriers or cognitive deficits. For example, patients with dementia can reliably use self-assessment pain scales, and this self-assessment is more accurate than observing the patient for signs of pain according to an observational pain scale.[159] Pain scales based on a child's expression and behavior are used to rate pain in very young children and infants (Table 3-1).

These types of scales are frequently used to assess the severity of a patient's clinical pain because they are quick and easy to administer and easily understood and provide readily quantifiable data.[158] However, visual analog and numeric scales reflect only the intensity of pain and lack information about the patient's response to pain or the effect of the pain on function and activity. Sometimes, combining a visual analog scale with quality of life questions can be an effective way to obtain more information about the impact of pain on a person's life.[160] The reliability of visual analog and numeric rating varies between individuals and with the patient group examined, although the two scales have a high degree of agreement between them.[161] These types of measures are most useful in the clinical setting for a quick estimate of a patient's perceived progress or change in symptoms over time or in response to different activities or interventions.

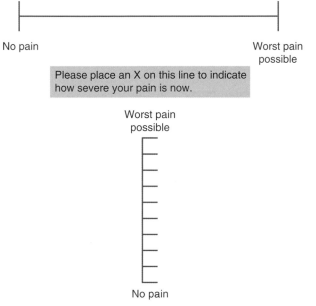

FIG 3-10 Visual analog scales for rating pain severity.

> **Ⓠ Clinical Pearl**
>
> Visual analog and numeric pain scales are best used for a quick estimate of pain severity.

COMPARISON WITH A PREDEFINED STIMULUS

Pain quantification methods that involve comparison with a predefined painful stimulus are intended to provide a greater degree of intersubject reliability than visual analog and numeric scales. For this type of assessment, the individual compares the severity of his or her symptoms with the same predefined stimulus, causing their rating scales to be more similar. Stimuli used for comparison

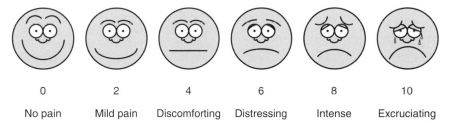

FIG 3-11 Face scale for rating pain severity in children age 3 years and older and others with limited numeric communication ability. The patient uses this tool by pointing to each face and using the brief word instructions under it to describe pain intensity. *Adapted from Wong DL, Perry SE, Hockenberry MJ: Maternal child nursing care, ed 3, St. Louis, 2006, Mosby.*

TABLE 3-1	Neonatal Infant Pain Scale (NIPS) Operational Definitions	
	Behavior and Score	**Description**
Facial expression	0: Relaxed muscles	Restful face, neutral expression
	1: Grimace	Tight facial muscles, furrowed brow, chin, jaw (negative facial expression—nose, mouth, and brow)
Cry	0: No cry	Quiet, not crying
	1: Whimper	Mild moaning, intermittent
	2: Vigorous cry	Loud screams, rising, shrill, continuous (Note: Silent cry may be scored if baby is intubated, as evidenced by obvious mouth, facial movement.)
Breathing patterns	0: Relaxed	Usual pattern for this baby
	1: Change in breathing	Indrawing, irregular, faster than usual, gagging, breath holding
Arms	0: Relaxed/restrained	No muscular rigidity, occasional random movements of arms
	1: Flexed/extended	Tense, straight arms, rigid or rapid extension, flexion
Legs	0: Relaxed/restrained	No muscular rigidity, occasional random leg movement
	1: Flexed/extended	Tense, straight legs, rigid or rapid extension, flexion
State of arousal	0: Sleeping/awake	Quiet, peaceful, sleeping, or alert and settled
	1: Fussy	Alert, restless, and thrashing

From Neonatal Infant Pain Scale, Children's Hospital of Eastern Ontario, Ottawa, Canada.
Score 0=no pain likely; maximum score 7 = severe pain likely.

include the application of a tourniquet to the upper extremity to produce ischemia and the application of electrical, thermal, or fingertip pressure stimuli.[162,163] The tourniquet pain test is reported to correlate well with pain assessments using a visual analog scale.[164] Matching the intensity of clinical pain with electrical, thermal, or fingertip pressure stimuli has also been reported to correlate well with other measures of pain and has been reported to have a high degree of intrasubject reliability.[165,166] However, these types of pain assessment tools have a number of limitations. They require that the patient experience clinical pain at the time at which the comparison stimulus is applied to make an accurate comparison. If a patient has severe pain, it may be both impractical and ethically unacceptable to induce a sufficiently intense pain to provide a comparison with the clinical pain. For patients with pain that is different in quality from the pain of the experimental stimulus; for example, burning or tingling rather than the ache of ischemic pain, a quantitative comparison may not be possible or meaningful. This type of pain measure also fails to take into account or report on the emotional, behavioral, or motivational components of a patient's clinical condition. Thus, although comparison pain measures may allow for a reliable gauge of some types of pain, particularly experimentally induced pain or clinical acute pain that is moderate or less severe, they are not well-suited for measuring clinical pain that is severe or chronic or that has a quality different from that of the comparison stimulus and therefore are rarely used in the clinical setting.

SEMANTIC DIFFERENTIAL SCALES

Semantic differential scales consist of word lists and categories that represent various aspects of the patient's pain experience. The patient is asked to select from these lists words that best describe his or her present experience of pain. These types of scales are designed to collect a broad range of information about the patient's pain experience and to provide quantifiable data for intrasubject and intersubject comparisons. The semantic differential scale included in the McGill Pain Questionnaire, or variations of this scale, are commonly used to assess pain[167-169] (Fig. 3-12). This scale includes descriptors of sensory, affective, and evaluative aspects of the patient's pain and groups the words into various categories within each of these aspects. The categories include temporal, spatial, pressure, and thermal to describe the sensory aspects of the pain; fear, anxiety, and tension to describe the affective aspects of the pain; and the cognitive experience of the pain based on past experience and learned behaviors to describe the evaluative aspects of the pain. The patient circles the one word in each of the applicable categories that best describes the present pain.[167,169]

Semantic differential scales have a number of advantages and disadvantages compared with other types of pain measures. They allow assessment and quantification of the pain's scope, quality, and intensity. Counting the total number of words chosen provides a quick gauge of the pain severity. A more sensitive assessment of pain severity can be obtained by adding the rank sums of all the words chosen to produce a pain rating index (PRI). For greater specificity with regard to the most problematic area, an index for the three major categories of the questionnaire can also be calculated.[169] The primary disadvantages of this scale are that it is time-consuming to administer and requires the patient to have an intact cognitive state and a high level of literacy. Given these advantages and limitations, the most appropriate use for this type of scale is when detailed information about a patient's pain is needed such as in a chronic pain treatment program or in clinical research. For example, in patients with chronic wounds, the McGill Pain Questionnaire was more sensitive to pain experience than a single rating of pain intensity and positively correlated with wound stage, affective stress, and symptoms of depression.[170]

> **◎ Clinical Pearl**
>
> Semantic differential pain scales should be used for a detailed pain description.

OTHER MEASURES

Other measures or indicators of pain that may provide additional useful information about the individual's pain complaint and clinical condition include daily activity/pain logs indicating which activities ease or aggravate the pain, body diagrams on which the patient can indicate the location and nature of the pain (Fig. 3-13), and open-ended, structured interviews.[171,173] Physical examination that includes observation of posture and assessment of strength, mobility, sensation, endurance, response to functional activity testing, and soft tissue tone and quality can also add valuable information to the evaluation of the severity and cause(s) of a patient's pain complaint.

In selecting the measures to assess pain, consider symptom duration, the patient's cognitive abilities, and the time needed to assess the patient's report of pain. Often, a simple visual analog scale may be sufficient, as when evaluating a progressive decrease in pain as a patient recovers from an acute injury. However, in more complex or prolonged cases, detailed measures such as semantic differential scales or a combination of several measures are more appropriate.

DOCUMENTING PAIN

To most clearly document pain, it is best to be as thorough as possible. Documentation should note the pain's location, quality, severity, and timing, as well as the factors that make it better or worse, the setting in which it occurs, and associated manifestations.[173,174] The pain should be quantified, and there should be an assessment of how the pain has affected a person's function, activities, and participation. An example of the documentation of pain follows:

JS reports 7/10 aching central low back pain when sitting for more than 15 minutes that improves to 5/10 with movement or ibuprofen. The pain began 1 week ago after bending to lift a heavy box, and since then JS has been unable to lift anything over 10 lb and has been unable to work in his construction job.

What does your pain feel like?

Some of the words below describe your *present* pain. Indicate which words describe it best. Leave out any word group that is not suitable. Use only a single word in each appropriate group—the one that applies *best*.

1	2	3	4
1 Flickering	1 Jumping	1 Pricking	1 Sharp
2 Quivering	2 Flashing	2 Boring	2 Cutting
3 Pulsing	3 Shooting	3 Drilling	3 Lacerating
4 Throbbing		4 Stabbing	
5 Beating		5 Lancinating	
6 Pounding			

5	6	7	8
1 Pinching	1 Tugging	1 Hot	1 Tingling
2 Pressing	2 Pulling	2 Burning	2 Itchy
3 Gnawing	3 Wrenching	3 Scalding	3 Smarting
4 Cramping		4 Searing	4 Stinging
5 Crushing			

9	10	11	12
1 Dull	1 Tender	1 Tiring	1 Sickening
2 Sore	2 Taut	2 Exhausting	2 Suffocating
3 Hurting	3 Rasping		
4 Aching	4 Splitting		
5 Heavy			

13	14	15	16
1 Fearful	1 Punishing	1 Wretched	1 Annoying
2 Frightful	2 Gruelling	2 Blinding	2 Troublesome
3 Terrifying	3 Cruel		3 Miserable
	4 Vicious		4 Intense
	5 Killing		5 Unbearable

17	18	19	20
1 Spreading	1 Tight	1 Cool	1 Nagging
2 Radiating	2 Numb	2 Cold	2 Nauseating
3 Penetrating	3 Drawing	3 Freezing	3 Agonizing
4 Piercing	4 Squeezing		4 Dreadful
	5 Tearing		5 Torturing

FIG 3-12 Semantic differential scale from the McGill Pain Questionnaire. *From Melzack R: The McGill Pain Questionnaire: major properties and scoring methods,* Pain *1(3):277-299, 1975.*

PAIN MANAGEMENT APPROACHES

Once the severity and nature of an individual's pain has been evaluated and ideally its source and nature determined, the goals of treatment include eliminating the cause of pain, controlling the nociceptor input, and improving patient function. A wide range of pain management approaches may help achieve these goals. These approaches are based on our current understanding of pain transmission and control mechanisms. They may act by controlling inflammation, altering nociceptor sensitivity, increasing binding to opiate receptors, modifying nerve conduction, modulating pain transmission at the spinal cord level, or altering higher-level aspects of pain perception. Some treatment approaches also address the psychological and social aspects of pain. Different approaches are appropriate for different situations and clinical presentations and are frequently most effective when used together.

The primary intervention used to alleviate pain is the administration of pharmacological agents. Although pharmacological agents often provide effective pain relief, they can also produce a variety of adverse effects. Therefore the use of physical agents, which also effectively control pain in many cases and produce fewer adverse effects, may be more appropriate. Some patients, particularly those with persistent pain, may need integrated multidisciplinary

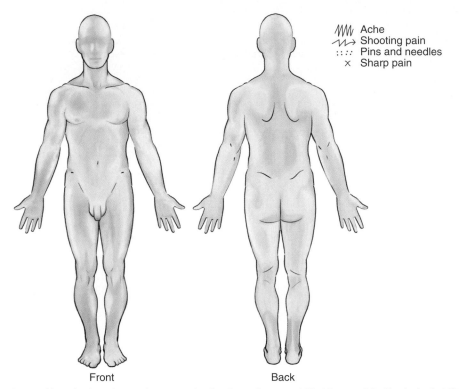

⁓⁓⁓	Ache
⁓↝	Shooting pain
∷∷	Pins and needles
×	Sharp pain

Front   Back

FIG 3-13 Body diagrams for marking the location and nature of pain. *From Cameron MH, Monroe, LG: Physical rehabilitation: evidence-based examination, evaluation, and intervention, St Louis, 2007, Saunders.*

treatment, which includes psychological and physiological therapies, to achieve pain relief or return to a more normal functional activity level.

PHARMACOLOGICAL APPROACHES

Pharmacological analgesic agents control pain by modifying inflammatory mediators at the periphery, altering pain transmission from the periphery to the cortex, or altering the central perception of pain. The selection of a particular pharmacological analgesic agent depends on the cause of the pain, the length of time the individual is expected to need the agent, and the side effects of the agent. Pharmacological agents may be administered systemically by mouth, injection, transdermally, or locally by injection into structures surrounding the spinal cord or into painful or inflamed areas. These different routes of administration allow concentration of the drug at different sites of pain transmission to optimize the control of symptoms with varying distributions.

Systemic Analgesics

Administration of a systemic analgesic is usually the primary method of pain management. This type of treatment is easy to administer and inexpensive and can be an effective and appropriate pain-relieving intervention for many patients. A wide range of analgesic medications can be systemically administered orally or by other routes. These medications include nonsteroidal antiinflammatory drugs (NSAIDs), acetaminophen, opiates and opioids, and antidepressants.

Nonsteroidal Antiinflammatory Drugs

NSAIDs have both analgesic and antiinflammatory properties and can therefore relieve pain from both inflammatory and noninflammatory sources. They inhibit peripheral pain and inflammation by inhibiting the conversion of arachidonic acid to prostaglandins by cyclooxygenase; however, much lower doses and blood levels are required to reduce pain than to reduce inflammation.[175]

> **◎ Clinical Pearl**
>
> Lower doses of NSAIDs are required to reduce pain than to reduce inflammation.

NSAIDs have been shown to reduce both spontaneous and mechanically evoked activity in C and A-delta fibers in acute and chronic models of joint inflammation. Evidence also exists that NSAIDs exert central analgesic effects at the spinal cord and at the thalamus.[176-180]

Although NSAIDs have excellent short- to medium-term application for the control of moderately severe pain caused by musculoskeletal disorders, particularly when the pain is associated with inflammation, side effects can limit their long-term use. The primary long-term complication of most NSAIDs is gastrointestinal irritation and bleeding.[181,182]

> **◎ Clinical Pearl**
>
> Gastrointestinal irritation and bleeding are the main long-term complications of NSAIDs.

NSAIDs also cause decreased platelet aggregation and thus prolonged bleeding time. They can cause kidney damage, edema, bone marrow suppression, rashes and anorexia, and decreased renal blood flow in dehydrated patients.[183,184] Using different NSAIDs together increases the risk of side effects.

The first NSAID was aspirin. Many other NSAIDs, such as ibuprofen (Motrin), naproxen sodium (Naprosyn, Aleve), and piroxicam (Feldene), are now available both over the counter (OTC) and by prescription. The principal advantages of these newer NSAIDs over aspirin are that some have a longer duration of action, allowing less frequent dosing and better compliance, and some cause fewer gastrointestinal side effects. However, for most patients, aspirin effectively relieves pain at considerably less expense, although with a slightly higher risk of gastrointestinal bleeding, than the newer NSAIDs.

More recently, specific cyclooxygenase type 2 (COX2) inhibitor NSAIDs, such as celecoxib (Celebrex) and rofecoxib (Vioxx), were developed with the goal of producing fewer gastrointestinal side effects than older NSAIDs that inhibit both COX1 and COX2. However, rofecoxib was voluntarily withdrawn from the market in September 2004 because of the increased risk of heart attack and stroke with long-term use (>18 months) seen in a study 4 years earlier.[185,186] A study shortly thereafter on the effect of celecoxib on colon adenoma also showed increased cardiovascular events.[187] Since then, placebo-controlled trials have confirmed that rofecoxib and valdecoxib use is associated with increased risk of stroke and myocardial infarction.[188,189] In April 2005, the FDA requested that valdecoxib be voluntarily taken off the market. Now, black box warnings restrict the use of these agents until their safety is properly evaluated.

NSAIDs are primarily administered orally, although one, ketorolac (Toradol), is available for administration by injection.[190] The mode of administration does not alter the analgesic or adverse effects of these drugs.

Acetaminophen

Acetaminophen (Tylenol) is an effective analgesic for mild to moderately severe pain; however, unlike an NSAID, it has no clinically significant antiinflammatory activity.[191] Taken in the same dosage as aspirin, it has analgesic and antipyretic effects comparable to those of aspirin.[191] Acetaminophen is administered primarily by the oral route, although administration by suppository is effective for patients who are unable to take medications by mouth. Acetaminophen is useful for patients who cannot tolerate NSAIDs because of gastric irritation or when prolonged bleeding time caused by NSAIDs would be a disadvantage. Prolonged use or large doses of acetaminophen can cause liver damage; this risk is elevated in the chronic alcoholic. When used in healthy adults for a short period, the suggested maximum daily dose is 4 gm.[192] If taken for more than 10 days, the recommended daily dose is 2.6 gm.[193] Elderly and ill patients should not exceed 2 gm daily, and those with significant liver disease should not take acetaminophen. Skin rashes are also an occasional side effect of this medication.

Opioids

Opioids are drugs that contain opium, derivatives of opium, or any of several semisynthetic or synthetic drugs with opium-like activity. Morphine, hydromorphone, fentanyl, meperidine, codeine, hydrocodone, oxycodone, and methadone are examples of opioids used clinically. Although these drugs have slightly different mechanisms of action, they all bind to opioid-specific receptors and their effects are reversed by naloxone.[194] The opioids differ primarily in their potency, duration of action, and restriction of use as a result of variations in pharmacodynamics and pharmacokinetics.

It has been proposed that opioids provide analgesia by mimicking the effects of endorphins and binding to opioid-specific receptor sites in the CNS.[195] They may also relieve pain by inhibiting the release of presynaptic neurotransmitters and inhibiting the activity of interneurons early in the nociceptive pathways to reduce or block C-fiber inputs into the dorsal horn.[143]

When given in sufficient doses, opioids will control even the most severe acute pain with tolerable side effects. They control pain that cannot be relieved by nonopioid analgesics and are most effective when the pain is dull and poorly localized. The side effects of opioids include nausea, vomiting, sedation, suppression of cough, gastrointestinal mobility, and respiration and a propensity to cause physical dependence and depression with long-term use. Respiratory depression also limits the dose that can be used even for short-term administration. People taking opioids can exhibit tolerance, dependence, and addicition. Tolerance is either the need for increasing drug doses to maintain the same level of pain control or decreasing pain control with the same dose. Physical dependence is a normal adaptation of the body to opioid use that causes withdrawal symptoms and a consequent rebound increase in pain when use of the drug is decreased or discontinued after long-term use. Addiction, on the other hand, is the compulsive use of a drug despite physical harm, and the presence of tolerance or dependence does not predict addiction.

Opioids are generally used to relieve postoperative pain or pain caused by malignancy, and in recent years, their use has increased greatly, a result primarily to the more aggressive treatment of chronic pain.[196] Approximately 90% of patients with chronic pain receive opioids.[197] Long-term opioid may result in tolerance, hyperalgesia, hormonal effects, and immunosuppression.[198] Unfortunately, concerns about tolerance and side effects frequently result in the administration of insufficient doses of these medications to patients with severe pain, resulting in unnecessarily high levels of pain.[199,200] The risk of psychological addiction or habituation should not prevent the appropriate use of opioids, particularly in the management of terminal illness.

Opioids can be delivered by mouth, nose, rectum, intravenously, transdermally, subcutaneously, epidurally, intrathecally, or by direct intraarticular injection. A popular and effective means of administration, particularly for hospitalized patients, is **patient-controlled analgesia** (PCA) (Fig. 3-14). With PCA, patients use a pump to self-administer small, repeated intravenous doses. The amount

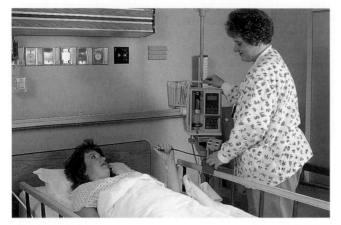

FIG 3-14 Patient-controlled analgesia. *From Potter P, Perry A: Fundamentals of nursing: fundamentals & skills, ed 6, St Louis, 2005, Mosby.*

of medication delivered is limited by preestablished dosing intervals and maximum doses within a defined period. Pain control is more effective and adverse effects are less common with this means of administration than with more conventional physician-controlled opioid administration methods.[203,204]

Antidepressants

Antidepressants, particularly the tricyclics such as amitryptiline (Elavil), have been found to be an effective adjunctive component of chronic pain treatment, with smaller doses being effective for this application than those typically used for the treatment of depression.[205,206] The efficacy of these drugs for the treatment of chronic pain is thought to be related to their effects on sleep, nerve function, and mood. Studies have shown that patients with chronic pain who are also depressed report much higher levels of pain and show more pain-related behaviors than those who are not depressed.[207-209] In addition, antidepressants may also exert an antinociceptive effect independent of the presence of depression,[210] it is still uncertain if the higher level of pain in patients with depression is the cause or the product of their depression, and the use of antidepressants in either situation may prove beneficial.

Spinal Analgesia

Pain relief may be achieved by the administration of drugs such as opioids, local anesthetics, and corticosteroids into the epidural or subarachnoid space of the spinal cord.[211] This route of administration provides analgesia to the areas innervated by the segments of the cord receiving the drug and is therefore most effective when the pain has a spinal distribution, such as a dermatomal distribution in a single limb. The primary advantages of this route of administration are that the drug bypasses the blood-brain barrier and that high concentrations reach the spinal cord at opiate receptors at sites of nociceptive transmission, thus increasing the analgesic effects while reducing adverse side effects.

Opioids administered spinally exert their effects by stimulating opiate receptors in the dorsal horn of the spinal cord.[212] When administered spinally, fat-soluble opioids have a rapid onset and a short duration of action, whereas water-soluble opioids have a slow onset and a more prolonged duration of action.[213] Local anesthetics delivered spinally have the unique ability to completely block nociceptive transmission; however, with increasing concentration, these drugs also block sensory and then motor transmission, causing numbness and weakness.[214] High doses of these drugs can also cause hypotension. These side effects of local anesthetics limit their application to the short-term control of pain and diagnostic purposes. Catabolic corticosteroids, such as cortisone and dexamethasone, can be administered to the epidural or subarachnoid space to relieve pain caused by inflammation of the spinal nerve roots or surrounding structures, although the safety of administering steroids intrathecally has yet to be determined.[215] These drugs inhibit the inflammatory response to tissue injury; however, because of the side effects of repeated or prolonged use, including fat and muscle wasting, osteoporosis, and symptoms of Cushing's syndrome, these drugs are not suitable for long-term application.

Local Injection

Local injection of a corticosteroid, opiate, or a local anesthetic can be particularly effective for relieving pain associated with local inflammation. Such injections can be administered into joints, bursae, trigger points, or around tendons and can be used for therapeutic purposes, to relieve pain, or for diagnostic purposes in identification of the structure(s) at fault.[216] Although this type of treatment can be very effective, repeated local injections of corticosteroids are not recommended because they can cause tissue breakdown and deterioration. Local injections of corticosteroids directly after acute trauma are also not recommended because these drugs reduce the inflammatory response and may thus impair healing. Local injections of anesthetics generally provide only short-term pain relief and are therefore used primarily during painful procedures or diagnostically.

Other

New and alternative medications to treat pain are continually being developed. These include anticonvulsants, nontricyclic antidepressants, blood pressure medications, and various topical agents. Anticonvulsants alter nerve conduction and are primarily used to treat neuropathic pain.[217] Gapapentin and carbamazepine are anticonvulsants that improve chronic neuropathic pain,[218,219] and pregabalin, another anticonvulsant, was specifically developed for the treatment of neuropathic pain and has been shown to relieve pain associated with postherpetic neuralgia.[215,220] Selective serotonin and norephinephrine reuptake inhibitors (SNRIs), including duloxetine and venlafaxine, are antidepressants thought to decrease pain by mediating descending inhibitory pathways of the brain stem and spinal cord. Duloxetine and venlafaxine have been shown to improve pain associated with diabetic peripheral neuropathy as well as other types of neuropathic pain.[220,221] It should be noted that although SNRIs can relieve neuropathic pain, data are limited, and it is uncertain which one of this antidepressant class works best.[222] Calcium channel blockers and alpha-adrenergic antagonists, which are antihypertensive medications, are useful for treating pain associated with CRPS.[217] Capsaicin, a botanical compound found in chile peppers, can be applied topically to reduce pain by depleting substance P and has been shown to be effective for diabetic neuropathy, osteoarthritis, and psoriasis.[223] Topical lidocaine has also been used successfully in the treatment of postherpetic neuralgia.[215]

PHYSICAL AGENTS

Physical agents can relieve pain directly by moderating the release of inflammatory mediators, modulating pain at the spinal cord level, altering nerve conduction, or increasing endorphin levels. They may indirectly reduce pain by decreasing the sensitivity of the muscle spindle system, thereby reducing muscle spasms, or by modifying vascular tone and the rate of blood flow, thereby reducing edema or ischemia.[224-226] In addition, physical agents may reduce pain by helping resolve the underlying cause of the painful sensation.

Different physical agents control pain in different ways. For example, cryotherapy, the application of cold, controls acute pain in part by reducing the metabolic rate and thus reducing the production and release of inflammatory mediators such as serotonin, histamine, bradykinin, substance P, and prostaglandins.[227] These chemicals cause pain directly by stimulating nociceptors and indirectly by impairing the local microcirculation and can damage tissue and impair tissue repair. Reducing the release of inflammatory mediators can thus directly relieve pain caused by acute inflammation and may indirectly limit pain by controlling edema and ischemia. These short-term benefits can also optimize the rate of tissue healing and recovery.

Cryotherapy, thermotherapy, ES, and traction, which provide thermal, mechanical, or other nonnociceptive sensory stimuli, are thought to alleviate pain in part by inhibiting pain transmission at the spinal cord. Physical agents that act by this mechanism can be used for the treatment of acute and chronic pain because they do not generally produce significant adverse effects or adverse interactions with drugs and do not produce physical dependence with prolonged use. They are also effective and appropriate for pain caused by conditions that cannot be directly modified, such as pain caused by malignancy or a recent fracture, and for pain caused by peripheral nervous system pathology, such as phantom limb pain and peripheral neuropathy.[228]

ES is also thought to control pain in part by stimulating the release of opiopeptins at the spinal cord and at higher levels.[155] Studies have shown that pain relief by certain types of ES is reversed by naloxone.[155]

Physical agents have many advantages over other pain-modifying interventions. They are associated with fewer and generally less severe side effects than pharmacological agents. The adverse effects of physical agents used to control pain are generally localized to the area of application and are easily avoided with care in applying the treatment. When used appropriately, attending to all contraindications and dose recommendations, the risk of

further injury from the use of physical agents is minimal. For example, an excessively warm hot pack may cause a burn in the area of application, but this risk can be minimized by carefully monitoring the hot pack's temperature, using adequate insulation between the hot pack and the patient, not applying hot packs to individuals with impaired sensation or an impaired ability to report pain, and by checking with the patient for any sensation of excessive heat. Patients also do not develop dependence on physical agents, although they may wish to continue to use them even after they are no longer effective because they enjoy the sensation or attention associated with their application. For example, patients may wish to continue to be treated with ultrasound even though they have reached a stage of recovery where they would benefit more from active exercise. Physical agents also do not generally cause a degree of sedation that would impair an individual's ability to work or drive safely.

Many physical agents can be used independently by patients to treat themselves. For example, a patient can learn to apply a pain-controlling agent, such as heat, cold, or ES, when needed and so become more independent of the health care practitioner and pharmacological agents. The application of such physical agents at home can be an effective component of the treatment of both acute and chronic pain.[229] This type of self-treatment can also help contain the costs of medical care.

Physical agents, used either alone or in conjunction with other interventions such as pharmacological agents, manual therapy, or exercises, can also help remediate the underlying cause of pain while controlling the pain itself. For example, cryotherapy applied to an acute injury controls pain; however, this treatment also controls inflammation, limiting further tissue damage and pain. In this case, the use of NSAIDs, rest, elevation, and compression in conjunction with cryotherapy could also prove beneficial, although it may make assessment of the benefits of any one of these interventions more difficult. The selection of physical agents and their specific mechanisms of action and modes of application for controlling pain are discussed in detail in Part II of this book.

MULTIDISCIPLINARY PAIN TREATMENT PROGRAMS

Over the past 2 to 3 decades, multidisciplinary programs have been developed specifically for the treatment of chronic pain.[4,230] These programs are based on a biopsychosocial model of pain and attempt to address the multiple facets of chronic pain with a multidisciplinary, coordinated program of care.[4,231] These programs attempt to address not only the physical and physiological aspects of the patients' pain but also the behavioral, cognitive-affective, and environmental factors contributing to their symptoms by the use of medical, psychological, and physical interventions. Examples of interventions that might be part of a multidisciplinary program include exercise, physical agents, education, counseling, occupational therapy, and cognitive behavioral therapy.

Psychological intervention is focused on improving the coping skills of patients and modifying their behavior, whereas physical activities are focused on reversing the adverse effects of the sedentary lifestyle adopted by most patients with chronic pain. Coping skills can be improved with relaxation training, activity pacing, distraction techniques, cognitive restructuring, and problem solving.[234,235] Behavior modification using the principles of operant conditioning can also alter the patient's perception of and response to pain.[236] Cognitive behavioral therapy can be tailored made to address concerns, such as pain, disability, fatigue, negative mood, and social relationships, and has been highly effective at reducing fatigue and depression in some patients with chronic pain.[237] Graded activation and exercise programs, in which the patient learns the difference between hurt and harm, can help patients with chronic pain return to a more functional, active lifestyle.[238] The patients' family members are generally involved in these programs by learning appropriate coping skills for themselves and the patient. Such involvement can assist family members to help individuals with chronic pain more effectively rather than reinforce pain-related behaviors.

In contrast with traditional treatment approaches to acute pain, in which the goal of care is to eliminate the sensation of pain, the goals of care in most multidisciplinary pain treatment programs also include learning to cope and function with pain that may not resolve, although frequently patients also report a reduction in pain after completing these programs.[239,240] Goals of treatment also generally include decreasing dependence on health care personnel and pain-relieving medications, particularly habit-forming opioids; increasing physical activities; and returning patients to their usual social roles. If necessary, opioid medications are replaced with non–habit-forming drugs or with nonchemical modes of pain relief such as exercise or physical agents.[4] These programs have also been shown to be cost effective.[241-243]

Studies have shown that multidisciplinary pain treatment programs do result in increased functional activity levels while reducing pain behaviors and the use of medical interventions in patients with chronic pain.[244-247] Various types of pain may be successfully treated with a multidisciplinary approach. In patients with chronic back pain, multidisciplinary programs have been found to improve function and pain, although they may or may not affect a patient's return to the workplace.[248] In patients with subacute back pain, multidisciplinary programs that include workplace visits can help patients to return to work faster, result in fewer sick leaves, and alleviate subjective disability.[249] One trial comparing multidisciplinary treatment with standard biomedical treatment of subacute low back pain found that although both approaches had a positive short-term effect, at 6 months the patients in the multidisciplinary program showed further improvement, whereas those on standard therapy were back to where they had started. During the 2 years after therapy, far fewer patients in the multidisciplinary program required sick leave.[250] A review of studies on neck and shoulder pain showed no evidence that a multidiscplinary approach helps, although few studies were included in this review and most studies were of poor quality.[251] Chronic musculoskeletal disorders, such as fibromyalgia, are often treated with multidisciplinary programs. Although high-quality studies are lacking, overall the evidence does suggest that behavioral treatment and stress management can help patients with chronic pain and that education combined with physical training has some positive long-term effects.[252]

CLINICAL CASE STUDIES

The following case studies summarize the concepts of pain discussed in this chapter. Based on the scenario presented, an evaluation of the clinical findings and goals of treatment are proposed. This is followed by a discussion of the factors to be considered in treatment selection.

CASE STUDY 3-1

Severe Central Low Back Pain
Examination
History

MP is a 45-year-old woman who has been referred to physical therapy with a diagnosis of low back pain and a physician's order to evaluate and treat. MP complains of severe central low back pain that is aggravated by any movement, particularly forward bending. She reports no radiation of pain or other symptoms into her extremities. Pain disturbs her sleep, and she is unable to work at her usual secretarial job or perform her usual household tasks such as grocery shopping and cleaning. She reports that the pain started about 4 days ago when she reached to pick up a suitcase and has gradually decreased since its initial onset from a severity of 8, on a scale of 1 to 10, to a severity of 5 or 6. Her only current treatment is 600 mg ibuprofen, which she is taking 3 times a day.

Tests and Measures

The objective examination is significant for restricted lumbar range of motion (ROM) in all planes. Forward bending is restricted to approximately 20% of normal, backward bending is restricted to approximately 50% of normal, and sidebending is restricted to approximately 30% of normal in both directions. Palpable muscle guarding and tenderness in the lower lumbar area occur when the patient is standing or prone. All neurological testing, including straight leg raise and lower extremity sensation, strength, and reflexes are within normal limits.

Does this patient have acute or chronic pain? Is inflammation contributing to this patient's pain?

CLINICAL CASE STUDIES—*cont'd*

Evaluation, Diagnosis, Prognosis, and Goals
Evaluation and Goals

ICF Level	Current Status	Goals
Body structure and function	Low back pain Limited lumbar ROM in all directions Muscle guarding and tenderness in the lower lumbar area	Decrease pain to zero in next week Increase lumbar ROM to 100% of normal Prevent recurrence of symptoms
Activity	Cannot sleep	Return to normal sleeping pattern
Participation	Unable to work, clean, or go grocery shopping	Return to secretarial job in 1 week Return to 100% of household activities in 2 weeks

Diagnosis

Preferred Practice Pattern 4F: Impaired joint mobility, motor function, muscle performance, ROM, and reflex integrity associated with spinal disorders.

Prognosis/Plan of Care

The optimal intervention would address the acute symptom of pain and the underlying inflammation and if possible, would help to resolve any underlying structural tissue damage or changes. Although a single treatment may not be able to address all of these issues, treatments that address as many of these issues as possible and that do not adversely affect the patient's progress are recommended. As is explained in greater detail in Part II, a number of physical agents, including cryotherapy and ES, may be used to control this patient's pain and reduce the probable acute inflammation of the lumbar structures, and lumbar traction may also help to relieve her pain while modifying the underlying spinal dysfunction.

CASE STUDY 3-2

Stiffness and Aching in Lower Back
Examination
History

TJ is a 45-year-old woman who has been referred for therapy with a diagnosis of low back pain and an order to evaluate and treat, with a focus on developing a home program. TJ complains of stiffness and general aching of her lower back that is aggravated by sitting for more than 30 minutes. She reports occasional radiation of pain into her left lateral leg but no other symptoms in her extremities. She states that the pain occasionally disturbs her sleep, and she is unable to work at her usual secretarial job because of her limited sitting tolerance. She can perform most of her usual household tasks, such as grocery shopping and cleaning, although she frequently receives help from her family. She reports that the pain started about 4 years ago, when she reached to pick up a suitcase, and although it was initially severe, at a level of 10 on a scale of 1 to 10, and subsided to some degree over the first few weeks, it has not changed significantly in the past 2 to 3 years and is now usually at a level of 9 or greater. She has had multiple diagnostic tests that have not revealed any significant anatomical pathology, and she has received multiple treatments, including narcotic analgesics and physical therapy consisting primarily of hot packs, ultrasonography, and massage, without significant benefit. Her only current treatment is 600 mg of ibuprofen, which she is taking 3 times a day.

Tests and Measures

The objective examination is significant for restricted lumbar ROM in all planes. Forward bending is restricted to approximately 40% of normal, backward bending is restricted to approximately 50% of normal, and sidebending is restricted to approximately 50% of normal in both directions. Palpation reveals stiffness of the lumbar facet joints at L3 through L5 and tenderness in the lower lumbar area. All neurological testing, including lower extremity sensation, strength, and reflexes are within normal limits, although straight leg raising is limited to 40 degrees bilaterally by hamstring tightness and prone knee bending is limited to 100 degrees bilaterally by quadriceps tightness. TJ is 5 feet 3 inches tall and reports her weight to be 180 lb. She reports that she has gained 50 lb since her initial back injury 4 years ago.

Does this patient have acute or chronic pain? What factors are contributing to the patient's pain?

Evaluation, Diagnosis, Prognosis, and Goals
Evaluation and Goals

ICF Level	Current Status	Goals
Body struture and function	Low back pain Restricted lumbar ROM Hamstring and quadriceps tightness	Reduce pain to a tolerable level Increase lumbar ROM Normalize hamstring and quadriceps length
Activity	Impaired sleep Cannot sit for >30 minutes	Improve to normal sleeping patterns in 1 month Improve sitting tolerance to 1 hour in 2 weeks
Participation	Unable to work Impaired ability to do cleaning and shopping	Return to at least 50% of work activities in 1 month Return to 100% ability to clean and grocery shop Reduce dependence on medical personnel and medical treatment

Continued

Diagnosis
Preferred Practice Pattern 4B: Impaired posture.

Prognosis/Plan of Care
Although further analysis may help identify the specific structures causing this patient's pain, the long duration of the pain is well beyond the normal time needed for a minor back injury to resolve. The lack of change in her pain over the previous years and its lack of response to multiple treatments indicate that her pain may have a variety of contributory factors beyond local tissue damage, including deconditioning, psychological dysfunction, or social problems.

The optimal intervention would ideally address the functional limitations caused by this patient's chronic pain and provide her with independent means to manage her symptoms without adverse consequences. Thus the focus of care should be on teaching TJ coping skills and improving her physical condition, including strength and flexibility. The use of physical agents would probably be restricted to independent use for pain management or as an adjunct to promote progression toward functional goals. As is explained in greater detail in Part II of this book, a number of physical agents, including cryotherapy, thermotherapy, and ES, may be used by patients independently to control pain, whereas thermotherapy may also be used to help increase the extensibility of soft tissues to allow for more effective and rapid recovery of flexibility.

CHAPTER REVIEW

1. Pain is the result of a complex interaction of physical and psychological processes that occur when tissue is damaged or at risk of being damaged. The sensation and experience of pain varies with the duration and source of the painful stimulus to produce acute, chronic, or referred pain. Pain is generally perceived when specialized pain receptors (nociceptors) at the periphery are stimulated by noxious thermal, chemical, or mechanical stimuli. Nociceptors cause transmission of the sensation of pain along C fibers and A-delta fibers to the dorsal horn of the spinal cord and thence, via the thalamus, to the cortex.

2. Pain transmission may be inhibited at the spinal cord level by activity of A-beta fibers that transmit innocuous sensations or, at the periphery, spinal cord, or higher levels by endogenous opioids. Pain may also be modified indirectly by disruption of the pain-spasm-pain cycle.

3. The severity and quality of an individual's pain can be assessed using a variety of measures, including visual analog and numeric scales, comparison with a predefined stimulus, or selection of words from a given list. These measures can help to direct care and indicate patient progress.

4. Approaches that relieve or control pain include pharmacological agents, physical agents, and multidisciplinary treatment programs. Pharmacological agents may alter inflammation or peripheral nociceptor activation or may act centrally to alter pain transmission. Physical agents can also modify nociceptor activation and may alter endogenous opiate levels. Multidisciplinary treatment programs integrate pharmacological, physical, and other medical approaches with psychological and social interventions to address the multifaceted dysfunction of chronic pain.

5. A good understanding of the mechanisms underlying pain transmission and control, the tools available for measuring pain, and the various approaches available for treating pain is required to select and direct the use of physical agents appropriately within a comprehensive treatment program for the patient with pain.

6. The reader is referred to the Evolve web site for further exercises and links to resources and references.

ADDITIONAL RESOURCES *evolve*
Web Sites

Mayday Pain Project: The web site for this organization lists online pain resources: http://www.painandhealth.org/index.html:

The National Foundation for the Treatment of Pain: Not-for-profit organization is dedicated to providing support for patients with intractable pain, their families, friends, and the physicians who treat them. The web site includes patient articles and advocacy information. www.paincare.org

National Pain Foundation: The web site for this organization provides education and support resources for people in pain, their families, and health care providers. It has information about different types of pain conditions and also has an online community. www.painconnection.org

Spine Health: Web site has in-depth, peer-reviewed information written by physicians specifically for patients with back pain and neck pain. www.spine-health.com

GLOSSARY *evolve*

Acute pain: Pain of less than 6 months' duration for which an underlying pathology can be identified

A-beta fibers: Relatively large myelinated nerve fibers with receptors located in the skin, bones, and joints that transmit sensation related to vibration, stretching of skin, and mechanoreception. When working abnormally, can contribute to the sensation of pain; also called wide dynamic-range neurons.

A-delta fibers: Small, myelinated nerve fibers that transmit pain quickly to the CNS in response to high-intensity mechanical stimulation, heat, or cold; pain transmitted by these fibers usually has a sharp quality; also called group III afferents.

Afferent nerves: Nerves that conduct impulses from the periphery toward the CNS.

Allodynia: Pain in response to stimuli that do not usually produce pain.

Analgesia: Insensibility to pain, as in the effect of pain killers.

Autonomic nervous system: The division of the nervous system that controls involuntary activities of smooth and cardiac muscles and glandular secretion. Composed of the sympathetic and parasympathetic systems.

C fibers: Small, unmyelinated nerve fibers that transmit pain slowly to the CNS in response to noxious levels of mechanical, thermal, and chemical stimulation. Pain transmitted by these fibers is usually dull, long-lasting, and aching; also called group IV afferents.

Central sensitization: Lowering of the firing threshold of spinal cord pain-transmitting neurons caused by increased input from peripheral nociceptors; central sensitization amplifies the response to both noxious (hyperalgesia) and innocuous (allodynia) inputs, causes neurons to fire after the initiating input has ceased, and expands sensitivity so that pain is experienced beyond the original site of damage. Central sensitization is also called wind-up.

Chronic pain: Pain that persists beyond the usual amount of time for tissue healing; also called persistent pain.

Complex regional pain syndrome (CRPS): Pain believed to involve sympathetic nervous system over-activation; previously called reflex sympathetic dystrophy and sympathetically maintained pain.

Efferent nerves: Nerves that conduct impulses from the CNS to the periphery.

Endogenous opiate theory: A theory of pain control and modulation that states that pain is modulated at the peripheral, spinal cord, and cortical levels by endogenous neurotransmitters that have the same effect as opiates.

Endorphins: See Opiopeptins.

Enkephalins: Pentapeptides that are naturally occurring in the brain and that bind to opiate receptors producing analgesic and other opiate-like effects.

Gamma-aminobutyric acid (GABA): An inhibitory neurotransmitter, GABA increases pain by inhibiting the activity of pain-controlling structures, including A-beta afferents, and neurons in the periaqueductal grey matter and the raphe nucleus.

Gate control theory of pain modulation: A theory of pain control and modulation that states that pain is modulated at the spinal cord level by inhibitory effects of innocuous afferent input.

Hyperalgesia: Increased sensitivity to a noxious stimuli.

Neurotransmitter: A substance released by presynaptic neurons that activates postsynaptic neurons.

Nociception: The sensory component of pain.

Nociceptors: Nerve endings that are activated by noxious stimuli, contributing to a sensation of pain.

Noxious stimulus: Anything that activates a nerve to cause pain.

Opiopeptins: Endogenous opiate-like peptides that reduce the perception of pain by binding to opiate receptors in the nervous system; previously called endorphins.

Pain: An unpleasant sensory and emotional experience associated with actual or threatened tissue damage.

Pain gating: The inhibition of pain by inputs from non-nociceptor afferents.

Pain-spasm-pain cycle: A cycle in which nociceptor activation results in transmission cell activation that stimulates anterior horn cells to cause muscles to contract. This produces compression of blood vessels and thus accumulation of fluid and tissue irritants and mechanical compression of the nociceptor which then further increases nociceptor activation.

Patient-controlled analgesia (PCA): A way of controlling pain in hospitalized patients in which patients use a pump to self-administer small, repeated intravenous doses of analgesic medication and which results in more effective pain control and fewer adverse effects than physician-controlled methods.

Peripheral sensitization: Lowering of the nociceptor firing threshold in response to the release of various substances, including substance P, neurokinin A, and calcitonin gene–related peptide (CGRP), from nociceptive afferent fibers; also causes an increased magnitude of response to stimuli, an increase in spontaneous activity, and an increase in the area from which stimuli can evoke action potentials.

Referred pain: Pain that is experienced in one area when the actual or threatened tissue damage is in another area.

Sensitization: A lowering of the pain threshold that increases the experience of pain.

Substance P: A chemical mediator thought to be involved in the transmission of neuropathic and inflammatory pain.

Sympathetic nervous system: The part of the autonomic nervous system involved in the "flight or fight" reaction of the body that causes increased heart rate, blood pressure, and sweating and dilation of the pupils.

Synapse: The site of functional connection between neurons where an impulse is transmitted from one neuron (the presynaptic neuron) to another (the postsynaptic neuron), usually by a chemical neurotransmitter.

Transduction: A process by which a chemical or mechanical stimulus is converted into electrical activity (i.e., action potentials).

Transmission cells (T cells): Second-order neurons located in the dorsal horn of the spinal cord that receive signals from pain fibers and make connections with other neurons in the spinal cord.

REFERENCES *evolve*

1. Sweet WH: Neurophysiology. In Field J, Magoun HW, Hall VE, eds: *Handbook of physiology: neurophysiology*, vol I, Washington, DC, 1959, American Physiological Society.
2. Bonica JJ: Pain: what is science doing about it? *Pain* 2:12-15, 1975.

3. Merskey H, ed: Classification of chronic pain: description of chronic pain syndromes and definition of pain terms, *Pain* 3(suppl):S1, 1986.

4. Vasudevan SV, Lynch NT: Pain centers: organization and outcome, *West J Med* 154(5):532-535, 1991.

5. Vasudevan SV: Rehabilitation of the patient with chronic pain: is it cost effective? *Pain Digest* 2:99-101, 1992.

6. Kazis LE, Meenan RF, Anderson J: Pain in the rheumatic diseases: investigation of a key health status component, *Arthritis Rheum* 26(8):1017-1022, 1986.

7. Strang P: Emotional and social aspects of cancer pain, *Acta Oncol* 31(3):323-326, 1992.

8. Stubble HG, Grubb BD: Afferent and spinal mechanisms of joint pain, *Pain* 55:5-54, 1993.

9. Sluka KA: Pain mechanisms involved in musculoskeletal disorders, *J Orthop Sport Phys Ther* 24(4):240-254, 1996.

10. Grigg P, Stubble HG, Schmidt RF: Mechanical sensitivity of group III and IV afferents from posterior articular nerve in normal and inflamed cat knee, *J Neurophysiol* 55:635-643, 1986.

11. Bonica JJ: *The management of pain,* ed 2, Philadelphia, 1990, Lea & Febiger.

12. Bonica JJ: Importance of the problem. In Aronoff GM, ed: *Evaluation and treatment of chronic pain,* Baltimore, 1985, Urban & Schwarzenberg.

13. Vasudevan SV: Management of chronic pain: what have we achieved in the last 25 years? In Ghia JN, ed: *The multidisciplinary pain center: organization and personnel functions for pain management,* Boston, 1988, Kluwer.

14. Melzack R, Dennis SG: Neurophysiological foundations of pain. In Sternbach RA, ed: *The psychology of pain,* New York, 1978, Raven Press.

15. Kellgren JH: Observations on referred pain arising from muscle, *Clin Sci* 3:175-190, 1938.

16. Staff PH: Clinical consideration in referred muscle pain and tenderness—connective tissue reactions, *Eur J Appl Physiol* 57:369-372, 1988.

17. Black RG: Evaluation of the pain patient, *J Disabil* 1:85-97, 1990.

18. International Association for the Study of Chronic Pain, Subcommittee on Taxonomy: Classification of chronic pain, *Pain* 3(suppl): S1-S225, 1986.

19. Crue BL, ed: *Pain: research and treatment,* New York, 1974, Academic Press.

20. Osterweis M, Kleinman A, Mechanic D, eds: *Pain and disability—clinical behavioral and public policy perspective: Committee on Pain, Disability and Chronic Illness Behavior,* Washington, DC, 1987, National Academy Press.

21. Magni G, Caldieron C, Luchini SR, et al: Chronic musculoskeletal pain and depressive symptoms in the general population: an analysis of the 1st National Health and Nutrition Examination Survey data, *Pain* 43:299-307, 1990.

22. Bernabei R, Gambassi G, Lapane K, et al: Management of pain in elderly patients with cancer. SAGE Study Group. Systematic assessment of geriatric drug use via epidemiology, *JAMA.* 279:1877-1882, 1998.

23. Garcia J, Altman RD: Chronic pain states: pathophysiology and medical therapy, *Semin Arthritis Rheum* 27:1, 1997.

24. AGS Panel on Chronic Pain in Older Persons: The management of chronic pain in older persons, *J Am Geriatr Soc* 46:635-651, 1998.

25. Ferrell B: Acute and chronic pain. In Cassel C, ed: *Geriatric medicine: an evidence-based approach,* ed 4, New York, 2003, Spring-Verlag.

26. Braky AJ, Klerman GL: Overview: hypochondriasis, bodily complaints, and somatic styles, *Am J Psychol* 140:273-283, 1983.

27. Brena SF: The mystery of pain: is pain a sensation? In Brena SF, Chapman SL: *Management of patients with chronic pain,* New York, 1983, SP Medical & Scientific Books.

28. Gildenberg PL, DeVaul RA: *The chronic pain patient: evaluation and management,* New York, 1985, Karger.

29. Leavitt F, Garron DC: Psychological disturbance and pain report differences in both organic and non-organic low back pain patients, *Pain* 7:65-68, 1979.

30. Nichols ML, Allen BJ, Rogers SD, et al: Transmission of chronic nociception by spinal neurons expressing the substance P receptor, *Science* 286:1558-1561, 1999.

31. Dickenson AH: NMDA receptor agonists as analgesics. In Fields HL, Liebeskind JC, eds: *Pharmacologic approaches to the treatment of chronic pain: new concepts and critical issues: progress in pain research,* vol 1, Seattle, 1994, IASP Press.

32. Price DD, Hayes RL, Ruda M, et al: Spatial and temporal transformation of input to the spinothalamic tract neurons and their relationship to somatic sensations, *J Neurophysiol* 41:933-947, 1978.

33. Woolf CJ: Evidence for a central component of post-injury pain hypersensitivity, *Nature* 41:686-688, 1983.

34. Dickenson AH, Sullivan AF: Evidence for a role of the NMDA receptor in the frequency dependent potentiation of deeper dorsal horn neurons following C-fiber stimulation, *Neuropharmacology* 26:1235-1238, 1987.

35. Gottschalk A, Smith DS, Jobes DR, et al: Preemptive epidural analgesia and recovery from radical prostatectomy: a randomized controlled trial, *JAMA* 279:1076-1082, 1998.

36. Carr DB: Preempting the memory of pain, *JAMA* 279:1114-1115, 1998.

37. Ji RR, Baba H, Brenner GJ, et al: Nociceptive-specific activation of ERK in spinal neurons contributes to pain hypersensitivity, *Nat Neurosci* 2:1114-1119, 1999.

38. Arnow BA, Hunkeler EM, Blasey CM, et al: Comorbid depression, chronic pain, and disability in primary care, Psychosom Med 68(2):262-268, 2006.

39. Lin EH, Katon W, Von Korf M, et al: Effect of improving depression care on pain and functional outcomes among older adults with arthritis: a randomized controlled trial, *JAMA* 290:2428-2429, 2003.

40. Edwards RR, Bingham CO 3rd, Bathon J, et al: Catastrophizing and pain in arthritis, fibromyalgia, and other rheumatic diseases, *Arthritis Rheum* 55(2):325-332, 2006.

41. Kato K, Sullivan PF, Evengard B, et al: Chronic widespread pain and its comorbidities: a population-based study, *Arch Intern Med* 166:1649-1654, 2006.

42. Breivik H, Collett B, Ventafridda V, et al: Survey of chronic pain in Europe: prevalence, impact on daily life, and treatment, *Eur J Pain* 10(4):287-333, 2006.

43. Gullacksen AC, Lidbeck J: The life adjustment process in chronic pain: psychosocial assessment and clinical implications, *Pain Res Manag* 9(3):145-153, 2004.

44. Wooley S, Blackwell B, Winger C: A learning theory model of chronic illness behavior: theory, treatment, and research, *Psychosom Med* 40:379-401, 1978.

45. Brena SF, Chapman SL: *Management of patients with chronic pain,* New York, 1983, SP Medical & Scientific Books.

46. Blackwell B, Galbraith JR, Dahl DS: Chronic pain management, *Hosp Community Psychiatry* 35:999-1008, 1984.

47. Kehlet H, Jensen TS, Woolf CJ: Persistent postsurgical pain: risk factors and prevention, *Lancet* 367(9522):1618-1625, 2006.

48. Tippett SR: Referred knee pain in a young athlete: a case study, *J Orthop Sports Phys Ther* 19(2):117-120, 1994.

49. Kendall FP, McCreary EK: *Muscles, testing and function,* ed 3, Baltimore, 1983, Williams & Wilkins.

50. Willis WD, Coggeshall RE: *Sensory mechanisms of the spinal cord,* New York, 1991, Plenum Press.

51. Von Frey J: Beitrage zur physiologica des schmerzsinns, *Ber Kgl Sachs Ges Wis* 46:185, 1894.

52. Perl ER: Pain and nociception. In Brookhart JM, Mountcastle VB, Darian-Smith I, et al: *Handbook of physiology,* vol III, Bethesda, MD, 1984, American Physiological Society.

53. Willis WD: *The pain system: the neural basis of nociceptive transmission in the mammalian nervous system,* Basel, 1985, Karger.

54. Goldscheider A: *Veber den Schmertz in Physiologischer und Klinischer Hensicht,* Berlin, 1894, Hirschwald.

55. Torebjork HE, Schady W, Ochoa J: Sensory correlates of somatic afferent fibre activation, *Hum Neurobiol* 3:15-20, 1984.

56. Zimmerman M: Basic concepts of pain and pain therapy, *Drug Res* 34(2):1053-1059, 1984.

57. Heppleman B, Meslinger K, Neiss WF, et al: Ultrastructural three-dimensional reconstruction of group III and IV sensory nerve endings ("free nerve endings") in the knee joint capsule of the cat: evidence for multiple receptive sites, *J Comp Neurol* 292:103-116, 1990.

58. Cavanaugh JM, Ozaktay AC, Yamashita T, et al: Mechanisms of low back pain: a neurophysiologic and neuroanatomic study, *Clin Orthop Relat Res* 335:166-180, 1997.

59. Peng B, Wu W, Hou S, et al: The pathogenesis of discogenic low back pain, *J Bone Joint Surg* 87B:62-67, 2005.

60. Polacek P: Receptors of joints: their structure, variability and classification, *Acta Facultat Med Univesitat Brunensis* 23:1-107, 1966.

61. Freeman MAR, Wyke B: The innervation of the knee joint: an anatomical and histological study in the cat, *J Anat* 101:505-532, 1967.

62. Halata Z, Groth HP: Innervation of the synovial membrane of the cat's joint capsule, *Cell Tissue Res* 169:415-418, 1976.

63. Halata Z, Badalamente ME, Dee R, et al: Ultrastructure of sensory nerve endings in monkeys' knee joint capsule, *J Orthop Res* 2:218-226, 1984.

64. Beck PW, Handwerker HO: Bradykinin and serotonin effects on various types of cutaneous nerve fibers, *Pflugers Arch* 347:209-222, 1974.

65. Berberich P, Hoheisel U, Mense S: Effects of a carrageenan-induced myositis on the discharge properties of group III and IV muscle receptors in the cat, *J Neurophysiol* 59:1395-1409, 1988.

66. Gilfoil TM, Klavins I: 5-Hydroxytryptamine, bradykinin and histamine as mediators of inflammatory hyperesthesia, *J Physiol* 208:867-876, 1965.

67. Stubble H, Schmidt RF: Effects of an experimental arthritis on the sensory properties of fine articular afferent units, *J Neurophysiol* 54:1109-1122, 1985.

68. Stubble H, Schmidt RF: Time course of mechanosensitivity changes in articular afferents during a developing experimental arthritis, *J Neurophysiol* 60:2180-2194, 1988.

69. Mense S, Stahnke M: Responses in muscle afferent fibres of slow conduction velocity to contraction and ischemia in the cat, *J Physiol (Lond)* 342:383-387, 1983.

70. Fields HL, Levine JD: Pain—mechanisms and management, *West J Med* 141:347-357, 1984.

71. Elliott KJ: Taxonomy and mechanisms of neuropathic pain, *Semin Neurol* 14(3):195-205, 1994.

72. Ochoa JL, Torebjork HE: Sensations by intraneural microstimulation of single mechanoreceptor units innervating the human hand, *J Physiol (Lond)* 342:633-654, 1983.

73. Torebjork HE, Ochoa JL, Schady W: Referred pain from intraneuronal stimulation of muscle fascicles in the median nerve, *Pain* 18:145-156, 1984.

74. Marchettini P, Cline M, Ochoa JL: Innervation territories for touch and pain afferents of single fascicles of the human ulnar nerve, *Brain* 113:1491-1500, 1990.

75. Gybels J, Handwerker HO, Van Hees J: A comparison between the discharges of human nociceptive fibers and the subject's rating of his sensations, *J Physiol (Lond)* 186:117-132, 1979.

76. Wood L: Physiology of pain. In Kitchen S, Bazin S, eds: *Clayton's electrotherapy*, ed 10, London, 1996, WB Saunders.

77. Watkins LR, Mayer D: Organization of endogenous opiate and nonopiate pain control systems, *Science* 216:1185-1192, 1982.

78. Heppleman B, Heuss C, Schmidt RF: Fiber size distribution of myelinated and unmyelinated axons in the medial and posterior articular nerves of the cat's knee joint, *Somatosens* Res 5:267-275, 1988.

79. Nolan MF: Anatomic and physiologic organization of neural structures involved in pain transmission, modulation, and perception. In Echternach JL, ed: *Pain*, New York, 1987, Churchill Livingstone.

80. Grevert P, Goldstein A: Endorphins: Naloxone fails to alter experimental pain or mood in humans, *Science* 199:1093-1095, 1978.

81. Schaible H-G, Richter F: Pathophysiology of pain, *Langenbecks Arch* Surg 389:237-243, 2004.

82. Woolf CJ, Shortland P, Coggeshall RE: Peripheral nerve injury triggers central sprouting of myelinated afferents, *Nature* 355:75-78, 1992.

83. Wu G, Ringkamp M, Hartke TV, et al: Early onset of spontaneous activity in uninjured C-fiber nociceptors after injury to neighboring nerve fibers, *J Neurosci* 21:1-5, 2001.

84. Lamotte C: Distribution of the tract of Lissauer and the dorsal root fibers in the primate spinal cord, *J Comp Neurol* 72:529-561, 1977.

85. Light AR, Perl ER: Spinal termination of functionally identified primary afferent neurons with slowly conducting myelinated fibers, *J Comp Neurol* 186:133-150, 1979.

86. Light AR, Perl ER: Re-examination of the dorsal root projection to the spinal dorsal horn including observations on the differential termination of course and fine fibers, *J Comp Neurol* 186:117-132, 1979.

87. Light AR, Perl ER: Differential termination of large-diameter and small-diameter primary afferent fibers in the spinal dorsal gray matter as indicated by labeling with horseradish peroxidase, *Neurosci Lett* 6:59-63, 1977.

88. Besson JM, Charouch A: Peripheral and spinal mechanisms of nociception, *Physiol Rev* 67(1):67-186, 1988.

89. Melzack JD, Wall PD: Pain mechanisms: a new theory, *Science* 150:971-979, 1965.

90. Hillman P, Wall PD: Inhibitory and excitatory factors influencing the receptive fields of lamina 5 spinal cord cells, *Exp Brain Res* 9:161-171, 1969.

91. Belcher G, Ryall RW, Schaffner R: The differential effects of 5-hydroxytryptamine, noradrenaline, and raphe stimulation on nociceptive and non-nociceptive dorsal horn interneurons in the cat, *Brain Res* 151:307-321, 1978.

92. Fleetwood-Walker SM, Mitchell R, Hope PJ, et al: An A2 receptor mediates the selective inhibition by noradrenaline of nociceptive responses of identified dorsal horn neurons, *Brain Res* 334:243-354, 1985.

93. Unnerstall JR, Kopajtic TA, Kuhar MJ: Distribution of A2 agonist binding sites in the rat and human central nervous system: analysis of some functional autonomic correlates of the pharmacologic effects of clonidine and related adrenergic agents, *Brain Res* 319:69-101, 1984.

94. Willis WD: Control of nociceptive transmission in the spinal cord. In Autrum H, Ottoson D, Perl ER, Schmidt RF, eds: *Progress in sensory physiology*, vol 3, Berlin, 1982, Springer-Verlag.

95. Janig W, Kollmann W: The involvement of the sympathetic nervous system in pain, *Drug Res* 34(2):1066-1073, 1984.

96. Gilman AG, Goodman L, Rall TW, et al, eds: *Goodman and Gilman's the pharmacologic basis of therapeutics*, ed 7, New York, 1985, Macmillan.

97. Janig W, McLachlan EM: The role of modification in noradrenergic peripheral pathways after nerve lesions in the generation of pain. In Fields HL, Liebeskind JC, eds: *Pharmacologic approaches to the treatment of chronic pain: new concepts and critical issues: progress in pain research and management*, vol 1, Seattle, 1994, IASP Press.

98. Bonica JJ, Liebeskind JC, Albe-Fessard DG: *Advances in pain research and therapy*, vol 3, New York, 1979, Raven Press.

99. Kleinert HE, Norberg H, McDonough JJ: Surgical sympathectomy: upper and lower extremity. In Omer GE, ed: *Management of peripheral nerve problems*, Philadelphia, 1980, WB Saunders.

100. Campbell JN, Raja SN, Selig DK, et al: Diagnosis and management of sympathetically maintained pain. In Fields HL, Liebeskind JC, eds: *Pharmacological approaches to the treatment of chronic pain: new concepts and critical issues: progress in pain research and management*, vol 1, Seattle, 1994, IASP Press.

101. Cepeda MS. Carr DB. Lau J: Local anesthetic sympathetic blockade for complex regional pain syndrome, *Cochrane Database of Syst Rev* 4:CD004598, 2005.

102. Cepeda MS, Lau J, Carr D: Defining the therapeutic role of local anesthetic sympathetic blockade in complex regional pain syndrome: a narrative and systematic review, *Clin J Pain* 18(4):216-223, 2002.

103. Price DD, Long S, Huitt C: Sensory testing of pathophysiological mechanisms of pain in patients with reflex sympathetic dystrophy, *Pain* 49:163-173, 1992.

104. Stanton-Hicks M, Janig W, Hassenbusch S, et al: Reflex sympathetic dystrophy: changing concepts and taxonomy, *Pain* 63:127-133, 1995.

105. Fields HL: *Pain: mechanisms and management,* New York, 1987, McGraw Hill.

106. Selkowitz DM: The sympathetic nervous system in neuromotor function and dysfunction and pain: a brief review and discussion, *Funct Neurol* 7:89-95, 1992.

107. White DM, Helme RD: Release of substance P from peripheral nerve terminals following electrical stimulation of the sciatic nerve, *Brain Res* 336:27-31, 1985.

108. Larsson J, Ekblom A, Henriksson K, et al: Concentration of substance P, neurokinin A, calcitonin gene-related peptide, neuropeptide Y and vasoactive intestinal polypeptide in synovial fluid from knee joints in patients suffering from rheumatoid arthritis, *Scand J Rheumatol* 20:326-335, 1991.

109. Marshall KW, Chiu B, Inman RD: Substance P and arthritis: analysis of plasma and synovial fluid levels, *Arthritis Rheum* 33:87-90, 1990.

110. Gamse R, Holzer P, Lembeck F: Decrease of substance P in primary afferent neurons and impairment of neurogenic plasma extravasation by capsaicin, *Br J Pharmacol* 68:207-213, 1980

111. Neugebauer V, Wieretter F, Stubble HG: Involvement of substance P and neurokinin-1 receptors in hyperexcitability of dorsal horn neurons during development of acute arthritis in rat's knee joint, *J Neurophysiol* 73:1574-1583, 1995.

112. Randic M, Miletic V: Effect of substance P in cat dorsal horn neurons activated by noxious stimuli, *Brain Res* 128:164-169, 1977.

113. Stubble HG, Jarrott B, Hope PJ, et al: Release of immunoreactive substance P in the spinal cord during development of acute arthritis in the knee joint of the cat: a study with antibody microprobes, *Brain Res* 529:214-223, 1990.

114. Lucas HJ, Brauch CM, Settas L, et al: Fibromyalgia—new concepts of pathogenesis and treatment, *Int J Immunopathol Pharmacol* 19(1):5-10, 2006.

115. Oku R, Satoh M, Tagaki H: Release of substance P from the spinal dorsal horn is enhanced in polyarthritic rats, *Neurosci Lett* 74:315-319, 1987.

116. Russell IJ, Orr MD, Littman B, et al: Elevated cerebrospinal fluid levels of substance P in patients with the fibromyalgia syndrome, *Arthritis Rheum* 37(11):1593-1601, 1994.

117. Vaeroy H, Helle R, Forre O, et al: Elevated CSF levels of substance P and high incidence of Raynaud phenomenon in patients with fibromyalgia: new features for diagnosis, *Pain* 32:21-26, 1988.

118. Radharkrishnan V, Henry JL: Antagonism of nociceptive responses of cat spinal dorsal horn neurons in vivo by the NK-1 receptor antagonists CP-96,345 and CP-99,994, but not by CP-96,344, *Neuroscience* 64:943-958, 1995.

119. Slake KA, Milton MA, Westlund KN, et al: Involvement of neurokinin receptors in the joint inflammation and heat hyperalgesia following acute inflammation in unanesthetized rats, *J Physiol (Lond)* 483P:152-153, 1995.

120. Schinkel C, Gaertner A, Zaspel J, et al: Inflammatory mediators are altered in the acute phase of posttraumatic complex regional pain syndrome. *Clin J Pain* 22(3):235-239, 2006.

121. Khalil Z, Hleme RD: Sequence of events in substance P mediated plasma extravasation in rat skin, *Brain Res* 500:256-262, 1989.

122. Vasko MR, Campbell WB, Waite KJ: Prostaglandin E2 enhances bradykinin-stimulated release of neuropeptides from rat sensory neurons in culture, *J Neurosci* 14:4987-4997, 1994.

123. Nakae K, Saito K, Iino T, et al: A prostacyclin receptor antagonist inhibits the sensitized release of substance P from rat sensory neurons, *J Pharmacol Exp Ther* 315(3):1136-1142, 2005.

124. Gerspacher M: Selective and combined neurokinin receptor antagonists. *Progr Med Chem* 43:49-103, 2005.

125. Keller M, Montgomery S, Ball W, et al: Lack of efficacy of the substance p (neurokinin1 receptor) antagonist aprepitant in the treatment of major depressive disorder, *Biol Psychiatr* 59(3):216-223, 2006.

126. Jessell TM, Iversen LL: Opiate analgesics inhibit substance P release from rat trigeminal nucleus, *Nature* 268:549-551, 1977.

127. Watanabe H, Mizoguchi H, Orito T, et al: Differential inhibitory effects of mu-opioids on substance P- and capsaicin-induced nociceptive behavior in mice, *Peptides* 27(4):760-768, 2006.

128. Wang X, Douglas SD, Commons KG, et al: A non-peptide substance P antagonist (CP-96,345) inhibits morphine-induced NF-kappa B promoter activation in human NT2-N neurons, *J Neurosci Res* 75(4):544-553, 2004.

129. Jasmin L, Tien D, Weinshenker D, et al: The NK1 receptor mediates both the hyperalgesia and the resistance to morphine in mice lacking in noradrenaline, *Proc Natl Acad Sci USA* 99:1029-1034, 2002.

130. Sakurada T, Komatsu T, Sakurada S: Mechanisms of nociception evoked by intrathecal high-dose morphine, *Neurotoxicology* 26(5):801-809, 2005.

131. Nathan PW, Wall PD: Treatment of post-herpetic neuralgia by prolonged electrical stimulation, *Br Med J* 3:645-657, 1974.

132. Wall PD, Sweet WH: Temporary abolition of pain in man, *Science* 155:108-109, 1967.

133. Nathan PW, Rudge P: Testing the gate control theory of pain in man, *J Neurol Neurosurg Psychiatry* 3:645-657, 1974.

134. Kerr FWL: Pain: a central inhibitory balance theory, *Mayo Clin Proc* 50:685-690, 1975.

135. Melzack R, Casey KL: Sensory, motivational, and central control determinants of pain. In Kenshalo DR, ed: *The skin senses,* Springfield, IL, 1968, Charles C Thomas.

136. Pert CB, Pasternak G, Snyder SH: Opiate agonists and antagonists discriminated by receptor binding in the brain, *Science* 182(119):1359-1361, 1973.

137. Simon EJ: In search of the opiate receptor, *Am J Med Sci* 266(3):160-168, 1973.

138. Terenius L: Characteristics of the "receptor" for narcotic analgesics in synaptic plasma membrane fraction from rat brain, *Acta Pharmacol Toxicol (Copenh)* 33(5):377-384, 1973.

139. Huges J, Smith TW, Kosterlitz HW, et al: Identification of two related pentapeptides from the brain with potent opiate agonist activity, *Nature* 258:577-579, 1975.

140. Mayer DJM, Price DD: Central nervous system mechanisms of analgesia, *Pain* 2:379-404, 1976.

141. Simon EJ, Hiller JM: The opiate receptors, *Annu Rev Pharmacol Toxicol* 18:371-377, 1978.

142. Willer JC: Endogenous, opioid, peptide-mediated analgesia, *Int Med* 9(8):100-111, 1988.

143. Mao J, Price DD, Mayer DJ: Mechanisms of hyperalgesia and morphine tolerance: a current view of their possible interactions: review article, *Pain* 62:259-274, 1995.

144. Hao JX, Xu XJ, Yu YX, et al: Baclofen reverses the hypersensitivity of dorsal horn wide dynamic range neurons to mechanical stimulation after transient spinal cord ischemia: implications for a tonic GABAergic inhibitory control of myelinated fiber input, *J Neurophysiol* 68:392-396, 1992.

145. Balagura S, Ralph T: The analgesic effect of electrical stimulation of the diencephalon and mesencepahlon, *Brain Res* 60:369-381, 1973.

146. Duggan AW, Griersmith BT: Inhibition of spinal transmission of nociceptive information by supraspinal stimulation in the cat, *Pain* 6:149-161, 1979.

147. Adams JE: Naloxone reversal of analgesia produced by brain stimulation in the human, *Pain* 2:161-166, 1976.

148. Akil H, Mayer DJ, Liebeskind JC: Antagonism of stimulation-produced analgesia by naloxone, a narcotic antagonist, *Science* 191:961-962, 1976.

149. Snyder SH: Opiate receptors and internal opiates, *Sci Am* 240(3):44-56, 1977.

150. Terman GW, Shavit Y, Lewis JW, et al: Intrinsic mechanisms of pain inhibition: activation by stress, *Science* 226:1270-1277, 1984.

151. Willer JC, Dehen H, Cambrier J: Stress-induced analgesia in humans: endogenous opioids and naloxone-reversible depression of pain reflexes, *Science* 212:689-691, 1981.

152. Willer JC, Roby A, Le Bars D: Psychophysical and electro-physiological approaches to the pain-relieving effects of heterotopic nociceptive stimuli, *Brain Res* 107:1095-1112, 1984.

153. Tricklebank MD, Curzon G: *Stress-induced analgesia,* Chichester, England, 1984, Wiley.

154. Mayer DJ, Price DD, Barber J, et al: Acupuncture analgesia: evidence for activation of a pain inhibitory system as a mechanism of action. In Bonica JJ, Albe-Fessard D, eds: *Advances in pain research and therapy,* New York, 1976, Raven Press.

155. Bassbaum AI, Fields HL: Endogenous pain control mechanisms: review and hypothesis, *Ann Neurol* 4:451-462, 1978.

156. Levine JD, Gordon NC, Fields HL: The mechanism of placebo analgesia, *Lancet* 2:654-657, 1978.

157. Bendetti F, Amanzio M, Baldi S, et al: Inducing placebo respiratory depressant responses in humans via opioid receptors, *Eur J Neurosci* 11:625-631, 1999.

158. Downie W, Leatham PA, Rhind VM, et al: Studies with pain rating scales, *Ann Rheum Dis* 37:378-388, 1978.

159. Pautex S, Herrmann F, Le Lous P, et al: Feasibility and reliability of four pain self-assessment scales and correlation with an observational rating scale in hospitalized elderly demented patients *J Gerontol A Biol Sci Med Sci* 60(4):524-529, 2005.

160. Ushijima S, Ukimura O, Okihara K, et al: Visual analog scale questionnaire to assess quality of life specific to each symptom of the International Prostate Symptom Score, *J Urology* 176(2):665-671, 2006.

161. Grossman SA, Shudler VR, McQuire DB, et al: A comparison of the Hopkins Pain Rating Instrument with standard visual analogue and verbal description scales in patients with chronic pain, *J Pain Symptom Mgmt* 7:196-203, 1992.

162. Sternbach RA: *Pain patients: traits and treatment,* New York, 1974, Academic Press.

163. Posner J: A modified submaximal effort tourniquet test for evaluation of analgesics in healthy volunteers, *Pain* 19:143-151, 1984.

164. Sternbach RA: The tourniquet pain test. In Melzack R, ed: *Pain measurement and assessment,* New York, 1983, Raven Press.

165. Kast EC: An understanding of pain and its measurement, *Med Times* 94:1501-1503, 1966.

166. Hardy JD, Wolff HG, Goodell H: *Pain sensations and reactions,* New York, 1952, Hafner.

167. Melzack R: The McGill Pain Questionnaire: major properties and scoring methods, *Pain* 1:277-299, 1975.

168. Byrne M, Troy A, Bradley LA, et al: Cross-validation of the factor structure of the McGill Pain Questionnaire, *Pain* 13(2):193-201, 1982.

169. Prieto EJ, Hopson L, Bradley LA, et al: The language of low back pain: factor structure of the McGill Pain Questionnaire, *Pain* 8(1):11-19, 1980.

170. Roth RS, Lowery JC, Hamill JB: Assessing persistent pain and its relation to affective distress, depressive symptoms, and pain catastrophizing in patients with chronic wounds: a pilot study, *Am J Phys Med Rehabil* 83(11):827-834, 2004 Nov.

171. Ransford AO, Cairns D, Mooney V: The pain drawing as an aid to the psychological evaluation of patients with low-back pain, *Spine* 1(2):127-134, 1976.

172. Grieve GP: Common patterns of clinical presentation. In Grieve GP: *Common vertebral joint problems,* ed 2, New York, 1988, Churchill Livingstone.

173. Quinn L, Gordon J: *Functional outcomes documentation for rehabilitation,* St Louis, 2003, Saunders.

174. Bickley LS, Hoekelman RA: *JG Bates' guide to physical examination and history taking,* ed 7, Philadelphia, 1999, Lippincott, Williams & Wilkins.

175. Tuman KJ, McCarthy RJ, March RJ, et al: Effects of epidural anesthesia and analgesia on coagulation and outcome after major vascular surgery, *Anesth Analg* 73:696-704, 1991.

176. Heppleman B, Pfeffer A, Stubble HG, et al: Effects of acetylsalicylic acid and indomethacin on single groups III and IV sensory units from acutely inflamed joints, *Pain* 26:337-351, 1986.

177. Grubb BD, Birrell J, McQueen DS, et al: The role of PGE2 in the sensitization of mechanoreceptors in normal and inflamed ankle joints of the rat, *Exp Brain Res* 84:383-392, 1991.

178. Malmberg AB, Yaksh TL: Hyperalgesia mediated by spinal glutamate or substance P receptor block by cyclo-oxygenase inhibition, *Science* 257:1276-1279, 1992.

179. Carlsson KH, Monzel W, Jurna I: Depression by morphine and the non-opioid analgesic agents, metamizol (dipyrone), lysine and acetylsalicylate, and paracetomol, of activity in rat thalamus neurons evoked by electrical stimulation of nociceptive afferents, *Pain* 32:313-326, 1988.

180. Jurna I, Spohrer B, Bock R: Intrathecal injection of acetylsalicylic acid, salicylic acid and indomethacin depresses C-fibre-evoked activity in the rat thalamus and spinal cord, *Pain* 49:249-256, 1992.

181. Semble EL, Wu WC: Anti-inflammatory drugs and gastric mucosal damage, *Semin Arthritis Rheum* 16:271-286, 1987.

182. Griffin MR, Piper JM, Daugherty JR, et al: Nonsteroidal anti-inflammatory drug use and increased risk for peptic ulcer disease in elderly persons, *Ann Intern Med* 114:257-259, 1991.

183. Ali M, McDonald JWD: Reversible and irreversible inhibition of platelet cyclo-oxygenase and serotonin release by nonsteroidal anti-inflammatory drugs, *Thromb Res* 13:1057-1065, 1978.

184. Patronon C, Dunn MJ: The clinical significance of inhibition of renal prostaglandin synthesis, *Kidney Int* 31:1-12, 1987.

185. Juni P, Nartey L, Reichenbach S, et al: Risk of cardiovascular events and rofecoxib: cumulative meta-analysis, *Lancet* 364(9450):2021-2029, 2004.

186. Bombardier C, Laine L, Reicin A, et al: Comparison of upper gastrointestinal toxicity of rofecoxib and naproxen in patients with rheumatoid arthritis, *N Engl J Med* 343:1520-1528, 2000.

187. Solomon SD, McMurray JV, Pfeffer MA, et al: Cardiovascular risk associated with celecoxib in a clinical trial for colorectal adenoma prevention, *N Engl J Med* 352:1071-1080, 2005.

188. Bresalier RS, Sandler RS, Quan H, et al: Cardiovascular events associated with rofecoxib in a colorectal adenoma chemoprevention trial, *N Engl J Med* 352:1092-1102, 2005.

189. Nussmeier NA, Whelton AA, Brown MT, et al: Complications of COX-2 inhibitors parecoxib and valdecoxib after cardiac surgery, *N Engl J Med* 352:1081-1091, 2005.

190. Package insert: Toradol, *Hoffmann-La Roche,* Nutley, NJ, July 1995.

191. Ameer B, Greenblatt DJ: Acetaminophen, *Ann Intern Med* 87:202-209, 1977.

192. McNeil: Regular Strength Tylenol acetaminophen Tablets; Extra Strength Tylenol acetaminophen Gelcaps, Geltabs, Caplets, Tablets; Extra Strength Tylenol acetaminophen Adult Liquid Pain Reliever; Tylenol acetaminophen Arthritis Pain Extended-Relief Caplets. In *Physicians desk reference,* ed 56, Montvale, NJ, 2002, Medical Economics Company.

193. USP DI: *Drug information for the health care professional,* ed 22, Englewood, CO, 2002, Micromedex.

194. Hyleden JLK, Nahin RL, Traub RJ, et al: Effects of spinal kappa-aged receptor agonists on the responsiveness of nociceptive superficial dorsal horn neurons, *Pain* 44:187-193, 1991.

195. Hudson AH, Thomson IR, Cannon JE, et al: Pharmacokinetics of fentanyl inpatients undergoing abdominal aortic surgery, *Anesthesiology* 64:334-338, 1986.

196. Trescot AM, Chopra P, Abdi S, et al: Opioid guidelines in the management of chronic non-cancer pain, *Pain Physician* 9(1):1-439, 2006.

197. Manchikanti L, Damron KS, McManus CD, et al: Patterns of illicit drug use and opioid abuse in patients with chronic pain at initial evaluation: a prospective, observational study, *Pain Physician* 7(4):431-437, 2004.

198. Anderson G, Sjøgren P, Hansen SH, et al: Pharmacological consequences of long-term morphine treatment in patients with cancer and chronic non-malignant pain, *Eur J Pain* 8(3):263-271, 2004.

199. D'Amours RH, Ferrante FM: Postoperative pain management, *J Orthop Sport Phys Ther* 24(4):227-236, 1996.

200. Dickey NW: Pain management at the end of life, *J Orthop Sport Phys Ther* 24(4):237-239, 1996.

201. Stein C, Comisel K, Haimerl E, et al: Analgesic effect of intraarticular morphine after arthroscopic surgery, *N Engl J Med* 325:1123-1126, 1991.

202. Likaar R, Schafer M, Paulak F, et al: Intra-articular morphine analgesia in chronic pain patients with osteoarthritis, *Anesth Analg* 84:1313-1317, 1997.

203. Camp JF: Patient-controlled analgesia, *Am Fam Physician* 44:2145-2149, 1991.

204. Egbert AM, Parks LH, Short LM, et al: Randomized trial of postoperative patient-controlled analgesia vs. intramuscular

narcotics in frail elderly men, *Arch Intern Med* 150:1897-1903, 1990.

205. Watson CP, Evans RJ, Reed K, et al: Amitriptyline versus placebo in postherpetic neuralgia, *Neurology (NY)* 32:671-673, 1983.

206. Von Korff M, Wagner EH, Dworkin SF, et al: Chronic pain and use of ambulatory health care, *Psychosom Med* 53(1):61-79, 1991.

207. Parmalee PA, Katz IB, Lawton MP: The relation of pain to depression among institutionalized aged, *J Gerontol* 46:15-21, 1991.

208. Keefe FJ, Wilkins RH, Cook WA, et al: Depression, pain, and pain behavior, *J Consult Clin Psychol* 54:665-669, 1986.

209. Kudoh A, Katagai H, Takazawa T: Increased postoperative pain scores in chronic depression patients who take antidepressants, *J Clin Anesth*, 14(6):421-425,2002.

210. Fishbain D: Evidence-based data on pain relief with anti-depressants, *Ann Med* 32(5):305-316, 2000.

211. Coombs DW, Danielson DR, Pagneau MG, et al: Epidurally administered morphine for postceasarean analgesia, *Surg Gynecol Obstet* 154:385-388, 1982.

212. Yaksh TL, Noveihed R: The physiology and pharmacology of spinal opiates, *Ann Rev Pharmacol* 25:443-462, 1975.

213. Sjostrum S, Hartvig P, Persson MP, et al: The pharmacokinetics of epidural morphine and meperidine in humans, *Anesthesiology* 67:877-888, 1987.

214. Gissen AJ, Covino BG, Gregus J: Differential sensitivity of fast and slow fibers in mammalian nerve. III. Effect of etidocaine and bupivicaine on fast/slow fibres, *Anesth Analg* 61:570-575, 1982.

215. Hempenstall K, Nurmikko TJ, Johnson RW, et al: Analgesic therapy in postherpetic neuralgia: a quantitative systematic review, *PLoS Med* 2(7):e164, 2005.

216. McAfee JH, Smith DL: Olecranon and prepatellar bursitis: diagnosis and treatment, *West J Med* 149:607-612, 1988.

217. Wheeler AH, Stubbart J, Hicks B: Pathophysiology of chronic back pain. Last updated: April 13, 2006. http://www.emedicine.com/neuro/topic516.htm. Accessed October 23, 2006.

218. Wiffen PJ, McQuay HJ, Edwards JE, et al: Gabapentin for acute and chronic pain, *Cochrane Database Syst Rev* 3:CD005452, 2005.

219. Wiffen PJ, McQuay HJ, Moore RA: Carbamazepine for acute and chronic pain, *Cochrane Database Syst Rev* 3:CD005451, 2005.

220. Attal N, Nurmikko TJ, Johnson RW, et al and EFNS Task Force: EFNS guidelines on pharmacological treatment of neuropathic pain, *Eur J Neurol* 13(11):1153-1169, 2006.

221. Raskin J, Pritchett YL, Wang F, et al: A double-blind, randomized multicenter trial comparing duloxetine with placebo in the management of diabetic peripheral neuropathic pain, *Pain Med* 6(5):346-356, 2005.

222. Saarto T, Wiffen PJ: Antidepressants for neuropathic pain, *Cochrane Database Syst Rev* 3:CD005454, 2005.

223. Zhang WY, Li Wan Po A: The effectiveness of topically applied capsaicin. A meta-analysis, *Eur J Clin Pharmacol* 46(6):517-522, 1994.

224. Ernst E, Fialka V: Ice freezes pain? A review of the clinical effectiveness of analgesic cold therapy, *J Pain Symp Mgmt* 9(1):56-59, 1994.

225. Crockford GW, Hellon RF, Parkhouse J: Thermal vasomotor response in human skin mediated by local mechanisms, *J Physiol* 161:10-15, 1962.

226. McMaster WC, Liddie S: Cryotherapy influence on posttraumatic limb edema, *Clin Orthop Relat Res* 150:283-287, 1980.

227. Hocutt JE, Jaffe R, Ryplander CR: Cryotherapy in ankle sprains, *Am J Sports Med* 10:316-319, 1982.

228. Winnem MF, Amundsen T: Treatment of phantom limb pain with transcutaneous electrical nerve stimulation, *Pain* 12:299-300, 1982.

229. Bigos S, Bowyer O, Braen G, et al: *Acute low back problems in adults,* Clinical Practice Guideline No 14. AHCPR Publication No. 95-0642, Rockville, MD, 1994, Agency for Health Care Policy and Research, Public Health Service, US Dept of Health and Human Services.

230. Aronoff AM: *Pain centers: a revolution in health care,* New York, 1988, Raven Press.

231. Fordyce WE: *The biopsychosocial model revisited.* Paper presented at the annual meeting of the American Pain Society, Los Angeles, November 1995.

232. Tollison CD, Kriegel ML, Satherwaite JR, et al: Comprehensive pain center treatment of low back workers compensation injuries—an industrial medicine clinical outcome follow-up comparison, *Orthop Res Suppl* 8:1115-1126, 1989.

233. Cicala RS, Wright H: Outpatient treatment of patients with chronic pain: an analysis of cost savings, *Clin J Pain* 5:223-226, 1989.

234. Keefe FJ, Beaupre PM, Gil KM: Group therapy for patients with chronic pain. In Turk DC, Gatchel RJ, eds: *Psychological factors in pain: critical perspectives,* New York, 1999, Guildford Press.

235. Keefe FJ, Kashikar-Zuck S, Opiteck J, et al: Pain in arthritis and musculoskeletal disorders: the role of coping skills training and exercise interventions, *J Orthop Sport Phys Ther* 24(4):279-290, 1996.

236. Wickramaskerra I: Biofeedback and behavior modification for chronic pain. In Echternach HL, ed: *Pain,* New York, 1987, Churchill Livingstone.

237. Evers AW, Kraaimaat FW, van Riel PL, et al: Tailored cognitive-behavioral therapy in early rheumatoid arthritis for patients at risk: a randomized controlled trial, *Pain* 100:141-153, 2002.

238. Linton LJ, Bradley LA, Jensen I, et al: The secondary prevention of low back pain: a controlled study with follow up, *Pain* 36:197-207, 1989.

239. Keefe FJ, Caldwell DS, Williams DA, et al: Pain coping skills training in the management of osteoarthritic knee pain: a comparative study, *Behav Ther* 21:49-62, 1990.

240. Keefe FJ, Caldwell DS, Williams DA, et al: Pain coping skills training in the management of osteoarthritic knee pain: follow-up results, *Behav Ther* 21:435-448, 1990.

241. Mayer TG, Gatchel RJ, Mayer H, et al: A prospective two-year study of functional restoration in industrial low back injury—an objective assessment procedure, *JAMA* 258:1763-1767, 1987.

242. Stieg RL, Williams RC, Timmermans-Williams G, et al: Cost benefits of interdisciplinary chronic pain treatment, *Clin J Pain* 1:189-193, 1986.

243. Simmons JW, Avant WS Jr, Demski J, et al: Determining successful pain clinic treatment through validation of cost effectiveness, *Spine* 13:342-344, 1988.

244. Swanson DW, Swenson WM, Maruta T, et al: Program for managing chronic pain. Program description and characteristics of patients, *Mayo Clin Proc* 51:401-408, 1976.

245. Seres JL, Newman RI: Results of treatment of chronic low-back pain at the Portland Pain Center, *J Neurosurg* 45:32-36, 1976.

246. Guck TP, Skultety FM, Meilman DW, et al: Multidisciplinary pain center follow-up study: evaluation with no-treatment control group, *Pain* 21:295-306, 1985.

247. Keefe FJ, Caldwell DS, Queen KT, et al: Pain coping strategies in osteoarthritis patients, *J Consult Clin Psychol* 55:208-212, 1987.

248. Guzman J, Esmail R, Karjalainen, K, et al: Multidisciplinary bio-psycho-social rehabilitation for chronic low back pain, *Cochrane Database Syst Rev* 1:CD000963, 2002.

249. Karjalainen K, Malmivaara A, van Tulder M, et al: Multidisciplinary biopsychosocial rehabilitation for subacute low back pain among working age adults: update, *Cochrane Database Syst Rev* 2:CD002193, 2003.

250. Schiltenwolf M, Buchner M, Heindl B, et al: Comparison of a biopsychosocial therapy (BT) with a conventional biomedical therapy (MT) of subacute low back pain in the first episode of sick leave: a randomized controlled trial, *Eur Spine J* 15(7):1083-1092, 2006.

251. Karjalainen K, Malmivaara A, van Tulder M, et al: Multidisciplinary biopsychosocial rehabilitation for neck and shoulder pain among working age adults: update, *Cochrane Database Syst Rev* 2:CD002194, 2003.

252. Karjalainen K, Malmivaara A, van Tulder M, et al: Multidisciplinary rehabilitation for fibromyalgia and musculoskeletal pain in working age adults, *Cochrane Database Syst Rev* 2:CD001984, 2000.

Chapter 4

Tone Abnormalities

Diane D. Allen and Gail L. Widener

Muscle contraction reveals itself through movement, and can be observed and measured. The force of a contraction is determined by measuring the net force or torque generated around a joint. In contrast, **muscle tone** reveals itself through the stiffness or slackness of muscles, conditions that can change both at rest and during muscle contraction based on a number of normally occurring or pathological factors. Extreme conditions and fluctuations within the normal range can be observed, but the changing nature of muscle tone makes it difficult to define and quantify. Because abnormalities of muscle tone can affect function, clinicians must define and assess muscle tone so that they can effect changes and ultimately improve function. This chapter describes accepted definitions of muscle tone and its related concepts, ways of measuring muscle tone, the anatomical and pathological factors that influence muscle tone, and some of the issues that arise when tone is abnormal. Examples, problems, and interventions arise from both neuromuscular and musculoskeletal diagnostic groups. As in the rest of this text, problems discussed focus on those that may be affected by physical agents.

MUSCLE TONE

Muscle tone is the underlying tension in the muscle that serves as a background for contraction. It has been variously described as muscle tension or stiffness at rest,[1] readiness to move or hold a position, priming or tuning of the muscles,[2] or the degree of activation before movement. It can also be described as the passive resistance in response to stretching of a muscle. Passive resistance means that a person does not actively contract against the applied stretch, so that the resistance noted can be attributed to muscle tone rather than to voluntary muscle contraction. Muscle tone includes the involuntary resistance generated by neurally activated muscle fibers and the passive, biomechanical tension inherent in the connective tissue and muscle at the length at which the muscle is tested.[3] Physical agents used in physical therapy may affect the neural or the biomechanical components of muscle tone, or both.

To visualize the concept of muscle tone, consider the following example. A runner's quadriceps muscles have lower tone when the runner is relaxed and sitting, with feet propped up, than when those same muscles are lengthened over a flexed knee and preparing for imminent contraction at the starting block of a race (Fig. 4-1). At the starting block, both biomechanical and neural components contribute to increased muscle tone. From the biomechanical standpoint, the muscle is stretched over the flexed knee, so any slack in the soft tissue is taken up, and the contractile elements are positioned for most efficient muscle shortening when the nerves signal the muscle to contract. From the neural standpoint, when the runner is poised at the starting block, neural activity increases in anticipation of the beginning of the race. This neural activation of the quadriceps is greater than when the runner was sitting and relaxed; it presets the muscle for imminent contraction. The difference between the lower tone and the higher tone can be palpated as a qualitative difference in the resistance to finger pressure over the muscle in each instance. In the relaxed condition, a pal-

High tone in quadriceps muscle

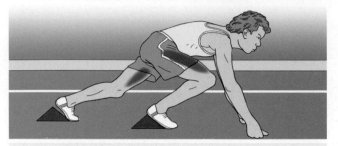

Low tone in quadriceps muscle

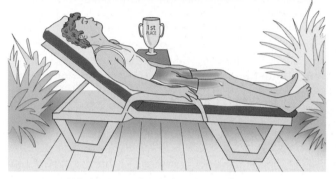

FIG 4-1 Normal variations in muscle tone.

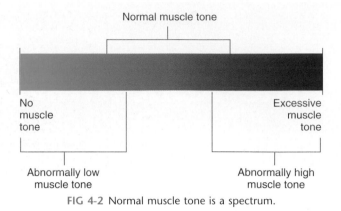

FIG 4-2 Normal muscle tone is a spectrum.

pating finger will sink into the muscle slightly because the muscle provides little resistance to that deforming pressure, which is a type of stretch on the surface muscle fibers. The finger will register relative softness compared with the hardness or resistance to deformation that is felt in the "ready" condition.

CHALLENGES TO ASSESSING MUSCLE TONE

One of the difficulties with tone assessment and description is the overlap between how a muscle looks and feels when it is subconsciously being prepared to move or hold and how it looks and feels when it is consciously ordered to contract. Note that the same qualitative difference in resistance to finger pressure from the relaxed state could be palpated whether the runner contracted the quadriceps voluntarily or prepared to contract them at the start of the race. A key to the assessment of muscle tone is that no active resistance to the muscle stretch occurs.

> **◎ Clinical Pearl**
>
> Assessment of muscle tone must occur when there is no active contraction or resistance to muscle stretch.

If a subject cannot avoid actively resisting, then the tonal quality assessed when the muscle is stretched will be a combination of tone and voluntary contraction. Even people who have normal control over their muscles sometimes have difficulty relaxing at will; therefore differentiating between muscle tone and voluntary muscle contraction can sometimes be difficult.

The continually changing nature of muscle tone under normal conditions can also make tone assessment difficult. The neural components of muscle tone can change with movement, posture, intention, and environment. The biomechanical components can change because body tissues are thixotropic, meaning that substances stiffen at rest and become less stiff with movement.[1] Initial stiffness noted when passively stretching muscles may ease with repeated movements, indicating an expected state change rather than a change in muscle properties. The runner in the example cited had differences in tone between the relaxed and imminent-contraction, or ready, states and is considered to have normal muscle tone in both instances. Normal is a spectrum rather than a precise point on a scale. Abnormal muscle tone may overlap with normal muscle tone at either end of the span (Fig. 4-2), but with abnormal tone the individual has reduced ability to change tone to prepare to move readily or to hold a position. Lower tone is not abnormal unless an individual cannot increase it sufficiently to prepare for movement or holding, and higher tone is not abnormal unless the individual cannot alter it at will, or unless it produces discomfort as in **muscle spasms** or cramps. Thus normal muscle tone is not a particular amount of passive resistance to stretch but rather a controllable range of tension that supports normal movement and posture.

TONE ABNORMALITIES

HYPOTONICITY

Hypotonicity, or low tone, describes decreased resistance to stretch compared with normal muscles. Down syndrome and poliomyelitis are examples of conditions that can result in hypotonicity. **Flaccidity** is the term used to denote total lack of tone or the absence of resistance to stretch within the middle range of the muscle's length. Flaccidity is an extreme case of hypotonicity and often occurs with total **paralysis** of the muscle. Paralysis describes a complete loss of voluntary muscle contraction. Paralysis is a movement disorder and not a tone disorder, although it may be associated with abnormalities of muscle tone.

HYPERTONICITY

Hypertonicity, or high tone, describes increased resistance to stretch compared with normal muscles. Hyperto-

TABLE 4-1	What Spasticity Is and Is Not
What Spasticity Is	**What Spasticity Is Not**
A type of abnormal muscle tone	Paralysis
One type of hypertonicity	Abnormal posturing
Velocity-dependent resistance to passive muscle stretch	A particular diagnosis or neural pathology
	Hyperactive stretch reflex
	Muscle spasm
	Voluntary movement restricted to movement in flexor or extensor synergy

Note: Spasticity, when present, does not always cause motor dysfunction.

nicity may be either rigid or spastic. **Rigidity** is an abnormal, hypertonic state in which muscles are stiff or immovable and resistant to stretch regardless of velocity. **Akinesia**, a movement disorder, is a lack or paucity of movement sometimes coincident with but distinct from rigidity. **Spasticity** is defined as velocity-dependent resistance to stretch.[4] The term spasticity has wide clinical use but causes confusion unless it is narrowly defined (Table 4-1). The term is sometimes paired with paralysis and has shared the blame for the loss of function noted in patient conditions labeled spastic paralysis or spastic hemiplegia.[5,6] However, spasticity itself does not necessarily inhibit function. Clinical assessment can help determine whether spasticity or other disorders affect function in a particular patient.

Clonus is the term used to describe multiple rhythmic oscillations or beats of muscle contraction in response to a quick stretch, observed particularly with stretching the ankle plantar flexors or wrist flexors. The **clasp-knife phenomenon** consists of initial resistance followed by a sudden release of resistance in response to a quick stretch of a hypertonic muscle, much like the resistance felt when closing a pocketknife. A muscle spasm is an involuntary, neurogenic contraction of a muscle, typically as the result of a noxious stimulus. A person who has pain in the low back may have muscle spasms in the paraspinal musculature that he or she cannot relax voluntarily. A contracture is a shortening of tissue resulting in loss of range of motion (ROM) at a particular joint; if the shortened tissue is within the muscle itself, whether because of nonneurogenic contraction of muscle fibers[1] or shortening of connective tissue around the fibers, hypertonicity may result.

TERMS CONFUSED WITH MUSCLE TONE

Muscle tone and voluntary muscle contraction are distinct from each other. Patients with hypertonic or hypotonic muscles, for example, may still be able to move voluntarily. Muscle tone and posture are also different entities. For example, an individual who presents with an adducted and internally rotated shoulder, a flexed elbow, and flexed wrist and fingers, holding the hand close to the chest, can be said to have a flexed posture of the arm. He or she cannot be said to have hypertonicity or spasticity until the passive resistance to stretch is assessed at different velocities for each of the involved muscle groups. Spasticity coexists with hyperactive **muscle stretch reflexes** in its

typical clinical presentation,[5,7] but because patients with rigidity can also have hyperactive stretch reflexes,[8] the two terms should not be equated. In addition, some confusion has arisen regarding the term spasticity because it has been applied to abnormal muscle tone resulting from different underlying neural pathologies, including spinal cord injury, stroke, and cerebral palsy. To clarify use in this text, the term spasticity is only applied to a particular type of abnormal muscle response, whatever the pathology, in which quicker passive muscle stretch elicits greater resistance than a slower stretch.[4]

FLUCTUATING ABNORMAL TONE

Qualitative terms are often used to describe fluctuating abnormal tone. Muscle tone is especially difficult to assess when it fluctuates widely, so it is common to describe visible movement rather than the tone itself. The common term used to describe any type of abnormal movement that is involuntary and has no purpose is **dyskinesia**. Some specific terms used to describe types of dyskinesia are choreiform movements or **chorea** (dancelike, sharp, jerky movements), **ballismus** (ballistic or large throwing-type movements), **tremor** (low-amplitude, high-frequency oscillating movements), **athetoid movements** (wormlike writhing motions), and **dystonia** (involuntary sustained muscle contraction usually resulting in abnormal postures or repetitive twisting movements[9]). Dystonia is seen in the condition called spasmodic torticollis, or wry neck, in which the individual's neck musculature is continuously contracted on one side and the individual involuntarily holds the head asymmetrically[10] (Fig. 4-3).

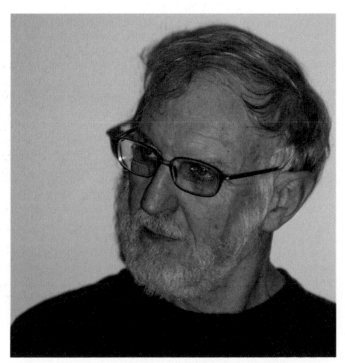

FIG 4-3 Torticollis.

MEASURING MUSCLE TONE

Several quantitative and qualitative methods have been used to assess muscle tone. Its variability with subtle intrasubject or environmental changes, however, limits the usefulness of static measures of muscle tone. In addition, measuring tone at one point in time during one movement or state of the muscle (at rest or during contraction) provides little information about how the muscle tone enhances or limits a different movement or state.[11] Therefore examiners must be careful to record the specific state of contraction or relaxation of the muscle group in question when they assess muscle tone and not interpret the results as true for all other states of the muscle group. In other words, ankle plantar flexor hypertonicity assessed at rest cannot be said to limit ankle dorsiflexion during the swing phase of gait unless testing is completed while the client is upright and moving the leg forward. The methods described in this section for measuring muscle tone should be used with two caveats in mind. First, the examiner should avoid generalizing the results of a single test, or even multiple tests, to all conditions of the muscle. Second, the examiner should include measures of movement or function to obtain a more complete picture of the subject's ability to use muscle tone appropriately.

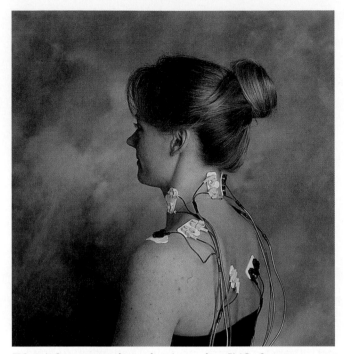

FIG 4-4 Components for performing surface EMG. *Courtesy Noromed, Kent, WA.*

> ◎ **Clinical Pearl**
>
> Assess movement and function with muscle tone to get a more complete picture.

QUANTITATIVE MEASURES

Passive resistance to stretch provided by muscle tone can be measured by tools similar to those used to measure the force generated by a voluntarily contracting muscle. When a voluntary contraction is measured, a subject is asked to "push against the device with all your strength." When muscle tone is measured, a subject is asked to "relax and let me move you." Such measures are restricted to the assessment of muscles that are both reasonably accessible to the examiner and easy to isolate by the subject to contract or relax on command. Muscles at the knee, elbow, wrist, and ankle, for example, are easier to position and to isolate than trunk muscles.

Dynamometer or Myometer

Boiteau et al described a protocol for quantifying muscle tone in the ankle plantar flexors using a hand-held dynamometer or myometer.[12] For this protocol, the subject is seated and positioned with the feet unsupported. The head of the dynamometer is placed at the metatarsal heads of the foot. The examiner passively dorsiflexes the ankle to a neutral position with pressure through the dynamometer several times at different velocities. The examiner controls the velocity by counting seconds: completing the movement in 3 seconds for a slow velocity and in less than half a second for a fast velocity. The authors reported high reproducibility (intraclass correlation coefficients = 0.79 and 0.90) for both the high- and low-velocity conditions.[12]

Comparing high- and low-velocity conditions enables the examiner to distinguish between neural and biomechanical components of spasticity. Greater resistance to high-velocity movement than low-velocity movement indicates increased tone. In contrast, high resistance at both low and high velocities indicates a biomechanical cause for the resistance such as a shortened muscle or tight joint capsule.

Isokinetic Testing Systems

Quantification of tone at the elbow in patients after stroke using an isokinetic machine adapted to allow the elbow to move with gravity eliminated has also been described.[13] Assessments of resistive torque at various speeds can be used to control for the biomechanical components of muscle tone and to determine the overall spasticity of the muscles crossing the elbow. In a small study, the reliability of this quantitative measure of biceps and triceps spasticity was 0.90 over 6 tests performed over 2 days.[13]

Electromyography

Electromyography (EMG) is a diagnostic tool frequently used in research for quantifying muscle tone (Fig. 4-4). EMG is a record of the electrical activity of muscles using surface, fine wire/needle electrodes (Fig. 4-5). During neurogenic muscle activation, the record will show deviations away from a straight isoelectric line (Fig. 4-6). The number and size of the deviations (peaks and valleys) give a measure of the amount of muscle tissue that is electrically active during the contraction. When a supposedly relaxed

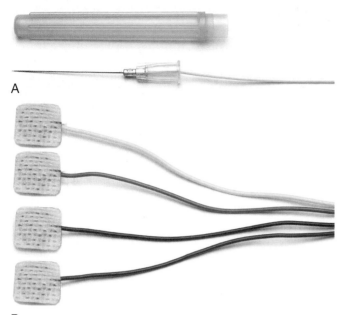

A

B

FIG 4-5 EMG electrodes. **A,** Fine wire/needle; **B,** surface. *Courtesy The Electrode Store, Enumclaw, WA.*

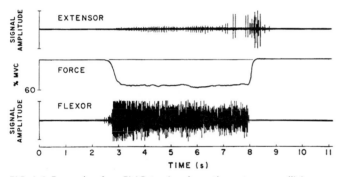

FIG 4-6 Example of an EMG tracing from the extensor pollicis longus *(upper tracing)* and flexor pollicis muscles *(lower tracing)* during an isometric contraction of the flexor pollicis longus muscle. The middle tracing is the force output produced with a 60% maximum voluntary contraction *(MVC). From Basmajian JV, De Luca CJ: Muscles alive: their functions revealed by electromyography, ed 5, Baltimore, 1985, Williams & Wilkins.*

muscle demonstrates electrical activity when stretched, that activity is a measure of the neurally derived muscle tone at that moment.

There are several advantages to using EMG to evaluate muscle tone. One advantage is its sensitivity to low levels of muscle activity that may not be readily palpable by an examiner. In addition, precise timing of muscle activation or relaxation can be detected by EMG and matched in time to a command to contract or relax. Because of these benefits, EMG can be used to provide **biofeedback** to a subject who is trying to learn how to initiate contraction or relaxation in a particular muscle group.[14] Another advantage of EMG is that in some cases it can differentiate between the neural and biomechanical components of muscle tone, which palpation alone is unable to do. If a

relaxed muscle shows no electrical activity via EMG when stretched but still provides resistance to passive stretch, then its tone can be attributed to the biomechanical rather than the neural components of the muscle involved.

Disadvantages of EMG include its ability to monitor only a local area of muscle tissue directly adjacent to (within about 1 cm from[1]) the electrode. It also requires specialized equipment and training that is beyond the resources of many clinical facilities. In addition, muscle tone and active muscle contraction cannot be distinguished from each other by looking at an EMG record. A label of some kind must state when the subject was told to contract and relax and when the muscle was stretched. Although EMG can record the amount of muscle activation, it measures force only indirectly via a complex relationship between activity and force output.[15]

Pendulum Test

Some measures of muscle tone have been developed to test particular types of abnormalities, not just tone in general. One of these is called the **pendulum test**,[1] which is intended to test spasticity. The test consists of holding an individual's limb so that when it is dropped, gravity provides a quick stretch to the spastic muscle. The resistance to that quick stretch will stop the limb from falling before it reaches the end of its range. The measurement of spasticity, sometimes quantified via an electrogoniometer[16] or isokinetic dynamometer,[17] is the difference between the angle at which the spastic muscle "catches" the movement and the angle the limb would reach at the end of its normal range. Bohannon reported the test-retest reliability as high when the quadriceps muscle was tested consecutively in 30 patients who had spasticity after experiencing a stroke or head injury.[17] A limitation of the pendulum test is that some muscle groups cannot be tested by dropping a limb and watching it swing specifically the muscles of the trunk and neck.

QUALITATIVE MEASURES
Clinical Tone Scale

Muscle tone is more often assessed qualitatively than quantitatively. The traditional clinical measure is a 5-point ordinal scale that places normal tone at 2+ (Table 4-2). No tone and hypotonicity are given scores of 0 and 1+, respectively, and moderate and severe hypertonicity are given scores of 3+ and 4+, respectively.[18] The clinician obtains an impression of the muscle tone relative to normal by passively moving the patient at varying speeds. When muscle tone is normal, movement is light and easy. When

TABLE 4-2	Commonly Used Clinical Tone Scale
Grade	Description
0	No tone
1+	Hypotonicity
2+	Normal tone
3+	Moderate hypertonicity
4+	Severe hypertonicity

muscle tone is decreased, movement is still easy or unrestricted, but the limbs are heavy, as if they are dead weight. When tone is increased for a particular muscle, the movement that mechanically stretches that muscle is stiff or unyielding. Various movements must be made at multiple joints to distinguish between normal variations of muscle tone in different muscle groups.

Muscle Stretch Reflex Test

Another commonly used qualitative method of assessing muscle tone is to observe the response elicited by tapping on the muscle's tendon, activating the muscle stretch reflex. As with the clinical tone scale, in this 5-point scale, 2+ is considered normal, 0 is absent reflexes, 1+ is diminished, 3+ is brisker than average, and 4+ is very brisk or hyperactive.[19] The normal responses for different tendons differ. For example, a tap on the patellar tendon will normally result in a slight swing of the free lower leg from the knee. In contrast, a biceps or triceps tendon tap is still considered normal if a small twitch of the muscle belly is observed or palpated; actual movement of the whole lower arm would generally be considered hyperactive. Normal responses are determined by what is typical for that tendon reflex. In addition, symmetry of reflexes, assessed by comparing the responses to stimulation of the left and right sides of the body, determines the degree of normalcy of the response.

Ashworth and Modified Ashworth Scale

The Ashworth Scale[20] and the Modified Ashworth Scale[21] are scales of spasticity. These scales have the advantages of known reliability but are limited to describing increased but not decreased muscle tone. Because there is no rigorously tested scale for quantifying or describing low muscle tone, clinicians commonly use the clinical scale presented in Table 4-2.

> ### ◎ Clinical Pearl
>
> The Modified Ashworth Scale is used to describe normal or increased tone, whereas the commonly used 5-point scale describes low, normal, and high tone.

The Ashworth Scale includes five ordinal grades from 0 (no increase in muscle tone) to 4 (rigidly held in flexion or extension). The intermediate grade of 1+ was added to the original Ashworth Scale to produce the Modified Ashworth Scale (Table 4-3). This grade is defined by a slight catch and continued minimal resistance through the range. Bohannon and Smith reported 86.7% interrater agreement for the Modified Ashworth Scale when used to test 30 patients with spasticity of the elbow flexor muscles.[21]

GENERAL CONSIDERATIONS WHEN MEASURING MUSCLE TONE

The relative positions of the limb, body, neck, and head with respect to one another and to gravity can all affect muscle tone. For example, the asymmetrical and sym-

TABLE 4-3	Modified Ashworth Scale for Grading Spasticity
Grade	**Description**
0	No increase in muscle tone
1	Slight increase in muscle tone manifested by a catch and release or by minimal resistance at the end of the ROM when the affected part(s) is moved in flexion or extension
1+	Slight increase in muscle tone manifested by a catch, followed by minimal resistance throughout the remainder (less than half) of the ROM
2	More marked increase in muscle tone through most of the ROM, but affected part(s) easily moved
3	Considerable increase in muscle tone, passive movement difficult
4	Affected part(s) rigid in flexion or extension

From Bohannon RW, Smith MB: Interrater reliability of a Modified Ashworth Scale of Muscle Spasticity, *Phys Ther* 67:207, 1987. *ROM,* Range of motion.

metrical tonic neck reflexes (ATNR and STNR, respectively) are known to influence the tone of the flexors and extensors of the arms and legs, depending on the position of the head (Fig. 4-7), both during infancy and in subjects who have neurological deficits.[22] Subtle differences in muscle tone as a result of these reflexes can be detected by palpation when the head position changes even in subjects with mature and intact nervous systems. Likewise, the pull of gravity on a limb to stretch muscles or on the **vestibular system** to trigger responses to keep the head upright will change muscle tone according to the position of the head and the body. Therefore the testing position must be reported for accurate interpretation and replication of any measurement of muscle tone.

> ### ◎ Clinical Pearl
>
> The testing position should be reported when documenting muscle tone measurement.

Additional general guidelines for measuring muscle tone include standardization of touch and consideration of the muscle length at which a group of muscles is to be tested. The examiner must be aware that touching the subject's skin, either with a hand or with an instrument, can influence muscle tone. Handholds and instrument placement must therefore be consistent for accurate interpretation and replication. The length at which a specific muscle's tone is tested must also be standardized. Because muscle tone differs with passive biomechanical differences at the extremes of range and ROM can be altered as a result of long-term changes in tone, the most consistent length to measure muscle tone is at the midrange of the available length of the muscle tested.

> ### ◎ Clinical Pearl
>
> Muscle tone is most accurately measured at the midrange of the muscle's length.

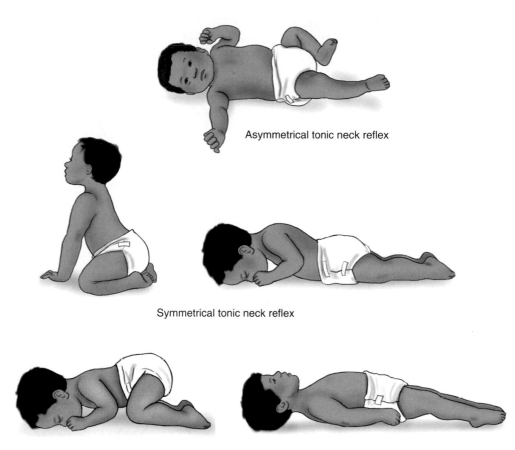

Asymmetrical tonic neck reflex

Symmetrical tonic neck reflex

Tonic labyrinthine reflex

FIG 4-7 Reflex responses to head or neck position.

THE ANATOMICAL BASES OF MUSCLE TONE AND ACTIVATION

Muscle tone and muscle activation originate from interactions between nervous system input and the biomechanical and biochemical properties of the muscle and its surrounding connective tissue. The practitioner must have an understanding of the anatomical basis for both tone and activation to determine appropriate physical agents to apply when either is dysfunctional. The anatomical contributions to muscle tone and activation are reviewed in this section.

MUSCULAR CONTRIBUTIONS TO MUSCLE TONE AND ACTIVATION

Muscle is composed of (1) contractile elements in the muscle fibers, (2) cellular elements providing structure, (3) connective tissue providing coverings for the fibers and the entire muscle, and (4) tendons attaching muscle to bone. When neural input signals the muscle to contract or relax, biochemical activity of the contractile elements shortens and lengthens muscle fibers. As the contractile elements work, they slide against each other, facilitated by the cellular elements to maintain structure and the connective tissue coverings to provide support and lubrication while the muscle changes length.

Myofilaments are the contractile elements of muscle. With neural stimulation of the muscle fiber, storage sites in the muscle release calcium ions that allow **actin** and **myosin** protein molecules on different myofilaments to bind together. The binding occurs at particular sites to form cross-bridges (Fig. 4-8). Breaking of these cross-bridges, so that new bonds can be formed at different sites, is mediated by energy derived from adenosine triphosphate (ATP). As bonds are formed, broken, and reformed, the length of the contractile unit, or **sarcomere**, changes. The cycle of binding and releasing continues as long as calcium ions and ATP are present. Calcium ions are taken back into storage when activation of muscle ceases. Sources within the muscle supply an adequate amount of ATP for short-duration activities, but the muscle must depend on fuel delivered by the circulatory system for long-duration activities.

Actin and myosin myofilaments must overlap for cross-bridges to form (Fig. 4-9). When the muscle is stretched too far, cross-bridges cannot form because there is no overlap. When the muscle is in its most shortened position, actin and myosin run into the structural elements of

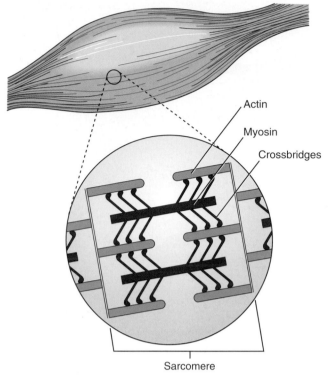

Actin

Myosin

Crossbridges

Sarcomere

FIG 4-8 Cross-bridge formation within muscle fibers.

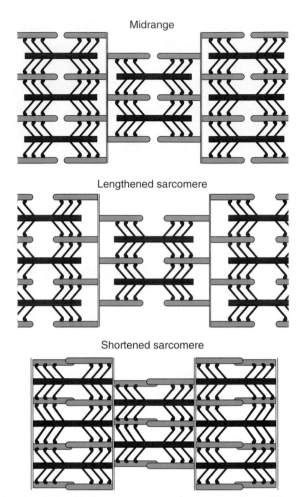

Midrange

Lengthened sarcomere

Shortened sarcomere

FIG 4-9 Relationship between actin and myosin at three different sarcomere lengths.

the muscle fiber and no further cross-bridges can be formed. In the midrange of the muscle, actin and myosin can form the greatest number of cross-bridges. The midrange is the length at which a muscle can generate the greatest amount of force, or tension. This length-tension relationship is one of the biomechanical properties of muscles.

Other biomechanical properties of muscles include friction and elasticity. Friction between connective tissue coverings as they slide past one another may be affected by pressure on the tissues and by the viscosity of the tissues and fluids in which they reside. Elasticity of connective tissue results in varying responses to stretch at different muscle lengths. When tissue becomes taut, as it is when a muscle is fully lengthened, connective tissue contributes more to the overall resistance of the muscle to stretch. When connective tissue is slack, it contributes very little to a muscle's tension. In fact, when muscle is stimulated to contract while it is shortened, there is a delay before movement can occur or force can be generated while the slack in the connective tissue is taken up. The runner's crouch in Fig. 4-1 takes up some initial slack in the quadriceps before the start of the race to reduce any delay in activation.

Both active contractile elements and passive properties of the tissues contribute to muscle tone and activation. However, muscle tone can be generated from the passive elements alone, whereas muscle activation requires both active and passive elements.

Physical agents can change both muscle tone and activation. Heat increases the accessibility of ATP to the myofilaments through improved circulation. Heat and cold can change the elasticity or friction of the tissues and physical agents such as electrical stimulation can also change the amount of neural stimulation of the muscle fibers.

NEURAL CONTRIBUTIONS TO MUSCLE TONE AND ACTIVATION

Neural sources of input that contribute to muscle tone and muscle activation come from the periphery, the spinal cord, and **supraspinal** brain centers (Fig. 4-10). Even though multiple areas of the nervous system may participate, all of them must work through the final common pathway, the **alpha motor neuron**, which ultimately stimulates muscle fibers to contract (Fig. 4-11). The generation, **summation**, and conduction of an activating signal in alpha motor **neurons** are critical components of muscle tone and activation. In this section, discussion of nerve structure and function is followed by an account of some significant influences on the alpha motor neuron. See a major neurophysiological text for a more complete description of known input to alpha motor neurons.

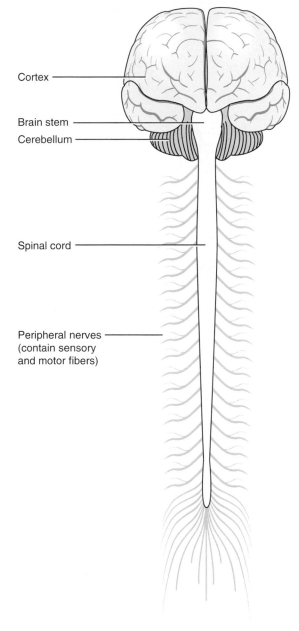

Cortex

Brain stem

Cerebellum

Spinal cord

Peripheral nerves
(contain sensory
and motor fibers)

FIG 4-10 Schematic drawing of the nervous system, front view.

Structure and Function of Nerves

Nerve cells, or neurons, include most of the components of other cells, including cell bodies with a cell membrane, nucleus, and multiple internal organelles that keep the cell alive. The distinguishing features of a neuron include the multiple projections, called **dendrites**, that receive stimuli—usually from other nerve cells—and the single **axon** that conducts stimuli toward a destination. The axon branches ends in multiple synaptic boutons (Fig. 4-12). These boutons transmit stimuli across the narrow gap, or **synapse**, between a bouton and its target muscle fibers, bodily organs, glands, or other neurons. Although a few specialized neurons can receive electrical, mechanical, chemical, or thermal stimuli, most neurons respond to and transmit signals via chemicals known as **neurotransmitters**.

Neurotransmitter molecules are manufactured and stored in the synaptic boutons (Fig. 4-13, *A*). An electrical signal conducted down an axon causes the release of these molecules into the synapse. The molecules cross the synapse and if the postsynaptic cell is another neuron, bind to one of the chemically specific receptor sites covering the dendrites, cell body, or axon (Fig. 4-13, *B*).

The neurotransmitter dopamine exemplifies the specificity of neurotransmitters and is significant to the study of muscle tone and activation. Dopamine is normally found in high concentration in the neurons of the substantia nigra, one of the **basal ganglia** discussed later in this chapter. Deficits in the production or use of dopamine result in rigidity, resting tremors, and difficulty initiating and executing movement,[23] all manifestations of Parkinson's disease. Examples of other neurotransmitters are acetylcholine, norepinephrine, and serotonin.

The binding of a specific neurotransmitter with its receptor site tends to either excite or inhibit the postsynaptic cell. Whether the postsynaptic cell responds by transmitting the signal from the receptor site to the rest of the cell depends on summation, or adding together, of many excitatory and inhibitory signals. Summation may be spatial or temporal (Fig. 4-14). Input to receptor sites from many different synaptic boutons at one time results in spatial summation. Sequential stimulation over time through the same receptor sites results in temporal summation. Excitatory input must exceed inhibitory input if the sum is to result in signal conduction down an axon. A single neuron typically receives input from hundreds or thousands of other neurons.

Once excitatory stimulation reaches a particular threshold level, the signal is conducted down the axon in an **action potential**. The action potential rapidly transforms the membrane of the neuron from its electrochemical state at rest. Membrane transformation occurs in a wave of electrochemical current that progresses rapidly from the cell body down the axon to the synaptic boutons.

At rest, the neuronal membrane separates the concentration of sodium (Na^+), chloride (Cl^-), and potassium (K^+) ions on the inside of the cell from the concentration on the outside. Na^+ and Cl^- are in greater concentration outside the cell, and K^+ and negatively charged protein molecules are in greater concentration inside the cell. In addition to the chemical difference across the membrane, an overall electrical difference exists immediately adjacent to the membrane of approximately -70 mV, with the inside of the membrane more negative than the outside. Biological systems with a difference in charge or concentration between two areas will come to equilibrium if possible. Because of the electrochemical difference, the membrane is said to have a **resting potential**, which is the potential for movement of ions toward equilibrium if the membrane allowed it.

Channels or holes in the membrane allow selective movement of ions from one side of the membrane to the other. Allowing movement of only some ions makes the membrane semipermeable. K^+ move freely across the membrane when the neuron is at rest. Some membrane channels open and close at specific times to allow certain

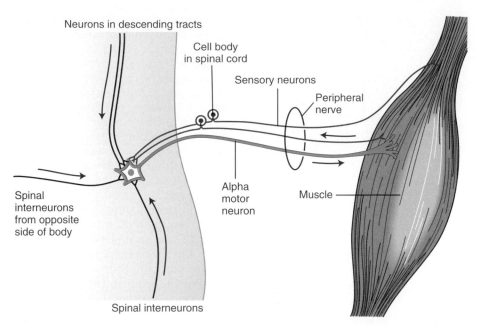

Neurons in descending tracts

Cell body
in spinal cord

Sensory neurons

Peripheral
nerve

Spinal
interneurons
from opposite
side of body

Alpha
motor
neuron

Muscle

Spinal interneurons

FIG 4-11 Alpha motor neuron: the final common pathway of neural signals to muscles.

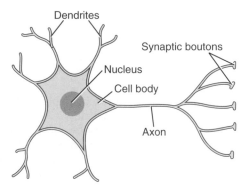

Dendrites

Synaptic boutons

Nucleus

Cell body

Axon

FIG 4-12 A typical alpha motor neuron.

other ions to move according to their **electrochemical gradients**. Still other ions are actively moved through the membrane from one side to the other in a biochemical pumping process. This process requires energy because these ions are moved against their electrochemical gradient (i.e., they move farther away from equilibrium of charge or concentration on the two sides of the membrane).

When an action potential sweeps down an axon, channels in the membrane open, allowing Na^+ ions to rush into the cell, thereby altering both the concentration and the electrical differences between the inside and outside of the membrane. During the action potential, the polar difference between the electrical charge inside and outside the membrane changes in that location (i.e., that section of membrane has depolarized), with an increase in positive charge on the inside. A Na^+/K^+ pump quickly restores the electrochemical difference between the inside and outside by transporting Na^+ ions back outside the cell and K^+ ions back inside. The end result of the Na^+/K^+

pump is **repolarization** of that section of the cell membrane.

The successive **depolarization** and repolarization of membrane sections continues down the axon until those changes stimulate the release of neurotransmitters from all of the axon's synaptic boutons (see Fig. 4-13, *B*). The speed of conduction of an action potential depends on the diameter of the neuron and the insulation available along the axon. Neurons with smaller diameters have slower conduction velocities. Larger-diameter neurons have faster conduction velocities.

◎ Clinical Pearl

Neurons with small diameter axons conduct more slowly than neurons with large-diameter axons.

Insulation speeds the transmission of a depolarizing wave by increasing the speed with which the ions move across the membrane. A fatty tissue called **myelin**, provided by Schwann cells in the **peripheral nervous system** (PNS) and oligodendrocytes in the **central nervous system** (CNS), is the source of insulation for neurons. Myelin wraps around the axons of neurons, leaving gaps at regular intervals (Fig. 4-15). When a depolarizing wave travels down an axon, it moves quickly down sections that have myelin and slows at gaps where no myelin is present, at the nodes of Ranvier. Because the signal slows at the nodes and travels very quickly between nodes, it appears to jump from one node to the next in rapid succession all the way to the end of all the axonal branches.[24] This jumping is referred to as **saltatory conduction** (Fig. 4-16).

The fastest conduction velocities recorded in human nerves are up to 70 to 80 m/sec.[25] Temperature changes

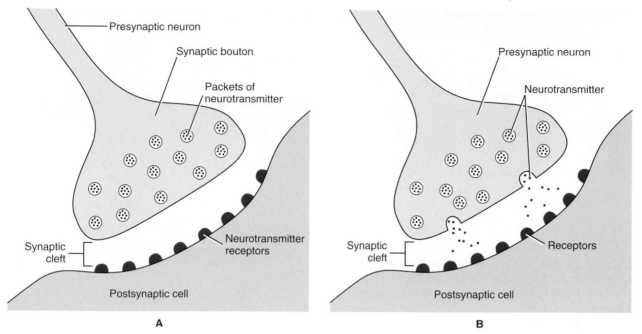

FIG 4-13 **A,** Synapse between presynaptic and postsynaptic neurons at rest. **B,** Synapse between presynaptic and postsynaptic neurons when activated.

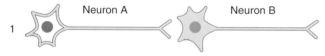

1

Multiple discharges from neuron A will activate neuron B temporally, or in time

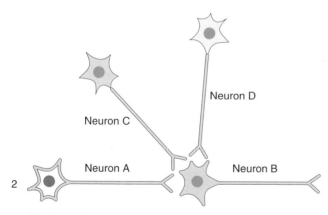

2

Discharges from neurons A, C, and D will activate neuron B spatially, or from multiple places on neuron B

FIG 4-14 Temporal and spatial summation of input to a neuron.

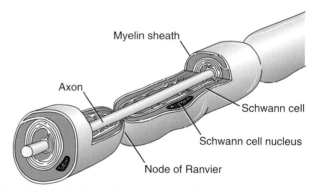

FIG 4-15 Myelin formed by Schwann cells on a peripheral neuron.

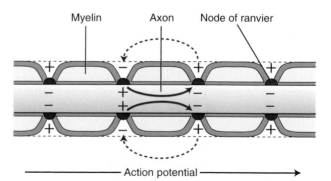

FIG 4-16 Saltatory conduction along a myelin-wrapped axon.

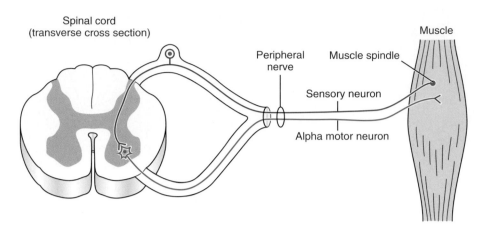

FIG 4-17 Monosynaptic muscle stretch reflex.

can alter these velocities. When axons are cooled, as with the application of ice packs, nerve conduction velocity slows by approximately 2 m/sec for every 1° C decrease in temperature.[26]

◎ **Clinical Pearl**

Cold slows nerve conduction velocities.

Once the signal reaches the synaptic boutons and neurotransmitters are released, there is a slight delay as the molecules move across the synaptic cleft. Even at 200 Ångstrom units (200×10^{-10} m), it takes time for diffusion and then reception by the next neuron or target tissue. In addition, the receiving neuron must sum all of its inputs, both excitatory and inhibitory, before an action potential can develop. Therefore larger numbers of connections between neurons take longer to transmit a signal than smaller numbers. The shortest connection known is the single monosynaptic connection of the muscle stretch reflex, observable when certain tendons are tapped (Fig. 4-17). It is called monosynaptic because there is only one synapse between the sensory neuron receiving the stretch stimulus and the motor neuron transmitting the signal to the muscle fibers to contract.

Monosynaptic transmission, as recorded from muscle stretch (tap) to initiation of muscle stretch reflex contraction, has been recorded in as little as 25 ms at the arm.[27] The length of time between stimulus and response when multiple synapses are involved is longer. For example, when the arm is working to move a load and visual input indicates a sudden change in the load, it takes approximately 300 ms for the arm muscles to respond to that input.[27] If a person unexpectedly saw a ball begin to drop off a shelf 1 m above her, the ball would fall approximately 44 cm before she could start to move to catch it.

SOURCES OF NEURAL STIMULATION OF MUSCLE

The Alpha Motor Neuron

Muscle tone and activation depend on alpha motor neurons for neural stimulation. An alpha motor neuron,

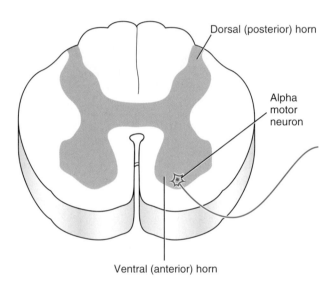

FIG 4-18 One motor unit: alpha motor neuron and muscle fibers innervated by it.

which is sometimes called an **anterior horn cell**, transmits signals from the CNS to muscles. With its cell body in the ventral or anterior grey matter or horn of the spinal cord (Fig. 4-17), its axon exits the spinal cord and thus the CNS through the ventral nerve root. Each axon eventually reaches muscle, where it branches and innervates between 6 (in the eye muscles) and 2000 (in the gastrocnemius muscle) muscle fibers at motor endplates.[28] The muscle fibers innervated by a single axon with its branches, which is one **motor unit** (Fig. 4-18), all contract at once whenever an action potential is transmitted down that axon. A single action potential generated by the alpha motor neuron cannot provide its motor unit with a graded signal; each action potential is "all or none." When sufficient motor units are recruited, the muscle visibly contracts. More forceful contraction of the muscle requires an increased number or rate of action potentials down the same axons or recruitment of additional motor units.

Activation of a particular motor unit depends on the sum of excitatory and inhibitory input to that alpha motor neuron (Fig. 4-19). Excitation or inhibition in turn depends on the sources and amounts of input from the

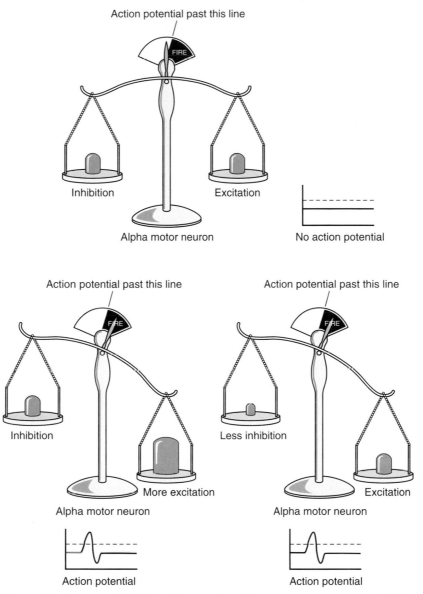

FIG 4-19 Balance of excitatory and inhibitory input to the alpha motor neuron at rest and when activated.

TABLE 4-4	Input to Alpha Motor Neurons (Simplified)	
From Peripheral Receptors	**From Spinal Sources**	**From Supraspinal Sources**
Muscle spindles via 1a sensory neurons	Propriospinal interneurons	Cortex, basal ganglia via corticospinal tract
GTOs via 1b sensory neurons	—	Cerebellum, red nucleus via rubrospinal tract
Cutaneous receptors via other sensory neurons	—	Vestibular system, cerebellum via vestibulospinal tracts
		Limbic system, autonomic nervous system via reticulospinal tracts

GTOs, Golgi tendon organs.

thousands of neurons that synapse on that one particular alpha motor neuron. An understanding of the sources of input to alpha motor neurons is essential to understanding control of motor unit activation and alteration of muscle tone by physical agents or other means (Table 4-4).

Input from the Periphery

The PNS includes all of the neurons that project outside of the CNS, even if the cell bodies are located within the CNS. The PNS is composed of the alpha motor neurons, **gamma motor neurons**, some autonomic nervous system effector neurons, and all of the sensory neurons that carry information from the periphery to the CNS.

Sensory neurons can stimulate neurons in the spinal cord directly and therefore generally have a quicker and less modulated effect on alpha motor neurons than other sources of input that must traverse the brain. Quick, relatively stereotyped motor responses, called reflexes,

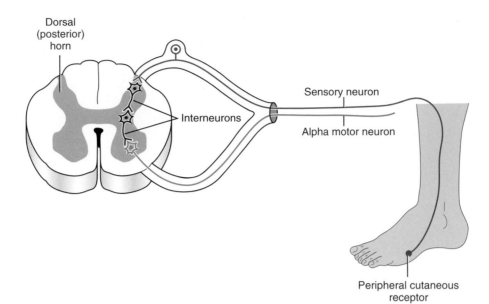

Dorsal (posterior) horn

Interneurons

Sensory neuron

Alpha motor neuron

Peripheral cutaneous receptor

FIG 4-20 Sensory input into spinal cord to alpha motor neurons.

commonly result from unmodulated peripheral input. At its simplest, a reflex involves only one synapse between a sensory neuron and a motor neuron, as in the monosynaptic stretch reflex defined previously (see Fig. 4-17). In this case, every action potential in the sensory neuron provides the same unmodulated input to the motor neuron. Most reflexes, however, involve multiple **interneurons** in the spinal cord between the sensory and motor neurons (Fig. 4-20). Because of the volume of input from multiple neurons and sources, the motor response to a specific sensory input can be modulated according to the context of the action.[29]

The presumed reason for multiple peripheral sources of input in the normally functioning nervous system is to protect the body, counter obstacles, or adapt to unexpected occurrences in the environment during volitional movement. Because of its direct connections in the spinal cord, peripheral input can assist function even before the brain has received or processed information about the success or failure of the movement. Peripheral input also influences muscle tone and is frequently the medium through which physical agents effect change.

Muscle Spindle. Inside the muscle, lying parallel to muscle fibers, are sensory organs called **muscle spindles** (Fig. 4-21). When a muscle is stretched, as it is when a tendon is tapped to stimulate a stretch reflex, the muscle spindles are also stretched. Receptors wrapped around the equatorial regions of the spindles sense the lengthening and send an action potential through **type Ia sensory neurons** into the spinal cord. A primary destination of this signal is the pool of alpha motor neurons for the muscle that was stretched (the agonist muscle). If the excitatory input of the Ia sensory neurons is sufficiently greater than inhibitory input from elsewhere, the alpha motor neurons will generate a signal to contract their associated muscle fibers. Several traditional facilitation techniques for increasing muscle tone, including quick

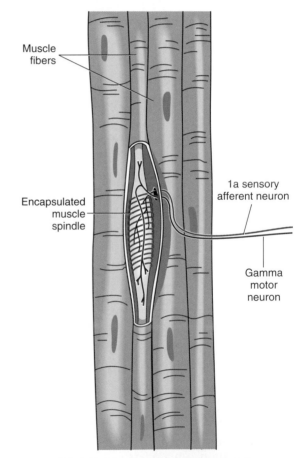

Muscle fibers

Encapsulated muscle spindle

1a sensory afferent neuron

Gamma motor neuron

FIG 4-21 Muscle spindle within a muscle.

stretch, tapping, resistance, high-frequency vibration, and positioning a limb so that gravity can provide stretch or resistance, take advantage of the stretch reflex.

Another destination for signals transmitted by type Ia sensory neurons from the muscle spindle is the pool of

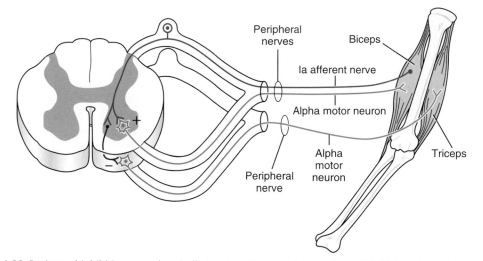

FIG 4-22 Reciprocal inhibition: muscle spindle input excites agonist muscles and inhibits antagonist muscles.

alpha motor neurons for the antagonist muscle to inhibit activity on the opposite side of the joint. For example, signals from the muscle spindles in the biceps excite alpha motor neurons of the biceps and inhibit those of the triceps (Fig. 4-22). This **reciprocal inhibition** prevents a muscle from working against its antagonist when activated.

Because muscles shorten as they contract and muscle spindles register muscle stretch only if they are taut, spindles must be continually reset to eliminate sagging in the center portion of the spindles. Gamma motor neurons innervate muscle spindles at the end regions and when stimulated, cause the equatorial region of the spindle to tighten (see Fig. 4-21). Thus gamma motor neurons sensitize the spindles to changes in muscle length.[30] Gamma motor neurons are typically activated at the same time as alpha motor neurons during voluntary movement, a process called **alpha-gamma coactivation**.[31] Gamma motor neurons can also be activated independently of alpha motor neurons via peripheral afferent nerves in the muscle, skin, and joints[32] and possibly via separate descending tracts from the brain stem.[33] Mechanoreceptors and chemoreceptors in the homonymous muscles send excitatory input to gamma motor neurons during contraction,[32] ensuring that the muscle spindles retain a high sensitivity to stretch as the muscle shortens. Another purpose of separate gamma motor neuron activation is to prepare the muscle spindle to sense expected changes in length that might occur during voluntary movement. For example, when someone walks across an icy sidewalk, knowing that a slip is probable, gamma motor neurons increase spindle sensitivity so that muscles can respond especially quickly if one foot starts to slip on the ice.

Golgi Tendon Organs. Golgi tendon organs (GTOs) are sensory organs located in the connective tissue at the junction between muscle fibers and tendons (Fig. 4-23). They function in series with muscle fibers, in contrast to muscle spindles, which function in parallel. Because of their location at the musculotendinous junction, GTOs

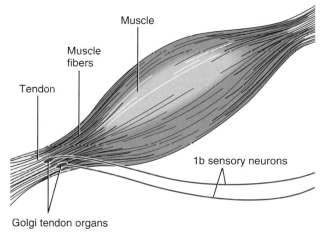

FIG 4-23 Golgi tendon organs (GTOs) within a muscle.

signal a maximal stretch of the muscle and are thus thought to protect against muscle damage.[34] GTOs are also extremely sensitive to active contraction, particularly small force contractions from as few as one or two muscle fibers in series with that GTO.[35] GTOs are limited in their ability to sense steady or larger levels of muscular tension, however, so they must be supplemented by other types of peripheral input in signaling overall muscle contraction.[36]

GTOs transmit signals to the alpha motor neuron pools of both the agonist and antagonist muscles via type Ib sensory neurons. The input to homonymous muscles is inhibitory to signal the muscle fibers not to contract. This spinal reflex response is called **autogenic inhibition**. The input to alpha motor neurons of antagonist muscles is excitatory to signal contraction. The purpose of the GTOs is to regulate active muscle contraction, possibly to help "put on the brakes" during activation.

Note that muscle stretch can provide contradictory input to an alpha motor neuron. Quick stretch stimulates the spindles to register a change in length, facilitating muscle contraction. Prolonged stretch may initially facilitate contraction but ultimately inhibits contraction perhaps because the GTOs register tension at the tendon and inhibit the homonymous alpha motor neurons. Prolonged stretch is thus traditionally used to inhibit abnormally high tone in agonists and facilitate antagonist muscle groups.[37] Inhibitory pressure on the tendon of a hypertonic muscle is also thought to stimulate the GTOs to inhibit abnormal muscle tone in the agonists while facilitating antagonists.[37]

> ### Ⓞ Clinical Pearl
>
> Prolonged stretch and pressure on the tendon of a hypertonic muscle can inhibit high tone in agonist muscles and facilitate antagonist muscles.

These techniques should be considered when positioning a patient for application of physical agents or other modalities.

Cutaneous Receptors. Stimulation of cutaneous sensory receptors occurs with every interaction of a person's skin with the external world. Temperature, texture, pressure, pain, and touch are all transmitted through these receptors. Cutaneous reflex responses tend to be more complex than muscle and tendon responses, involving multiple muscles. Painful stimuli at the skin, like stepping on a tack or touching a hot iron, will ultimately facilitate alpha motor neurons of withdrawal muscles. In a flexor withdrawal reflex, the hip and knee flexors or elbow flexors are signaled to pull the foot or hand away from the painful stimulus. If the body is upright when the painful stimulus occurs, a crossed extension reflex occurs. Alpha motor neurons of the opposite leg's hip and knee extensor muscles will be facilitated so that when the foot is withdrawn from the painful stimulus, the other leg can support the individual's weight (Fig. 4-24).

Because muscles are linked to each other neurally via spinal interneurons for more efficient functioning, activation of an agonist frequently affects additional muscles. For example, when the biceps muscle is facilitated during a withdrawal reflex, the triceps muscle of the same arm is inhibited. Likewise, if a muscle is contracting strongly, many of its synergists will also be facilitated to contract to help the function of the original muscle.

Intervention techniques that use cutaneous receptors to increase muscle tone include quick, light touch; manual contact; brushing; and quick icing. Techniques that use cutaneous receptors to decrease muscle tone include slow stroking, maintained holding, neutral warmth, and prolonged icing. These facilitative and inhibitory techniques take advantage of the motor responses to cutaneous stimulation reported by Hagbarth[38] and developed for clinical use by sensorimotor therapists.[39-41] The difference between facilitative and inhibitory techniques in clinical use usually lies in the speed and novelty of the stimulation. The nervous system stays alert when rapid changes are perceived, preparing the body to respond with movement, which necessitates increases in muscle tone. The inhibitory techniques begin in a similar way to the facilitative techniques, but the slow, repetitive, or maintained nature

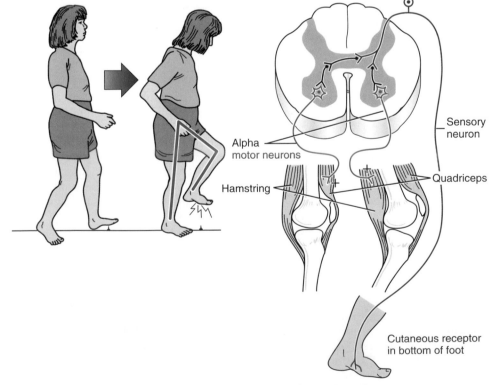

FIG 4-24 Flexor withdrawal and crossed extension reflexes.

of the stimuli leads to adaptation by the cutaneous receptors. The nervous system ignores what it already knows is there, and general relaxation is possible, with a diminution of muscle tone.

Because cutaneous receptors can affect muscle tone, any physical agent that touches the skin can change tone, whether the touch is intentional or incidental.

> ### ◎ Clinical Pearl
> Any physical agent that touches the skin can affect muscle tone.

Thus it is necessary to consider the location and type of cutaneous input provided whenever using physical agents, especially because the effect on muscle tone may counter the effect desired from the agent itself.

Input from Spinal Sources

In addition to the sensory information from the periphery that signals alpha motor neurons, circuits of neurons within the spinal cord also contribute to excitation and inhibition. These circuits are composed of interneurons, neurons that connect two other neurons. Propriospinal pathways are one type of neural circuit that communicates intersegmentally, between different levels within the spinal cord. They receive input from peripheral afferents, as well as from many of the descending pathways that are discussed in the next section, and help produce **synergies** or particular patterns of movements.[42]

For example, when a person flexes the elbow forcefully against resistance, propriospinal pathways assist in the communication between neurons at multiple spinal levels. The result is coordinated recruitment of synergistic muscles that add force to the movement. That same resisted arm movement also facilitates flexor muscle activity in the opposite arm via the propriospinal pathways. Both of these principles have been used in therapeutic exercises to increase the tone and force output from muscles in persons with neurological dysfunction.[39,40,43]

Input from Supraspinal Sources

Supraspinal refers to CNS areas that originate above the spinal cord in the upright human (see Fig. 4-10). Ultimately, these brain areas influence alpha motor neurons by sending signals down axons in a variety of descending pathways. Any voluntary, subconscious, or pathological change in the amount of input from descending pathways alters the excitatory and inhibitory input to alpha motor neurons. Such changes in turn alter muscle tone and activation, depending on the individual and the pathway or tract involved. Several of the major descending pathways and their influence on motor neurons are discussed in relation to the brain areas to which they are most closely related.

Sensorimotor Cortical Contributions. Volitional movement originates in response to a sensation, an idea, a memory, or an external stimulus to move, act, or respond. The decision to move is initiated in the cortex, with signals

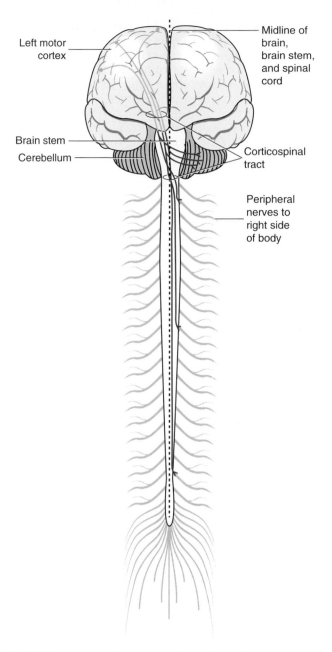

FIG 4-25 Corticospinal tract: schematic pathway from cortex to cerebellum and spinal cord.

moving rapidly among neurons in various brain areas until they reach the motor cortex. Axons from many of the neurons in the motor cortex form a corticospinal tract (from cortex to spinal cord) that runs through the brain, mostly crosses at the pyramids at the base of the brain stem, and descends to synapse on appropriate alpha motor neurons on the opposite side of the spinal cord (Fig. 4-25). When the alpha motor neurons have sufficient excitatory input, action potentials signal all the associated muscle fibers to contract. Corticospinal input to alpha motor neurons in the spinal cord is primarily responsible for voluntary contraction, particularly distal fine motor functions.

Cerebellum. For every set of instructions that descends through the corticospinal tract to signal posture or movement, a copy is routed to the **cerebellum** (see Fig. 4-25). Neurons in the cerebellum compare the intended movement with the sensory input received about the actual movement. The cerebellum registers any discrepancies between the signal from the motor cortex and the accumulated sensory input from muscle spindles, tendons, joints, and skin of the body during the movement. Cerebellar output helps correct for movement errors or unexpected obstacles to movement via the cortex and the red nuclei in the brain stem. The red nuclei in turn can send signals to the alpha motor neurons through the rubrospinal tracts (RuSTs). Ongoing correction is successful only during slower movements; if a movement is completed too quickly to alter, information about the success or failure of the movement can improve subsequent trials. Both corticospinal and rubrospinal inputs to alpha motor neurons function primarily to activate musculature. Direct influences of the cerebellum on muscle tone and posture are mediated through connections with the vestibulospinal tracts (VSTs).

Basal Ganglia. The basal ganglia modulate movement and tone. Any volitional movement involves processing through connections in the basal ganglia, which are composed of five nuclei or groups of neurons: putamen, caudate, globus pallidus, subthalamic nucleus, and substantia nigra (Fig. 4-26). Multiple chains of neurons looping through these nuclei, back and forth to the brain stem and back to motor cortical areas, influence the planning and postural adaptation of motor behavior.[33] Dysfunction of any of the nuclei of the basal ganglia is associated with abnormal tone and disordered movement. The rigidity and akinesia associated with Parkinson's disease, for example, are a result of basal ganglion pathology.

Other Descending Input. The VSTs help regulate posture by transmitting signals from the vestibular system to the alpha motor neuron pools in the spinal cord. The vestibular system receives ongoing information about the position of the head and the way it moves in space with respect to gravity. The vestibular nuclei also integrate and transmit responses to information received about the movement of the head via the joint, muscle, and skin receptors of the head and neck. The VSTs and related tracts generally facilitate the extensor (antigravity) alpha motor neurons of the lower extremity and trunk to keep the body and head upright against gravity. The muscle tone of antigravity muscles tends to be higher than the tone of other muscle groups when a person has a neurological deficit, partly because of the stretch that gravity places on them and partly because of the increased effort required to stay upright.

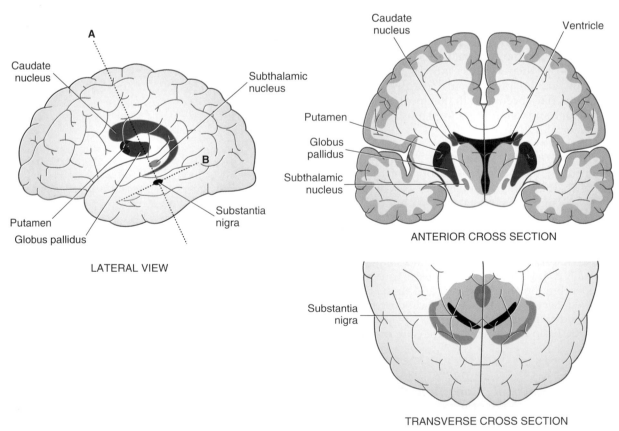

FIG 4-26 Basal ganglia within the brain: lateral and cross-sectional views.

The reticulospinal tracts (RSTs) transmit signals from the reticular system, which is a group of neuron cell bodies located in the central region of the brain stem, to the spinal cord. The **reticular-activating system** receives a rich supply of input from multiple sensory systems, including the vision, auditory, vestibular, and somatosensory systems, and the motor cortex. In addition, it receives input from the autonomic nervous system (ANS) and hypothalamus, reflecting the individual's emotions, motivation, and alertness. Muscle tone differences between someone who is slumped because of sadness or lethargy and someone who is happy and energetic is mediated through these tracts. The RSTs can also help regulate responses to reflexes according to the context of the current movement. For example, while walking, someone may step on a sharp object with the right foot, noticing it only as the left foot is leaving the ground. Instead of allowing the expected flexor withdrawal reflex on the right (which would cause the person to fall), the RSTs help increase input to the alpha motor neurons of extensor muscles on the right, momentarily permitting weight bearing on that sharp object until the left foot can be positioned to bear weight.

Limbic System. The **limbic system** influences movement and muscle tone via the RSTs and through connections with the basal ganglia. Circuits of neurons in the limbic system provide the ability to generate memories and attach meaning to them. Changes in muscle tone or activation can occur as a result of emotions recalled with particular memories of real or imagined events. For example, fear may heighten one's awareness when walking into a dark parking lot, activating the sympathetic nervous system (SNS) to start planning for fight or flight. The SNS activates the heart and lungs to work faster, dilates the pupils, and decreases the amount of blood pulsing through the internal organs, diverting that blood flow to the muscles. Muscle tone is increased to get ready to fight or flee from any potential danger in the parking lot. Muscle tone may further increase with a sudden unexpected noise but then decrease again to an almost limp state when the noise is quickly identified as two good friends approaching from behind. Patients may have similar changes in muscle tone with emotional responses to fears of falling or of increased pain.

SUMMARY OF NORMAL MUSCLE TONE

Muscle tone and muscle activation depend on the normal composition and functioning of the muscles, the PNS, and the CNS. Although both biomechanical and neural factors influence muscular responses, neural stimulation through the alpha motor neurons is the most powerful influence on both muscle tone and activation, especially when the muscle is in the midrange of its length. Multiple sources of neural input, both excitatory and inhibitory, are required for normal functioning of the alpha motor neurons (see Table 4-4). Ultimately, the sum of all the input determines the amount of muscle tone and activation.

The assumption in this section is that the body is intact. The motor units, with both the alpha motor neurons and the muscle fibers, are all functioning normally and receiving normal input from all sources. When pathology or injury affects the muscles, alpha motor neurons, or any of the sources of input to the alpha motor neurons, abnormalities in muscle tone and activation may result.

ABNORMAL MUSCLE TONE AND ITS CONSEQUENCES

Various injuries or pathologies can result in abnormal muscle tone, and some of these are considered in this section. An example, nerve root compression with its potential effects on muscle tone and function, is depicted in Fig. 4-27. When present, abnormal muscle tone is considered an impairment that may or may not lead to functional changes. Examination of muscle tone before and after an intervention can indicate the effectiveness of the intervention in reducing muscle tone or in changing its precipitating condition. Management decisions will depend on the role abnormal muscle tone plays in exacerbating limitations of function, activity, or participation or whether it is likely to result in future problems such as adverse shortening of soft tissue.

In this section, some consequences of muscle tone abnormalities are listed and rehabilitation interventions are discussed. The consequences of abnormal tone depend

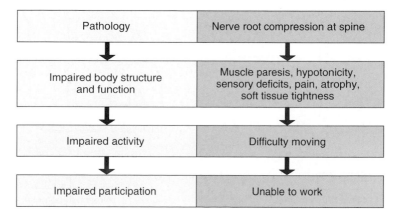

FIG 4-27 Example of the effect of pathology on body structure and function, activity, and participation.

on individual circumstances, and these must also be assessed when examining muscle tone. Circumstances could include any additional impairments the patient has and the psychological, physiological, and environmental resources available to the patient. A young, active, optimistic patient tends to have less severe functional limitations than an older, sedentary, depressed patient with the same degree of impairment. The results of intervention also depend on individual circumstances. Unfortunately for the study of muscle tone, research results generally focus on change in muscle activation or function rather than changes in muscle tone. The suggestions for interventions to influence abnormal muscle tone generally stem from clinical observations of immediate change that enhances subsequent muscle activation and functional training.

Although some muscle or motor endplate diseases may result in abnormal muscle tone, this discussion is limited to abnormalities of neurological origin. Observed changes in muscle tone may ultimately include both neural and biomechanical components, but any changes resulting from pathology of input to the nervous system depends on the remaining input available to that muscle's alpha motor neurons. The remaining input may include partial or aberrant information from sources damaged by the pathology, normal information from undamaged sources, and altered input from undamaged sources in response to the pathology. When an individual has a movement problem, he or she will use whatever resources are most available to solve it. For example, high muscle tone may be useful for some patients if increased quadriceps tone allows weight bearing on an otherwise weak leg.

LOW MUSCLE TONE

Abnormally low muscle tone, or hypotonicity, generally results from loss of normal alpha motor neuron input to otherwise normal muscle fibers.

> **◎ Clinical Pearl**
>
> Abnormally low muscle tone is usually caused by decreased neural stimulation of the muscles.

Losses may result from damage to the alpha motor neurons themselves, so that the related motor units cannot be activated. Loss of neural stimulation of the muscles may also result from conditions that either increase inhibitory input or decrease excitatory input to the alpha motor neurons (Fig. 4-28).

Hypotonicity means there is insufficient activation of the motor units to prepare for holding or movement. Consequences include (1) difficulty developing enough force to maintain posture or movement and (2) poor posture caused by frequent supporting of weight through taut ligaments, as in a hyperextended knee. Poor posture results in cosmetically undesirable changes in appearance, especially with a slumped spine or drooping facial muscles. Stretched ligaments can compromise joint integrity and lead to pain (Box 4-1).

Alpha Motor Neuron Damage

If alpha motor neurons are damaged, electrochemical impulses will not reach the muscle fibers of those motor units. If all the motor units of a muscle are involved, the muscle tone is flaccid and muscle activation is not possible; the muscle is paralyzed. Sometimes the term **flaccid paralysis** is used to describe such a muscle's tone and loss of activation. When disease or injury of the alpha motor neurons removes neuronal input from the muscle, **denervation** results. Denervation of a muscle or group of muscles may be whole or partial. Examples of processes that may result in symptoms of denervation include poliomyelitis, which affects the cell bodies; Guillain-Barré syndrome, which attacks the Schwann cells so that the axons

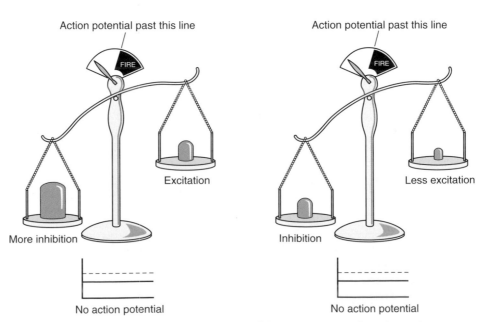

Action potential past this line

FIRE

Excitation

More inhibition

No action potential

Action potential past this line

FIRE

Less excitation

Inhibition

No action potential

FIG 4-28 Inhibition of alpha motor neuron: inhibitory input exceeds excitatory input.

are essentially demyelinated; crush or cutting types of trauma to the nerves; and nerve compression.

When poliomyelitis eliminates functioning alpha motor neurons, recovery is limited by the number of intact motor units remaining. Each remaining alpha motor neuron may increase the number of muscle fibers it innervates by increasing its number of axonal branches. This process is known as **rearborizing**. Intact neurons may thereby reinnervate muscle fibers that lost their innervation with the destruction of associated alpha motor neurons (Fig. 4-29). Such muscles would be expected to have larger-than-normal motor units, with more muscle fibers being innervated by a single alpha motor neuron.[44] Denervated muscle fibers that are not close enough to an intact alpha motor neuron for reinnervation will die, and loss of muscle bulk (atrophy) will occur. Maintaining the length and viability of the muscle fibers while potential rearborization takes place is advocated.[44,45]

Recovery after injury that cuts or compresses the axons of alpha motor neurons also includes the possibility of regrowth of the axons from an intact cell body, through any remaining myelin sheaths toward the muscle fibers.[23] Regrowth is slow, however, proceeding at a rate of 1 to 8 mm/day[45] and may not be able to continue if the distance is too far. Again, maintaining the viability of muscle fibers while regrowth takes place is advocated.[44] Recovery after Guillain-Barré syndrome depends both on remyelination of the axons, which can be fairly rapid, and on regrowth of any axons that were secondarily damaged during the demyelinated period.[46]

Rehabilitation After Alpha Motor Neuron Damage. Rehabilitation of patients with denervation includes interventions that help activate alpha motor neurons. In the past, electrical stimulation was used to facilitate muscle fiber viability while axons regrew or rearborized. Electrical stimulation (ES) for this purpose has become controversial, with evidence that the quiescence of denervated muscle may actually trigger regrowth of neurons (see Chapter 8). Alternative physical agents that are used after alpha motor neuron damage include hydrotherapy and quick ice.[37,47]

Hydrotherapy may be used to support the body or limbs and resist movement with ROM exercises in the water.[47] The combination of buoyancy and resistance can help strengthen remaining or returning musculature (see Chapter 9). Quick ice (see Chapter 6) or light touch on the skin over a particular muscle group adds excitatory input to any intact alpha motor neurons via cutaneous sensory neurons.[37]

| **BOX 4-1** | **Possible Consequences of Abnormally Low Muscle Tone** |

1. Difficulty developing adequate force output for normal posture and movement
   • Motor dysfunction
   • Secondary problems resulting from lack of movement (e.g., pressure sores, loss of cardiorespiratory endurance)
2. Poor posture
   • Reliance on ligaments to substitute for muscle holding—eventual stretching of ligaments, compromised joint integrity, pain
   • Cosmetically undesirable changes in appearance (e.g., slumping of spine, drooping of facial muscles)
   • Pain

◎ **Clinical Pearl**

Physical agents used for hypotonicity caused by alpha motor neuron damage include hydrotherapy and quick ice.

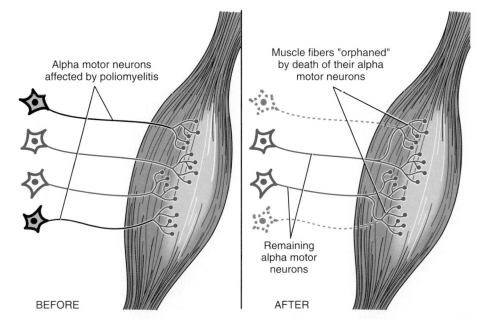

BEFORE   AFTER

FIG 4-29 Rearborization of remaining axons to innervate orphaned muscle fibers after polio eliminates some alpha motor neurons.

Other interventions include ROM exercise and therapeutic exercise to maintain muscle length and joint mobility and to strengthen the remaining musculature. Management also includes functional training that teaches patients to compensate for the movement losses they have experienced. Orthotic devices may be prescribed to support a limb for function while the muscle is flaccid or to protect the nerve from being overstretched.

Note that excitatory input to an alpha motor neuron that is not intact will be ineffective. The alpha motor neuron that is not intact cannot transmit information to its related muscle fibers, either to change tone or to contract voluntarily. Also, if alpha motor neurons are damaged in a cut or crush injury or by compression, local sensory neurons bringing information in the same nerve could also be damaged and unable to provide sensory input.

Insufficient Excitation of Alpha Motor Neurons

If pathology affects peripheral, spinal, or supraspinal sources of input to alpha motor neurons but does not affect the alpha motor neurons or muscle fibers themselves, hypotonicity may result. The alpha motor neurons may be stimulated to transmit information causing muscle fibers to contract if excitatory input can be raised to a higher level than inhibitory input. Any condition, however, that prohibits alpha motor neurons from receiving sufficient excitatory input to activate the muscle fibers will result in decreased muscle tone.

Altered Peripheral Input: Immobilization. One condition that alters peripheral sources of input to the alpha motor neuron is the application of a cast to maintain a position during fracture healing. The cast applies a fairly constant stimulus to cutaneous receptors but inhibits reception of the variety of cutaneous input ordinarily encountered. The cast also inhibits movement at one or more joints, restricting lengthening or shortening of the local muscles. Alpha motor neurons are thus deprived of normal alterations in muscle spindle, GTO, or joint receptor input. When the cast is removed, the result is typically a measurable loss of strength in the muscles and a loss of ROM in the joints. Muscle tone is also affected, with decreased activation of the motor units and increased biomechanical stiffness. Because the neural and biomechanical components of muscle tone counter one another in this case, the actual change in resistance to passive stretch must be carefully assessed. The known effects of immobilization in decreasing muscle tone have been used deliberately to lower hypertonicity in severe cases.[48]

Altered Supraspinal Input: Stroke or Head Injury. Supraspinal input to the alpha motor neurons may be affected by loss of blood supply or direct injury to cortical or subcortical neurons, as occurs with stroke or head injury. The resulting muscle tone changes depend on the remaining proportion of excitatory and inhibitory input to the alpha motor neurons. For example, if all of the descending tracts are destroyed, volitional movement and muscle tone may be lost in the associated muscles.

However, few if any pathologies affect all tracts equally, so most of the alpha motor neuron groups will not lose all descending input. Those alpha motor neurons with loss of any descending input must adapt to a new proportion of excitatory and inhibitory input. The usual progression from flaccidity to increased tone after a stroke[40] may be a result of adaptation to new levels of inhibitory and excitatory input.

The prediction of muscle tone changes in a particular individual after a stroke is complicated by the fact that lesions within the supraspinal areas do not always completely eliminate the corticospinal tract. The portion of the tract that remains can still be used to signal voluntary movement. In addition, although most of the fibers of the corticospinal tract cross to synapse on the opposite side of the body, some of the fibers do not cross. Therefore, even if all of one corticospinal tract is destroyed, some fibers of the opposite corticospinal tract may provide enough input to alpha motor neurons for the tone in some of the muscles to remain relatively normal.

Rehabilitation to Increase Muscle Tone. Physical agents are not often used for the rehabilitation of patients who have had a stroke, head injury, or other supraspinal lesions, particularly addressing hypotonicity. However, they can be a valuable adjunct to the therapeutic exercises, orthotics, and functional training of traditional neurorehabilitation.[6,40] ES, hydrotherapy, and quick ice may all be used in this context.[37]

◎ **Clinical Pearl**

Physical agents used for hypotonicity caused by decreased input to the alpha motor neuron include ES, hydrotherapy, and quick ice.

The intent of any of these is to affect the alpha motor neurons via the remaining intact peripheral, spinal, and supraspinal sources of input. Quick icing and tapping, for example, are facilitative techniques that can increase tone via cutaneous and muscle spindle receptors, respectively, and when paired with voluntary movement, can increase functional motor output. ES might be combined with resistance of the muscle being stimulated or of synergistic muscles to increase tone and activation via interneurons of the spinal cord. Many authors have described in detail the options available to the rehabilitation specialist for increasing muscle tone and motor output in patients who have had a stroke or head injury.[6,37,40,49,50] Box 4-2 summarizes management options to increase low muscle tone and improve functional activation.

HIGH MUSCLE TONE

Many pathological conditions result in abnormally high muscle tone. Any of the supraspinal lesions mentioned in the previous section could ultimately result in hypertonicity, even though they begin with some form of low muscle tone. Only the loss of alpha motor neurons will cause hypotonicity; lesions affecting only the alpha motor

BOX 4-2	Interventions for Low Muscle Tone

- Hydrotherapy
- Quick ice
- Electrical stimulation (when muscle fibers are innervated)
- Biofeedback
- Light touch
- Tapping
- Resistive exercises
- Range-of-motion exercises
- Therapeutic exercises
- Functional training
- Orthotics

BOX 4-3	Possible Consequences of Abnormally High Muscle Tone

- Discomfort or pain from muscle spasms
- Contractures
- Abnormal posture
- Skin breakdown
- Increased effort by caregivers to assist with bathing, dressing, transfers
- Development of stereotyped movement patterns that may inhibit development of movement alternatives
- May inhibit function

neurons do not cause hypertonicity. Hypertonicity is a result of abnormally high excitatory input compared to the inhibitory input to an otherwise intact alpha motor neuron (see Fig. 4-19).

Researchers have argued about the effects of hypertonicity, particularly spasticity, on function. Some have pointed out that spasticity of the antagonist does not necessarily interfere with voluntary movement of the agonist.[5,51] During walking, for example, it has been assumed that spasticity in the ankle plantar flexors prevents adequate dorsiflexion during the swing phase of gait, resulting in toe drag. However, EMG studies of patients with hypertonicity have shown essentially absent activity in the plantar flexors during swing, as in normal gait.[8] Another study of upper extremity function found deficits resulting from inadequate recruitment of the agonists, not by increased activity in the spastic antagonist muscles.[52] Instead, voluntary movement is hindered by slowed and inadequate recruitment of the agonist and delayed termination of agonist contraction.[5] In addition, hypertonicity in patients with CNS lesions can be caused by biomechanical changes within the muscles, as well as by inappropriate activation of muscles as a result of the CNS dysfunction.[53]

On the other side of the argument, some researchers have shown that coactivation of spastic antagonists increases with faster movements, substantiating the claim that abnormal activation inhibits voluntary motor control.[54] Additionally, a review of multiple drug studies has revealed improved function in 60% to 70% of patients receiving intrathecally administered baclofen, a drug that reduces spasticity. The authors state that "spasticity reduction can be associated with improved voluntary movement," although it is also possible that a decrease in tone will have no measurable effect or even a negative effect on function.[55]

Because of this controversy, it cannot be stated unequivocally that hypertonicity itself inhibits voluntary movement. However, other effects of hypertonicity must not be ignored. These include the potential for (1) muscle spasms that contribute to discomfort; (2) contractures (shortened resting length) or other soft tissue changes caused by hypertonicity in a muscle group on one side of a joint; (3) abnormal postures that can lead to skin breakdown or pressure ulcers; (4) resistance to passive movement of a nonfunctioning limb that results in difficulties with assisted dressing, transfers, hygiene, and other activities; and (5) possibly a stereotyped movement pattern that could inhibit alternative movement solutions (Box 4-3).

Pain, Cold, and Stress

Pain is an example of a peripheral source of input that can lead to hypertonicity. Cutaneous reception of painful stimuli and the consequent withdrawal and crossed-extension reflexes have already been discussed. Painful stimuli to the muscles or joints can result in increased muscle tension in the muscles around the painful area, although not necessarily in the muscle in which the pain originates, which may show no heightened EMG activity.[1] The build-up of muscle tension may manifest as muscle spasms in the paraspinal musculature of a person with back pain, for example. Such muscle spasms are called **guarding** and are thought to be a way to avoid further pain. Guarding probably has a supraspinal, as well as a peripheral, component because the emotions and thus the limbic system are so heavily involved in the interpretation of and response to pain.

The human body also responds to cold via peripheral and supraspinal systems. When homeostasis is threatened, muscle tone increases and the body may begin to shiver. Muscle tone also tends to increase with other threats, registered as stress. Hypertonicity may be palpable in various muscle groups, such as those in the shoulders and neck, when an individual registers more general pain or perceives a situation as threatening to the body or to self-esteem. The muscles prepare for fight or flight as the rest of the body engages in other SNS responses.

Managing Hypertonicity as a Result of Pain, Cold, or Stress. Patients with hypertonicity resulting from pain, cold, or stress can be managed in several ways. The first and most effective measure is to remove the source of the hypertonicity, including eliminating biomechanical causes of pain, warming the patient, and alleviating stress. When these measures are not possible, not applicable, or otherwise ineffective, management to decrease muscle tone may include education in relaxation techniques, EMG biofeedback, the use of neutral warmth or heat (see Chapter 6), hydrotherapy (see Chapter 9), or cold after painful stimuli.

Spinal Cord Injury

After a complete spinal cord injury (SCI), the alpha motor neurons below the level of the lesion lack both inhibitory and excitatory input from supraspinal sources. They still receive input from propriospinal and other neurons below the level of the lesion. Immediately after the injury, however, the nervous system is typically in a state called spinal shock, in which the nerves shut down at and below the level of the injury. The condition may last for hours or weeks and is marked by the flaccid tone of the affected muscles and the loss of spinal level reflex activity such as the muscle stretch reflex. When spinal shock resolves, the lack of inhibitory input from supraspinal areas as a result of the SCI allows alpha motor neurons below the level of the injury to respond especially easily to muscle spindle, GTO, or cutaneous input. The hypertonicity thus apparent is known as spasticity because quick stretch elicits greater resistance than slow stretch.

Quick stretch may occur not only when the muscles are specifically tested for tone but also whenever the patient moves and gravity suddenly exerts a different pull on the muscles, depending on the mass of the limb. For example, a patient who has a complete thoracic level injury may use his arms to pick up his legs and place his feet on the foot pedals of his wheelchair. When the leg is lifted, the foot hangs down with the ankle plantarflexed. When the leg is placed, the weight lands on the ball of the foot and the ankle moves passively into relative dorsiflexion. If the foot placement is quick, the plantar flexors are quickly stretched and clonus may be seen.

Frequently, the hypertonicity is greater on one side of a joint than on the other because the force of gravity is unidirectional on the mass of a limb. Because the patient with a complete SCI has no active movement that can counter the hypertonicity, muscle shortening tends to occur in the muscles that are relatively more hypertonic. The biomechanical stiffness of the hypertonic muscles thus increases, and contractures can develop. Such contractures can inhibit functions such as dressing, transfers, and positioning for pressure relief.

Managing Hypertonicity After Spinal Cord Injury. Selective ROM exercises,[56,57] prolonged stretch,[37] positioning or orthotics to maintain functional muscle length, local or systemic medications, and surgery[57] have been used to counter either hypertonicity or contractures that interfere with function after SCI. Heat could be used before stretching of shortened muscles (see Chapter 6), but it must be carefully monitored because of the patient's decreased or absent sensation below the level of the SCI. Other locally applied tone-inhibiting therapies, such as prolonged icing, could theoretically alleviate hypertonicity in patients with SCI. However, research is lacking either to confirm or to reject the usefulness of these agents in this population. Functional electrical stimulation (FES) has also been used to increase the function of paretic muscles in this population (see Chapter 8) but not for changing muscle tone.

Patients with SCI may also have muscle spasms generally attributable to painful stimuli, except that patients may be unaware of the pain because sensory signals arising from below the level of the injury do not reach the cerebral cortex. Muscle spasms may also be caused by visceral stimuli such as a urinary tract infection, distended bladder, or some other internal irritation.[57] Identification and removal of the painful stimuli are the first steps in alleviating muscle spasms. When muscle spasms are persistent, frequent, or inhibit function and are without identifiable and removable causes, systemic or locally injected medications are sometimes prescribed to alleviate them.[57] Careful evaluation of the source of a muscle spasm must occur before any physical agent or other intervention is applied.

Cerebral Lesions

CNS lesions from cerebral vascular disorders (stroke), cerebral palsy, tumors, CNS infection, or head injury may result in hypertonicity. In addition, conditions that affect transmission of neural impulses in the CNS, such as multiple sclerosis (MS), can result in hypertonicity. Hypertonicity in patients after all of these pathologies results from a change in input to alpha motor neurons (see Fig. 4-19). The extent of the pathology determines whether many muscle groups are affected or only a few and whether alpha motor neurons to a particular muscle group lose all or only some of a particular source of supraspinal input.

Hypertonicity: Primary Impairment or Adaptive Response? The neurophysiological mechanism of hypertonicity is in some dispute. Various management approaches address hypertonicity based on assumptions about its significance. In one approach, developed by Bobath,[6] the nervous system is assumed to function as a hierarchy in which the supraspinal centers control the spinal centers of movement and "abnormal tonus" results from loss of inhibitory control from higher centers. The resultant therapeutic sequence is to normalize the hypertonicity before facilitating normal movement. In another approach, the task-oriented approach, which is based on a systems model of the nervous system, the primary goal of the nervous system in producing movement is to accomplish the desired task.[58] After a lesion develops, the nervous system uses its remaining resources to perform movement tasks. Hypertonicity may be the best adaptive response the nervous system can make given its available resources after injury rather than a primary result of the injury itself.

An example of task-oriented reasoning is as follows: patients with paresis are sometimes able to use trunk and lower extremity extensor hypertonicity to hold an upright posture. In this case, hypertonicity is an adaptive response to accomplish the task of maintaining an upright posture.[58,59] Eliminating the hypertonicity in such a case would decrease function unless concurrent increases in controlled voluntary movement are elicited. On the other hand, controlled movement is always preferable to hypertonicity if it can be elicited. Control implies the ability to make changes in a response according to environmental demands, whereas the hypertonic extensor response mentioned previously is relatively stereotyped. The use of a

stereotyped hypertonic response for function seems to block spontaneous development of more normal control.[6,60]

Evidence that hypertonicity may be an adaptive response includes the fact that it is not an immediate sequela of injury but instead develops over time. After a cortical stroke, recovery of muscle tone and voluntary movement follows a fairly predictable course.[40,48] At first, muscles are flaccid and paralyzed on the side of the body opposite the lesion, without elicitable stretch reflexes. The next stage of recovery is characterized by increasing response of the muscles to quick stretch and the beginning of voluntary motor output that is limited to movement in flexor or extensor patterns called synergies. Because muscle tone and synergy patterns of movement appear at approximately the same time, clinicians tend to equate the two, but spasticity and synergy are distinct from each other (see Table 4-1). Further recovery stages include progression to full-blown spasticity and ultimately the gradual normalization of muscle tone. At the same time, voluntary movement shows full-blown synergy dependence, progressing to the mixing of synergies, and finally resolving in controlled movement of isolated musculature.[40] A particular patient's course of recovery may stall, skip, or plateau anywhere along the way, but it does not regress. An argument against spasticity as an adaptive response is that changes in muscle tone in patients with complete SCI occur without any supraspinal input, so no cerebral adaptation to motor task requirements can be occurring, at least in this population.[53]

Managing Hypertonicity After Stroke. Rehabilitation to address hypertonicity after a stroke depends on whether the clinician believes that hypertonicity inhibits function or is a product of adaptive motor control. In either case, the emphasis is on return of independent function, whether that necessitates tone reduction or the reeducation of controlled voluntary movement patterns.

Management to reduce hypertonicity after a stroke could include prolonged icing, inhibitory pressure, prolonged stretch,[37] inhibitory casting,[61] or positioning. Biofeedback and task training can improve passive ROM, thus addressing biomechanical components of hypertonicity.[62] Reeducation of controlled voluntary movement patterns could include weight bearing to facilitate normal postural responses or training with directed practice of functional movement patterns.[49] Reduction of hypertonicity may be a product of improved motor control in the following example. If a patient feels insecure standing upright, muscle tone will increase commensurate with the anxiety level. If balance and motor control are improved so that the patient feels more confident in the upright position, hypertonicity will also be reduced.[49] Positioning for comfort and to reduce anxiety is a critical adjunct to any intervention intended to reduce muscle tone.

Knott and Voss describe a twofold approach to decreasing tone of a particular muscle group.[39] Muscles can be approached directly, with verbal cues to relax or application of cold towels to elicit muscle relaxation. Alternatively, muscles can be approached indirectly, by stimulating the antagonists, which results in reciprocal inhibition of agonists and lowers agonist muscle tone. Antagonists can be stimulated with resisted exercise or electrical stimulation (see Chapter 8).

If a patient has severe hypertonicity or if many muscle groups are affected, techniques that influence the ANS to decrease arousal or calm the individual generally might be used. Such techniques include soft lighting or music, slow rocking, neutral warmth, slow stroking, maintained touch,[37] rotation of the trunk, or hydrotherapy (see Chapter 9), as long as the patient feels safely supported. For example, hydrotherapy in a cool water pool is particularly advocated for patients with MS to reduce spasticity.[39] Stretching and cold packs are also of benefit in temporarily reducing the spasticity of MS, but they lack hydrotherapy's added benefit of allowing gentle ROM exercises with a diminished pull of gravity.[59]

Rigidity: a Consequence of Central Nervous System Pathology. Some cerebral lesions are associated with rigidity rather than spasticity. Head injuries, for example, may result in one of two specific patterns of rigidity that may be either constant or intermittent. Both patterns include hypertonicity in the neck and back extensors; the hip extensors, adductors, and internal rotators; the knee extensors; and the ankle plantar flexors and invertors. The elbows are held rigidly at the sides, with the wrists and fingers flexed in both patterns, but in decorticate rigidity the elbows are flexed and in decerebrate rigidity they are extended (Fig. 4-30). The two types of posture are thought to indicate the level of the lesion: above (decorticate) or below (decerebrate) the red nucleus in the brain stem. In most patients with head injury, however, the lesion is diffuse and this designation is not helpful. Two positioning principles can diminish rigidity in either case and

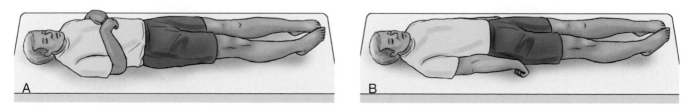

FIG 4-30 **A,** Decorticate posture. **B,** Decerebrate posture.

should be considered along with any other therapies: (1) reposition the patient in postures opposite to those listed, with emphasis on slight neck and trunk flexion and hip flexion past 90 degrees, and (2) avoid the supine position, which promotes extension in the trunk and limbs via the symmetrical tonic labyrinthine response (see Fig. 4-7).

Rigidity, like spasticity, can result in biomechanical muscle stiffness after sustained placement in the shortened position. The longer the period of time without ROM exercises or positioning to elongate a muscle group, the greater the biomechanical changes that occur. Prevention is the best cure for biomechanical components of hypertonicity, but orthotics[63] or serial casting[61] have also been useful in reducing the muscle stiffness related to hypertonicity. Heat may be used to increase ROM temporarily before applying a cast or orthotic.

Parkinson's disease typically causes rigidity throughout the skeletal musculature rather than just of the extensors. In addition to pharmacological replacement of dopamine,[64] management can include temporary reduction of hypertonicity through heat and other general inhibiting techniques to allow patients to accomplish particular functions. Table 4-5 summarizes management suggestions to decrease high muscle tone.

FLUCTUATING MUSCLE TONE

Commonly, pathology of the basal ganglia results in disorders of muscle tone and activation. Not only is voluntary motor output difficult to initiate, execute, and control, but the variations in muscle tone seen in this population can be so extreme as to be visible with movement. The resting tremor of a patient with Parkinson's disease is an example of fluctuating tone that results in involuntary movement. A child with athetoid-type cerebral palsy, for whom movement is a series of involuntary writhings, also demonstrates fluctuating tone.

When an individual has fluctuating tone that moves the limbs through large ROMs, contractures are usually not a problem, but inadvertent self-inflicted injuries sometimes occur. As a hand or foot flails around, it will sometimes run into a hard, immovable object. Patients and caregivers can be educated to alter the environment, padding necessary objects or removing unnecessary ones to avoid harm. If the fluctuating tone does not result in movement of large amplitude, then positioning and ROM interventions should be considered. Neutral warmth has been advocated to reduce excessive movement resulting from muscle tone fluctuations in athetosis.[41]

TABLE 4-5	Interventions for High Muscle Tone
High Muscle Tone Association	**Interventions**
Pain, cold, or stress	Remove the source: • Eliminate pain • Warm the patient • Alleviate stress Relaxation techniques EMG biofeedback Neutral warmth Heat Hydrotherapy Cold towels Stimulation of antagonists • Resisted exercise • Electrical stimulation
Spinal cord injury	Selective ROM exercises Prolonged stretch Positioning Orthotics Medication Surgery Heat Prolonged ice
Cerebral lesions	Prolonged ice Inhibitory pressure Prolonged stretch Inhibitory casting Positioning Reeducation of voluntary movement patterns Stimulation of antagonists • Resisted exercise • Electrical stimulation General relaxation techniques • Soft lighting or music • Slow rocking • Neutral warmth • Slow stroking • Maintained touch • Rotation of the trunk • Hydrotherapy
Rigidity	Positioning ROM exercises Orthotics Serial casting after head injury Heat Medication General relaxation techniques (as listed above)

EMG, Electromyography; *ROM*, range of motion.

CLINICAL CASE STUDIES

The following case studies summarize the concepts of tone abnormalities discussed in this chapter and are not intended to be exhaustive. Based on the scenarios presented, an evaluation of the clinical findings and goals of management are proposed. These are followed by a discussion of the factors to be considered in intervention selection. Note that any technique used to alter tone abnormalities must be followed with functional use of the musculature involved if the patient is to improve the ability to hold or move.

CASE STUDY 4-1

Bell's Palsy
Examination
History
GM is a 37-year-old businessman who states that the first signs of his Bell's palsy appeared 2 days ago after a long airplane flight when he slept with his head against the window. He had a cold and in addition to drooping on the left side of his face, he is having trouble controlling saliva and eating properly because he cannot close his lips. GM states that the left side of his face feels as though it is being pulled downward. He is concerned that this may not go away and it may impact his ability to interact with others in his business.

Tests and Measures
On examination, a noticeable droop is visible on the left side of his face, and he is unable to close his lips or his left eye tightly. The left corneal reflex is absent.

What is the muscle tone in the left facial muscles? What techniques would be appropriate for changing the tone for this patient?

Evaluation, Diagnosis, Prognosis, and Goals
Evaluation and Goals

ICF Level	Current Status	Goals
Body structure and function	Left facial hypotonicity	Prevent overstretching of soft tissues Protect left eye Strengthen facial muscles as reinnervation occurs in 1 to 3 months
Activity	Unable to close lips and eat normally	Normalize function of lips
Participation	Difficulty conducting normal business transactions	Return to normal business activity

Diagnosis
Preferred Practice Pattern 5D: Impaired motor function and sensory integrity associated with nonprogressive disorders of the central nervous system—acquired in adolescence or adulthood.

Prognosis/Plan of Care
Bell's palsy is any disorder of the facial nerve, usually only on one side, with varied etiologies. The sudden onset of GM's symptoms may have been instigated by the chilling of the side of his face while on the airplane or by his cold virus. If the entire facial nerve is affected on the left, then none of the muscle fibers on the left side of the face will be able to receive signals from any alpha motor neurons, and the muscles will be flaccid. If the facial nerve is only partially affected, then some muscles might be hypotonic. Fortunately, reinnervation of the muscle fibers is common after a facial palsy, usually within 1 to 3 months. Muscle tone can be expected to normalize as reinnervation occurs if the muscle and connective tissues have been maintained so that secondary biomechanical changes do not interfere.

Intervention
Gentle passive movement of the facial musculature may be indicated to counter soft tissue changes resulting from lack of active movement. Otherwise, GM may be left with a cosmetically unacceptable facial droop when the muscles are reinnervated. A patch or other form of protection over the left eye may be required to prevent eye injury while the motor component of the corneal reflex is paralyzed. As the muscle fibers are reinnervated, the emphasis will be on exercises to elicit voluntary contraction rather than on improving muscle tone. Quick icing or light touch on the skin over a particular muscle that is beginning to be innervated may help GM isolate a muscle to move it voluntarily. Practice of facial movements while looking in a mirror may provide extra feedback for GM as he is attempting to reestablish normal activation of the facial muscles. ES with biofeedback may be used to help GM resume function once muscles are reinnervated.

CASE STUDY 4-2

Arthritic Hip Damage
Examination
History
EL is a 42-year-old woman with severe arthritic damage in her right hip. She has had abnormal use of her right leg for almost her entire life, after a case of polio when she was an infant. Several surgeries in childhood to stabilize the foot and to transfer a hamstring tendon anteriorly to function for the quadriceps allowed her independent ambulation, but her limp worsened over the last several years. When the head of the femur slipped out of the acetabulum and moved farther up toward her trunk, EL's right leg became several inches shorter than the left and she walked on her right toes. After a successful total hip replacement to even the leg lengths, EL is now learning to walk again. Her gait training has been more complex than is typical after total hip replacement

Continued

surgery because of her prior condition. She currently relies on a friend to do her grocery shopping, moves around her house with a wheelchair, and needs assistance with transfers.

Tests and Measures

The patient has an incision site over her right lateral hip covered by a bandage, and the area is mildly tender to palpation, with no erythema. The patient rates her right hip pain 5/10. During supine passive ROM of the right leg (within the limits allowed by her postoperative total hip precautions), the ankle plantar flexors resist stretch. Passive right ankle flexion reveals resistance in the middle of the available range and tone is 3+. Her right hip and knee move easily but the leg feels heavy. Right hip flexor and knee extensor tone is 1+.

Based on the information presented, how should EL's muscle tone be described in the hip flexors? The knee extensors? The ankle plantar flexors? What intervention techniques would be appropriate to alter the muscle tone labeled in the preceding question?

Evaluation, Diagnosis, Prognosis, and Goals
Evaluation and Goals

ICF Level	Current Status	Goals
Body structure and function	Right hip pain Right lateral hip incision Limited right LE ROM	Decrease pain Facilitate incision healing Improve right LE ROM, especially ankle flexion
Activity	Unable to walk and transfer without assistance	Transfer independently Ambulate independently
Participation	Difficulty performing daily activities such as grocery shopping	Return to performing all usual daily activities

Diagnosis

Preferred Practice Patterns 4H: Impaired joint mobility, motor function, muscle performance and range of motion associated with joint arthroplasty; or 5G: Impaired motor function and sensory integrity associated with acute or chronic polyneuropathies.

Prognosis/Plan of Care

The quadriceps muscle was presumably affected by the polio because the hamstring tendon was transferred many years ago. The quadriceps would have been hypotonic after loss of the affected alpha motor neurons: no activation would have been possible via those neurons, either for passive resistance to stretch or for voluntary contraction. EL's present knee extensor, the hamstring muscle, will probably exhibit normal tone once the hip heals further and pain resolves.

Having no information about EL's muscle tone or strength before the total hip replacement surgery, the clinician must palpate for activation of the muscles during voluntary contraction. EMG testing of the quadriceps, hip flexors, ankle plantar flexors, and hamstrings may also provide information about the number and size of active motor units in each muscle group. Such information could differentiate between muscles that were more or less affected by poliomyelitis. Muscles that were more affected do not have the same capacity for motor unit recruitment during strength training as muscles that were less affected. The goals for strengthening would be reduced in muscles that were more affected.

Intervention

Pain control could be accomplished with physical agents, soft tissue mobilization, and positioning. (See Chapter 6 for instructions on the use of heat or cold or Chapter 8 for instructions on the use of electrical stimulation.) Gait training and functional training with appropriate feedback and practice will be necessary. Gait training in a pool will take advantage of buoyancy and the resistance the water provides against movement and could begin as soon as the surgical incision is well healed (see Chapter 9). The hypotonicity is expected to become less apparent as EL is better able to contract at will.

Management of the ankle plantar flexors must include prolonged stretch, preferably with prior heat or thermal-level ultrasound (see Chapters 6 and 7) for soft tissue remodeling. Stretch could be accomplished with exercise or weight bearing on the whole foot. Some would advocate serial casting if functional dorsiflexion ROM cannot be obtained in any other way.

CASE STUDY 4-3

Intermittent Low Back Pain
Examination
History

SP is a 24-year-old woman who has had intermittent back pain over the last several months. The pain began when her lifestyle changed from that of an athlete training regularly to that of a student sitting for long periods. The pain in her lower back increased dramatically yesterday while she was bowling for the first time in 2 years. The pain is exacerbated by movement and long periods of sitting and alleviated somewhat by ibuprofen and ice. SP is distressed because she has been unable to study for her final examinations because of pain.

Tests and Measures

The patient rates her pain as 8/10. She has palpable muscle spasm in the paraspinal muscles at the lumbar level. Spinal ROM is limited in all directions because of pain.

What is the underlying stimulus causing the muscle spasm? What intervention is appropriate to alleviate the spasm?

Evaluation, Diagnosis, Prognosis, and Goals
Evaluation and Goals

ICF Level	Current Status	Goals
Body structure and function	Low back pain Lumbar paraspinal muscle spasm Limited spinal ROM	Identify and remove painful stimulus Alleviate muscle spasm Regain normal spinal ROM
Activity	Limited movement Unable to sit for prolonged periods	Return to normal movement Regain ability to sit for at least 1 hour at a time
Participation	Unable to study for examinations	Return to studies

Diagnosis

Preferred Practice Patterns 4D: Impaired joint mobility, motor function, muscle performance, and range of motion associated with connective tissue dysfunction; 4E: Impaired joint mobility, motor function, muscle performance, and range of motion associated with localized inflammation; 4F: Impaired joint mobility, motor function, muscle performance, range of motion, and reflex integrity associated with spinal disorders; 4B: Impaired posture.

Prognosis/Plan of Care

Muscle spasms typically originate from painful stimuli, even if the stimuli are subtle. Possible stimuli in SP's case include injury to muscle fibers or other tissue while engaging in vigorous but unaccustomed activity, pain signals from a facet joint, or nerve root irritation. The consequent tension in surrounding muscles may hold or splint the injured area to avoid local movement that could irritate and exacerbate the pain. If persistent, the muscle spasm itself can contribute to the pain and discomfort by inhibiting local circulation and setting up its own painful feedback loop.

Intervention

Diagnosing the source of the painful stimulus is beyond the scope of this chapter, but many texts are devoted to the subject.[65-67] Once stimulus identification and removal occurs, the muscle spasm may diminish by itself or it may require separate intervention. Heat, ultrasound, or massage can increase local circulation (see Chapters 6 and 7). Prolonged icing, neutral warmth, or slow stroking could be used to diminish the hypertonicity directly and thus allow restoration of more normal local circulation. Once the painful feedback loop of the muscle spasm is broken, patient education is necessary. Education should include instructions on strengthening of local musculature and avoidance of postures and movements that aggravate the initial injury. Other stretching and strengthening exercises have been identified but will not be discussed in this text.

Recent Stroke
Examination
History

RB is a 74-year-old man who recently had a stroke. He initially had left hemiplegia, which has progressed from an initial flaccid paralysis to his current status of hypertonicity in the biceps brachii and ankle plantar flexors. He has little control of movement on the left side of his body and requires assistance with movement in bed and transfers. He is able to stand with assistance but has difficulty maintaining his balance or taking steps with a quad-cane. He is highly motivated to regain function and spend time with his several grandchildren.

Tests and Measures

During clinical observation, RB rests his left forearm in his lap while sitting with his back supported, but with standing, RB gravity quick stretches his biceps once the weight of his forearm is unsupported, and the left elbow flexes to approximately 80 degrees. During bed mobility, transfers, or standing, full elbow extension is never observed. His left ankle bounces with plantar flexion clonus when he first stands up, ending with weight mostly on the ball of his foot unless care is taken to position the foot before standing to facilitate weight bearing through the heel.

On examination, RB has a hyperactive stretch reflex in both the left biceps and the triceps, but muscle tone in the triceps is hypotonic, with a 1+ on the clinical tone scale. The left biceps and plantar flexors are a 1+ on the Modified Ashworth Scale, equal to a 3+ on the clinical tone scale. During quick stretch of the left plantar flexors, clonus was apparent, lasting for three beats. When asked to lift his left arm, he is unable to do so without elevating and retracting his scapula, abducting and externally rotating his shoulder, and flexing and supinating at the elbow, all consistent with a flexor synergy. When standing, he tends to rotate internally and adduct his left hip, with a retracted pelvis and a hyperextended knee, consistent with the lower extremity extensor synergy pattern.

What measures of muscle tone are appropriate in evaluating RB? What intervention is appropriate considering RB's hypertonicity?

Continued

CLINICAL CASE STUDIES—*cont'd*

Evaluation, Diagnosis, Prognosis, and Goals

Evaluation and Goals

ICF Level	Current Status	Goals
Body structure and function	Changes in muscle tone on the left side	Improve muscle tone
Activity	Abnormal voluntary movement of left upper extremity and left lower extremity Unable to stand without assistance	Regain ability to move voluntarily Able to stand independently
Participation	Cannot play with grandchildren	Return to playing with grandchildren

Diagnosis

Preferred Practice Pattern 5D: Impaired motor function and sensory integrity associated with nonprogressive disorders of the central nervous system—acquired in adolescence or adulthood.

Prognosis/Plan of Care

Goals are focused on improving RB's function and preventing secondary problems. Other possible tests for RB's muscle tone include the pendulum test for the biceps, a dynamometer or myometer test for the plantar flexors, or EMG studies to compare muscle activity on the two sides of RB's body. These quantitative measures would be especially useful for research that requires more precise measurement than the qualitative measures described previously.

Intervention

Appropriate interventions for RB may come from multiple sources and theoretical backgrounds. Only a few techniques that influence muscle tone are discussed here. Prolonged stretch of the biceps or the plantar flexors may be incorporated into functional activities like standing or weight bearing on the hand to normalize muscle tone. Prolonged icing (see Chapter 6) may be added if soft tissue shortening is inhibiting full passive ROM. Exercises to facilitate activity of the antagonists to inhibit the biceps or plantar flexors may be used. Electrical stimulation of the triceps and dorsiflexors would have the dual benefit of inhibiting hypertonic musculature and strengthening muscles that are currently weak (see Chapter 8). EMG biofeedback might be used during a specific task to train RB in more appropriate activation patterns for the biceps or plantar flexors.

The hypertonicity increase seen during standing could be alleviated with techniques to increase RB's alignment, balance, and confidence while standing. If he is better able to relax in this posture, his muscle tone will decrease as well. Discussion of specific therapeutic exercises to enhance RB's balance is beyond the scope of this chapter.

CHAPTER REVIEW

1. Muscle tone is a muscle's passive resistance to stretch. This resistance is affected by neural, biomechanical, and chemical phenomena. Neural input involves subconscious or involuntary activation of motor units via alpha motor neurons. Biomechanical properties of muscle that affect muscle tone include the stiffness of the muscle and surrounding connective tissue. Biochemical changes, such as those caused by inflammation, may also affect muscle tone.

2. Normal muscle tone and activation depend on normal functioning of the muscles, the PNS, and the CNS. The neural component of muscle tone is a result of input from peripheral, spinal, and supraspinal neurons. The summation of their excitatory and inhibitory signals determines whether an alpha motor neuron will send a signal to the muscle to contract or to increase tone.

3. Neurally mediated tone abnormalities (hypotonicity, hypertonicity, and fluctuating tone) result from abnormal inhibitory or excitatory input to the alpha motor neuron. Abnormal input may occur as a result of pathologies that affect either the alpha motor neuron itself or input to the alpha motor neuron.

4. Hypotonicity is low muscle tone. For patients with hypotonicity, rehabilitation interventions are directed to increase tone to promote easier activation of muscles, improve posture, and restore an acceptable cosmetic appearance. Physical agents that may be used to assist with this include hydrotherapy and quick ice.

5. Hypertonicity is high muscle tone. For patients with hypertonicity, rehabilitation interventions are often directed to decreasing tone to decrease discomfort, increase ROM, allow normal positioning, and prevent contractures. Physical agents used to achieve these goals include heat, prolonged ice, hydrotherapy, biofeedback, and ES.

6. For patients with fluctuating muscle tone, rehabilitation interventions are directed to normalizing tone to maximize function and prevent injuries.

7. The reader is referred to the Evolve web site for further exercises and links to resources and references.

ADDITIONAL RESOURCES *evolve*

Web Sites

American Stroke Association: The goal of this organization, a division of the American Heart Association, is to reduce the incidence of strokes. The web site includes information on warning signs of stroke, what to expect after a stroke, how to prevent strokes, and terminology and information for health care professionals. www.strokeassociation.org

GLOSSARY *evolve*

Actin: A cellular protein found in myofilaments that participates in muscle contraction, cellular movement, and maintenance of cell shape.

Action potential: A momentary change in electrical potential between the inside of a nerve cell and the extracellular medium that occurs in response to a stimulus and transmits along the axon.

Akinesia: A lack of movement that may be permanent or intermittent.

Alpha motor neuron: A nerve cell that stimulates muscle cells to contract.

Alpha-gamma coactivation: The activation of gamma motor neurons at the same time as alpha motor neurons during voluntary movement. Alpha-gamma coactivation sensitizes the muscle spindle to changes in muscle length.

Anterior horn cell: Another term for alpha motor neuron; named because the cell's body is located in the anterior horn of the spinal cord.

Athetoid movements: A type of dyskinesia that consists of wormlike writhing movements.

Autogenic inhibition: The mechanism by which type Ib sensory fibers from the Golgi tendon organs send simultaneous signals to inhibit agonist (homonymous) muscles while stimulating antagonist muscles to contract.

Axon: The part of a neuron that conducts stimuli toward other cells.

Ballismus: A type of dyskinesia that consists of large throwing-type movements.

Basal ganglia: Groups of neurons (nuclei) located in the brain that modulate volitional movement, tone, and cognition.

Biofeedback: The technique of making unconscious or involuntary body processes perceptible to the senses to manipulate them by conscious mental control.

Central nervous system (CNS): The part of the nervous system consisting of the brain and spinal cord.

Cerebellum: The part of the brain that coordinates movement by comparing intended movements to actual movements and correcting for movement errors or unexpected obstacles to movement.

Chorea: A type of dyskinesia that consists of dancelike, sharp, jerky movements.

Clasp-knife phenomenon: Initial resistance followed by a sudden release of resistance in response to a quick stretch of a hypertonic muscle.

Clonus: Multiple rhythmic oscillations or beats in the resistance of a muscle responding to quick stretch.

Dendrites: Projections of a neuron that receive stimuli.

Denervation: The removal of neural input to an end organ.

Depolarization: The reversal of the resting potential in excitable cell membranes, with a tendency of the inside of the cell to become positive relative to the outside.

Dyskinesia: Any abnormal movement that is involuntary and without purpose.

Dystonia: A type of dyskinesia that consists of involuntary sustained muscle contraction.

Electrochemical gradient: The difference in charge or concentration of a particular ion inside the cell compared to outside the cell.

Electromyography (EMG): Record of the electrical activity of muscles using surface or fine wire/needle electrodes.

Flaccid paralysis: A state characterized by loss of both muscle movement (paralysis) and muscle tone (flaccidity).

Flaccidity: Lack of tone or absence of resistance to passive stretch within the middle range of the muscle's length.

Gamma motor neurons: Nerves that innervate muscle spindles at the polar end regions and when stimulated, cause the central region of the spindle to tighten, thus making the muscle spindles more sensitive to muscle stretch.

Golgi tendon organs (GTOs): Sensory organs located at the junction between muscle fibers and tendons that detect active contraction.

Guarding: A protective, involuntary increase in muscle tension in response to pain that manifests itself as muscle spasms.

Hypertonicity: High tone or increased resistance to stretch compared with normal muscles.

Hypotonicity: Low tone or decreased resistance to stretch compared with normal muscles.

Interneurons: Neurons that connect other neurons.

Limbic system: A collection of neurons in the brain involved in generating emotions, memories, and motivation; can affect muscle tone through connections with the hypothalamus, reticular system, and the basal ganglia.

Monosynaptic transmission: Movement of a nerve signal through a single synapse; for example, the muscle stretch reflex.

Motor unit: Muscle fibers innervated by all the branches of a single alpha motor neuron.

Muscle spasm: An involuntary, strong contraction of a muscle.

Muscle spindles: Sensory organs that lie within muscle; they sense when muscle is stretched and send sensory signals via type Ia sensory nerves.

Muscle stretch reflexes: Fast contractions of the muscle in response to stretch, mediated by the monosynaptic connection between a sensory nerve and an alpha motor nerve; usually tested by tapping on the tendon; also called the deep tendon reflex.

Muscle tone: The underlying tension in a muscle that serves as a background for contraction.

Myelin: A fatty tissue that surrounds the axons of neurons in both the peripheral and central nervous system, allowing electrical signals to travel quickly.

Myofilaments: Structural components of the contractile units of muscles, made up of many proteins including actin and myosin.

Myosin: A fibrous globulin (protein) of muscle that can split ATP and react with actin to contract a muscle fibril.

Neuron: A nerve cell.

Neurotransmitters: Chemicals released from neurons that transmit signals to and from nerves.

Paralysis: Loss of voluntary movement.

Pendulum test: A test for spasticity that uses gravity to provide a quick stretch for a particular muscle group and measured by observing the resistance to stretch in the swing of the limb after the stretch.

Peripheral nervous system (PNS): The part of the nervous system that lies outside the brain and spinal cord.

Rearborizing: A response to destruction of alpha motor neurons in which a remaining neuron increases the number of muscle fibers it innervates by increasing its number of axonal branches.

Reciprocal inhibition: A mechanism by which agonist muscles are excited while antagonist muscles are simultaneously inhibited so that they do not work against each other; also called reciprocal innervations.

Repolarization: The return of cell membrane potential to resting potential after depolarization.

Resting potential: The difference in charge between the inside and outside of the cell at rest.

Reticular-activating system: A group of neurons located in the central brain stem that receives sensory, autonomic, and hypothalamic input and influences muscle tone to reflect the individual's emotions, motivation, and alertness.

Rigidity: An abnormal, hypertonic state in which muscles are stiff or immovable and in which they are resistant to all stretch regardless of velocity or direction.

Saltatory conduction: The movement of an electrical signal down a nerve axon that has myelin coating; as the signal travels quickly through myelin-coated regions of the axon and slowly at unmyelinated regions (nodes of Ranvier), it appears to jump from one node to the next.

Sarcomere: The contractile unit of muscle cells, consisting of actin and myosin myofilaments that slide by each other causing contraction.

Spasticity: An abnormal, hypertonic muscle response in which quicker passive muscle stretches elicit greater resistance than slower stretches.

Stereotyped hypertonic response: A pattern of muscle response to stimuli that is involuntary and is the same each time a stimulus occurs.

Summation: The adding together of excitatory and inhibitory signals that takes place in a postsynaptic cell.

Supraspinal: CNS areas that originate above the spinal cord in the upright human.

Synapse: The gap between a synaptic bouton (nerve ending) and its target (muscles, bodily organs, glands, or other neurons); also called synaptic cleft.

Synergies: Patterns of contraction in which several muscles work together to produce a movement.

Tremor: A type of dyskinesia that consists of low-amplitude, high-frequency oscillating movements.

Type Ia sensory neurons: Afferent nerves that carry stretch signals from muscle spindles to the alpha motor neuron and that cause the stretched muscle to contract.

Vestibular system: The parts of the inner ear and brain stem that receive, integrate, and transmit information about the position of the head in relation to gravity and rotation of the head and contribute to maintenance of upright posture.

REFERENCES *evolve*

1. Simons DG, Mense S: Understanding and measurement of muscle tone as related to clinical muscle pain, *Pain* 75:1-17, 1998.
2. Keshner EA: Reevaluating the theoretical model underlying the neurodevelopmental theory: a literature review, *Phys Ther* 61:1035-1040, 1981.
3. Brooks VB: Motor control: how posture and movements are governed, *Phys Ther* 63:664-673, 1983.
4. Lance JW: The control of muscle tone, reflexes, and movement: Robert Wartenberg lecture, *Neurology* 30:1303-1313, 1980.
5. Sahrmann SA, Norton BJ: The relationship of voluntary movement to spasticity in the upper motor neuron syndrome, *Ann Neurol* 2:460-465, 1977.
6. Bobath B: *Adult hemiplegia: evaluation and treatment,* ed 2, London, 1978, Heinemann.
7. Teasell R: Musculoskeletal complications of hemiplegia following stroke, *Semin Arthritis Rheum* 20(6):385-395, 1991.
8. Dietz V, Quintern J, Berger W: Electrophysiological studies of gait in spasticity and rigidity: evidence that altered mechanical properties of muscle contribute to hypertonicity, *Brain* 104:431-449, 1981.
9. Albanese A: The clinical expression of primary dystonia, *J Neurol* 250:1145-1151, 2003.
10. Claypool DW, Duane DD, Ilstrup DM, et al: Epidemiology and outcome of cervical dystonia (spasmodic torticollis) in Rochester, Minnesota, *Movement Disorders* 10(5):608-614, 1995.
11. Giuliani C: Dorsal rhizotomy for children with cerebral palsy: support for concepts of motor control, *Phys Ther* 71:248-259, 1991.
12. Boiteau M, Malouin F, Richards CL: Use of a hand-held dynamometer and a Kin-ComR dynamometer for evaluating spastic hypertonicity in children: a reliability study, *Phys Ther* 75:796-802, 1995.
13. Starsky AJ, Sangani SG, McGuire JR, et al: Reliability of biomechanical spasticity measurements at the elbow of people poststroke, *Arch Phys Med Rehabil* 86:1648-1654, 2005.
14. Wolf SL, Catlin PA, Blanton S, et al: Overcoming limitations in elbow movement in the presence of antagonist hyperactivity, *Phys Ther* 74:826-835, 1994.
15. Basmajian JV, De Luca CJ: *Muscles alive: their functions revealed by electromyography,* ed 5, Baltimore, 1985, Williams & Wilkins.
16. Bajd T, Vodovnik L: Pendulum testing of spasticity, *J Biomed Eng* 6:9-16, 1984.
17. Bohannon RW: Variability and reliability of the pendulum test for spasticity using a Cybex II Isokinetic Dynamometer, *Phys Ther* 67:659-661, 1987.
18. O'Sullivan SB: Assessment of motor function. In O'Sullivan SB, Schmitz TJ, eds: *Physical rehabilitation: assessment and treatment,* ed 4, Philadelphia, 2001, FA Davis.
19. Bates B: *A guide to physical examination,* ed 4, Philadelphia, 1987, JB Lippincott.
20. Ashworth B: Preliminary trial of carisoprodol in multiple sclerosis, *Practitioner* 192:540-542, 1964.
21. Bohannon RW, Smith MB: Interrater reliability of a modified Ashworth scale of muscle spasticity, *Phys Ther* 67:206-207, 1987.

22. Bohannon RW, Andrews AW: Influence of head-neck rotation on static elbow flexion force of paretic side in patients with hemiparesis, *Phys Ther* 69:135-137, 1989.
23. DeLong MR: The basal ganglia. In Kandel ER, Schwartz JH, Jessell TM, eds: *Principles of neural science*, ed 4, New York, 2000, McGraw-Hill.
24. Koester J, Siegelbaum SA: Local signaling: passive membrane properties of the neuron. In Kandel ER, Schwartz JH, Jessell TM, eds: *Principles of neural science*, ed 4, New York, 2000, McGraw-Hill.
25. Rothwell J: *Control of human voluntary movement*, ed 2, New York, 1994, Chapman and Hall.
26. De Jesus P, Housmanowa-Petrusewicz I, Barchi R: The effect of cold on nerve conduction of human slow and fast nerve fibers, *Neurology* 23:1182-1189, 1973.
27. Dewhurst DJ: Neuromuscular control system, *IEEE Trans Bio-Med Eng* 14:167-171, 1967.
28. Rowland LP: Diseases of the motor unit. In Kandel ER, Schwartz JH, Jessell TM, eds: *Principles of neural science*, ed 4, New York, 2000, McGraw-Hill.
29. Nashner LM: Adapting reflexes controlling the human posture, *Exp Brain Res* 26:59-72, 1976.
30. Vallbo AB: Afferent discharge from human muscle spindles in non-contracting muscles: steady state impulse frequency as a function of joint angle, *Acta Physiol Scand* 90:303-318, 1974a.
31. Vallbo AB: Human muscle spindle discharge during isometric voluntary contractions: amplitude relations between spindle frequency and torque, *Acta Physiol Scand* 90:319-336, 1974b.
32. Knutson GA: The role of the gamma-motor system in increasing muscle tone and muscle pain syndromes: a review of the Johansson/Sojka Hypothesis, *J Manip Physiol Ther* 23(8):564-573, 2000.
33. Takakusaki K, Saitoh K, Harada H, et al: Role of basal ganglia-brainstem pathways in the control of motor behaviors, *Neurosci Res* 50:137-151, 2004.
34. Matthews PBC: *Mammalian muscle receptors and their central actions*, London, 1972, Arnold.
35. Houk J, Henneman E: Responses of Golgi tendon organs to active contractions of the soleus muscle of the cat, *J Neurophysiol* 30:466-481, 1967.
36. Jami L: Golgi tendon organs in mammalian skeletal muscle: functional properties and central actions, *Physiol Rev* 72:623-666, 1992.
37. O'Sullivan SB: Strategies to improve motor control and motor learning. In O'Sullivan SB, Schmitz TJ, eds: *Physical rehabilitation: assessment and treatment*, ed 4, Philadelphia, 2001, FA Davis.
38. Hagbarth KE: Spinal withdrawal reflexes in human lower limb. In Brunnstrom S: *Movement therapy in hemiplegia*, Hagerstown, MD, 1970, Harper and Row.
39. Gracies JM, Meunier S, Pierrot-Deseilligny E, et al: Patterns of propriospinal-like excitation to different species of human upper limb motor neurons, *J Physiol* 434:151-167, 1990.
40. Knott M, Voss DE: *Proprioceptive neuromuscular facilitation: patterns and techniques*, ed 2, New York, 1968, Harper & Row.
41. Brunnstrom S: *Movement therapy in hemiplegia: a neurophysiological approach*, Hagerstown, MD, 1970, Harper & Row.
42. Sawner KA, LaVigne JM: *Brunnstrom's movement therapy in hemiplegia: a neurophysiological approach*, ed 2, Philadelphia, 1992, JB Lippincott.
43. McDonald-Williams MF: Exercise and postpolio syndrome, *Neurol Rep* 20(2):37-44, 1996.
44. Stockert BW: Peripheral neuropathies. In Umphred DA, ed: *Neurological rehabilitation*, ed 3, St Louis, 1995, Mosby.
45. Bassile CC: Guillain-Barré syndrome and exercise guidelines, *Neurol Rep* 20(2):31-36, 1996.
46. Morris DM: Aquatic neurorehabilitation, *Neurol Rep* 19(3):22-28, 1995.
47. Barnard P, Dill H, Eldredge P, et al: Reduction of hypertonicity by early casting in a comatose head-injured individual, *Phys Ther* 64:1540-1542, 1984.
48. Duncan PW, Badke MB: Therapeutic strategies for rehabilitation of motor deficits. In Duncan PW, Badke MB, eds: *Stroke rehabilitation: the recovery of motor control*, Chicago, 1987, Year Book Medical Publishers.
49. Lehmkuhl LD, Krawczyk L: Physical therapy management of the minimally-responsive patient following traumatic brain injury: coma stimulation, *Neurol Rep* 17(1):10-17, 1993.
50. Dietz V: Supraspinal pathways and the development of muscle-tone dysregulation, *Dev Med Child Neurol* 41:708-715, 1999.
51. Gowland C, deBruin H, Basmajian JV, et al: Agonist and antagonist activity during voluntary upper-limb movement in patients with stroke, *Phys Ther* 72:624-633, 1992.
52. Dietz V: Spastic movement disorder, *Spinal Cord* 38:389-393, 2000.
53. Knutsson E, Martensson A: Dynamic motor capacity in spastic paresis and its relation to prime mover dysfunction, spastic reflexes and antagonist co-activation, *Scand J Rehab Med* 12:93-106, 1980.
54. Campbell SK, Almeida GL, Penn RD, et al: The effects of intrathecally administered baclofen on function in patients with spasticity, *Phys Ther* 75:352-362, 1995.
55. Somers MF: *Spinal cord injury: functional rehabilitation*, Norwalk, CT, 1992, Appleton & Lange.
56. Schmitz TJ: Traumatic spinal cord injury. In O'Sullivan SB, Schmitz TJ, eds: *Physical rehabilitation: assessment and treatment*, ed 3, Philadelphia, 1994, FA Davis.
57. Shumway-Cook A, Woollacott MH: *Motor control: theory and practical applications*, ed 2, Philadelphia, 2001, Lippincott, Williams & Wilkins.
58. Rosner LJ, Ross S: *Multiple sclerosis*, New York, 1987, Prentice Hall Press.
59. Bobath B: *Abnormal postural reflex activity caused by brain lesions*, ed 2, London, 1971, Heinemann.
60. Giorgetti MM: Serial and inhibitory casting: implications for acute care physical therapy management, *Neurol Rep* 17(1):18-21, 1993.
61. Wolf SL, Catlin PA, Blanton S, et al: Overcoming limitations in elbow movement in the presence of antagonist hyperactivity, *Phys Ther* 74:826-835, 1994.
62. McClure PW, Blackburn LG, Dusold C: The use of splints in the treatment of joint stiffness: biologic rationale and an algorithm for making clinical decisions, *Phys Ther* 74:1101-1107, 1994.
63. Cutson TM, Laub KC, Schenkman M: Pharmacological and nonpharmacological interventions in the treatment of Parkinson's disease, *Phys Ther* 75:363-373, 1995.
64. Stockmeyer SA: An interpretation of the approach of Rood to the treatment of neuromuscular dysfunction, *Am J Phys Med* 46(1):900-956, 1967.
65. Maitland GD: *Vertebral manipulation*, ed 6, London, 2000, Butterworth-Heinemann.
66. Grieve GP: *Common vertebral joint problems*, ed 2, Edinburgh, 1988, Churchill Livingstone.
67. Saunders HD, Saunders R: *Evaluation, treatment and prevention of musculoskeletal disorders*, vol 1, ed 3, Bloomington, MN, 1993, Educational Opportunities.

Motion Restrictions

Linda G. Monroe

This chapter discusses motion between body segments and the factors that can restrict such motion. The amount of motion that occurs when one segment of the body moves in relation to an adjacent segment is known as **range of motion** (ROM). When a segment of the body moves through its available ROM all tissues in that region, including the bones, joint capsule, ligaments, tendons, intraarticular structures, muscles, nerves, fascia, and skin, may be affected. If all of these tissues function normally, full, normal ROM can be achieved; however, dysfunction of any of these tissues may contribute to a restriction of the available ROM. Many patients in rehabilitation seek medical treatment for motion restrictions. To restore motion most effectively, the therapist must understand the factors that influence normal motion and the factors that may contribute to motion restrictions.

Motion restriction is an impairment that may directly or indirectly contribute to patient functional limitation and disability. For example, restricted shoulder ROM may stop an individual from raising the arm above shoulder height and may prevent him or her from performing a job that involves overhead lifting. This impairment may also contribute indirectly to further pathology by causing impingement of the rotator cuff tendons, resulting in pain, weakness, and further limitation of lifting ability.

In the absence of pathology, ROM is generally constrained by tissue length or approximation of anatomical structures. The integrity and flexibility of the soft tissues surrounding a joint and the shape and relationship of the articular structures affect the amount of motion that can occur. When a joint is in the middle of its range it can generally be moved with the application of a small force. This is because the collagen fibers in the connective tissue surrounding the joint are in a relaxed state, loosely oriented in various directions, and only sparsely cross-linked with other fibers, allowing them to distend readily. As the joint approaches the end of its range the collagen fibers begin to align in the direction of the stress and start to straighten. Motion ceases at the normal terminal range when the fibers have achieved their maximum alignment, or when soft or bony tissues approximate. For example, ankle dorsiflexion normally ends when the fibers of the calf muscles have achieved maximum alignment and are fully lengthened (Fig. 5-1, *A*), whereas elbow flexion normally ends when the soft tissues of the anterior arm approximate with the soft tissues of the anterior forearm (Fig 5-1, *B*) and elbow extension ends when the olecranon process of the ulna approximates with the olecranon fossa of the humerus (Fig. 5-1, *C*).

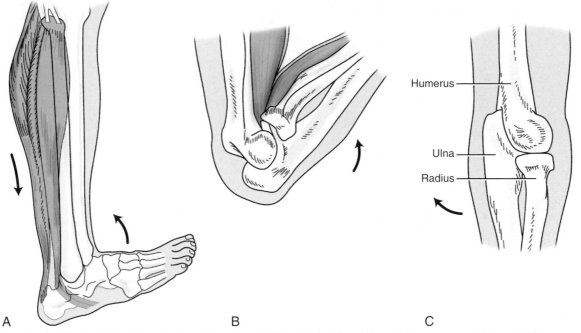

FIG 5-1 A, Ankle dorsiflexion limited by soft tissue distention. **B,** Elbow flexion limited by soft tissue approximation. **C,** Elbow extension limited by bone approximation.

The normal ROM for all human joints has been measured and documented.[1-3] However, these measures vary with the individual's age, gender, and health status.[4-6] ROM generally decreases with age and is greater in women than in men, although these differences vary with different motions and joints and are not consistent for all individuals.[7-13] Because of this variability, normal ROM is generally determined by comparison to the motion of the contralateral limb, if available, rather than by comparison with normative data. A motion is considered to be restricted when it is less than that of the same segment on the contralateral side of the same individual. When a normal contralateral side is not available—as occurs, for example, with the spine or when both shoulders are affected—motion is considered to be restricted when it is less than normal for the individual's age and gender.

TYPES OF MOTION

The motion of body segments can be classified as active or passive.

ACTIVE MOTION

Active motion is the movement produced by contraction of the muscles crossing a joint. Examination of active ROM can provide information about an individual's functional abilities. Active motion may be restricted by muscle weakness, abnormal muscle tone, pain originating from the musculotendinous unit or other local structures, an inability or unwillingness of the subject to follow directions, or as the result of restrictions in passive ROM.[14]

PASSIVE MOTION

Passive motion is movement produced entirely by an external force without voluntary muscle contraction by the subject. The external force may be produced by gravity, a machine, another individual, or another part of the subject's own body. Passive motion may be restricted by soft tissue shortening, edema, **adhesion**, mechanical block, spinal disc herniation, or adverse neural tension.

Normal passive ROM is greater than normal active ROM when motion is limited by the lengthening or approximation of soft tissue, but both types of motion are equal when motion is limited by approximation of bone. For example, a few degrees of passive ankle dorsiflexion motion are available beyond the limit of active motion because the limiting tissues are elastic and may be lengthened by an external force that is greater than that of the active muscles when at terminal active ROM. A few degrees of additional passive elbow flexion are available beyond the limit of active range because the limiting tissues are compressible by an external force greater than that of the active muscles in that position and because the approximating muscles may be less bulky when relaxed. This additional passive ROM may protect joint structures by absorbing external forces during activities performed at or close to the end of active range.

PHYSIOLOGICAL AND ACCESSORY MOTION

Physiological motion is the motion of one segment of the body relative to another segment. For example, physiological knee extension is the straightening of the knee that occurs when the leg moves away from the thigh. **Accessory motion**, also called joint play, is the motion that occurs between the joint surfaces during normal physiological motion.[15,16] For example, anterior gliding of the tibia on the femur is the accessory motion that occurs during physiological knee extension (Fig. 5-2). Accessory

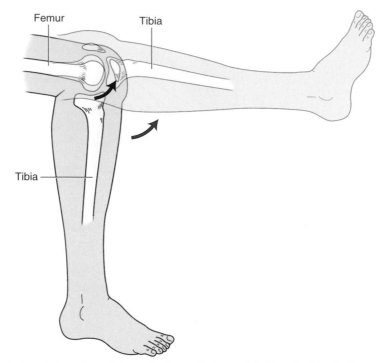

Femur   Tibia

Tibia

FIG 5-2 Accessory anterior gliding of the tibia on the femur *(red arrow)* during physiological knee extension *(blue arrow)*.

motions may be intraarticular, as in the prior example of anterior tibial gliding during knee extension, or extraarticular, as with the upward rotation of the scapula during physiological shoulder flexion (Fig. 5-3). Although accessory motions cannot be performed actively in isolation from their associated physiological movement, they may be performed passively in isolation from their associated physiological movement.

Normal accessory motion is required for normal active and passive joint motion to occur. The direction of normal accessory motion depends on the shape of the articular surfaces and the direction of physiological motion. Concave joint surfaces require accessory gliding to be available in the direction of the associated physiological motion of the segment, whereas convex joint surfaces require accessory gliding to be available in the opposite direction of the associated physiological motion of the segment.[15]

Clinical Pearl

With concave joint surfaces, accessory gliding occurs in the direction of the associated physiological joint motion. With convex joint surface, accessory gliding occurs in the opposite direction to the associated physiological joint motion.

For example, the tibial plateau, which has a concave surface at the knee, glides anteriorly during knee extension when the tibia is moving anteriorly, and the femoral condyles, which have convex surfaces at the knee, glide posteriorly during knee extension when the femur is moving anteriorly.

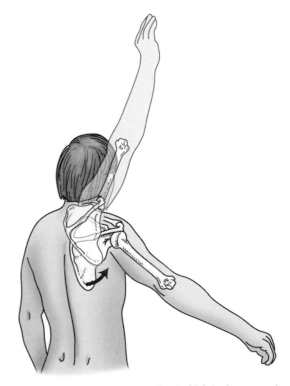

FIG 5-3 Extraarticular accessory motion, which is the upward rotation of the scapula that accompanies shoulder flexion.

PATTERNS OF MOTION RESTRICTION

The restriction of motion at a joint can be classified as having either a capsular or a noncapsular pattern.

CAPSULAR PATTERN OF MOTION RESTRICTION

A **capsular pattern of restriction** is the specific combination of motion loss that is caused by shortening of the joint capsule surrounding a joint. Each synovial joint has a unique capsular pattern of restriction.[17] Capsular patterns generally include restrictions of motion in multiple directions. For example, the capsular pattern for the glenohumeral joint involves restriction of external rotation, abduction, internal rotation, and flexion to progressively smaller degrees. Capsular patterns of restriction may be caused by the effusion, fibrosis, or inflammation commonly associated with degenerative joint disease, arthritis, immobilization, and acute trauma.

> ### ◎ Clinical Pearl
>
> Causes of capsular patterns of restriction include effusion, fibrosis, or inflammation of the joint capsule.

NONCAPSULAR PATTERN OF MOTION RESTRICTION

A **noncapsular pattern of restriction** is a combination of motion loss that does not follow the capsular pattern. A noncapsular pattern of motion loss may be caused by ligamentous adhesion, an internal derangement, or an extraarticular lesion.

> ### ◎ Clinical Pearl
>
> Causes of noncapsular patterns of restriction include ligamentous adhesion, internal derangements, or extraarticular lesions in the region of a joint.

Ligamentous adhesion will limit motion in the directions that stretch the adhered ligament. For example, an adhesion of the talofibular ligament after an ankle sprain will restrict ankle inversion because this motion places the adhered ligament on stretch; however, this adhesion will not alter the motion of the ankle in other directions. Internal derangement, the displacement of loose fragments within a joint, will generally limit motion only in the direction that compresses the fragment. For example, a cartilage fragment in the knee will generally limit knee extension but will not limit knee flexion. Extraarticular lesions, such as muscle adhesions, hematomas, cysts, or inflamed bursae, may limit motion in the direction of either stretch or compression, depending on the nature of the lesion. For example, adhesion of the quadriceps muscle to the shaft of the femur will limit stretching of the muscle, whereas a popliteal cyst will limit compression of the popliteal area. Both of these lesions will restrict motion in the noncapsular pattern of restricted knee flexion, with full, painless knee extension.

TISSUES THAT CAN RESTRICT MOTION

Any of the musculoskeletal tissues in the area of a motion restriction may contribute to that restriction. These tissues

BOX 5-1	Contractile and Noncontractile Sources of Motion Restrictions
Contractile Tissue	**Noncontractile Tissue**
Muscle	Skin
Musculotendinous junction	Ligament
Tendon	Bursa
Tendinous interface with bone	Capsule
	Articular cartilage
	Intervertebral disc
	Peripheral nerve
	Dura mater

are most readily classified as contractile or noncontractile (Box 5-1).

CONTRACTILE TISSUES

Contractile tissue is composed of the musculotendinous unit, which includes the muscle, the musculotendinous junction, the tendon, and the tendon's interface with bone. Skeletal muscle is considered to be contractile because it can contract by forming cross-bridges of the myosin proteins with the actin proteins within its fibers. Tendons and their attachments to bone are considered contractile because contracting muscles apply tension directly to these structures. When a muscle contracts it applies tension to its tendons causing the bones to which it is attached and the surrounding tissues to move through the available active ROM. When all the components of the musculotendinous unit and the **noncontractile tissues** are functioning normally, the available active ROM will be within normal limits. Injury or dysfunction of contractile tissue generally results in a restriction of active ROM in the direction of movement produced by contraction of the musculotendinous unit. Dysfunction of contractile tissue may also result in pain or weakness on resisted testing of the musculotendinous unit. For example, a tear in the anterior tibialis muscle or tendon can restrict active dorsiflexion at the ankle and reduce the force generated by resisted testing of ankle dorsiflexion, but this lesion is not likely to alter passive plantarflexion or dorsiflexion ROM or active plantarflexion strength.

NONCONTRACTILE TISSUES

All tissues that are not components of the musculotendinous unit are considered noncontractile. Noncontractile tissues include skin, fascia, scar tissue, ligament, bursa, capsule, articular cartilage, bone, intervertebral disc, nerve, and dura mater. When the noncontractile tissues in an area are functioning normally, the passive ROM of the segments in that area will be within normal limits. Injury or dysfunction of noncontractile tissue can cause a restriction of the passive ROM of the joints in the area of the tissue in question and may also contribute to restriction of active ROM. The direction, degree, and nature of the motion restriction depend on the type of noncontractile tissue involved, the type of tissue dysfunction, and the severity of involvement. For example, adhesive capsulitis of the shoulder, which involves shortening of the glenohumeral joint capsule and elimination of the inferior axillary fold, will restrict both passive and active shoulder ROM (Fig. 5-4).[18-23]

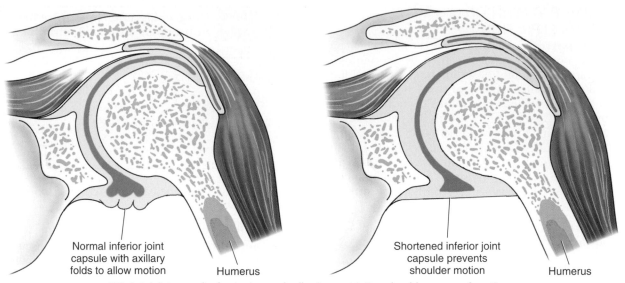

Normal inferior joint capsule with axillary folds to allow motion

Humerus

Shortened inferior joint capsule prevents shoulder motion

Humerus

FIG 5-4 Joint capsule shortening and adhesion restricting shoulder range of motion.

PATHOLOGIES THAT CAN CAUSE MOTION RESTRICTIONS

CONTRACTURE

Motion may be restricted if any of the soft tissue structures in an area have become shortened. Such soft tissue shortening, known as a **contracture**, may occur in contractile or noncontractile tissues.[24,25] A contracture may be a consequence of external immobilization or lack of use. External immobilization is usually produced with a splint or a cast. Lack of use is usually the result of weakness, as may occur after poliomyelitis; poor motor control, as may occur after a stroke; or pain, as may occur after trauma.[24,25] It is believed that immobilization results in contracture because it allows anomalous cross-links to form between collagen fibers and because it causes fluid to be lost from fibrous connective tissue, including tendon, capsule, ligament, and fascia.[26-28] Anomalous cross-links can develop when tissues remain stationary because, in the absence of normal stress and motion, fibers remain in contact with each other for prolonged periods and start to adhere at their points of interception. These cross-links may prevent normal alignment of the collagen fibers when motion is attempted. They also increase the stress required to stretch the tissue, limit tissue extension, and result in contracture (Fig. 5-5). Fluid loss can also impair normal fiber gliding, causing collagen fibrils to have closer contact and limiting tissue extension.[24]

The risk of contracture formation in response to immobilization is increased when the tissue has been injured because scar tissue, which is formed during the proliferation phase of healing, tends to have poor fiber alignment and a high degree of cross-linking between its fibers. Restriction of motion after an injury may be further aggravated if a concurrent problem, such as sepsis or ongoing trauma, amplifies the inflammatory response and causes excessive scarring.[25]

A permanent shortening of a muscle producing deformity or distortion is known as a muscle contracture. A

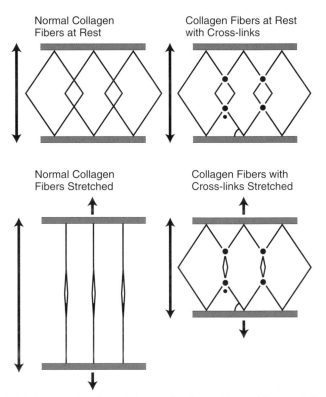

Normal Collagen Fibers at Rest

Collagen Fibers at Rest with Cross-links

Normal Collagen Fibers Stretched

Collagen Fibers with Cross-links Stretched

FIG 5-5 Normal collagen fibers and collagen fibers with cross-links. *Adapted from Woo SL, Matthews JV, Akeson WH, et al: Connective tissue response to immobility. Correlative study of biomechanical measurements of normal and immobilized rabbit knees,* Arthritis Rheum *18(3):262, 1975.*

muscle contracture can be caused by prolonged muscle spasm, guarding, muscle imbalance, muscle disease, ischemic muscle necrosis, or immobilization.[25] A muscle contracture may limit active and passive motion of the joint(s) that the muscle crosses and can also cause deformity of the joint(s) normally controlled by the muscle.

When a joint is immobilized over time, the structures that contribute to the limitation in ROM may change. Trudel et al reported that restrictions in ROM during immobilization in an animal model were initially caused by changes in muscle, but articular structures from week 2 to 32 contributed more to limitations in ROM.[29]

EDEMA

Normally, a joint capsule contains fluid and is not fully distended when the joint is in midrange. This allows the capsule to fold or distend, altering its size and shape as needed for movement through full ROM. If excessive fluid forms inside a joint capsule, a condition known as **intraarticular edema**, the joint capsule distends, limiting its folding and further distention and potentially restricting both passive and active joint motion in a capsular pattern. For example, intraarticular edema in the knee will limit knee flexion and extension, with flexion being most affected.

Accumulation of fluid outside the joint, a condition known as **extraarticular edema**, may also restrict active and passive motion by causing soft tissue approximation to occur earlier in the range. Extraarticular edema generally restricts motion in a noncapsular pattern. For example, edema in the calf muscle may restrict knee flexion ROM but have no effect on knee extension ROM.

> ◎ **Clinical Pearl**
>
> Intraarticular edema restricts motion in a capsular pattern. Extraarticular edema restricts motion in a noncapsular pattern.

ADHESION

Adhesion is the abnormal joining of parts to each other.[30] Adhesion may occur between different types of tissue and frequently causes restriction of motion. During the healing process, scar tissue can adhere to surrounding structures. Fibrofatty tissue may also proliferate inside joints and, as it matures into scar tissue, adhere between intraarticular structures.[31] Prolonged joint immobilization, even in the absence of local injury, can also cause the synovial membrane surrounding the joint to adhere to the cartilage inside the joint. Adhesions can affect both the quality and the quantity of joint motion. For example, with adhesive capsulitis, adhesion of the joint capsule to the synovial membrane limits the quantity of motion. This adhesion also reduces, or even obliterates, the space between the cartilage and the synovial membrane, blocking normal synovial fluid nutrition and causing articular cartilage degeneration that can alter the quality of joint motion.[25]

MECHANICAL BLOCK

Motion can be mechanically blocked by bone or fragments of articular cartilage, or by tears in intraarticular discs or menisci. Degenerative joint disease (and associated **osteophyte** formation) or malunion of bony segments after fracture healing frequently results in formation of a bony block that restricts joint motion in one or more directions (Fig. 5-6). These pathologies cause extra bone

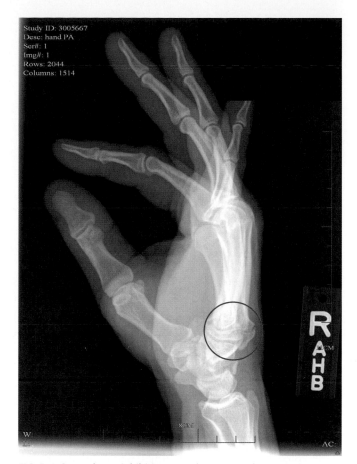

FIG 5-6 Osteophytes inhibiting carpal-metacarpal movement. *Courtesy J. Michael Pearson, MD, Oregon Health & Science University, Portland, OR.*

to form in or around the joints. Loose bodies or fragments of articular cartilage, caused by avascular necrosis or trauma, can also alter the mechanics of the joint, causing "locking" in various positions, pain, and other dysfunctions.[25] Tears in intraarticular fibrocartilaginous discs and menisci caused by high-force traumatic injury or by repetitive low-force strain generally block motion in one direction only.

SPINAL DISC HERNIATION

Spinal disc herniation may result in direct blockage of spinal motion if a portion of the discal material becomes trapped in a facet joint or if the disc compresses a spinal nerve root where it passes through the vertebral foramen. Other pathologies associated with spinal disc herniation, including inflammation, hypertrophic changes, decreased disc height, and pain, may further limit spinal motion. Inflammation about the spinal facet joint or herniated segment can limit motion by narrowing the vertebral foramen and compressing the nerve root. Hypertrophic changes at the vertebral margins and facet joints, as well as decreased disc height, also narrow the vertebral foramen, making the nerve root more vulnerable to compression. Pain may limit motion by causing involuntary muscle spasms or by causing the individual to restrict movements voluntarily.

ADVERSE NEURAL TENSION

Under normal circumstances, the nervous system, including the spinal cord and the peripheral nerves, must adapt to both mechanical and physiological stresses.[32] For example, during forward flexion of the trunk, the nervous system must adapt to the increased length of the spinal column without interruption of transmission.[33] Adverse neural tension is the presence of abnormal responses produced from peripheral nervous system structures when their ROM and stretch capabilities are tested.[34] Adverse neural tension may result from major or minor nerve injury or may be caused indirectly by extraneural adhesions that result in tethering of the nerve to surrounding structures. Nerve injury may be the result of trauma caused by friction, compression, or stretch. It may also be caused by disease, ischemia, inflammation, or a disruption in the axonal transport system. Ischemia can be caused by pressure from extravascular fluid, blood, disc material, or soft tissues.

Adverse neural tension is most commonly caused by restriction of nerve motion. A number of structural features predispose nerve motion to restriction. Nerve motion is commonly restricted where nerves pass through tunnels; for example, where the median nerve passes through the carpal tunnel or where the spinal nerves pass through the intervertebral foramina. Peripheral nerve motion is also likely to be restricted at points where the nerves branch; for example, where the ulnar nerve splits at the hook of the hammate or where the sciatic nerve splits into the peroneal and tibial nerves in the thigh. Places where the system is relatively fixed are also points of vulnerability; for example, at the dura mater at L4 or where the common peroneal nerve passes the head of the fibula. The system is also relatively fixed where nerves are close to unyielding interfaces; for example, where the cords of the brachial plexus pass over the first rib or the greater occipital nerve passes through the fascia in the posterior skull.[34]

WEAKNESS

When muscles are too weak to generate the force required to move a segment of the body through its normal ROM, active ROM will be restricted. Muscle weakness may be the result of contractile tissue changes such as atrophy or injury, poor transmission to or along the motor nerves, or poor synaptic transmission at the neuromuscular junction.

OTHER FACTORS

Motion restrictions may also be caused by many other factors, including pain, psychological factors, and tone. Pain may restrict active or passive motion, depending on whether contractile or noncontractile structures are the source of the pain. Psychological factors, such as fear, poor motivation, or poor comprehension, are most likely to cause restriction of only active ROM. Tone abnormalities, particularly hypotonia or flaccidity, may also impair the control of active muscle contractions and may thus limit active ROM.

EXAMINATION AND EVALUATION OF MOTION RESTRICTIONS

When a patient seeks medical treatment for limited motion, mobility of all the structures in the area of the restriction, including the joints, muscles, intraarticular and extraarticular structures, and nerves, should be examined. Examination of all these structures is required to determine the pathophysiology underlying the motion restriction, identify the tissues limiting motion, and evaluate the severity and irritability of the dysfunction. This complete examination and evaluation will direct treatment to the appropriate structure(s) and will facilitate selection of the optimal intervention to meet goals. Ongoing examination and evaluation of outcomes is required so that treatment is modified appropriately in response to changes in the dysfunction. This approach will accelerate and optimize progress toward the treatment goals. A variety of tools and methods are available for quantitative and qualitative examination of motion and motion restrictions.

QUANTITATIVE MEASURES

Goniometers, tape measures, and various types of inclinometers are commonly used in the clinical setting for quantitative measurement of ROM (Fig. 5-7). These tools provide objective and moderately reliable measures of ROM and are practical and convenient for clinical use. Radiographs, photographs, electrogoniometers, flexometers, and plumb lines may be used to increase the accuracy and reliability of ROM measurement. These additional tools are often used for research purposes but are not available in most clinical settings. The different tools provide different information about the available or demonstrated ROM. Most tools, including goniometers, inclinometers, and electrogoniometers, provide measures of the angle, or change in angle, between body segments, whereas other tools, such as the tape measure, provide measures of the change in length of body segments.[35]

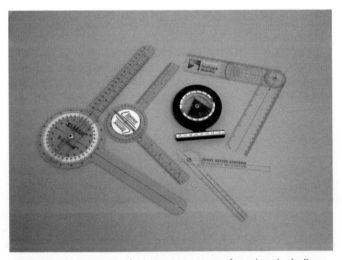

FIG 5-7 Instruments used to measure range of motion, including goniometers and an inclinometer.

QUALITATIVE MEASURES

Qualitative assessment techniques, such as soft tissue palpation, accessory motion testing, and **end-feel,** provide valuable information about motion restrictions that can help guide treatment. Soft tissue palpation may be used to assess the mobility of skin or scar tissue, local tenderness, the presence of muscle spasm, skin temperature, and the quality of edema. It is also used to identify bony landmarks before quantitative measurement of ROM.

TEST METHODS AND RATIONALE

Active, resisted, passive, and accessory motion and neural tension testing can be used to determine which tissues are restricting motion and the nature of the pathologies contributing to a motion restriction.

Active Range of Motion

Active ROM is tested by asking the subject to move the desired segment to its limit in a given direction. The subject is asked to report any symptoms or sensations, such as pain or tingling, experienced during this activity. The maximum motion is measured, and the quality or coordination of the motion and any associated symptoms are noted. Testing of active ROM yields information about the subject's ability and willingness to move functionally and is generally most useful for evaluating the integrity of contractile structures.

The following questions should be noted when testing active ROM:
- Is the subject's ROM symmetrical, normal, restricted, or excessive?
- What is the quality of the available motion?
- Are any signs or symptoms associated with the motion?

Resisted Muscle Testing

Resisted muscle testing is performed by having the subject contract his or her muscle against a resistance strong enough to prevent movement.[3] Resisted muscle tests provide information about the ability of a muscle to produce force. This information may help determine whether contractile or noncontractile tissues are the source of a motion restriction because muscle weakness is commonly the cause of a loss of active ROM.

Cyriax[17] identified four possible responses to resisted muscle testing and proposed interpretations for each of these responses (Table 5-1). When the force is strong and there is no pain with testing, no pathology of contractile or nervous tissues is indicated. When the force is strong but pain is produced with testing, a minor structural lesion of the musculotendinous unit is usually indicated. When the force is weak and there is no pain with testing, a complete rupture of the musculotendinous unit or a neurological deficit is indicated. When the force is weak but pain is produced with testing, a minor structural lesion of the musculotendinous unit with a concurrent neurological deficit or inhibition of contraction resulting from pain caused by pathology, such as inflammation, fracture, or neoplasm, is indicated.

TABLE 5-1	Cyriax's Interpretation of Resisted Muscle Tests
Finding	**Interpretation**
Strong and painless	No apparent pathology of contractile or nervous tissue
Strong and painful	Minor lesion of musculotendinous unit
Weak and painless	Complete rupture of the musculotendinous unit
Weak and painful	Partial disruption of the musculotendinous unit Inhibition by pain as a result of pathology such as inflammation, fracture, or neoplasm Concurrent neurological deficit

From Cyriax J: *Textbook of orthopedic medicine,* ed 6, Baltimore, 1975, Lippincott, Williams and Wilkins.

Passive Range of Motion

Passive ROM is assessed by the tester moving the segment to its limit in a given direction. During passive ROM testing, the quantity of available motion is measured and the quality of motion and symptoms associated with motion and the end-feel are noted. End-feel is the quality of the resistance at the limit of passive motion felt by the clinician. An end-feel may be physiological (normal) or pathological (abnormal). A physiological end-feel exists when passive ROM is full and the normal anatomy of the joint stops movement. Certain end-feels are normal for some joints but may be pathological at other joints or at abnormal points in the range. Other end-feels are pathological if felt at any point in the motion of any joint. Physiological and pathological end-feels for most joints are listed in Table 5-2.[14,36] Passive ROM is normally limited by stretching of soft tissues or by the opposition of soft tissues or bone and may be restricted as a result of soft tissue contracture, mechanical block, or edema. The amount of passive motion available and the quality of the end-feel can assist in the determination of the structures at fault and the nature of the pathologies contributing to the motion restriction.

Combining the Findings of Active Range of Motion, Resisted Muscle Contraction, and Passive Range of Motion Testing. Combining the findings of active ROM, resisted muscle contraction, and passive ROM testing can help differentiate motion restrictions caused by contractile structures from those caused by noncontractile structures. For example, if active elbow flexion is restricted, contraction of the elbow flexors is weak, and passive elbow flexion range is normal, then the structures limiting motion are most likely to be contractile. In contrast, if both active and passive elbow flexion ROM are restricted but contraction of the elbow flexors is of normal strength, then noncontractile tissues are probably involved. Other combinations of motion and contraction strength findings may indicate muscle substitution during active ROM testing, psychological factors limiting motion, the use of poor testing technique, or pain that inhibits muscle contraction (Table 5-3). To definitely implicate a particular

TABLE 5-2	Descriptions and Examples of Different Types of End-Feels		
Type	**Description**	**Examples**	**Comments**
Hard	Abrupt halt to movement when two hard surfaces meet	Physiological: elbow extension Pathological: result of malunion fracture or heterotrophic ossification	May be physiological or pathological
Firm	Leathery, firm resistance when range is limited by joint capsule	Physiological: shoulder rotation Pathological: result of adhesive capsulitis	May be physiological or pathological
Soft	Gradual onset of resistance when soft tissue approximates or when range is limited by length of muscle	Approximation: knee flexion Muscle length: cervical sidebending	May be physiological or pathological, depending on tissue bulk and muscle length
Empty	Movement is stopped by subject before tester's feeling resistance	Passive shoulder abduction stopped by subject because of pain	Always pathological
Spasm	Movement stopped abruptly by reflex muscle contraction	Passive ankle dorsiflexion in subject with spasticity as a result of upper motor neuron lesion Active trunk flexion in subject with acute low back injury	Always pathological
Springy block	Rebound felt and seen at end of range	Caused by loose body or displaced meniscus	Always pathological
Boggy	Resistance by fluid	Knee joint effusion	Always pathological
Extended	No resistance felt within the normal range expected for the particular joint	Joint instability or hypermobility	Always pathological

From Kaltenborn FM: *Mobilization of the extremity joints: examination and basic treatment techniques,* ed 3, Oslo, 1980, Olaf Norlis Bokhandel.

TABLE 5-3	Combining the Findings of Active Range of Motion, Resisted Muscle Testing, and Passive Range of Motion Assessment		
Active ROM	**Resisted Testing**	**Passive ROM**	**Probable Cause**
Full	Strong	Full	No pathology restricting motion
Full	Strong	Restricted	Pathology beyond terminal active ROM Poor testing technique for passive ROM
Full	Weak	Restricted	Poor testing technique for passive ROM Strength at least 3/5 but less than 5/5
Full	Weak	Full	Strength at least 3/5 but less than 5/5
Restricted	Strong	Restricted	Noncontractile tissue restricting motion
Restricted	Weak	Full	Contractile tissue injury restricting motion
Restricted	Strong	Full	Poor testing techniques for active ROM or psychological factors limiting active ROM
Restricted	Weak	Restricted	Contractile and noncontractile tissues restricting motion

ROM, Range of motion.

pathology or structure, the findings of these noninvasive tests may need to be correlated with the findings of other diagnostic procedures such as radiographic imaging, diagnostic injection, and surgical exploration.

Passive Accessory Motion

Passive accessory motion is tested using joint mobilization treatment techniques. The clinician can use these techniques to assess the motion of joint surfaces and the extensibility of major ligaments and portions of the joint capsule. During accessory motion testing the clinician notes qualitatively if the motion felt is greater than, less than, or similar to the normal accessory motion expected for that joint in that plane in the particular individual and if pain is produced with testing.[16,37,38] Accessory motion

testing may provide information about joint mechanics not available from other tests. For example, a reduction of accessory gliding of the glenohumeral joint when passive shoulder flexion ROM is normal may indicate that glenohumeral joint motion is restricted and that motion of the scapulothoracic joint is excessive.

Muscle Length

Muscle length is tested by passively positioning muscle attachments as far apart as possible to elongate the muscle in the direction opposite to its action.[3] The testing of muscle length by this technique will produce valid results only if pathology of the noncontractile structures or muscle tone does not limit joint motion. When testing the length of muscles that cross only one joint, the passive

ROM available at that joint will indicate the length of the muscle. For example, the length of the soleus muscle can be assessed by measurement of passive dorsiflexion ROM at the ankle. To test the length of a muscle that crosses two or more joints, the muscle must first be elongated across one of the joints and then that joint must be held in that position while the muscle is elongated as far as possible across the other joint that it crosses.[3] The passive ROM available at the second joint will indicate the length of the muscle. For example, the length of the gastrocnemius muscle can be tested by first elongating it across the knee by placing the knee in full extension and then measuring the amount of passive dorsiflexion available at the ankle. It is essential that multijoint muscles be fully extended across one joint before measurement at the other joint to obtain a valid test of muscle length.

> ### Ⓒ Clinical Pearl
>
> When measuring muscle length in a muscle that crosses two joints, first extend the muscle fully across one joint then, while holding that joint in place, extend the muscle across the other joint.

Adverse Neural Tension

Adverse neural tension is usually tested for by passively placing neural structures in their position of maximum length. Evaluation is based on comparison with the contralateral side, comparison with norms, and assessment of the symptoms produced in the position of maximum length.

Adverse neural tension tests include the passive straight-leg raise (PSLR, or Lasègue's sign), prone knee bend, passive neck flexion, and upper limb tension tests. The PSLR is the most commonly used neural tension test and is intended to test for adverse neural tension in the sciatic nerve.

Because adverse neural tension tests may also provoke symptoms in the presence of pathologies associated with the muscles or joints, it is recommended that maneuvers that apply tension to the nervous system but do not additionally stress the muscles or joints be used to differentiate the source of symptoms with this type of test. For example, the PSLR test can provoke symptoms in the presence of pathologies associated with the hamstring muscles or the sacroiliac, iliofemoral, or lumbar spinal facet joints. Therefore, at the onset of symptoms with this test, additional tension can be applied to the nervous system by passively dorsiflexing the ankle to increase the tension on the sciatic nerve distally or by passively flexing the neck to tighten the dura proximally. If these maneuvers increase the patient's symptoms, adverse neural tension rather than joint or muscle pathology is probably the cause of symptoms.[34]

CONTRAINDICATIONS AND PRECAUTIONS TO RANGE OF MOTION TECHNIQUES

Range of motion techniques are contraindicated when motion may disrupt the healing process. However, some controlled motion within the range, speed, and tolerance of the patient may be beneficial during the acute recovery stage or immediately after acute tears, fractures, and surgery. Limited, controlled motion is recommended to reduce the severity of adhesion, contracture, as well as the decreased circulation and loss of strength associated with complete immobilization.[39,40]

CONTRAINDICATIONS

for the Use of Active and Passive ROM Examination Techniques

Active and passive ROM examination techniques are contraindicated with the following:
- In the region of a dislocation or an unhealed fracture.
- Immediately after surgical procedures to tendons, ligaments, muscle, joint capsule, or skin.

PRECAUTIONS

for the Use of Active or Passive ROM Techniques

Caution should be observed when performing active or passive ROM techniques when motion to the part might aggravate the condition. This may occur with the following:
- When there is an infection or an inflammatory process in or around the joint.
- In patients taking analgesic medication that may cloud perception or communication of pain.
- In the presence of osteoporosis or any condition that causes bone fragility.
- With hypermobile joints or joints prone to subluxation.
- In painful conditions where the techniques might reinforce the severity of the symptoms.
- In patients with hemophilia.
- In the region of a hematoma.
- If bony ankylosis is suspected.
- Immediately after an injury where there has been a disruption of soft tissue.
- In the presence of myositis ossificans.

In addition, neural tension testing should be performed with caution in the presence of inflammatory conditions; spinal cord symptoms; tumors; signs of nerve root compression; unrelenting night pain; neurological signs such as weakness, reflex changes, or loss of sensation; recent paresthesia or anesthesia; and reflex sympathetic dystrophy.[32,34] Detailed contraindications and precautions for each specific neural tension test are provided in other texts devoted to the assessment and treatment of adverse neural tension.[34]

TREATMENT APPROACHES FOR MOTION RESTRICTIONS

STRETCHING

Currently, most noninvasive interventions for reestablishing soft tissue ROM involve stretching. Clinical and experimental evidence demonstrates that stretching can increase

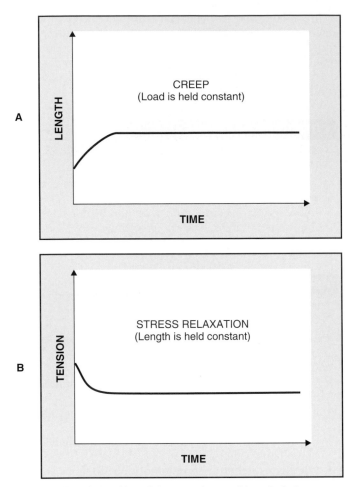

A

CREEP
(Load is held constant)

LENGTH

TIME

B

STRESS RELAXATION
(Length is held constant)

TENSION

TIME

FIG 5-8 The relationships of time, tension, and length during
A, creep and **B,** stress relaxation.

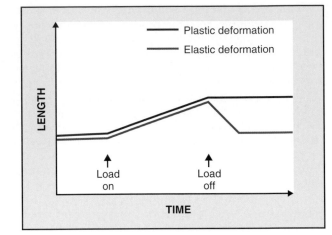

— Plastic deformation
— Elastic deformation

LENGTH

Load
on

Load
off

TIME

FIG 5-9 Plastic and elastic deformation.

motion; however, the results may not be consistent and the recommended protocols vary. When a stretch is applied to connective tissues within the elastic limit, over time the tissues may demonstrate **creep**, **stress relaxation**, and **plastic deformation**.[41] Creep is transient lengthening or deformation with the application of a fixed load. Stress relaxation is a decrease in the amount of force required over time to hold a given length (Fig. 5-8). Creep and stress relaxation can occur in soft tissue in a short time and are thought to depend on the viscous components of the tissue.[42,43,44] Plastic deformation is the elongation produced under loading that remains after the load is removed (Fig. 5-9). After plastic deformation, tissue will have a permanent increase in length. A controlled stretch must be applied for a prolonged time to cause plastic deformation. The length of time necessary to determine that no further ROM gains are possible is not known and probably varies with different pathologies[45] and tissues causing the restriction, as well as the duration of the restriction. In addition to time, the force, direction, and speed of the stretch must be controlled to produce optimal lengthening of the appropriate structures without damaging tissue or causing hypermobility.

There are many stretching techniques to increase soft tissue length. The most common are **passive stretching**, **proprioceptive neuromuscular facilitation** (PNF), and **ballistic stretching** (Table 5-4). To perform a passive stretch, the limb is held passively in a position in which the subject feels a mild stretch. The force of gravity on the involved body part, the force of other limbs, or another individual can apply passive stretch. External devices, such as progressive end range splints, serial casts, or dynamic splints, may also be used to passively stretch tissue. Although optimal parameters for passively stretching normal and pathological tissues have not been established, it is generally recommended that low-load, prolonged forces be applied to minimize the risk of adverse effects. Studies with adult subjects under 40 years old and without lower extremity pathology found that passive hamstring muscle stretching performed for 30 or 60 seconds, 5 times a week for 6 weeks, increased passive ROM more than equally frequent stretching performed for only 15 seconds, with the 30- and 60-second stretching producing equivalent effects.[46,47] However, in people over 65 years of age, who stretched their hamstring muscles 5 times a week for 6 weeks, stretching for 60 seconds increased passive ROM more than 15 or 30 seconds of stretching.[48] Table 5-5 summarizes some of the protocols and findings of static stretching programs.[46-49]

Manipulation of a joint while the subject is anesthetized involves high-force passive stretching of the soft tissues to increase ROM. Manipulation under anesthesia can produce a rapid increase in ROM because high forces that would otherwise be painful or cause muscles to spasm may be applied. These forces may cause greater increases in soft tissue length and may tear adhesions to increase motion; however, the risk of damaging structures or exacerbating inflammation may be greater with such techniques than with stretching while the subject is awake.

PNF techniques for muscle stretching inhibit contraction of the muscle being stretched and facilitate contraction of its opponent.[51] This is achieved by having the subject actively contract and then voluntarily relax the muscles to be stretched before the application of the

TABLE 5-4	Types of Stretching		
Method	Description	Examples	Comments
Passive	Limb held passively in a position in which the subject feels a mild stretch.	Manual progressive stretching Progressive end-range splinting Dynamic splinting	Pain perception is a factor. Results in no motor learning. Optimal parameters have not been established.
PNF	Active muscle contraction followed by muscle relaxation in conjunction with passive stretch.	Contract-relax Hold-relax Subject resists and aids	Requires the assistance of an individual proficient in the technique. May result in motor learning.
Ballistic	Active, quick, short-amplitude movements at the end of the subject's available ROM.	Active stretching with "bounce" at end of range	Not generally used or recommended because this may increase tissue tightness by activating the stretch reflex in normal and spastic muscles.

Data from Magnusson SP, Simonsen EB, Aagaard P, et al: A mechanism for altered flexibility in human skeletal muscle, *J Physiol* 497(1):291-298, 1996; Zito M, Driver D, Parker C, et al: Lasting effects of one bout of two 15-second passive stretches on ankle dorsiflexion range of motion, *JOSPT* 26:214-221, 1997; Bandy WD, Irion JM, Briggler M: The effect of time and frequency of static stretching on flexibility of the hamstring muscles, *Phys Ther* 77:1090-1096, 1997.
PNF, Proprioceptive neuromuscular facilitation; *ROM,* range of motion.

TABLE 5-5	Summary of Studies on Different Types of Stretching		
Citation	Subjects	Intervention	Findings
Bandy et al[46]	57 men and women Ages 21-37	Static stretching to hamstring muscles 5 days/week for 6 weeks Group 1: 15 sec stretches Group 2: 30 sec stretches Group 3: 60 sec stretches Group 4: CG	Both 30 and 60 sec of static stretch increased ROM more than 15 sec or no stretch. No significant difference between 30 and 60 sec of stretching.
Bandy et al[47]	93 men and women Ages 21-39	Static stretching to hamstring muscles 5 days/week for 6 weeks Group 1: 1 min stretch ×3 Group 2: 30 sec stretch ×3 Group 3: 1 min stretch ×1 Group 4: 30 sec stretch ×1 Group 5: CG	ROM for all stretching groups improved. No significant differences between stretching groups.
Feland et al[48]	62 men and women Ages 65-97	Static stretching to hamstring muscles 5 days/week for 6 weeks Group 1: 15 sec ×4 Group 2: 30 sec ×4 Group 3: 60 sec ×4 Group 4: CG	60-sec group had a greater rate of gain and more sustained changes in ROM.
Roberts et al[49]	24 men and women Ages 19-22	Static stretching to hamstring, quadriceps and lower leg muscles 3 days/week for 5 weeks Group 1: 5 sec stretch ×9 Group 2: 15 sec stretch ×3 Group 3: CG	15-sec group had significantly greater active ROM. No significant difference in passive ROM increase between stretching groups.
Davis et al[50]	19 men and women Ages 21-35	30 sec stretches to hamstrings 3 days/week for 4 weeks Group 1: Active self stretch Group 2: Static stretch Group 3: PNF reciprocal inhibition Group 4: CG	Only static stretch group showed significantly greater ROM.

CG, Control group, no stretching; *ROM,* range of motion; *PNF,* proprioceptive neuromuscular facilitation.

stretching force. PNF techniques have the advantage over other stretching techniques of including a motor learning component from the repeated active muscle contractions; however, their use is frequently limited by the requirement that a skilled individual must help the patient perform the technique.

Ballistic stretching is a technique in which the subject performs short, bouncing movements at the end of the available range. Although some people attempt to stretch in this manner, ballistic stretching is not generally used or recommended because it may increase tissue tightness by activating the stretch reflex.[52]

MOTION

The formation of contractures is a time-related process that may be inhibited by motion.[27] Motion can inhibit contracture formation by physically disrupting the adhesions between gross structures and/or by limiting intermolecular cross-linking. Active or passive motion also stretches tissues, promotes their lubrication and may also alter their metabolic activity.[26] Because active ROM may be contraindicated during early stages of healing, particularly after contractile tissue injury or surgery, gentle passive motion may be used to limit contracture formation at this stage. For example, continuous passive motion (CPM) can be used to prevent motion loss after joint trauma or surgery. Research and clinical protocols for the use of CPM vary considerably, but it has been found that adding CPM to physical therapy after total knee arthroplasty results in greater active knee flexion ROM and reduced length of stay and need for postoperative manipulation.[53] In addition to inhibiting the formation of contractures and adhesions, CPM has been shown to accelerate healing, improve the orientation of collagen fibers, and inhibit edema formation.[54,55]

SURGERY

Although the noninvasive approaches of stretching and motion frequently resolve or prevent motion restrictions, in some cases these approaches are not effective and surgery may be required to optimize motion. Surgery will be necessary if motion is restricted by a mechanical block, particularly if the mechanical block is bony. In such cases, the surgical procedure removes some or all of the tissue blocking motion. Surgery may also be required if stretching techniques cannot lengthen a contracture adequately or if the functional length of a tendon is decreased because of hypertonicity. For example, Z-plasty procedures are frequently performed to lengthen the Achilles tendon in children with limited dorsiflexion caused by congenital plantar flexion contractures or by hypertonicity of the plantar flexor muscles. Z-plasty is generally performed when it can be expected to permit a more functional gait than is achieved with noninvasive techniques alone. Surgical procedures to increase ROM are also frequently performed in adults. For example, surgical release may be performed to restore motion limited by a Dupuytren's contracture, and tenotomy may be performed when tendon length limits motion. Surgery may also be performed to release adhesions and lengthen scars that have formed after prolonged immobilization. For example, patients with extensive burns who have received limited medical intervention frequently develop contractures that cannot be stretched sufficiently to allow full function and therefore require surgical release. Surgery is more commonly required to release adhesions that form after injury if scarring is exaggerated by prolonged inflammation or infection.

THE ROLE OF PHYSICAL AGENTS IN THE TREATMENT OF MOTION RESTRICTIONS

Although physical agents alone are generally not sufficient to reverse or prevent motion restrictions, they may be used as adjuncts to the treatment of such impairments.

Physical agents combined with other interventions can enhance the functional recovery associated with regaining normal motion. Physical agents are generally used as components of the treatment of motion restrictions because they can increase soft tissue extensibility, control inflammation, control pain, and facilitate motion.

INCREASE SOFT TISSUE EXTENSIBILITY

Physical agents that increase tissue temperature may be used as components of the treatment of motion restriction because they can increase soft tissue extensibility, thereby decreasing the force required to increase tissue length and decreasing the risk of injury during the stretching procedure.[56,57] Applying physical agents to soft tissue before prolonged stretching can alter the viscoelasticity of the fibers, allowing more plastic deformation to occur.[58] To achieve the maximum benefit from physical agents that increase soft tissue extensibility, agents that increase superficial tissue temperature, such as those described in Chapter 6, should be used before stretching superficial tissues. Agents that increase deep tissue temperature, such as ultrasound and diathermy, should be used before stretching deep soft tissues.[59,60,61]

CONTROL INFLAMMATION AND ADHESION FORMATION

A number of physical agents, particularly cryotherapy and certain types of electrical currents, are thought to control inflammation and its associated signs and symptoms after tissue injury.[62-65] Controlling inflammation may help prevent the development of motion restrictions by limiting edema during the acute inflammatory stage, thereby limiting the degree of immobilization. Controlling the severity and duration of inflammation also limits the duration and extent of the proliferative response and may thus limit adhesion formation during tissue healing.

CONTROL PAIN DURING STRETCHING

Many physical agents, including thermotherapy, cryotherapy, and electrical currents, can help control pain. Pain control may assist in the treatment of motion restrictions because, if pain is decreased, tissues may be stretched for a longer period, which may increase tissue length more effectively. If pain is controlled, motion may also be initiated sooner after injury, limiting the loss of motion caused by immobilization.

FACILITATE MOTION

Some physical agents facilitate motion to assist in the treatment of motion restrictions. Electrical stimulation of the motor nerves of innervated muscles or direct electrical stimulation of denervated muscle can make muscles contract. These muscle contractions may complement motion produced by normal physiological contractions or substitute for such contractions if the subject does not or cannot move independently. Water may also facilitate motion since it provides buoyancy to an immersed body to assist with motion against gravity. The buoyancy of water may prove particularly beneficial in assisting patients with active ROM restrictions caused by contractile tissue weakness.

CLINICAL CASE STUDIES

The following case studies summarize the concepts of motion restrictions discussed in this chapter. Based on the scenario presented, an evaluation of the clinical findings and goals of treatment are proposed. These are followed by a discussion of the factors to be considered in treatment selection.

CASE STUDY 5-1

Radiating Low Back Pain
Examination
History

TR is a 45-year-old man who has been referred to physical therapy with a diagnosis of a right L5, S1 radiculopathy. He reports constant mild to moderately severe (4-7/10) right low back pain that radiates to his right buttock and lateral thigh after sitting for more than 20 minutes and that is relieved to some degree by walking or lying down. He reports no numbness, tingling, or weakness of the lower extremities. The pain started about 6 weeks ago, the morning after TR spent a day stacking firewood, at which time he woke up with severe low back and right lower extremity pain down to his lateral calf. He also had difficulty standing up straight. He has had similar problems in the past; however, they have always fully resolved after a couple of days of bed rest and a few aspirins. TR first saw his doctor regarding his present problem 5 weeks ago, and at that time he was prescribed a nonsteroidal antiinflammatory drug and a muscle relaxant and was told to take it easy. His symptoms improved to their current level over the following 2 weeks but have not changed since that time. He has also been unable to return to his job as a telephone installer since the onset of symptoms 6 weeks ago. A magnetic resonance imaging (MRI) scan last week showed a mild posterolateral disc bulge at L5-S1 on the right. The patient has had no prior physical therapy for his back problem.

Tests and Measures

TR weighs 91 kg (200 lb). He has a 50% restriction of lumbar active ROM in forward bending and right side-bending, both of which cause increased right low back and lower extremity pain. Left side bending decreases the patient's pain. Passive straight leg raising is 35 degrees on the right, limited by right lower extremity pain, and 60 degrees on the left, limited by hamstring tightness. Palpation reveals stiffness and tenderness to right unilateral posterior-anterior pressure at L5-S1 and no notable areas of hypermobility. All other tests, including lower extremity sensation, strength, and reflexes, are within normal limits.

What should be the goals of therapy for this patient? What is the best physical agent to use at this time and why?

Evaluation, Diagnosis, Prognosis, and Goals
Evaluation and Goals

ICF Level	Current Status	Goals
Body structure and function	Right low back pain with radiation to right buttock and lateral thigh Restricted lumbar ROM Restricted lumbar nerve root mobility on the right (limited right straight leg raise) Bulging L5-S1 disc	Decrease pain to 1/10-3/10 in 1 week Eliminate pain completely in 3 weeks Return lumbar ROM and straight leg raise to normal
Activity	Decreased sitting tolerance Unable to stand straight or lift	Increase sitting tolerance to 1 hour in 1 week Stand straight in 1 week Lift 20 lbs in 2 weeks
Participation	Unable to work	Return to limited work duties within 2 weeks

Diagnosis

Preferred Practice Pattern 4F: Impaired joint mobility, motor function, muscle performance, ROM, and reflex integrity associated with spinal disorders

Prognosis/Plan of Care

The distribution of this patient's pain and its response to changes in loading indicate that his symptoms are probably related to the mild posterolateral disc bulge at L5-S1 on the right noted on his MRI scan. The patient has a good prognosis for a full functional recovery. The plan is for him to receive physical therapy 2 to 3 times per week for 4 to 6 weeks.

Intervention

The optimal treatment for this patient would include interventions that could increase the intervertebral disc spaces or reduce disc protrusion, thus decreasing compression on the nerve roots and allowing improved, pain-free motion. Therefore an intervention of choice at this time would be spinal traction. The appropriate type of traction and the parameters of treatment are discussed in Chapter 10, and this patient's case is discussed in Case Study 10-1.

Continued

CLINICAL CASE STUDIES—*cont'd*

CASE STUDY 5-2

Adhesive Capsulitis

Examination

History

MP is a 45-year-old female physical therapist. She has been diagnosed with adhesive capsulitis of the right shoulder and has been referred to physical therapy. She reports that her shoulder first began to hurt about 6 months ago without any apparent cause. Although the pain has almost completely resolved since that time, her shoulder has gradually become more stiff, with a tight sensation at the end of range. Although she is able to perform most of her work functions, she has difficulty reaching overhead, which interferes with placing objects on high shelves and with serving when playing tennis, and she has difficulty reaching behind her to fasten clothing. MP has had no prior treatment for this problem.

Tests and Measures

MP has significantly restricted ROM of the right shoulder as follows:

Active ROM	Right	Left
Flexion	120°	170°
Abduction	170°	80°
Hand behind back	Central thoracolumbar junction	Left sacroiliac joint

Passive ROM	Right	Left
Internal rotation	90°	50°
External rotation	80°	10°

Glenohumeral passive inferior and posterior glide are both restricted on the left.

Is this patient's condition acute or chronic? Why is her shoulder movement restricted? What physical agents will best address this restriction?

Evaluation, Diagnosis, Prognosis, and Goals

Evaluation and Goals

ICF level	Current status	Goals
Body structure and function	Capsular pattern of restricted left shoulder active and passive motion	Restore normal active and passive motion of left shoulder
Activity	Unable to reach overhead, behind back	Improve ability to reach overhead and behind back
Participation	Decreased ability to dress and groom herself	Perform all activities of daily living (ADLs) as she did before injury

Diagnosis

Preferred Practice Pattern 4D: Impaired joint mobility, motor function, muscle performance, and range of motion associated with connective tissue dysfunction.

Prognosis/Plan of Care

This patient's signs and symptoms and their duration indicate that the problem has probably progressed to the remodeling stage of healing, with some possibility of chronic inflammation. MP's signs and symptoms are consistent with the diagnosis of adhesive capsulitis, which occurs most often in the shoulder. The onset of this problem is frequently reported to be insidious, although it may be associated with other pathology such as local trauma, tendinitis, cerebrovascular accident, or surgery of the neck and thorax. Predisposing factors include female gender, history of diabetes, immobilization, and age over 40 years.[20,21,66]

Since MP's shoulder ROM is probably restricted by soft tissue shortening, intervention should be directed at increasing the extensibility and length of the shortened tissues, particularly the anterior-inferior capsule of the glenohumeral joint. Other appropriate goals for this late stage of healing are to control scar tissue formation and to ensure adequate circulation. Although no strength abnormalities were noted on this initial examination, the patient's strength should be retested as she regains ROM because she may have strength deficits at these end-ranges from disuse. If strength deficits become apparent, an additional goal of treatment would be to restore normal strength to the left shoulder muscles.

Intervention

Although there is disagreement concerning the optimal intervention for adhesive capsulitis, it has been suggested that treatments that increase the extensibility and length of the restricted soft tissues around the glenohumeral joint and decrease local inflammation facilitate the resolution of this problem.[21,67,68] As is explained in greater detail in Part II of this book, a number of physical agents that provide localized deep heating may increase soft tissue extensibility, whereas other physical agents, such as ice or low-dose ultrasound, may facilitate resolution of inflammation. Thermotherapy could be used in conjunction with stretching and ROM activities to lengthen the shortened tissues. Joint mobilization and later strengthening may also be necessary to regain full function of the shoulder.

CHAPTER REVIEW

1. The musculoskeletal and neural structures of the body are normally able to move. Active movement occurs when muscles contract, and passive movement occurs when the body is acted on by an outside force. Physiological joint motion is the motion of one segment of the body relative to another, and accessory motion is the motion that occurs between the joint surfaces during normal physiological motion.

2. The amount of motion that is normal is different for different joints and may vary with the subject's age, gender, and health status.

3. Motion may be restricted by a variety of pathologies, including contractures, edema, adhesions, mechanical blocks, spinal disc herniation, adverse neural tension, and weakness.

4. Motion may be restricted in a capsular pattern if the capsule surrounding a joint is the primary structure affected. A capsular pattern of motion restriction usually produces limitations of motion in more than one direction. Patterns of motion restriction that do not fit a capsular pattern are called noncapsular.

5. Various tests and measures may be used to determine the degree of motion restriction, the tissue involved, and the nature of the pathology contributing to a motion restriction. Motion restrictions can be measured quantitatively using goniometers, tape measures, and inclinometers. Qualitative measures of motion restrictions include manual tests of active, passive, resisted, and accessory motion and neural tension testing.

6. Motion restrictions may be treated conservatively by stretching and motion or, sometimes may require invasive surgery to resolve. Physical agents may serve as adjuncts to these interventions by increasing soft tissue extensibility before stretching, controlling inflammation and adhesion formation during tissue healing, controlling pain during stretching or motion, or by facillitating motion.

7. The reader is referred to the Evolve web site for further exercises and links to resources and references.

ADDITIONAL RESOURCES `evolve`

Textbooks

Norkin CC, White DJ: *Measurement of joint motion: a guide to goniometry*, ed 3, Philadelphia, 2003, FA Davis.

Reese NB, Bandy WB: *Joint range of motion and muscle length testing*, Philadelphia, 2002, Elsevier.

GLOSSARY `evolve`

Accessory motion: The motion that occurs between joint surfaces during normal physiological motion; also called joint play.

Active motion: Movement produced by contraction of the muscles crossing a joint.

Adhesion: Binding together of normally separate anatomical structures by scar tissue.

Ballistic stretching: A type of muscle stretching in which the subject performs short, bouncing movements at the end of the available range.

Capsular pattern of restriction: A pattern of motion loss that is caused by shortening of the joint capsule.

Contractile tissue: Tissue, such as muscle and tendon, that is able to shorten.

Contracture: Fixed shortening of soft tissue structures that restricts passive and active motion and that can cause permanent deformity.

Creep: Transient lengthening or deformation of connective tissues with the application of a fixed load.

End-feel: The quality of resistance at the limit of passive motion as felt by the clinician.

Extraarticular edema: Excessive fluid outside of a joint.

Goniometer: A tool used to measure joint ROM.

Intraarticular edema: Excessive fluid within a joint capsule.

Noncapsular pattern of restriction: A pattern of motion loss that does not follow the capsular pattern.

Noncontractile tissue: Tissue that cannot actively shorten; for example, skin, ligament, and cartilage.

Osteophyte: An abnormal bony outgrowth, as seen in arthritis.

Passive accessory motion: The motion between joint surfaces produced by an external force without voluntary muscle contraction.

Passive motion: Movement produced entirely by an external force without voluntary muscle contraction.

Passive stretching: A type of muscle stretching in which the limb is moved passively.

Physiological motion: The motion of one segment of the body relative to another segment.

Plastic deformation: The elongation of connective tissue produced under loading that remains after the load is removed.

Proprioceptive neuromuscular facilitation (PNF): Muscle stretching achieved by active muscle contraction followed by muscle relaxation in conjunction with passive stretch.

Range of motion (ROM): The amount of motion that occurs when one segment of the body moves in relation to an adjacent segment.

Stress relaxation: A decrease in the amount of force required over time to maintain a certain length of connective tissue.

REFERENCES `evolve`

1. American Academy of Orthopaedic Surgeons: *Joint motion: methods of measuring and recording*, Edinburgh, 1965, Churchill Livingstone.

2. Hoppenfeld S: *Physical examination of the spine and extremities*, Norwalk, CT, 1976, Prentice-Hall, Inc.

3. Kendall FP, McCreary EK, Provance PG: *Muscles: testing and function*, ed 4, Philadelphia, 1995, Lippincott Williams & Wilkins.

4. Kilgour GM, McNair PJ, Stott NS: Range of motion in children with spastic diplegia, GMFCS I-II compared to age and gender matched controls, *Phys Occup Ther Pediatr* 25:61-79, 2005.

5. Sauseng S, Kastenbauer T, Irsigler K: Limoted joint mobility in selected hand and foot joints in patients with type 1 diabetes mellitus: a methodology comparison, *Diabetes Nutr Metab* 15:1-6, 2002.

6. Libby AK, Sherry DD, Dudgeon BJ: Shoulder limitation in juvenile rheumatoid arthritis, *Arch Phys Med Rehabil* 72:382-384, 1991.

7. Simoneau GG, Hoenig KJ, Lepley JE, et al: Influence of hip position and gender on active hip internal and external rotation, *J Orthop Sports Phys Ther* 28:158-164, 1998.

8. Doriot N, Wang X: Effects of age and gender on maximum voluntary range of motion of the upper body joints, *Ergonomics* 49:269-281, 2006.

9. Roach KE, Miles TP: Normal hip and knee active range of motion: the relationship to age, *Phys Ther* 71:656-665, 1991.

10. Sullivan MS, Dickinsin CE, Troup JD: The influence of age and gender on lumbar spine sagittal plane range of motion, *Spine* 19:682-686, 1994.

11. Kuhlman KA: Cervical range of motion in the elderly, *Arch Phys Med Rehabil* 74:1071-1079, 1993.

12. Einkauf DK, Gohdes ML, Jensen GM, et al: Changes in spinal mobility with increasing age in women, *Phys Ther* 67:370-375, 1987.

13. Lind B, Sihlbom H, Nordwall A, et al: Normal range of motion of the cervical spine, *Arch Phys Med Rehabil* 70:692-695, 1989.

14. Kessler RM, Hertling D: *Management of common musculoskeletal disorders, physical therapy principles and methods,* Philadelphia, 1983, Harper & Row.

15. Kaltenborn FM: *Mobilization of the extremity joints: examination and basic treatment techniques,* ed 3, Oslo, Norway, 1980, Olaf Norlis Bokhandel.

16. Maitland GD: *Vertebral manipulation,* ed 5, London, 1986, Butterworth-Heinemann.

17. Cyriax J: *Textbook of orthopaedic medicine,* ed 6, Baltimore, 1975, Williams & Wilkins.

18. Neviaser RJ, Neviaser TJ: The frozen shoulder: diagnosis and management, *Clin Orthop* 223:59-64, 1987.

19. Rizk TE, Pinals RS: Frozen shoulder, *Semin Arthritis Rheum* 11:440-452, 1982.

20. Bunker TD, Anthony PP: The pathology of frozen shoulder: a Dupuytren-like disease, *J Bone Joint Surg* 77B:677-683, 1995.

21. Parker RD, Froimson AI, Winsberg DD, et al: Frozen shoulder. 1. Chronology, pathogenesis, clinical picture, and treatment, *Orthopedics* 12:869-873, 1989.

22. Grubbs N: Frozen shoulder syndrome: a review of literature, *J Orthop Sports Phys Ther* 18:479-487, 1993.

23. Rundquist PJ, Ludewig PM: Patterns of motion loss in subjects with idiopathic loss of shoulder range of motion, *Clin Biomech* 19:810-818, 2004.

24. Akeson WH, Amiel D, Woo SL-Y: Immobility effects on synovial joints, the pathomechanics of joint contracture, *Biorheology* 17:95-110, 1980.

25. Salter RB: *Textbook of disorders and injuries of the musculoskeletal system,* ed 2, Baltimore, 1983, Williams & Wilkins.

26. Frank C, Akeson WH, Woo SL-Y, et al: Physiology and therapeutic value of passive joint motion, *Clin Orthop* 185:113-125, 1984.

27. Woo SL, Matthews JV, Akeson WH, et al: Connective tissue response to immobility. Correlative study of biomechanical and biochemical measurements of normal and immobilized rabbit knees, *Arthritis Rheum* 18:257-264, 1975.

28. Akeson WH, Amiel D, Abel MF, et al: Effects of immobilization on joints, *Clin Orthop* 219:28-37, 1987.

29. Trudel G, Uhthoff HK: Contractures secondary to immobility: is the restriction articular or muscular? An experimental longitudinal study in the rat knee, *Arch Phys Med Rehabil* 81:6-13, 2000.

30. *Dorland's illustrated medical dictionary,* ed 29, Philadelphia, 2000, WB Saunders.

31. Enneking WF: The intraarticular effects of immobilization on the human knee, *J Bone Joint Surg* 54A:973, 1972.

32. Slater H, Butler DS: The dynamic central nervous system. In *Grieve's modern manual,* ed 2, New York, 1994, Churchill Livingstone.

33. Oliver J, Middleditch A: *Functional anatomy of the spine,* London, 1991, Butterworth-Heinemann.

34. Butler DS: *Mobilization of the nervous system,* Edinburgh, 1991, Churchill Livingstone.

35. Norkin CC, White DJ: *Measurement of joint motion: a guide to goniometry,* Philadelphia, 1985, FA Davis.

36. Magee DJ: *Orthopedic physical assessment,* ed 4, Philadelphia, 2002, WB Saunders.

37. Riddle DL: Measurement of accessory motion: critical issues and related concepts, *Phys Ther* 72:865-874, 1992.

38. Binkley J, Stratford PW, Gill C: Interrater reliability of lumbar accessory motion mobility testing, *Phys Ther* 75:786-795, 1995.

39. Hwang JH, Lee KM, Lee JY: Therapeutic effect of passive mobilization exercise on improvement of muscle regeneration and prevention of fibrosis after laceration injury of rat, *Arch Phys Med Rehabil* 87:20-26, 2006.

40. Kaariainen M, Kaariainen J, Jarvinen TL: Correlation between biomechanical and structural changes during the regeneration of skeletal muscle after laceration injury, *J Orthop Res* 16:197-206, 1998.

41. Taylor DC, Dalton JD, Seaber AV, et al: Viscoelastic properties of muscle-tendon units: the biomechanics of stretching, *Am J Sports Med* 18:300, 1990.

42. Fung YC: *Biomechanics: mechanical properties of living tissues,* ed 2, New York, 1993, Springer-Verlag.

43. McClure PW, Blackburn LG, Dusold C: The use of splints in the treatment of stiffness: biologic rationale and an algorithm for making clinical decisions, *Phys Ther* 74:1101-1107, 1994.

44. Norkin CC, Levangie PK: *Joint structure and function: a comprehensive analysis,* ed 2, Philadelphia, 1990, FA Davis.

45. Farmer SE, James M: Contractures in orthopaedic and neurological conditions: a review of causes and treatment, *Disabil Rehabil* 23:549-558, 2001.

46. Bandy WD, Irion JM: The effect of time on static stretch on the flexibility of the hamstring muscles, *Phys Ther* 74:845-850, 1994.

47. Bandy WD, Irion JM, Briggler M: The effect of time and frequency of static stretching on flexibility of the hamstring muscles, *Phys Ther* 77:1090-1096, 1997.

48. Feland JB, Myrer JW, Schulthies SS: The effect of duration of stretching of the hamstring muscle group for increasing range of motion in people aged 65 years or older, *Phys Ther* 81:1110-1117, 2001.

49. Roberts JM, Wilson K: Effect of stretching duration on active and passive range of motion in the lower extremity, *Br J Sports Med* 33:259-263, 1999.

50. Davis DS, Ashby PE, McCale KL et al: The effectiveness of 3 stretching techniques on hamstring flexibility using consistent stretching parameters, *J Strength Cond Res* 19(1):27-32, 2005.

51. Voss DE, Ionta MK, Myers BJ: *Proprioceptive neuromuscular facilitation,* ed 3, Philadelphia, 1985, Harper & Row.

52. Lamontagne A, Maloun F, Richards CL: Viscoelastic behavior of plantar flexor muscle-tendon unit at rest, *J Orthop Sports Phys Ther* 26:244-252, 1997.

53. Milne S, Brosseau L, Robinson V: Continuous passive motion following total knee arthroplasty, *Cochrane Database Syst Rev* CD004260, 2003.

54. Salter RB, Bell RS, Keeley FW: The protective effect of continuous passive motion on living articular cartilage in acute septic arthritis: an experimental investigation in the rabbit, *Clin Orthop* 159:223-247, 1981.

55. Frank C, Akeson W, Woo S, et al: Physiology and therapeutic value of passive joint motion, *Clin Orthop* 185:113-125, 1984.

56. Lentell G, Hetherington T, Eagan J, et al: The use of thermal agents to influence the effectiveness of low load prolonged stretch, *J Orthop Sport Phys Ther* 16(5):200-207, 1992.

57. Warren C, Lehmann J, Koblanski J: Heat and stretch procedures: an evaluation using rat tail tendon, *Arch Phys Med Rehabil* 57:122-126, 1976.

58. Lehmann J, Masock A, Warren C, et al: Effect of therapeutic temperatures on tendon extensibility, *Arch Phys Med Rehabil* 51:481-487, 1970.

59. Ushuba M, Miyanaga Y, Miyakawa S, et al: Effect of heat in increasing the range of knee motion after the development if a joint contracture: an experiment with an animal model, *Arch Phys Med Rehabil* 87:247-253, 2006.

60. Robertson VJ, Ward AR, Jung P: The effects of heat on tissue extensibility: a comparison of deep and superficial heating, *Arch Phys Med Rehabil* 86:819-825, 2005.

61. Knight CA, Rutledge CR, Cox ME, et al: Effect of superficial heat, deep heat and active exercise warm-up on the extensibility of the plantar flexors, *Phys Ther* 81:1206-1214, 2001.

62. Hocutt JE, Jaffe R, Ryplander CR: Cryotherapy in ankle sprains, *Am J Sports Med* 10:316-319, 1982.

63. Cote DJ, Prentice WE, Hooker DN, et al: Comparison of three treatment procedures for minimizing ankle sprain swelling, *Phys Ther* 68(7):1072-1076, 1988.
64. Mendel FC, Wylegala JA, Fish DR: Influence of high voltage pulsed current in edema formation following impact injury in rats, *Phys Ther* 72:668-673, 1992.
65. Dolan MG, Mychaskiw AM, Mendel FC: Cool-water immersion and high-voltage electrical stimulation curb edema formation in rats, *J Athl Train* 38:225-230, 2003.
66. Kozin F: Two unique shoulders: adhesive capsulitis and sympathetic dystrophy syndrome of motion, *Postgrad Med* 73:207-216, 1983.
67. Rizk TE, Morris L, Gavant ML: Treatment of adhesive capsulitis (frozen shoulder) with arthrographic capsular distension and rupture, *Arch Phys Med Rehabil* 75:803-807, 1994.
68. Rizk TE, Pinals RS, Talaiver AS: Corticosteroid injections in adhesive capsulitis: investigation of their value and site, *Arch Phys Med Rehabil* 72:20-22, 1991.

PART II

The Physical Agents

Chapter 6

Thermal Agents: Cold and Heat

This chapter discusses the basic physical principles and physiological effects of transferring heat to or from patients using thermal agents. The clinical applications of cold and superficial heating agents are also addressed. Superficial heating agents are those that primarily increase the temperature of the skin and superficial subcutaneous tissues. In contrast, deep-heating agents also increase the temperature of deeper tissues, including large muscles and periarticular structures, and generally reach to a depth of about 5 cm. The clinical applications of deep-heating agents are not covered in this chapter but are discussed in Chapters 7 and 14.

The therapeutic application of thermal agents results in the transfer of heat to or from a patient's body and between the tissues and fluids of the body. Heat transfer occurs by **conduction, convection, conversion, radiation,** or evaporation. Heating agents transfer heat to the body, whereas cooling agents transfer heat away from the body. Thermoregulation by the body also uses the aforementioned processes to maintain core body temperature and to maintain equilibrium between internal metabolic heat production and heat loss or gain at the skin surface. The following section of this chapter discusses the physical principles of heat transfer to or from the body and within the body. This section is followed by discussions of the physiological effects of cooling and heating and directions for the clinical application of superficial cooling and heating modalities.

PHYSICAL PRINCIPLES OF THERMAL ENERGY

SPECIFIC HEAT

Specific heat is the amount of energy required to raise the temperature of a given weight of a material by a given number of degrees. The specific heat of different materials and body tissues differ (Table 6-1). For example, skin has higher specific heat than fat or bone, and water has a higher specific heat than air. Materials with a high specific heat require more energy to achieve the same temperature increase than materials with a low specific heat.

> ◎ **Clinical Pearl**
>
> Materials with a high specific heat require more energy to heat up and hold more energy at a given temperature than materials with a low specific heat.

Materials with a high specific heat also hold more energy than materials with a low specific heat when both are at the same temperature. Therefore, to transfer the same amount of heat to a patient, thermal agents with a high specific heat, such as water, are applied at lower temperatures than air-based thermal agents such as **fluidotherapy**. The specific heat of a material is generally expressed in Joules per gram per degree Celsius (J/gm/° C).

MODES OF HEAT TRANSFER

Heat can be transferred to, from, or within the body by conduction, convection, conversion, radiation, or evaporation.

Conduction

Heating by conduction is the result of energy exchange by direct collision between the molecules of two materials at different temperatures. Heat is conducted from the material at the higher temperature to the material at the lower temperature as the faster-moving molecules in the warmer material collide with the molecules in the cooler material and cause them to accelerate. Heat transfer continues until the temperature and the speed of molecular movement of both materials become equal. Heat may be transferred to or from a patient by conduction. If the physical agent used has a higher temperature than the patient's skin, for example, a hot pack or warm **paraffin**, heat will be transferred from the agent to the patient, and the temperature of the superficial tissues in contact with the heating agent will rise. If the physical agent used is colder than the patient's skin, for example, an ice pack, heat will be transferred from the patient to the agent, and the temperature of the superficial tissues in contact with the cooling agent will fall.

Heat can also be transferred from one area of the body to another by conduction. For example, when one area of the body is heated by an external thermal agent, the tissues adjacent to and in contact with that area will increase in temperature because of heating by conduction.

> ◎ **Clinical Pearl**
>
> Heat transfer by conduction occurs only between materials of different temperatures that are in direct contact with each other.

If there is any air between a conductive thermal agent and the patient, the heat is first conducted from the thermal agent to the air and then from the air to the patient.

Rate of Heat Transfer by Conduction. The rate at which heat is transferred by conduction between two materials depends on the temperature difference between the materials, their **thermal conductivity**, and their area of contact. The relationship among these variables is expressed by the following formula:

Rate of heat transfer = area of contact × thermal conductivity × temperature difference/tissue thickness

The thermal conductivity of a material describes the rate at which it transfers heat by conduction and is generally expressed in (cal/sec)/(cm² × [° C/cm]) (Table 6-2). Note that this is not the same as a material's specific heat.

TABLE 6-1	Specific Heat of Various Materials
Material	**Specific Heat in J/gm/° C**
Water	4.19
Air	1.01
Average for human body	3.56
Skin	3.77
Muscle	3.75
Fat	2.30
Bone	1.59

TABLE 6-2	Thermal Conductivity of Various Materials
Material	**Thermal Conductivity (Cal/Sec)/ (cm² × ° C/cm)**
Silver	1.01
Aluminum	0.50
Ice	0.005
Water at 20° C	0.0014
Bone	0.0011
Muscle	0.0011
Fat	0.0005
Air at 0° C	0.000057

A number of guidelines can be derived from the preceding formula.

Guidelines for Heat Transfer by Conduction

1. The greater the temperature difference between a heating or cooling agent and the body part it is applied to, the faster the rate of heat transfer. For example, the higher the temperature of a hot pack, the more rapidly the temperature of the area of the patient's skin in contact with the hot pack will increase. Generally, the temperatures of conductive physical agents are selected to achieve a fast but safe rate of temperature change. If a heating agent is only a few degrees warmer than the patient, heating will take too long; by contrast, if the temperature difference is large, heat transfer could be so rapid as to quickly burn the patient.

2. Materials with high thermal conductivity transfer heat faster than those with low thermal conductivity. Metals have high thermal conductivity, water has moderate thermal conductivity and air has low thermal conductivity.

Heating and cooling agents are generally composed of materials with moderate thermal conductivity to provide a safe and effective rate of heat transfer. Materials with low thermal conductivity can be used as insulators to limit the rate of heat transfer. For example, some types of hot packs are kept hot by soaking in and absorbing water that is kept at approximately 70° C (175° F). The high temperature, high specific heat, and moderate thermal conductivity of the water allow efficient heat transfer; however, if the pack is applied directly to a patient's skin, the patient will probably soon feel uncomfortably hot and could easily be burned. Therefore towels or terry cloth hot pack covers that trap air, which has low thermal conductivity, are placed between the pack and the patient to limit the rate of heat transfer. In general, six to eight layers of toweling are placed between a hot pack and a patient.

> ### ◎ Clinical Pearl
>
> Place six to eight layers of toweling between a hot pack and the patient to limit the rate of heat transfer and avoid burns. Additional layers of toweling can be added to further limit the rate of heat conduction.

If the patient gets too hot, additional layers of toweling can be added to further limit the rate of heat conduction. Note that newer towels and covers are generally thicker and therefore act as more effective insulators than older ones. Since subcutaneous fat has low thermal conductivity, it also acts as an insulator, limiting the conduction of heat to or from the deeper tissues.

Because metal has high thermal conductivity, metal jewelry should be removed from any area that will be in contact with a conductive thermal agent.

> ### ◎ Clinical Pearl
>
> Jewelry should be removed from any area that will be in contact with a conductive thermal agent to avoid overheating or cooling the skin in contact with the metal.

If metal jewelry is not removed, heat will rapidly transfer to the metal, with the potential to burn the skin that is in contact with it.

Ice causes more rapid cooling than water even at the same temperature, in part because it has a higher thermal conductivity than water and in part because of the amount of energy it takes to convert ice to water. The thermal conductivities of different commercially available cold packs vary, some are higher than water or ice and others are lower. Therefore, when changing the brand or type of cold pack used, one should not assume that the new pack can be applied in the same manner, for the same amount of time, or with the same number of layers of insulating material as the old pack.

3. The larger the area of contact between a thermal agent and the patient, the greater the total heat transfer. For example, when a hot pack is applied to the entire back, or when a patient is immersed up to the neck in a whirlpool or a **Hubbard tank**, the total amount of heat transferred will be greater than if a hot pack is applied only to a small area overlying the calf.

4. The rate of temperature rise decreases in proportion to tissue thickness. When a thermal agent is in contact with a patient's skin, the skin temperature increases the most and deeper tissues are progressively less affected. The deeper the tissue, the less its temperature will change. Therefore conductive thermal agents are well-suited to heating or cooling superficial tissues but should not be used when the goal is to change the temperature of deeper tissues.

Convection

Heat transfer by convection occurs as the result of direct contact between a circulating medium and another material of a different temperature. This is in contrast to heating by conduction in which there is constant contact between a stationary thermal agent and the patient. During heating or cooling by convection the thermal agent is in motion, so new parts of the agent at the initial treatment temperature keep coming into contact with the patient's body part. As a result, heat transfer by convection transfers more heat in the same period of time than heat transfer by conduction when the same material at the same initial temperature is used. For example, immersion in a whirlpool will heat a patient's skin more rapidly than immersion in a bowl of water of the same temperature, and the faster the water moves, the more rapid the rate of heat transfer will be.

> ### ◎ Clinical Pearl
>
> Whirlpools and fluidotherapy transfer heat by convection.

Blood circulating in the body also transfers heat by convection to reduce local changes in tissue temperature. For example, when a thermal agent is applied to an area of the body and produces a local change in tissue temperature, the circulation constantly moves the heated blood out of the area and moves cooler blood into the area to return the local tissue temperature to a normal level. This local cooling by convection reduces the impact of superficial heating agents on the local tissue temperature. **Vasodilation** increases the rate of circulation, increasing the rate at which the tissue temperature returns to normal.[1] Thus the vasodilation that occurs in response to heat protects the tissues by reducing the risk of burning.

> ◎ **Clinical Pearl**
>
> Circulating blood helps to keep local body temperature at baseline. The risk of thermal injury is increased when circulation is impaired.

Conversion

Heat transfer by conversion involves the conversion of a nonthermal form of energy, such as mechanical, electrical, or chemical energy, into heat. For example, **ultrasound**, which is a mechanical form of energy, is converted into heat when applied at a sufficient intensity to a tissue that absorbs ultrasound waves. Ultrasound causes vibration of molecules in the tissue, thereby generating friction between the molecules, resulting in an increase in tissue temperature. When **diathermy**, an electromagnetic form of energy, is applied to the body, it causes rotation of polar molecules, which also results in friction between the molecules and an increase in tissue temperature. Some types of cold packs cool by converting heat into chemical energy. Striking these chemical cold packs initiates a chemical reaction that extracts heat from the pack, causing it to become cold. Thermal energy is converted into chemical energy to drive this reaction.

> ◎ **Clinical Pearl**
>
> Diathermy and ultrasound heat patients by conversion.

Unlike heating by conduction or convection, heating by conversion is not affected by the temperature of the thermal agent. When transferring heat by conversion, the rate of heat transfer depends on the power of the energy source. The power of ultrasound and diathermy is usually measured in Watts, which is the amount of energy in Joules output per second. The amount of energy output by a chemical reaction depends on the reacting chemicals and is usually measured in Joules. The rate of tissue temperature increase also depends on the size of the area being treated, the size of the applicator, the efficiency of transmission from the applicator to the patient, and the type of tissue being treated. Different types of tissues absorb different forms of energy to different extents and therefore heat differently.[2]

Heat transfer by conversion does not require direct contact between the thermal agent and the body; however, it does require any intervening material to be a good transmitter of that type of energy. For example, a transmission gel, lotion, or water must be used between an ultrasound transducer and the patient to transmit the ultrasound because air, which might otherwise come between the transducer and the patient, transmits ultrasound poorly.

Physical agents that heat by conversion may also have other nonthermal physiological effects. For example,

although the mechanical energy of ultrasound and the electrical energy of diathermy can produce heat by conversion, they are also thought to have direct mechanical or electrical effects on tissue. A full discussion of absorption and the thermal and nonthermal effects of ultrasound and diathermy can be found in Chapters 7 and 14, respectively.

Radiation

Heating by radiation involves the direct transfer of energy from a material with a higher temperature to one with a lower temperature without the need for an intervening medium or contact. This is in contrast to heat transfer by conversion, in which the medium and the patient may be at the same temperature. It is also different from heat transfer by conduction or convection, which both require the thermal agent to be in contact with the tissue being heated. The rate of temperature increase caused by radiation depends on the intensity of the radiation, the relative sizes of the radiation source and the area being treated, the distance of the source from the treatment area, and the angle of the radiation to the tissue.

> ◎ **Clinical Pearl**
>
> Infrared lamps transfer heat by radiation.

Evaporation

A material must absorb energy to evaporate and thus change form from a liquid to a gas or vapor. This energy is absorbed in the form of heat, either from the material itself or from an adjoining material, resulting in a decrease in temperature. For example, when a **vapocoolant spray** is heated by the warm skin of the body, it changes from its liquid form to a vapor at its specific evaporation temperature. During this process, the spray absorbs heat and thus cools the skin.

> ◎ **Clinical Pearl**
>
> Vapocoolant sprays transfer heat from the patient by evaporation.

The evaporation of sweat also acts to cool the body. The temperature of evaporation for sweat is a few degrees higher than the normal skin temperature; therefore, if the skin temperature increases as the result of exercise or an external source and the humidity of the environment is low enough, the sweat produced in response to the increased temperature will evaporate, reducing the local body temperature. If the ambient humidity is high, evaporation will be impaired. Sweating is a homeostatic mechanism that serves to cool the body when it is overheated to help return body temperature toward the normal range.

CRYOTHERAPY

Cryotherapy, the therapeutic use of cold, has clinical applications in rehabilitation and other areas of medicine. Cryotherapy is primarily used outside of rehabilitation for the destruction of malignant and nonmalignant tissue growths; very low temperatures are used and the cooling

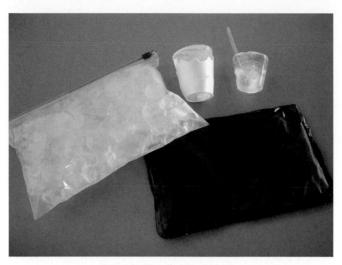

FIG 6-1 Cryotherapy agents.

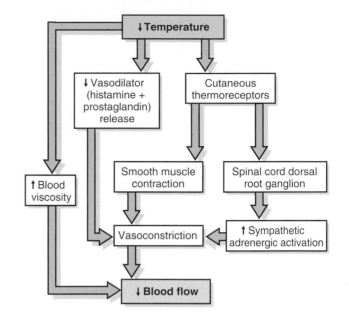

FIG 6-2 How cryotherapy decreases blood flow.

is generally applied directly to the tissue being treated. In rehabilitation, mild cooling is used to control inflammation, pain, and **edema**; to reduce **spasticity**; to control symptoms of multiple sclerosis; and to facilitate movement (Fig. 6-1). This type of cryotherapy is applied to the skin but can decrease tissue temperature deep to the area of application, including intraarticular areas.[3,4] Cryotherapy exerts its therapeutic effects by influencing hemodynamic, neuromuscular, and metabolic processes; the mechanisms of which are explained in detail in the next sections.

EFFECTS OF COLD

HEMODYNAMIC EFFECTS

Initial Decrease in Blood Flow

Generally, if cold is applied to the skin, it causes an immediate constriction of the cutaneous vessels and a reduction in blood flow. This **vasoconstriction** persists as long as the duration of the cold application is limited to less than 15 to 20 minutes.[5] Studies show that repeating ice application after an initial 20-minute application for 2 repetitions of 10 minutes off and 10 minutes on lowers blood flow significantly more than a single 20-minute ice application.[6] The vasoconstriction and reduction in blood flow produced by cryotherapy is most pronounced in the area where the cold is applied because this is where the tissue temperature decrease is greatest.

Cold causes cutaneous vasoconstriction both directly and indirectly (Fig. 6-2). Activation of the cutaneous cold receptors by cold directly stimulates the smooth muscles of the blood vessel walls to contract. Cooling of the tissue decreases the production and release of vasodilator mediators, such as histamine and prostaglandins, resulting in reduced vasodilation. Decreasing the tissue temperature also causes a reflex activation of sympathetic adrenergic neurons, resulting in cutaneous vasoconstriction in the area that is cooled and to a lesser extent, in areas distant from the site of cold application.[7] Cold is also thought to reduce the circulatory rate by increasing blood viscosity, thereby increasing the resistance to flow.

It is thought that the body reduces blood flow in response to decreased tissue temperature to protect other areas from excessive decreases in temperature and to stabilize the core body temperature.[8] The less blood that flows through an area being cooled, the smaller the amount of blood that is cooled and the less other areas in the circulatory system are affected. Reducing circulation results in a greater decrease in the temperature of the area to which a cooling agent is applied because warmer blood is not being brought into the area to raise its temperature by convection. Correspondingly, there is a smaller decrease in temperature in other areas of the body because little of the cold blood is circulated to these areas.

Later Increase in Blood Flow

The immediate vasoconstriction response to cold is a consistent and well-documented phenomenon; however, when cold is applied for longer periods of time or when the tissue temperature reaches less than 10° C (50° F), vasodilation may occur. This phenomenon is known as **cold-induced vasodilation** (CIVD) and was first reported by Lewis in 1930.[9] His findings were replicated in a number of later studies[10-12]; however, vasodilation has not been found to be a consistent response to prolonged cold application.[5,13]

Lewis reported that when an individual's fingers were immersed in an ice bath, his or her temperature initially decreased; however, after 15 minutes, his or her temperature cyclically increased and decreased (Fig. 6-3). Lewis correlated this temperature cycling with alternating vasoconstriction and vasodilation and called this the hunting response. It is proposed that the hunting response is mediated by an axon reflex in response to the pain of prolonged cold or very low temperatures, or that it is caused by inhibition of contraction of the smooth muscles of the blood vessel walls by extreme cold.[14] Maintained

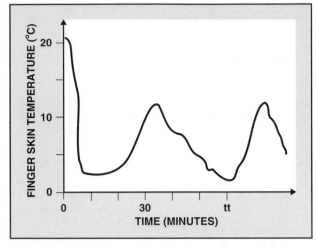

FIG 6-3 Hunting response, cold-induced vasodilation of finger immersed in ice water, measured by skin temperature change. *Adapted from Lewis T: Observations upon the reactions of the vessels of the human skin to cold, Heart 15:177-208, 1930.*

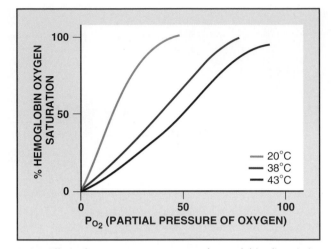

FIG 6-4 Effect of temperature on oxygen-hemoglobin dissociation curve. *Adapted from Barcroft J, King W: The effect of temperature on the dissociation curve of blood, J Physiol 39:374-384, 1909.*

vasodilation, without cycling, has also been observed with cooling human forearms at 1° C (35° F) for 15 minutes.[10]

CIVD is most likely to occur in the distal extremities, such as the fingers or toes, with applications of cold for more than 15 minutes at temperatures below 1° C. Although the amount of vasodilation is usually small, in clinical situations where vasodilation should be avoided, it is generally recommended that cold application be limited to 15 minutes or less, particularly when treating the distal extremities. When vasodilation is the intended goal of the intervention, cryotherapy is not recommended because it does not consistently have this effect.

Although the increase in skin redness seen with the application of cold may appear to be a sign of CIVD, it is actually thought to be primarily the result of an increase in the oxyhemoglobin concentration of the blood as a result of the decrease in oxygen-hemoglobin dissociation that occurs at lower temperatures (Fig. 6-4).[15] Since cooling decreases oxygen-hemoglobin dissociation, making less oxygen available to the tissues, CIVD is not considered to be an effective means of increasing oxygen delivery to an area.

NEUROMUSCULAR EFFECTS

Cold has a variety of effects on neuromuscular function, including decreasing nerve conduction velocity, elevating the pain threshold, altering muscle force generation, decreasing spasticity, and facilitating muscle contraction.

Decreased Nerve Conduction Velocity

When nerve temperature is decreased, nerve conduction velocity decreases in proportion to the degree and duration of the temperature change.[16] Decreased nerve conduction velocity has been documented in response to the application of a superficial cooling agent to the skin for 5 minutes or longer.[17] The decrease in nerve conduction velocity that occurs with 5 minutes of cooling fully reverses within 15 minutes in individuals with normal circulation. However, after 20 minutes of cooling, nerve conduction

velocity may take 30 minutes or longer to recover as a result of the greater reduction in temperature caused by the longer duration of cooling.[18]

Cold can decrease the conduction velocity of both sensory and motor nerves. It has the greatest effect on conduction by myelinated and small fibers and the least effect on conduction by unmyelinated and large fibers.[18] A-delta fibers, which are small-diameter, myelinated, pain-transmitting fibers, demonstrate the greatest decrease in conduction velocity in response to cooling. Reversible total nerve conduction block can also occur with the application of ice over superficially located major nerve branches such as the peroneal nerve at the lateral aspect of the knee.[19]

Increased Pain Threshold

Applying cryotherapy can increase the pain threshold and decrease the sensation of pain. The proposed mechanisms for these effects include counter-irritation via the gate control mechanism and the reduction of muscle spasm, sensory nerve conduction velocity, or postinjury edema.[20]

Stimulation of the cutaneous cold receptors by cold may provide sufficient sensory input to fully or partially block the transmission of painful stimuli to the brain cortex, producing an increase in pain threshold and a decrease in pain sensation. Such gating of the sensation of pain can also reduce muscle spasm by interrupting the pain-spasm-pain cycle, as described in Chapter 3. Cryotherapy may also reduce the pain associated with an acute injury by reducing the rate of blood flow in an area and by decreasing the rate of reactions related to acute inflammation, thus controlling postinjury edema formation.[21] Reducing edema can also alleviate pain produced by compression of nerves or other pressure-sensitive structures.

Altered Muscle Strength

Depending on the duration of the intervention and the timing of measurement, cryotherapy has been associated with both increases and decreases in muscle strength. Iso-

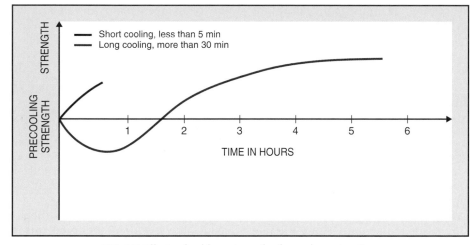

FIG 6-5 Effects of cold on strength of muscle contraction.

metric muscle strength has been found to increase directly after the application of ice massage for 5 minutes or less; however, the duration of this effect has not been documented.[22] The proposed mechanisms for this response to brief cooling include facilitation of motor nerve excitability and an increased psychological motivation to perform. In contrast, after cooling for 30 minutes or longer, isometric muscle strength has been found to decrease initially and then to increase an hour later, to reach greater than precooling strength for the following 3 hours or longer (Fig. 6-5).[23-25] The proposed mechanisms for the reduced strength after prolonged cooling include reduction of blood flow to the muscles, slowed motor nerve conduction, increased muscle viscosity, and increased joint or soft tissue stiffness.

It is important to be aware of these changes in muscle strength in response to the application of cryotherapy since they can obscure accurate, objective assessment of muscle strength and patient progress. It is therefore recommended that muscle strength be consistently measured before the application of cryotherapy and that precooling strength not be compared with postcooling strength when trying to assess patient progress.

> ⊚ **Clinical Pearl**
>
> Since muscle strength can be temporarily influenced by cryotherapy, strength testing should be performed before rather than after cryotherapy application.

Decreased Spasticity

When applied appropriately, cryotherapy can temporarily decrease spasticity. Two mechanisms are proposed to act sequentially to produce this effect: first, a decrease in gamma motor neuron activity and later, a decrease in afferent spindle and Golgi tendon organ (GTO) activity. A decrease in the amplitude of the Achilles tendon reflex and integrated electromyography (EMG) activity have been observed within a few seconds of the application of cold to the skin.[26,27] These changes are thought to be related to a decrease in the activity of the gamma motor

neurons as a reflex reaction to stimulation of the cutaneous cold receptors. This fast response must be related to stimulation of cutaneous structures because the temperature of the muscles cannot decrease after such a brief period of cooling.

After more prolonged cooling, lasting for 10 to 30 minutes, a temporary decrease or elimination of spasticity and clonus, depression of the Achilles tendon reflex, and a reduction in resistance to passive motion have also been observed in some patients with spasticity.[27-31] These changes are thought to be caused by a decrease in the discharge from the afferent spindles and GTOs as a result of decreased muscle temperature.[32] These later effects generally persist for 1 to 1½ hours and can therefore be taken advantage of in treatment by applying cryotherapy to hypertonic areas for up to 30 minutes before other interventions to reduce spasticity during functional or therapeutic activities.

Facilitation of Muscle Contraction

Brief application of cryotherapy is thought to facilitate alpha motor neuron activity to produce a contraction in a muscle that is flaccid because of upper motor neuron dysfunction.[27] This effect is observed in response to a few seconds of cooling and lasts for only a short time. With prolonged cooling of even a few minutes, a decrease in gamma motor neuron activity reduces the force of muscle contraction. This brief facilitation effect of cryotherapy is occasionally used clinically when trying to stimulate the production of appropriate motor patterns in patients with upper motor neuron lesions.

METABOLIC EFFECTS
Decreased Metabolic Rate

Cold decreases the rate of all metabolic reactions, including those involved in inflammation and healing. Thus cryotherapy can be used to control acute inflammation but is not recommended when healing is delayed because it may further impair recovery. The activity of cartilage-degrading enzymes, including collagenase, elastase, hyaluronidase, and protease, is inhibited by decreases in joint temperature, almost ceasing at joint temperatures of 30° C (86° F) or lower.[33] Thus cryotherapy is recommended as an intervention for the prevention or reduction of collagen destruction in inflammatory joint diseases such as osteoarthritis and rheumatoid arthritis.

USES OF CRYOTHERAPY

INFLAMMATION CONTROL

Cryotherapy can be used to control acute inflammation and thereby accelerate recovery from injury or trauma.[34] A recent critical review of studies on various treatment modalities for soft tissue injuries of the ankle found that cryotherapy reduced pain and edema and shortened recovery time if it was applied within the first 2 days after an injury.[35] Decreasing tissue temperature slows the rate of the chemical reactions that occur during the acute inflammatory response and also reduces the heat, redness, edema, pain, and loss of function associated with this phase of tissue healing. Cryotherapy directly reduces the heat associated with inflammation by decreasing the temperature of the area to which it is applied. The decrease in blood flow caused by vasoconstriction and increased blood viscosity and the decrease in capillary permeability associated with cryotherapy impede the movement of fluid from the capillaries to the interstitial tissue, thereby controlling bleeding and fluid loss after acute trauma. It is thought that in soft tissue injury cryotherapy also in part prevents microvascular damage by decreasing the activity of leukocytes, which damage vessel walls and increase capillary permeability.[36,37] These effects reduce the redness and edema associated with inflammation. As described in more detail in the next section, cryotherapy is thought to control pain by decreasing the activity of the A-delta pain fibers and by gating at the spinal cord level. Controlling the edema and pain associated with inflammation limits the loss of function associated with this phase of tissue healing.

It is recommended that cryotherapy be applied immediately after an injury and throughout the acute inflammatory phase.

> ◎ **Clinical Pearl**
>
> Apply cryotherapy immediately after injury and during the acute inflammatory phase of healing to help control bleeding, edema, and pain and to accelerate recovery.

Immediate application helps to control bleeding and edema; therefore the sooner the intervention is applied, the greater and more immediate the potential benefit.[38] Local skin temperature can be used to estimate the stage of healing and determine if cryotherapy is indicated. If the temperature of an area is elevated, the area is probably still inflamed and cryotherapy is likely to be beneficial. Once the local temperature returns to normal, the acute inflammation has probably resolved and cryotherapy should be discontinued. Acute inflammation usually resolves within 48 to 72 hours of acute trauma but may be prolonged with severe trauma, inflammatory diseases such as rheumatoid arthritis, or with chronic recurrent injuries. If the tempera-

ture of an area remains elevated for longer than expected, infection is a possibility and the patient should be referred to a physician for further evaluation. Cryotherapy should be discontinued when acute inflammation has resolved to avoid impeding recovery during the later stages of healing by slowing chemical reactions or impairing circulation.

Studies have also shown that applying low-level cryotherapy continuously for a number of days can reduce inflammation and pain after orthopedic surgery (hip replacement, shoulder surgery).[39-41] Although evidence in favor of this modality is mounting, prolonged cryotherapy is not currently routinely applied after surgical procedures.

The prophylactic use of cryotherapy after exercise can reduce the severity of **delayed-onset muscle soreness** (DOMS).[42] DOMS is thought to be the result of inflammation from muscle and connective tissue damage caused by exercise.[43,44] The prophylactic use of cryotherapy after aggressive joint or soft tissue mobilization, or after light activity in an area with a preexisting inflammation, can decrease postactivity soreness.

Cryotherapy is often recommended for the treatment of acute inflammation and may also be helpful in patients with chronic inflammatory conditions such as osteoarthritis and rheumatoid arthritis.[45-47] One study found that ice massage resulted in increased knee strength, ROM, and function in patients with osteoarthritis but did not affect pain in these subjects.[45] Another study found that brief application of whole-body cryotherapy (sitting in a room at −60° or −110° C [−76° or −166° F] for 2 to 3 minutes) provided more pain relief than local cryotherapy (cold air or ice packs at −30° C [−22° F]) applied to inflamed joints in patients with rheumatoid arthitis.[47] However, the expense and inconvenience of whole-body cryotherapy limit its practical use.

Although cryotherapy can help to control inflammation and its associated signs and symptoms, the cause of the inflammation must also be addressed directly to prevent recurrence. For example, if inflammation is caused by overuse of a tendon, the patient's use of that tendon must be modified if recurrence of symptoms is to be avoided.

When cryotherapy is applied with the goal of controlling inflammation, the treatment time is generally limited to 15 minutes or less because longer application has been associated with vasodilation and increased circulation.[9-12] However, since reflex vasodilation in response to cold has not been shown to occur outside of the distal extremities, longer treatment durations may be used for areas other than the distal extremities.[5,13] To limit the probability of excessive decreases in tissue temperature and cold-induced injury, cryotherapy applications should be at least 1 hour apart so that the tissue temperature can return to normal between treatments.

> ◎ **Clinical Pearl**
>
> When using cryotherapy to control inflammation on the extremities, apply for no longer than 20 minutes at least 1 hour apart.

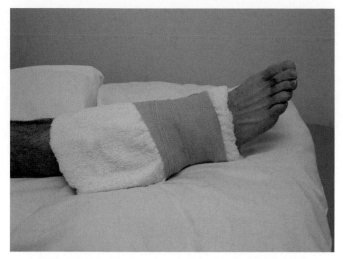

FIG 6-6 Cryotherapy with compression and elevation.

EDEMA CONTROL

Cryotherapy can be used to control the formation of edema, particularly when the edema is associated with acute inflammation.[45,48] During acute inflammation, edema is caused by extravasation of fluid into the interstitium as a result of increased intravascular fluid pressure and increased vascular permeability. Cryotherapy reduces the intravascular fluid pressure by reducing blood flow into the area via vasoconstriction and increased blood viscosity. Cryotherapy also controls increases in capillary permeability by reducing the release of vasoactive substances such as histamine.

To minimize edema formation, cryotherapy should be applied as soon as possible after an acute trauma. The formation of edema associated with inflammation will be most effectively controlled if the cryotherapy is applied in conjunction with compression and elevation of the affected area.[49,50] Compression can easily be applied with an elastic wrap, and elevation should be above the level of the heart (Fig. 6-6). Compression and elevation reduce edema by driving extravascular fluid out of the swollen area into the venous and lymphatic drainage systems. The combined intervention of rest, ice, compression, and elevation is frequently referred to by the acronym **RICE**.

> ### Clinical Pearl
> Cryotherapy, along with compression and elevation, reduces postinjury edema.

Although cryotherapy can reduce the edema associated with acute inflammation it is not effective for controlling edema caused by immobility and poor circulation. In such cases, increased rather than decreased venous or lymphatic circulation is required to move fluid out of the affected area. This is best accomplished with compression, elevation, heat, exercise, and massage.[51] The mechanisms of action of this combination of treatments are discussed in detail in Chapter 11 in the section on compression.

PAIN CONTROL

The decrease in tissue temperature produced by cryotherapy may directly or indirectly reduce the sensation of pain. Cryotherapy directly and rapidly modifies the sensation of pain by gating pain transmission with activity of the cutaneous thermal receptors. This immediate analgesic effect of cold is exploited when vapocoolant sprays or ice massage are used to cool the skin before stretching the muscles below. The reduced sensation of pain allows the stretch to be more forceful and thus potentially more effective.

Applying cryotherapy for 10 to 15 minutes or longer can control pain for 1 or more hours. This prolonged effect is thought to be the result of blocking conduction by deep pain-transmitting A-delta fibers and by gating of pain transmission by the cutaneous thermal receptors.[18] The effect is thought to be prolonged because the temperature of the area remains lower than normal for 1 or 2 hours after removal of the cooling modality. Rewarming of the area is slow because cold-induced vasoconstriction limits the flow of warm blood into the area, and subcutaneous fat insulates the deeper tissues from rewarming by conduction from the ambient air.

The reduction of pain by cryotherapy can also interrupt the pain-spasm-pain cycle, resulting in reduced muscle spasm and prolonged alleviation of pain even after the temperature of the treated area has returned to normal. Cryotherapy can also reduce pain indirectly by alleviating the underlying cause of this symptom such as inflammation or edema.

MODIFICATION OF SPASTICITY

Cryotherapy can be used to temporarily reduce spasticity in patients with upper motor neuron dysfunctions. As explained previously, brief applications of cold, lasting for about 5 minutes, cause an almost immediate decrease in deep tendon reflexes. Longer applications, for 10 to 30 minutes, also decrease or eliminate clonus and decrease the resistance of muscles to passive stretch.[26] Because longer applications of cryotherapy control more of the signs of spasticity, cryotherapy should be applied for up to 30 minutes when this is the goal of the intervention. The decrease in spasticity produced by prolonged cooling generally lasts for 1 hour or longer after the intervention, which is sufficient to allow for a variety of therapeutic interventions, including active exercise, stretching, functional activities, or hygiene.

SYMPTOM MANAGEMENT IN MULTIPLE SCLEROSIS

The symptoms of some patients with multiple sclerosis are aggravated by generalized heating such as occurs in warm environments or with activity. This group of patients can respond well to generalized cooling, with improvements in electrophysiological measures and in clinical symptoms and function.[52] Cooling with a vest has been shown to improve fatigue, muscle strength, visual function, and postural stability in a group of patients with heat-sensitive multiple sclerosis when compared with a sham noncooling vest.[53,54] Peripheral cooling has also been found to decrease tremor in some patients with multiple sclerosis.[55]

FACILITATION

The rapid application of ice as a stimulus to elicit desired motor patterns, known as **quick icing**, is a technique developed by Rood. Although this technique may be used effectively in the rehabilitation of patients with flaccidity resulting from upper motor neuron dysfunction, it tends to have unreliable results and is therefore not commonly used.[56] The results of quick icing are unreliable because the initial phasic withdrawal pattern stimulated in the agonist muscles may lower the resting potential of the antagonists, so that a second stimulus elicits activity in the antagonist muscles rather than in the agonists.[57] This produces motion first in the desired direction, followed by a rebound movement in the opposite direction. It has also been proposed that icing may adversely impact motor control caused by dyssynchronization of the cortex as a result of increased sympathetic tone.[58]

CRYOKINETICS AND CRYOSTRETCH

Cryokinetics is a technique that combines the use of cold and exercise in the treatment of pathology or disease.[59] This technique involves applying a cooling agent to the point of numbness shortly after any injury to reduce the sensation of pain and thus allow the patient to exercise and work toward regaining range of motion (ROM) as early as possible in the recovery process.[60] This approach is most commonly used in the rehabilitation of athletes. Cold is applied first for up to 20 minutes, or until the patient reports numbing of the area; then the patient performs strengthening and stretching exercises for 3 to 5 minutes until sensation returns.[61] The cooling agent is then reapplied until analgesia is regained. This sequence of cooling, exercise, and recooling is repeated approximately five times. Because the numbness produced by the cryotherapy masks the pain related to the injury and to avoid further trauma and tissue damage, it is essential that before applying this technique, the exact nature of the injury is known and the therapist is certain that it is safe to exercise the area involved.

Cryostretch is the application of a cooling agent before stretching. The purpose of this sequence of treatments is to reduce muscle spasm and thus allow greater ROM increases with stretching.[62] It has also been found that application of a cold pack after a hot pack is more effective than hot pack alone in improving passive ROM (PROM) in people with restricted knee ROM.[63]

Some recommend that elite athletes precool the entire body with cold water, air, or a cooling vest before exercising in hot conditions. This is thought to delay elevation of core body temperature and thereby delay exercise fatigue and reduced performance associated with hyperthermia. A number of small studies (n = 8-10) have found that precooling the entire body improves performance of exercise lasting at least 30 to 40 minutes.[64]

CONTRAINDICATIONS AND PRECAUTIONS FOR CRYOTHERAPY

Although cryotherapy is a relatively safe intervention, its use is contraindicated in some circumstances and it should be applied with caution in others. Cryotherapy may be applied by a qualified clinician or by a properly instructed patient. Rehabilitation clinicians may use all forms of cryotherapy that are noninvasive and do not destroy tissue. Patients may use cold packs or ice packs, ice massage, or **contrast baths** to treat themselves.

If the patient's condition is worsening or is not improving after two or three treatments, the treatment approach should be reevaluated and changed or the patient should be referred to a physician for further evaluation even when cryotherapy is not contraindicated.

CONTRAINDICATIONS FOR THE USE OF CRYOTHERAPY

> **CONTRAINDICATIONS**
> **for the Use of Cryotherapy**
> * Cold hypersensitivity (cold-induced urticaria)
> * Cold intolerance
> * Cryoglobulinemia
> * Paroxysmal cold hemoglobinuria
> * Raynaud's disease or phenomenon
> * Over regenerating peripheral nerves
> * Over an area with circulatory compromise or peripheral vascular disease

Cold Hypersensitivity (Cold-Induced Urticaria)

Some individuals have a familial or acquired hypersensitivity to cold that causes them to develop a vascular skin reaction in response to cold exposure.[65] This reaction is marked by the transient appearance of smooth, slightly elevated patches, which are redder or more pale than the surrounding skin and are often attended by severe itching. This response is known as cold hypersensitivity or cold-induced urticaria. These symptoms can occur only in the area of cold application or all over the body.

Cold Intolerance

Cold intolerance, in the form of severe pain, numbness, and color changes in response to cold, can occur in patients with some types of rheumatic diseases or after severe accidental or surgical trauma to the digits.

Cryoglobulinemia

Cryoglobulinemia is an uncommon disorder characterized by the aggregation of serum proteins in the distal circulation when the distal extremities are cooled. These aggregated proteins form a precipitate or gel that can impair circulation, causing local ischemia and then gangrene. This disorder may be idiopathic or may be associated with multiple myeloma, systemic lupus erythematosus, rheumatoid arthritis, or other hyperglobulinemic states. Therefore the therapist should check with the referring physician before applying cryotherapy to the distal extremities of any patient with these predisposing disorders.

Paroxysmal Cold Hemoglobinuria

Paroxysmal cold hemoglobinuria is a condition in which hemoglobin from lysed red blood cells is released into the urine in response to local or general exposure to cold.

Raynaud's Disease and Phenomenon

Raynaud's disease is the primary or idiopathic form of paroxysmal digital cyanosis. Raynaud's phenomenon, which is more common, is paroxysmal digital cyanosis that results from some other regional or systemic disorder. Both conditions are characterized by sudden pallor and cyanosis followed by redness of the skin of the digits precipitated by cold or emotional upset and relieved by warmth. These disorders occur primarily in young women. In Raynaud's disease the symptoms are bilateral and symmetrical even when cold is applied to only one area, whereas in Raynaud's phenomenon, the symptoms generally occur only in the cooled extremity. Raynaud's phenomenon may be associated with thoracic outlet syndrome, carpal tunnel syndrome, or trauma.

Ask the Patient

- Do you have any unusual responses to cold? If the patient answers "yes" to this question, ask for further details, and include the following questions:
- Do you develop a rash when cold? (A sign of cold hypersensitivity)
- Do you have severe pain, numbness, and color changes in your fingers when exposed to cold? (Signs of Raynaud's disease or Raynaud's phenomenon)
- Do you get blood in your urine after being cold? (A sign of paroxysmal cold hemoglobinuria)

If the responses indicate that the patient may have cold hypersensitivity, cold intolerance, cryoglobulinemia, paroxysmal cold hemoglobinuria, Raynaud's disease, or Raynaud's phenomenon, cryotherapy should not be applied.

Over Regenerating Peripheral Nerves

Cryotherapy should not be applied directly over a regenerating peripheral nerve because local vasoconstriction or altered nerve conduction may delay nerve regeneration.

Ask the Patient

- Do you have any nerve damage in this area?
- Do you have any numbness or tingling in this limb? If so, where?

Assess

- Test sensation

In the presence of sensory impairment or other signs of nerve dysfunction, cryotherapy should not be applied directly over the affected nerve.

Over an Area with Circulatory Compromise or Peripheral Vascular Disease

Cryotherapy should not be applied over an area with impaired circulation because it may aggravate the condition by causing vasoconstriction and increasing blood viscosity. Circulatory impairment may be the result of peripheral vascular disease, trauma to the vessels, or early healing and is often associated with edema. When edema is present, it is important that its cause be determined because edema that results from inflammation can benefit from cryotherapy, whereas edema that results from impaired circulation may be increased. These causes of edema can be distinguished by observation of local skin color and temperature. Edema caused by inflammation is characterized by warmth and redness, whereas edema caused by poor circulation is characterized by coolness and pallor.

> ### ⊚ Clinical Pearl
>
> In general, when edema is caused by poor circulation, the area is cool and pale, and when edema is caused by inflammation, the area is warm and red.

Ask the Patient

- Do you have poor circulation in this limb?

Assess

- Skin temperature and color

If the patient has signs of impaired circulation, such as pallor and coolness of the skin, in the area being considered for treatment, cryotherapy should not be applied.

PRECAUTIONS FOR THE USE OF CRYOTHERAPY

> ### PRECAUTIONS
> #### for the Use of Cryotherapy
>
> - Over a superficial main branch of a nerve
> - Over an open wound
> - Hypertension
> - Poor sensation or poor mentation
> - Very young and very old patients

Over a Superficial Main Branch of a Nerve

Applying cold directly over the superficial main branch of a nerve, such as the peroneal nerve at the lateral knee or the radial nerve at the posterolateral elbow, may cause a nerve conduction block.[16,19,66,67] Therefore, when applying cryotherapy to such an area, one should monitor for signs of changes in nerve conduction, such as distal numbness or tingling, and discontinue cryotherapy if these occur.

Over an Open Wound

Cryotherapy should not be applied directly over any deep open wound because it can delay wound healing by reducing circulation and metabolic rate.[68] Cryotherapy may be applied in areas of superficial skin damage; however, it is important to realize that this can reduce the efficacy and safety of the intervention because when there is superficial skin damage the cutaneous thermal receptors may also be damaged or absent. These receptors play a part in activating the vasoconstriction, pain control, and spasticity reduction produced by cryotherapy; therefore these responses are likely to be less pronounced when cryotherapy is applied to areas with superficial skin damage.

Caution should also be used if cryotherapy is applied to such areas because the absence of skin reduces the insulating protection of the subcutaneous layers and increases the risk of excessive cooling of these tissues.

Assess
• Inspect the skin closely for deep wounds, cuts, or abrasions.

Do not apply cryotherapy in the area of a deep wound. Use less intense cooling if cuts or abrasions are present.

Hypertension
Because cold can cause transient increases in systolic or diastolic blood pressure, patients with hypertension should be carefully monitored during the application of cryotherapy.[69] Treatment should be discontinued if blood pressure increases beyond safe levels during treatment. Guidelines for safe blood pressures for individual patients should be obtained from the physician.

Poor Sensation or Mentation
Although adverse effects with cryotherapy are rare, if the patient cannot sense or report discomfort or other abnormal responses, the clinician should monitor the patient's response directly. The clinician should check for adverse responses to cold, such as wheals or abnormal changes in color or strength, in the area of cold application and generally.

Very Young and Very Old Patients
Caution should be used when applying cryotherapy to the very young or the very old because these individuals frequently have impaired thermal regulation and a limited ability to communicate.

ADVERSE EFFECTS OF CRYOTHERAPY

A variety of adverse effects have been reported when cold is applied incorrectly or when contraindicated. The most severe adverse effect from the improper application of cryotherapy is tissue death caused by prolonged vasoconstriction, ischemia, and thromboses in the smaller vessels. Tissue death may also result from freezing of the tissue. Tissue damage can occur when the tissue temperature reaches 15° C (59° F); however, freezing (frostbite) does not occur until the skin temperature drops to between –4° and –10° C (39° to 14° F) or lower. Excessive exposure to cold may also cause temporary or permanent nerve damage, resulting in pain, numbness, tingling, hyperhidrosis, or nerve conduction abnormalities.[70] To avoid soft tissue or nerve damage, the duration of cold application should be limited to under 45 minutes, and the tissue temperature should be maintained above 15° C (59° F).

Because the prolonged application of cryotherapy to the distal extremities may cause reflex vasodilation and increased blood flow, cryotherapy should be applied for only 10 to 20 minutes when the goal of the intervention is vasoconstriction.

APPLICATION TECHNIQUES

GENERAL CRYOTHERAPY
Cryotherapy may be applied using a variety of materials, including cold or ice packs, ice cups, **controlled cold compression** units, vapocoolant sprays, frozen towels, ice water, cold whirlpools, and contrast baths.

> ◎ **Clinical Pearl**
>
> Cool cold packs for at least 2 hours before initial use and for 30 minutes between uses.

Different materials cool at different rates and to different degrees and depths. Ice packs and a water/alcohol mixture cool the skin more, and more quickly, than do gel packs or frozen peas at the same initial temperature.[71] Although frozen peas applied for 20 minutes can reduce skin temperatures sufficiently to cause localized skin analgesia, reduce nerve conduction velocity, and reduce metabolic enzyme activity, flexible frozen gel packs applied for the same length of time have been found not to cool to this level.[72] In general, applying a frozen gel packs or ice packs for 20 minutes reduces the temperature of the skin and tissues up to 2 cm deep.[73] However, overlying adipose tissue and exercising while the ice is applied can lessen the cooling effect of this type of cryotherapy.[74,75] Continuous cryotherapy applied for 23 hours can cause deeper cooling and has been shown to reduce temperatures within the shoulder joint.[39] In addition, submersion of the leg in a 10° C (50° F) whirlpool for 20 minutes has been found to more effectively maintain prolonged tissue cooling than application of crushed ice to the calf muscle area for the same amount of time.[76]

During the application of cryotherapy by any means the patient will usually experience the following sequence of sensations: intense cold followed by burning, then aching, and finally analgesia and numbness.

> ◎ **Clinical Pearl**
>
> The typical sequence of sensations in response to cryotherapy is: 1, intense cold; 2, burning; 3, aching; 4, analgesia; 5, numbness.

These sensations are thought to correspond to increasing stimulation of the thermal receptors and pain receptors followed by blocking of sensory nerve conduction as the tissue temperature decreases.

APPLICATION TECHNIQUE 6-1	**GENERAL CRYOTHERAPY**

1. Evaluate the patient and set the goals of treatment.
2. Determine if cryotherapy is the most appropriate intervention.
3. Determine that cryotherapy is not contraindicated for this patient or condition.

   Inspect the area to be treated for open wounds and rashes and assess sensation. Check the patient's chart for any record of previous adverse responses to cold and for any diseases that would predispose the patient to an adverse response. Ask the appropriate questions of the patient as described in the preceding sections on contraindications and precautions.
4. Select the appropriate cooling agent according to the body part to be treated and the desired response.

   Select an agent that provides the desired intensity of cold, best fits the location and size of the area to be treated, is easily applied for the desired duration and in the desired position, is readily available, and is reasonably priced. An agent that conforms to the contours of the area being treated should be used to maintain good contact with the patient's skin. With agents that cool by conduction or convection, such as cold packs or a cold whirlpool, good contact must be maintained between the agent and the patient's body at all times to maximize the rate of cooling. For brief cooling the best choice is an agent that is quick to apply and remove. Any of the cooling agents described in this text may be available for use in a clinical setting, and the patient can readily use ice packs, ice cups, and cold packs at home. Ice packs and ice massage are the least expensive means of providing cryotherapy, whereas controlled cold compression units are the most expensive.

5. Explain the procedure and reason for applying cryotherapy and the sensations the patient can expect to feel, as described previously.
6. Apply the appropriate cooling agent.

   Select from the following list (see applications for each cooling agent on the next pages):
   - Cold packs or ice packs
   - Ice cups for ice massage
   - Controlled cold compression units
   - Vapocoolant sprays or brief icing
   - Frozen towels
   - Ice water immersion
   - Cold whirlpool
   - Contrast bath

   The next section of this chapter gives details on application techniques for different cooling agents and the decisions to be made when selecting a specific agent and an application technique.
7. Assess the outcome of the intervention.

   After completing cryotherapy with any of the preceding agents, reassess the patient, checking particularly for progress toward the set goals of treatment and for any adverse effects of the intervention. Remeasure quantifiable subjective conditions and objective limitations, and reassess function and activity.
8. Document the intervention.

COLD PACKS OR ICE PACKS

Cold packs are usually filled with a gel composed of silica or a mixture of saline and gelatin and are usually covered with vinyl (Fig. 6-7). The gel is formulated to be semisolid at between 0° and 5° C (32° to 41° F) so the pack conforms to the body contours when it is within this temperature range. The temperature of a cold pack is maintained by storing it in specialized cooling units (Fig. 6-8) or in a freezer at –5° C (23° F). Cold packs should be cooled for at least 30 minutes between uses and for 2 hours or longer before initial use.

Patients can use plastic bags of frozen vegetables at home as a substitute for cold packs, or they can make their own cold packs from plastic bags filled with a 4:1 ratio mixture of water and rubbing alcohol cooled in a home freezer. The addition of alcohol to the water decreases the freezing temperature of the mixture so that it is semisolid and flexible at –5° C (23° F).

Ice packs are made of crushed ice placed in a plastic bag. Ice packs provide more aggressive cooling than cold packs at the same temperature because ice has a higher specific heat than most gels and ice absorbs a large amount of energy when it melts and changes from a solid to a liquid.[77] Both cold packs and ice packs are applied in a similar manner; however, more insulation should be used when applying an ice pack because it provides more aggressive cooling (Fig. 6-9).

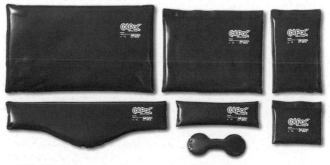

FIG 6-7 Cold packs. *Courtesy Chattanooga Group, Hixson, TN.*

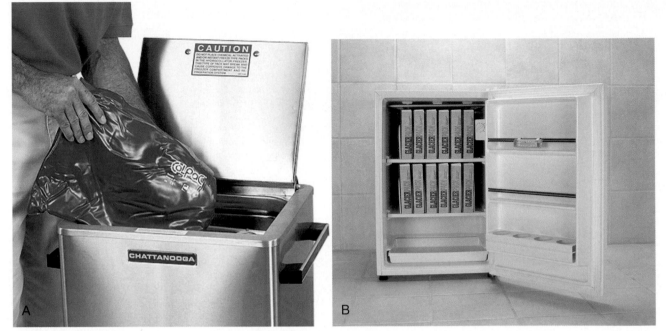

FIG 6-8 Cooling units for cold packs. **A**, *Courtesy Chattanooga Group, Hixson, TN;* **B**, *courtesy Whitehall Manufacturing, City of Industry, CA.*

APPLICATION TECHNIQUE 6-2 COLD PACKS OR ICE PACKS

Equipment Required

- Towels or pillow cases for hygiene and/or insulation
- AND, for cold packs
- Cold packs in a variety of sizes and shapes appropriate for different areas of the body
- Freezer or specialized cooling unit
- OR, for ice packs
- Plastic bags
- Ice chips
- Ice chip machine or freezer

Procedure

1. Remove all jewelry and clothing from the area to be treated and inspect the area.
2. Wrap the cold pack or ice pack in a towel. Use a damp towel if a maximal rate of tissue cooling is desired. It is recommended that warm water be used to dampen the towel to allow the patient to gradually become accustomed to the cold sensation. A thin, dry towel can be used if slower, less intense cooling is desired. A damp towel is generally appropriate for a cold pack, whereas a dry towel should be used for an ice pack because ice provides more intense cooling.
3. Position the patient comfortably, elevating the area to be treated if edema is present.
4. Place the wrapped pack on the area to be treated and secure it well. Packs can be secured with elastic bandages or towels to ensure good contact with the patient's skin.
5. Leave the pack in place for 10 to 20 minutes to control pain, inflammation, or edema. When cold is applied over bandages or a cast, the application time should be increased to allow the cold to penetrate through these insulating layers to the skin.[78] In this circumstance, the cold pack should be replaced with a newly frozen pack if the original pack melts during the course of the intervention.

If cryotherapy is being used to control spasticity, the pack should be left in place for up to 30 minutes. With these longer applications, check every 10 to 15 minutes for any signs of adverse effects.
6. Provide the patient with a bell or other means to call for assistance.
7. When the intervention is completed, remove the pack and inspect the treatment area for any signs of adverse effects such as wheals or a rash. It is normal for the skin to be red or dark pink after icing.
8. Cold or ice pack application can be repeated every 1 to 2 hours to control pain and inflammation.[79]

Advantages

- Easy to use.
- Inexpensive materials and equipment.
- Short use of clinician's time.
- Low level of skill required for application.
- Covers moderate to large areas.
- Can be applied to an elevated limb.

Disadvantages

- Pack must be removed to visualize the treatment area during treatment.
- Patient may not tolerate weight of the pack.
- Pack may not be able to maintain good contact on small or contoured areas.
- Long duration of treatment compared to massage with an ice cup.

Ice Pack Versus Cold Pack

- Ice pack provides more intense cooling.
- Ice pack is less expensive.
- Cold pack is quicker to apply.

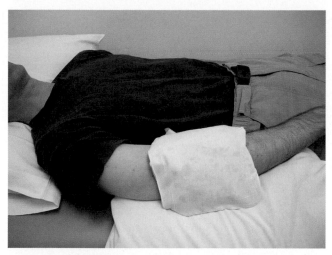

FIG 6-9 Application of a cold pack.

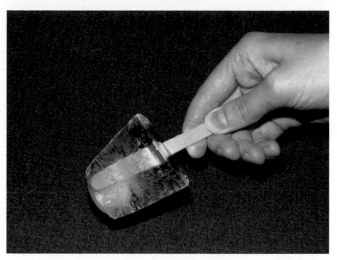

FIG 6-11 Water popsicle.

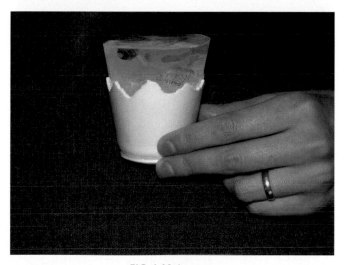

FIG 6-10 Ice cup.

ICE MASSAGE

Ice cups (Fig. 6-10) or frozen water popsicles[80] (Fig. 6-11) can be used to apply ice massage. Frozen ice cups are made by freezing small paper or Styrofoam cups of water. To use these, the therapist holds on to the bottom of the cup and gradually peels back the edge to expose the surface of the ice and puts it in direct contact with the patient's skin (Fig. 6-12). Water popsicles are made by placing a stick or tongue depressor into the water cup before freezing. When frozen the ice can be completely removed from the cup and the stick used as a handle for applying the ice. Patients can easily make ice cups or popsicles for home use.

| **APPLICATION TECHNIQUE 6-3** | **ICE MASSAGE** |

Equipment Required

- Small paper or Styrofoam cups
- Freezer
- Tongue depressors or popsicle sticks (optional)
- Towels to absorb water

Procedure

1. Remove all jewelry and clothing from the area to be treated and inspect the area.
2. Place towels around the treatment area to absorb any dripping water and to wipe away water on the skin during treatment.
3. Rub the ice over the treatment area using small, overlapping circles. Wipe away any water as it melts on the skin.
4. Continue ice massage application for 5 to 10 minutes or until the patient experiences analgesia at the site of application.
5. When the intervention is completed, inspect the treatment area for any signs of adverse effects such as wheals or a rash. It is normal for the skin to be red or dark pink after the

application of ice massage. Ice massage may be applied in the above manner for the local control of pain, inflammation, or edema. Ice massage can also be used as a stimulus for facilitating the production of desired motor patterns in patients with impaired motor control. When applied for this purpose, the ice is either rubbed with pressure for 3 to 5 seconds or quickly stroked over the muscle bellies to be facilitated. This technique is known as quick icing.

Advantages

- Treatment area can be observed during application.
- Can be used for small and irregular areas.
- Short duration of treatment.
- Inexpensive.
- Can be applied to an elevated limb.

Disadvantages

- Too time-consuming for large areas.
- Requires active participation by the clinician or patient throughout application.

APPLICATION TECHNIQUE 6-4   CONTROLLED COLD COMPRESSION

Equipment Required

- Controlled cold compression unit
- Sleeves appropriate for area(s) to be treated
- Stockinette for hygiene

Procedure

1. Remove all jewelry and clothing from the area to be treated and inspect the area.
2. Cover the limb with a stockinette before applying the sleeve.
3. Wrap the sleeve around the area to be treated (Fig. 6-13).
4. Elevate the area to be treated.
5. Set the temperature at 10° to 15° C (50° to 59° F).
6. Cooling can be applied continuously or intermittently. For intermittent treatment, apply cooling for 15 minutes every 2 hours.
7. Cycling intermittent compression may be applied at all times when the area is elevated.
8. When the intervention is completed, remove the sleeve and inspect the treatment area.

Advantages

- Allows simultaneous application of cold and compression.
- Temperature and compression force are easily and accurately controlled.
- Can be applied to large joints.

Disadvantages

- Treatment site cannot be visualized during treatment.
- Expensive.
- Usable only for extremities.
- Cannot be used for trunk or digits.

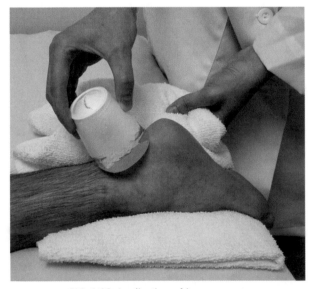

FIG 6-12 Application of ice massage.

CONTROLLED COLD COMPRESSION UNIT

Controlled cold compression units alternately pump cold water and air into a sleeve that is wrapped around a patient's limb (Fig. 6-13). The temperature of the water can be set at between 10° and 25° C (50° to 77° F) to provide cooling. Compression is applied by intermittent inflation of the sleeve with air. Controlled cold compression units are most commonly used directly after surgery for the control of postoperative inflammation and edema; however, they may also be used to control inflammation and related edema in other circumstances. A small study found that cold compression decreased capillary blood flow, preserved deep tendon oxygen saturation, and facilitated venous capillary outflow in the Achilles tendon when applied to this region.[81]

When applied postoperatively, the sleeve is put on the patient's affected limb immediately after completion of the surgery while the patient is in the recovery room, and the unit is sent home with the patient so that it can be used for a few days or weeks after surgery. The application of cold with compression in this manner has been shown to be more effective than ice or compression alone in controlling swelling, pain, and blood loss after surgery and in assisting the patient in regaining ROM.[82,83]

VAPOCOOLANT SPRAYS AND BRIEF ICING

The vapocoolant sprays ethyl chloride and Fluori-Methane (a commercially produced combination of 15% dichloro-difluoromethane and 85% trichloromonofluoromethane) were used for many years to achieve brief and rapid cutaneous cooling. These products cool by evaporation. Ethyl chloride was first used for this purpose; however, because it is volatile and flammable, can cause excessive temperature decreases, and can have anesthetic effects when inhaled,[84] Fluori-Methane, which also effectively cools the skin but is nonflammable and causes less reduction in temperature, was introduced.[85] However, because Fluori-Methane is a volatile chlorofluorocarbon that can damage the ozone layer, its production was discontinued and the company that manufactured it developed a vapocoolant spray that is nonflammable and does not deplete the ozone layer (Fig. 6-14). This product is made of a combina-

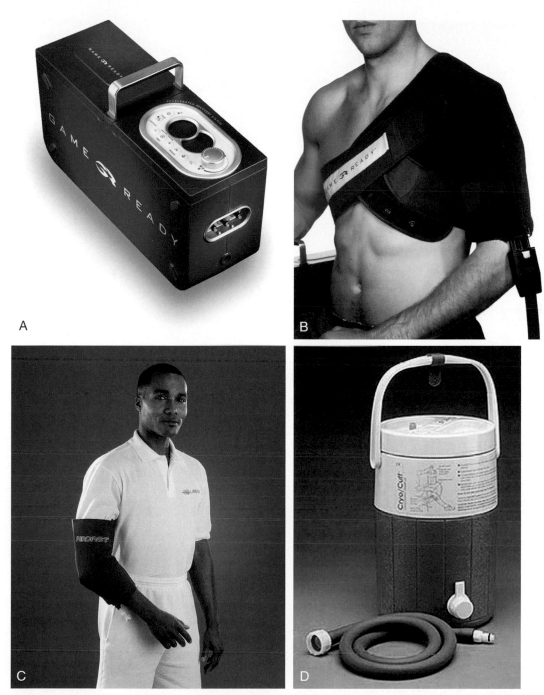

FIG 6-13 Controlled cold compression units and their applications. *A and B, Courtesy Game Ready, Inc. Berkeley, CA. C and D, Courtesy Aircast, Vista, CA.*

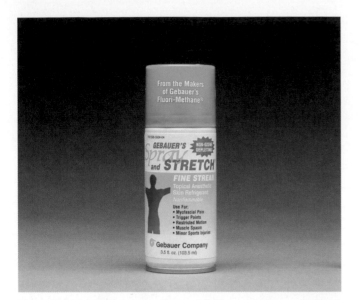

FIG 6-14 Vapocoolant spray. *Courtesy Gebauer Company, Cleveland, OH.*

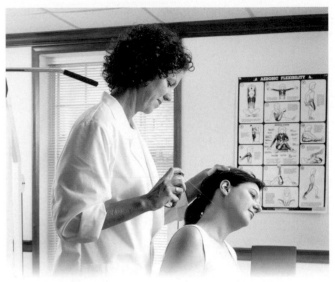

FIG 6-15 Application of vapocoolant spray. *Courtesy Gebauer Company, Cleveland, OH.*

tion of 1,1,1,3,3-pentafluoropropane and 1,1,1,2-tetrafluoroethane and is marketed under the trade names Spray and Stretch, Instant Ice, and Pain Ease (Gebauer Company, Cleveland, OH). Although each product contains the same chemical components, their delivery systems and FDA-approved indications are different. Spray and Stretch has a fine stream spray and is the product indicated for treatment of myofascial pain syndromes, trigger points, restricted motion, and minor sports injuries.

Rapid cutaneous cooling with a vapocoolant spray is generally used as a component of an approach to the treatment of trigger points known as spray and stretch. This technique was developed by Janet Travell, who describes this combination with the phrase "Stretch is the action; spray is the distraction."[86] For this application, the vapocoolant spray is applied in parallel strokes along the skin overlying the muscles with trigger points immediately before stretching these muscles (Fig. 6-15).[87] Ice may also be stroked along the skin in the same area for this purpose (Fig. 6-16). This type of intervention is frequently applied directly after trigger point injection. The purpose of the rapid cooling is to provide a counterirritant stimulus to the cutaneous thermal afferents overlying the muscles to cause a reflex reduction in motor neuron activity and thus a reduction in the resistance to stretch.[88] The "distraction" of rapid cutaneous cooling is intended to promote greater elongation of the muscle with passive stretching.

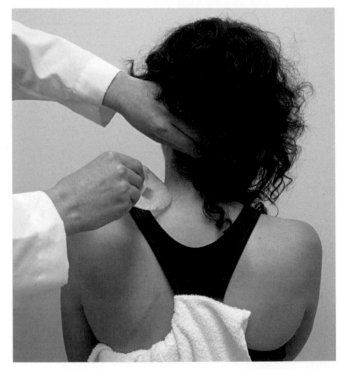

FIG 6-16 Quick stroking with ice popsicle.

Cryotherapy may also be applied using frozen wet towels, a bucket of ice or cold water, a cold whirlpool, or a contrast bath. Frozen wet towels are rarely used because they are inconvenient and messy. The use of cold water, cold whirlpools, and contrast baths is discussed in detail in Chapter 9.

APPLICATION TECHNIQUE 6-5	**VAPOCOOLANT SPRAYS AND BRIEF ICING**[89,90]

Procedure

1. Identify trigger points and their related tight muscles.
2. Position the patient comfortably, with all limbs and the back well supported and the area to be treated exposed and accessible. Inspect the area to be treated. Cover the patient's eyes, nose and mouth if spraying near the face, in order to minimize the patient's inhalation of the spray.
3. Apply two to five parallel sweeps of the spray or strokes of the ice 1.5 to 2 cm (0.5 to 1 inch) apart at a speed of approximately 10 cm (4 inches) per second along the direction of the muscle fibers. When using a spray, hold the can upright about 30 to 46 cm (12 to 18 inches) from the skin and angled so that the spray hits the skin at an angle of about 30 degrees. Continue until the entire muscle has been covered, including the muscle attachment and the trigger point.
4. During the cooling, maintain gentle, smooth, steady tension on the muscle to take up any slack that may develop.

5. Immediately after the cooling, have the patient take a deep breath and then perform a gentle passive stretch while exhaling. Contraction/relaxation techniques may also be used to enhance the ROM increases obtained with this procedure.
6. Following this procedure, the skin should be rewarmed with moist heat, and then the muscles should be moved through their full active ROM (AROM).

Advantages

- Brief duration of cooling.
- Very localized area of application.

Disadvantages

- Limited to use for brief, localized, superficial application of cold before stretching.
- Other means of applying cryotherapy.

DOCUMENTATION

The following should be documented:

- Area of the body treated
- Type of cooling agent used
- Treatment duration
- Patient positioning
- Response to the intervention

Documentation is typically written in the SOAP note (Subjective, Objective, Assessment, Plan) format. The following examples only summarize the modality component of the intervention and are not intended to represent a comprehensive plan of care.

EXAMPLES

When applying an ice pack (IP) to the left (L) knee to control postoperative (postop) swelling, document the following:

S: Pt reports postop L knee pain and swelling that increases with walking.

O: Pretreatment: Midpatellar girth 16½ in. Gait "step to" when ascending stairs.

Intervention: IP L anterior knee ×15 min, L LE elevated.

Posttreatment: Midpatellar girth 15 in. Gait "step through" when ascending stairs.

A: Decreased midpatellar girth, improved gait.

P: Instruct pt in home program of IP to L anterior knee, 15 min, with L LE elevated, 3× each day until next treatment session.

When applying ice massage (IM) to the area of the right (R) lateral (lat) epicondyle to treat epicondylitis, document the following:

S: Pt reports pain in R lat elbow.

O: Pretreatment: 8/10 R lat elbow pain. R elbow unable to fully extend.

Intervention: IM R lat elbow ×5 min.

Posttreatment: Pain 6/10. Full elbow extension.

A: Pain decreased and elbow ROM improved.

P: Continue IM at end of treatment sessions until pt has pain-free elbow function.

CLINICAL CASE STUDIES

The following case studies summarize the concepts of cryotherapy discussed in this chapter. Based on the scenario presented, an evaluation of the clinical findings and goals of treatment are proposed. These are followed by a discussion of the factors to be considered in the selection of cryotherapy as an indicated intervention and in the selection of the ideal cryotherapy agent to promote progress toward the set goals.

CASE STUDY 6-1

Post-operative Pain and Edema
Examination
History

TF is a 20-year-old male accountant. He injured his right knee 4 months ago while playing football and was

Continued

treated conservatively with nonsteroidal antiinflammatory drugs (NSAIDs) and physical therapy for 8 weeks, with moderate improvement in symptoms; however, he was not able to return to sports due to continued medial knee pain. A magnetic resonance imaging (MRI) scan 3 weeks ago revealed a tear of the medial meniscus, and the patient underwent arthroscopic partial medial meniscectomy of his right knee 4 days ago. He has been referred to physical therapy with an order to evaluate and treat. TF reports pain in his knee that has decreased in intensity from 9/10 to 7/10 since the surgery but that increases with weight bearing on the right lower extremity. He therefore limits his ambulation to essential tasks only. He also reports knee stiffness.

Tests and Measures

The objective examination reveals moderate warmth of the skin of the right knee, particularly at the anteromedial aspect, and ROM restricted to −10 degrees of extension and 85 degrees of flexion. The patient is ambulating without any assistive device but with a decreased stance phase on the right lower extremity and with his right knee held stiffly in approximately 30 degrees of flexion throughout the gait cycle. Knee girth at the midpatellar level is 17 inches on the right and 15½ inches on the left.

What signs and symptoms in this patient can be addressed by cryotherapy? Which cryotherapy applications would be appropriate for this patient? Which would not be appropriate?

Evaluation, Diagnosis, Prognosis, and Goals
Evaluation and Goals

ICF Level	Current Status	Goals
Body structure and function	R knee pain	Control pain
	Decreased R knee ROM	Increase R knee ROM to full
	Increased R knee girth	Control edema
		Accelerate resolution of the acute inflammation phase of healing
Activity	Limited ambulation	Tolerates ambulation up to ½ block in 2 weeks
Participation	Inability to play football	Return patient to playing noncontact sports in one month

Diagnosis

Preferred Practice Pattern 4I: Impaired joint mobility, motor function, muscle performance, and ROM associated with bony or soft tissue surgery.

Prognosis/Plan of Care

Cryotherapy is an indicated intervention for the control of pain, edema, and inflammation. It can control the formation of edema, and compression and elevation can reduce edema already present in the patient's knee.

The application of cryotherapy early during the recovery from articular surgery has also been associated with an acceleration of functional recovery.[91] Since the peroneal nerve is superficial at the lateral knee, the patient should be monitored for signs of nerve conduction block, such as tingling or numbness in his lateral leg, during the intervention. The presence of any contraindications, such as Raynaud's phenomenon or disease, should be ruled out before the application of cryotherapy. Cryotherapy also should not be applied if infection is suspected. Although this patient does have signs of inflammation, including heat, redness, pain, swelling, and loss of function, the fact that his signs and symptoms have decreased since surgery indicates an appropriate course of recovery and the probable absence of infection. A progressive increase in the signs and symptoms of inflammation or complaints of fever and general malaise would suggest the presence of infection, requiring physician evaluation before the initiation of rehabilitation.

Intervention

To obtain maximum cooling of the knee, cryotherapy should be applied to all skin surfaces surrounding the knee joint. A cold pack, ice pack, or controlled cold compression unit could adequately cover this area. In choosing among these agents, one should consider the convenience and ease of application of a cold pack, the low expense and ready availability of an ice pack, and the additional benefits (although greater cost) of intermittent compression provided by a controlled cold compression unit. Ice massage would not be an appropriate intervention because it would take too long to apply to such a large area. Immersion in ice or cold water would also not be appropriate because this would require the swollen knee to be in a dependent position, potentially aggravating the edema, and the additional discomfort of immersing the entire distal lower extremity in cold water. Whether using a cold pack, ice pack, or controlled cold compression unit, cryotherapy should generally be applied for approximately 15 minutes to ensure adequate cooling of the tissues and minimize the probability of excessive cooling or reactive vasodilation. This intervention should be reapplied by the patient at home every 2 to 3 hours while signs of inflammation are still present (Fig. 6-17).

Documentation

S: Pt reports R knee stiffness and pain that increases with weight bearing.

O: Pretreatment: R knee pain 7/10. Warm skin anteromedial R knee. R knee ROM −10 degrees extension and 85 degrees flexion. Gait: decreased stance phase on R LE and with R knee held at 30 degrees of flexion throughout gait cycle. R knee midpatellar girth 17 in, L knee 15½ in.

Intervention: IP R anterior knee ×15 min, R LE elevated.

CLINICAL CASE STUDIES—*cont'd*

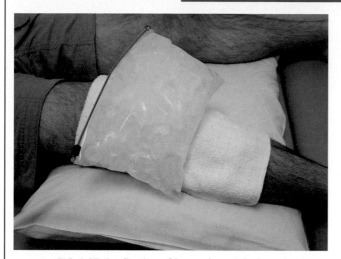

FIG 6-17 Application of ice pack to right knee.

Posttreatment: R knee pain 5/10. R midpatellar girth 16 in. R knee ROM −10 degrees extension and 85 degrees flexion. Ambulates with knee moving through approximately 10-30 degrees of flexion.

A: Pt tolerated treatment well, with decreased pain and edema.

P: Pt to apply IP at home, every 3 hours while edema and warmth of R knee remain.

CASE STUDY 6-2

Lateral Epicondylitis
Examination

History
SG is a 40-year-old female office worker. She has been referred to therapy with a diagnosis of lateral epicondylitis and an order to evaluate and treat. SG complains of constant moderate to severe pain (5 to 8/10) at her right lateral elbow that prevents her from playing tennis. The pain started about 1 month ago on a morning after she spent a whole day pulling weeds and remained unchanged in severity or frequency until 3 days ago. She reports a slight decrease in pain severity over the last 3 days, which she associates with starting to take an NSAID prescribed by her physician. She has had similar symptoms previously, after gardening or playing tennis, but these have always resolved within a couple of days without any medical intervention.

Tests and Measures
Objective examination reveals tenderness and mild swelling at the right lateral epicondyle and pain without weakness with resisted wrist extension. All other tests, including upper extremity sensation, ROM, and strength, are within normal limits.

What other interventions should be used with cryotherapy for this patient? What should you monitor for during cryotherapy application? How can she prevent a recurrence of her lateral epicondylitis?

Evaluation, Diagnosis, Prognosis, and Goals
Evaluation and Goals

ICF Level	Current Status	Goals
Body structure and function	R elbow pain, tenderness, and swelling	Resolve inflammation Control pain Prevent recurrence
Activity	Difficulty using R arm when wrist extension is required	Able to extend R wrist against resistance without pain
Participation	Unable to play tennis	Return to playing tennis

Diagnosis
Preferred Practice Pattern 4E: Impaired joint mobility, motor function, muscle performance, and ROM associated with localized inflammation.

Prognosis/Plan of Care
Cryotherapy is an indicated intervention for inflammation and pain and can also be used prophylactically after exercise to prevent the onset of inflammation and soreness. The advantages of cryotherapy over other interventions indicated for these applications, such as ultrasound or electrical stimulation, are that it is quick, easy, and inexpensive to apply and the patient can apply it at home. Cryotherapy alone may not resolve the present symptoms and may therefore need to be applied in conjunction with other physical agents, activity modification, manual therapy techniques, and/or exercises to achieve the proposed goals of treatment. Because the radial nerve is superficial at the lateral elbow, the patient should be monitored for signs of nerve conduction blockage during treatment such as tingling or numbness in her dorsal arm. The presence of any contraindications to the application of cryotherapy, such as Raynaud's phenomenon or disease, should be ruled out before the application of cryotherapy.

Intervention
Ice massage, an ice pack, or a cold pack can be used to provide cryotherapy to the area of the lateral epicondyle (Fig. 6-18). Because ice massage has the advantages of taking little time to apply to this small area while allowing visualization of the treatment area and assessment of signs and symptoms throughout the intervention, this would be the most appropriate agent to use for this patient, although an ice pack or cold pack could also be used. An ice pack or cold pack would be more appropriate if the symptomatic area was larger (e.g., if the area extended into the dorsal forearm). Cryotherapy should be applied until the treatment area is numb, which usually takes 5 to 10 minutes when using ice massage or about 15 minutes when using an ice pack or a cold pack. Treatment should be discontinued sooner if numbness extends into the hand in the distribution of the radial

Continued

CLINICAL CASE STUDIES—*cont'd*

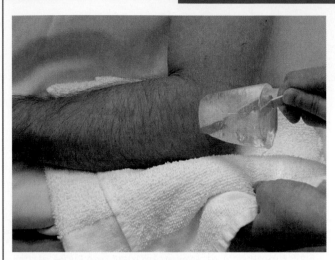

FIG 6-18 Application of ice massage to elbow.

nerve. Cryotherapy treatments should continue to be applied until the signs and symptoms of inflammation have resolved. Treatments should be discontinued thereafter because the vasoconstriction produced by cryotherapy may retard the later stages of tissue healing. The patient should also be instructed to apply cryotherapy prophylactically after activities that have previously resulted in elbow pain, such as tennis or gardening, to reduce the risk of a recurrence of her present symptoms.

Documentation

S: Pt reports R elbow pain, improved somewhat with NSAIDs.

O: Pretreatment: R lat epicondyle tenderness, mild edema, 8/10 pain with resisted wrist extension.

Intervention: IM to R lat epicondyle ×8 min.

Posttreatment: Decreased tenderness and edema. Pain 5/10 with resisted wrist extension.

A: Pt tolerated treatment well, with decreased pain and edema.

P: Pt to continue IM at home, as described, every 3 hours until edema and pain resolve. Pt educated on prevention of future symptoms by applying IP or IM after gardening or tennis.

CASE STUDY 6-3

Delayed-onset Muscle Soreness (DOMS)
Examination
History

FB is a 60-year-old male truck driver. He has been referred to physical therapy with a diagnosis of osteoarthritis of the left knee and an order to evaluate and treat. He reports that he has had arthritis in left knee for the last 5 years and that he recently started performing exercises that have increased the strength, stability, and endurance of his legs but cause knee pain and thigh muscle soreness the next day. His goals in therapy are to control this postexercise discomfort to allow continuation of his exercise program. He performed his exercises yesterday.

Tests and Measures

Palpation reveals a mild increase in the temperature of the left knee and tenderness of the anterior thigh. The patient reports 3/10 pain with resisted left knee extension. Knee girth and ROM are equal bilaterally.

In addition to using cryotherapy, how can this patient's postexercise pain be reduced? What should you monitor for during application of cryotherapy in this patient?

Evaluation, Diagnosis, Prognosis, and Goals
Evaluation and Goals

ICF Level	Current Status	Goals
Body structure and function	L knee and thigh pain after exercise	Control postexercise pain
Activity	Pain with resisted L knee extension	Pain-free resisted L knee extension
Participation	Decreased ability to do leg strengthening exercises	Return to full exercise program

Diagnosis

Preferred Practice Pattern 4E: impaired joint mobility, motor function, muscle performance, and ROM associated with localized inflammation.

Prognosis/Plan of Care

Cryotherapy is an indicated treatment for DOMS and joint inflammation; however, the patient's exercise program should also be evaluated and modified as appropriate to reduce his discomfort after exercising. The presence of any contraindications to the application of cryotherapy, such as Raynaud's phenomenon or disease, should be ruled out before the application of cryotherapy.

Intervention

As in Case Study 6-1, the application of cryotherapy for 15 minutes with an ice pack or cold pack would be appropriate for treatment of this patient's knee. The additional expense of a controlled cold compression unit is not justified in this case because there is no edema and therefore compression is not needed. The patient should apply the pack immediately after completing his exercise program. Because the peroneal nerve is superficial at the lateral knee, the patient should be monitored for signs of nerve conduction blockage, such as tingling or numbness in his lateral leg, during treatment.

Documentation

S: Pt reports knee and thigh pain lasting 1 day after performing leg strengthening exercises.

O: Pretreatment: L knee mild warmth. L anterior thigh tenderness. 3/10 pain with resisted L knee extension. Bilaterally equal knee girth and ROM.

Intervention: IP to L anterior thigh and knee ×15 min.

Posttreatment: Decreased L anterior thigh tenderness, 1/10 pain with L knee extension.

A: Pt tolerated treatment well, with decreased pain and tenderness.

P: Pt to apply IP immediately after completing exercise program. Exercise program should be reassessed and modified as needed to prevent pain.

THERMOTHERAPY

The therapeutic application of heat is called **thermotherapy**. Outside of the rehabilitation setting, thermotherapy is used primarily to destroy malignant tissue or to treat cold-related injuries. Within rehabilitation, thermotherapy is used primarily to control pain, increase soft tissue extensibility and circulation, and accelerate healing. Heat has these therapeutic effects because of its influence on hemodynamic, neuromuscular, and metabolic processes, the mechanisms of which are explained in detail in the following.

EFFECTS OF HEAT

HEMODYNAMIC EFFECTS

Vasodilation

Heat causes vasodilation and thus an increase in the rate of blood flow.[92] When heat is applied to one area of the body, there is vasodilation where the heat is applied and to a lesser degree, systemically, in areas distant from the site of heat application. Superficial heating agents produce more pronounced vasodilation in the local cutaneous blood vessels, where they cause the greatest change in temperature, and less pronounced dilation in the deeper vessels that run through muscles, where they cause little if any change in temperature. Thermotherapy applied to the whole body can also cause generalized vasodilation and may improve vascular endothelial function in the setting of cardiac risk factors and in chronic heart failure.[93-95] In rats, whole body hyperthermia was associated with the growth of new blood vessels in the heart.[96]

Thermotherapy may cause vasodilation by a variety of mechanisms, including direct reflex activation of the smooth muscles of the blood vessels by the cutaneous thermoreceptors, indirect activation of local spinal cord reflexes by the cutaneous thermoreceptors, or by increasing the local release of chemical mediators of inflammation (Fig. 6-19).[97,98] One study demonstrated that at least two independent mechanisms contribute to the rise in skin blood flow during local heating: a fast-responding vasodilator system mediated by the axon reflexes and a more slowly responding vasodilator system that relies on local production of nitrous oxide.[99]

Superficial heating agents stimulate activity of the cutaneous thermoreceptors. It is proposed that transmission from these cutaneous thermoreceptors via their axons directly to nearby cutaneous blood vessels causes the release of bradykinin and nitrous oxide and that bradykinin and nitrous oxide then stimulate relaxation of the smooth muscles of the vessel walls to cause vasodilation in the area where the heat is applied.[98-100] However, the role of bradykinin in heat-mediated vasodilation was recently called into question when it was found that blocking bradykinin receptors during whole-body heating did not alter the amount of cutaneous vasodilation.[101] This finding suggests that nitrous oxide is the primary chemical mediator of heat-induced vasodilation.

Cutaneous thermoreceptors also project via the dorsal root ganglion to synapse with interneurons in the dorsal horn of the gray matter of the spinal cord. These interneurons synapse with sympathetic neurons in the lateral grey horn of the thoracolumbar segments of the spinal cord to inhibit their firing and thus decrease sympathetic output.[102] This decrease in sympathetic activity causes a reduction in smooth muscle contraction, resulting in vasodilation at the site of heat application, as well as in the cutaneous vessels of the distal extremities.[103] This distant vasodilative effect of thermotherapy may be used to increase cutaneous

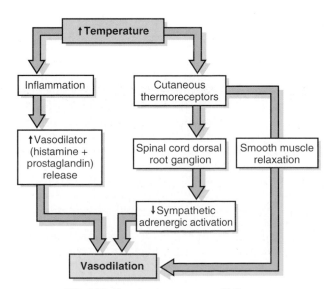

FIG 6-19 How heat causes vasodilation.

blood flow to an area where it is difficult or unsafe to apply a heating agent directly.[104] For example, if a patient has an ulcer on his leg as the result of arterial insufficiency in the extremity, thermotherapy may be applied to his lower back to increase the circulation to his lower extremity and thereby facilitate wound healing. This would be most appropriate if the ulcer was bandaged or did not tolerate pressure, or if the area lacked sufficient circulation or sensation to safely tolerate the direct application of heat.

Because blood flow in the skeletal muscles is primarily influenced by metabolic factors rather than by changes in sympathetic activity and superficial heating agents do not increase the temperature to the depth of most muscles, skeletal muscle blood flow is much less affected by superficial heating modalities than is skin blood flow.[105,106] The use of exercise or deep heating modalities, such as ultrasound or diathermy, or a combination of these interventions, is therefore recommended when the goal of treatment is to increase skeletal muscle blood flow.

> **◎ Clinical Pearl**
>
> Superficial heating agents do not heat to the depth of most muscles. To heat deep muscles, use exercise or deep heating modalities such as ultrasound or diathermy.

Cutaneous vasodilation and the increase in blood flow that occurs in response to increased tissue temperature act to protect the body from excessive heating and tissue damage. The increased rate of blood flow increases the rate at which an area is cooled by convection. Thus, when an area is heated with a thermal agent, it is simultaneously cooled by circulating blood, and as the temperature of the area increases, the rates of circulation and cooling both increase to reduce the impact of the thermal agent on tissue temperature, thereby reducing the risk of burning.

NEUROMUSCULAR EFFECTS

Changes in Nerve Conduction Velocity and Firing Rate

Increased temperature increases nerve conduction velocity and decreases the conduction latency of sensory and motor nerves.[107-109] Nerve conduction velocity increases by approximately 2 m/sec for every 1° C (1.8° F) increase in temperature. Although the clinical implications of these effects are not well understood, they may contribute to the reduced pain perception or improved circulation that occurs in response to increasing tissue temperature. Although conduction velocity in normal nerves increases with heat, demyelinated peripheral nerves treated with heat can undergo conduction block.[110,111] This occurs because heat shortens the duration of sodium channel opening at the nodes of Ranvier during neuronal depolarization.[112] In demyelinated nerves, less current reaches the nodes of Ranvier. If heat is added, the shortened opening time of the sodium channel can prevent the node from depolarizing, leading to conduction block. Therefore heat should be applied with caution to patients with demyelin-

ating conditions such as carpal tunnel syndrome or multiple sclerosis.

Nerve firing rate (frequency) has also been found to change in response to changes in temperature. Elevation of muscle temperature to 42° C (108° F) has been shown to result in a decreased firing rate of type II muscle spindle efferents and gamma efferents and an increased firing rate of type Ib fibers from GTOs.[113,114] These changes in nerve firing rates are thought to contribute to a reduction in the firing rate of alpha motor neurons and thus to a reduction in muscle spasm.[115] The decrease in gamma neuron activity causes the stretch on the muscle spindles to decrease, reducing afferent firing from the spindles.[116] The decreased spindle afferent activity results in decreased alpha motor neuron activity and thus in relaxation of muscle contraction.

Increased Pain Threshold

Several studies demonstrate that the application of local heat can increase pain threshold.[117,118] The proposed mechanisms of this effect include a direct and immediate reduction of pain by activation of the spinal gating mechanism and an indirect, later, and more prolonged reduction of pain by reduction of ischemia and muscle spasm or facilitation of tissue healing. Heat increases the activity of the cutaneous thermoreceptors, which can have an immediate inhibitory gating effect on the transmission of the sensation of pain at the spinal cord level. Stimulation of the thermoreceptors can also result in vasodilation, as described previously, causing an increase in blood flow and thus potentially reducing pain caused by ischemia. Ischemia may also be decreased as a result of reduction of spasm in muscles that compress blood vessels. The vasodilation produced by thermotherapy may also accelerate the recovery of the local pain threshold to a normal level by speeding tissue healing.

Changes in Muscle Strength

Muscle strength and endurance have been found to decrease during the initial 30 minutes after the application of deep or superficial heating agents.[119-121] It is proposed that this initial decrease in muscle strength is the result of changes in the firing rates of type II muscle spindle efferent, gamma efferent, and type Ib fibers from Golgi tendon organs caused by heating of the motor nerves. In turn, this decreases the firing rate of alpha motor neurons. Beyond 30 minutes after the application of heat and for the next 2 hours, muscle strength gradually recovers and then increases to above pretreatment levels. This delayed increase in strength is thought to be caused by an increase in pain threshold.

Because the changes in muscle strength produced by heating are temporary, heat is not used for strengthening. However, it is important to be aware of the effects of heat on strength when muscle strength is being used as a measure of patient progress. Because comparing preheating strength with postheating strength from the same session or another session can provide misleading information, it is recommended that muscle strength and endurance always be measured before and not after applying a heating modality.

Clinical Pearl

Measure muscle strength before applying heat, not after.

METABOLIC EFFECTS
Increased Metabolic Rate

Heat increases the rate of endothermic chemical reactions, including the rate of enzymatic biological reactions. Increased enzymatic activity has been observed in tissues at 39° to 43° C (102°° to 109° F), with the reaction rate increasing by approximately 13% for every 1.0° C (1.8° F) increase in temperature and doubling for every 10° C (18° F) increase in temperature.[34] Enzymatic and metabolic activity rates continue to increase up to a temperature of 45° C (113° F). Beyond this temperature, the protein constituents of enzymes begin to denature and enzyme activity rates decrease, ceasing completely at about 50° C (122° F).[122]

Any increase in enzymatic activity will result in an increase in the rate of cellular biochemical reactions. This can increase oxygen uptake and accelerate healing but may also increase the rate of destructive processes. For example, heat may accelerate the healing of a chronic wound; however, it has also been shown to increase the activity of collagenase and may thus accelerate the destruction of articular cartilage in patients with rheumatoid arthritis.[33] Therefore thermotherapy should be used with caution in patients with acute inflammatory disorders.

Clinical Pearl

Use thermotherapy with caution in patients with acute inflammatory disorders.

Increasing tissue temperature also shifts the oxygen-hemoglobin dissociation curve to the right, making more oxygen available for tissue repair (see Fig. 6-4). It has been shown that hemoglobin releases twice as much oxygen at 41° C (106° F) as it does at 36° C (97° F).[123] In conjunction with the increased rate of blood flow stimulated by increased temperature and the increased enzymatic reaction rate, this increased oxygen availability may contribute to acceleration of tissue healing by thermotherapy.

ALTERED TISSUE EXTENSIBILITY
Increased Collagen Extensibility

Increasing the temperature of soft tissue increases its extensibility.[124] When soft tissue is heated before stretching, it maintains a greater increase in length after the stretching force is applied, less force is required to achieve the increase in length, and the risk of tissue tearing is reduced.[125,126] If heat is applied to collagenous soft tissue, such as tendon, ligament, scar tissue, or joint capsule, before prolonged stretching, plastic deformation, in which the tissue increases in length and maintains most of the increase after cooling, can be achieved.[127,128] In contrast, if collagenous tissue is stretched without prior heating, elastic deformation, in which the tissue increases in length while the force is applied but loses most of the increase

when the force is removed, generally occurs. The maintained elongation of collagenous tissue that occurs after heating and stretching is caused by changes in the organization of the collagen fibers and by changes in the viscoelasticity of the fibers.

For heat to increase the extensibility of soft tissue, the appropriate temperature range and structures must be reached. A maximum increase in residual length is achieved when the tissue temperature is maintained at 40° to 45° C (104° to 113° F) for 5 to 10 minutes.[113,128] The superficial heating agents described in the next sections can cause this level of temperature increase in superficial structures such as cutaneous scar tissue or superficial tendons. However, to adequately heat deeper structures, such as the joint capsules of large joints or deep tendons, deep-heating agents, such as ultrasound or diathermy, must be used.

USES OF SUPERFICIAL HEAT
PAIN CONTROL

Thermotherapy can be used clinically to control pain. This therapeutic effect may be mediated by gating of pain transmission by activation of cutaneous thermoreceptors or may indirectly result from improved healing, decreased muscle spasm, or reduced ischemia.[129] Increasing skin temperature may also reduce the sensation of pain by altering nerve conduction or transmission.[130] For example, it is likely that the analgesia produced in the sensory distribution of the ulnar nerve (the volar and medial forearm), when infrared radiation is applied over the ulnar nerve at the elbow, is caused by altered nerve conduction.[117] The indirect effects of thermotherapy on tissue healing and ischemia are primarily attributable to vasodilation and increased blood flow. It has also been proposed that the psychological experience of heat as comfortable and relaxing may also influence the patient's perception of pain.

Although thermotherapy may reduce pain of any etiology, it is generally not recommended as an intervention for pain caused by acute inflammation because an increase in tissue temperature may aggravate other signs and symptoms of inflammation, including heat, redness, and edema.[131] However, recent studies have found that heat can reduce the pain associated with acute low back pain, pelvic pain, and renal colic (the pain associated with kidney stones).

A systematic review found moderate evidence that continuous low level local heat (using a commercially available disposable pack inside a Velcro closure belt that heats up to 40° C [104° F] when exposed to air and maintains this heat for 8 hours) reduces pain and disability for patients with back pain lasting less than 3 months.[132] However, the relief lasts for a short time and the effect is relatively small. Adding exercise to heat therapy appears to provide additional benefit, based on this review.

In two trials with a total of 258 participants with acute or subacute low-back pain, application of a heated back wrap for 8 hours a day for 3 consecutive days was associated with significantly reduced pain at 5 days compared with oral placebo.[133,134] One trial with 90 subjects with acute low back pain found that a heated blanket significantly decreased acute (<6 hours' duration) low back pain 25 minutes after application when compared with a nonheated blanket.[135] Another trial of 100 participants with back pain of less than 3 months' duration combined a heated back wrap with exercise and compared this to heat alone, exercise alone, or providing the subjects with an educational booklet and found that heat plus exercise provided significantly more pain relief and improvement in function than either heat or exercise alone.[136] When a blanket heated to 42° C (106° F) is used during emergency transport for patients with acute pelvic pain, low back pain, or renal colic, patients had less pain than with an unheated blanket.[135,137,138] Additionally, warming with an electric blanket decreased anxiety and nausea in patients with acute pelvic pain or renal colic when compared with an unheated blanket during emergency transport.[137,138]

The application of at least 8 hours of continuous low-level heat has also been shown to decrease pain in various other conditions, including DOMS when compared with a cold pack, acute low back pain when compared with placebo, and wrist pain when compared with placebo.[134,139,140] Interestingly, submersion of the affected body part in water at 45° C (113° F) for 20 minutes was more effective than ice for the reduction of pain from jelly fish–type stings.[141] Given these findings, current evidence suggests that heat may be used to control pain in patients with certain acute conditions. However, heat should be discontinued if there are signs of worsening inflammation, including increased pain, edema, or erythema.

INCREASED RANGE OF MOTION AND DECREASED JOINT STIFFNESS

Thermotherapy can be used clinically when the goals are to increase joint ROM and decrease joint stiffness.[142-144] Both of these effects are thought to be the result of the increase in soft tissue extensibility that occurs with increasing soft tissue temperature. Increasing soft tissue extensibility contributes to increasing joint ROM because it results in greater increases in soft tissue length and less injury when a passive stretch is applied. A maximum increase in length, with the lowest risk of injury, is obtained if the tissue temperature is maintained at 40° to 45° C (104° to 113° F) for 5 to 10 minutes and if a low-load, prolonged stretch is applied during the heating period and while the tissue is cooling (Fig. 6-20).[113,128] Therefore it is recommended that stretching be performed during and immediately after the application of thermotherapy because, if the tissues are allowed to cool before being stretched, the effects of the prior heating on tissue extensibility will be lost.

Thermotherapy can decrease joint stiffness, which is a quality related to the amount of force and the time required to move a joint; as joint stiffness decreases, less force and time are required to produce joint motion.[145-147] For example, increasing tissue temperature by placing the hands in a warm water bath or warm paraffin, or heating the surface with an **infrared (IR) lamp**, have all been shown to decrease finger joint stiffness.[148] The proposed mechanisms of this effect are increased extensibility and

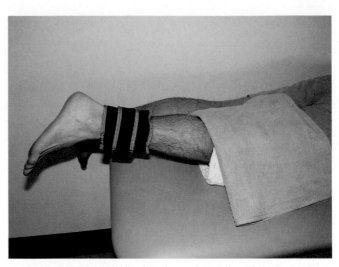

FIG 6-20 Low-load prolonged stretch with heat.

viscoelasticity of the periarticular structures, including the joint capsule and surrounding ligaments.

When using a heating agent to increase soft tissue extensibility before stretching, an agent that can reach the shortened tissue must be used. Thus superficial agents, such as hot packs, paraffin, or infrared lamps, are appropriate for use before stretching skin, superficial muscle, joints, or fascia, whereas deep-heating agents, such as ultrasound or diathermy, should be used before stretching deeper joint capsules, muscles, or tendons.

> **◎ Clinical Pearl**
>
> To increase soft tissue extensibility before stretching, use an agent that will heat the tissue that needs stretching.

ACCELERATED HEALING

Thermotherapy can accelerate tissue healing by increasing circulation and enzymatic activity rate and by increasing the availability of oxygen to the tissues. Increasing the rate of circulation accelerates the delivery of blood to the tissues, bringing in oxygen and other nutrients and removing waste products. The application of any physical agent that increases circulation can be beneficial during the proliferative or remodeling stages of healing or when chronic inflammation is present. However, since increasing circulation can increase edema, thermotherapy should be applied with caution during the acute inflammation phase to avoid prolonging this phase and delaying healing.

By increasing the enzymatic activity rate, thermotherapy also increases the rate of metabolic reactions, thus allowing the processes of inflammation and healing to proceed more rapidly. Increasing the temperature of the blood also increases the dissociation of oxygen from hemoglobin, making more oxygen available for the processes of tissue repair.

Because superficial heating agents only increase the temperature of the superficial few millimeters of tissue, they are most likely to only accelerate the healing of superficial structures, such as the skin, or deeper tissue layers exposed because of skin ulceration. Deeper effects may also occur as the result of consensual vasodilation in areas distant from or deep to the area of increased temperature.

INFRARED RADIATION FOR PSORIASIS

Although the ultraviolet (UV) frequency range of electro-magnetic radiation is used most commonly in the treatment of psoriasis (see Chapter 13), the IR range is also occasionally used for this application.[149,150] The increased temperature of the upper epidermis and dermis in the region of psoriatic plaques produced by IR radiation has been proposed as the mechanism for the reduction in psoriatic plaques that occurs in some individuals exposed to IR radiation.[150] Other applications of IR not related to heat are covered in Chapter 12.

CONTRAINDICATIONS AND PRECAUTIONS FOR THERMOTHERAPY

Although thermotherapy is a relatively safe intervention, its use is contraindicated in some circumstances and it should be applied with caution in others. Thermotherapy may be applied by a qualified clinician or by a properly instructed patient. Clinicians may use all forms of thermotherapy, and patients may be instructed to use hot packs, paraffin, or IR lamps at home to treat themselves. When patients are taught to use these modalities at home, they should be instructed how to use the modality, including the location it should be applied, the temperature to be used, safety precautions, and the duration and frequency of treatment. Patients must also be taught how to identify possible adverse effects and must be told to discontinue treatment should any of these occur.

Even when thermotherapy is not contraindicated, as with all interventions, if the patient's condition is worsening or not improving after two to three treatments, the treatment approach should be reevaluated or the patient should be referred to a physician for reevaluation.

CONTRAINDICATIONS FOR THE USE OF THERMOTHERAPY

CONTRAINDICATIONS

for the Use of Thermotherapy

- Recent or potential hemorrhage
- Thrombophlebitis
- Impaired sensation
- Impaired mentation
- Malignant tumor
- IR irradiation of the eyes[151]

Recent or Potential Hemorrhage

Heat causes vasodilation and an increased rate of blood flow. Because vasodilation may cause reopening of a vascular lesion, increasing the rate of blood flow in an area of recent hemorrhage can restart or worsen the bleeding. In addition, increasing blood flow in an area of potential hemorrhage can cause hemorrhage to start. Therefore it is recommended that heat not be applied to areas of recent or potential hemorrhage.

Ask the Patient
- When did this injury occur?
- Did you have any bruising or bleeding?

Assess
- Visually inspect for ecchymosis

Thermotherapy should not be applied if the patient reports bruising or bleeding in the previous 48 to 72 hours or if recently formed red, purple, or blue ecchymosis is present.

Thrombophlebitis

The vasodilation and increased rate of circulation caused by increased tissue temperature may cause a thrombus or a blood clot to become dislodged from the area being treated and to be moved to the vessels of vital organs, resulting in morbidity or even death.

Ask the Patient
- Do you have a blood clot in this area?

Assess
- Check for calf swelling and tenderness (Homan's sign) before applying heat to the leg.

Thermotherapy should not be applied if the patient says that there is a blood clot in the area. Thermotherapy to the leg should not be applied if there is tenderness and swelling of the calf until the presence of a thrombus in the lower extremity has been ruled out.

Impaired Sensation or Impaired Mentation

A patient's sensation and a report of heat or pain are used as the primary indicators of the maximum safe temperature for thermotherapy; thus a patient who cannot feel or report the sensation of heat can easily be burned before the clinician realizes that there is a problem. Therefore heat should not be applied to areas where sensation is impaired or to patients who may have any other difficulty letting the therapist know when they are too hot.

◎ Clinical Pearl

Sensation is often impaired in the distal extremities of patients with diabetes.

Ask the Patient
- Do you have normal feeling in this area?

Assess
- Sensation in the area: Test tubes containing hot and cold water can be used to test thermal sensation. If sensation is impaired only in the treatment area, heat may be applied proximally to increase peripheral circulation via the spinal cord reflex, as described previously. Note that sensation in the distal extremities is frequently impaired in patients with neuropathy as a result of diabetes mellitus.

• Alertness and orientation: Thermotherapy should not be applied if the patient is unresponsive or confused.

Malignant Tissue

Thermotherapy may increase the growth rate or rate of metastasis of malignant tissue, either by increasing circulation to the area or by increasing the metabolic rate.

Because a patient may not know that he or she has cancer or may be uncomfortable discussing this diagnosis directly, the therapist should first check the chart for a diagnosis of cancer. Then ask the patient the following questions.

Ask the Patient

• Are you under the care of a physician for any major medical problem? If so, what is the problem?
• Have you experienced any recent unexplained weight loss or gain?
• Do you have constant pain that does not change? Note: If the patient has experienced recent unexplained changes in body weight or has constant pain that does not change, defer thermotherapy until a physician has performed a follow-up evaluation to rule out malignancy. If the patient is known to have cancer, ask the following question:
• Do you know if you have a tumor in this area? Note: Thermotherapy should generally not be applied in the area of a known or possible malignancy; however, such treatment may be given, with informed consent, to provide relief of pain for the terminally ill patient.

Infrared Irradiation of the Eyes

IR irradiation of the eyes should be avoided because such treatment may cause optical damage. To avoid irradiation of the eyes, IR opaque goggles should be worn by the patient throughout treatment using an IR lamp and by the therapist when near the lamp, as occurs when setting up the treatment.

PRECAUTIONS FOR THE USE OF THERMOTHERAPY

PRECAUTIONS

for the Use of Thermotherapy

• Acute injury or inflammation
• Pregnancy
• Impaired circulation
• Poor thermal regulation
• Edema
• Cardiac insufficiency
• Metal in the area
• Over an open wound
• Over areas where topical counterirritants have recently been applied
• Demyelinated nerves

Acute Injury or Inflammation

Heat should be applied with caution to the area of an acute injury or acute inflammation because increasing tissue temperature can increase edema and bleeding as a result of vasodilation and increased blood flow.[152] This may aggravate the injury, increase pain, and delay recovery.

Ask the Patient

• When did this injury occur?

Assess

• Skin temperature and color and local edema

Heat should not be applied within the first 48 to 72 hours after an injury. Elevation of skin temperature, rubor, and local edema demonstrate the presence of acute inflammation and indicate that heat should not be applied to the area.

Pregnancy

A fetus may be damaged by maternal hyperthermia; however, because this is unlikely to occur with superficial heating of the limbs, thermotherapy may be applied to such areas, but full body heating, as occurs with immersion of most of the body in a whirlpool, should be avoided during pregnancy. Although maternal hyperthermia has not been demonstrated with application of hot packs to the low back or abdomen, such application is also generally not recommended.

Ask the Patient

• Are you pregnant?
• Do you think you may be pregnant?
• Are you trying to get pregnant?

If the patient is or may be pregnant, heat should not be applied to the abdomen or low back and the patient should not be immersed in a warm or hot whirlpool.

Impaired Circulation or Poor Thermal Regulation

Areas with impaired circulation and patients with poor thermal regulation may not vasodilate to a normal degree in response to an increase in tissue temperature and therefore may not have a sufficient increase in blood flow when tissue temperature increases to protect the tissues from burning. In general, poor thermal regulation is encountered in the elderly and very young.

Assess

• Check skin temperature and quality and nail quality, and look for tissue swelling or ulceration.

Decreased skin temperature, thin skin, poor nails, tissue swelling, and ulceration are all signs of impaired circulation. Milder superficial heat should be used in areas with poor circulation or in elderly or very young patients. Heat should be applied at a lower temperature or with more insulation, and these patients should be checked frequently for any discomfort or signs of burning.

Edema

The application of thermotherapy to a dependent extremity has been shown to increase edema.[131] This effect is thought to be the result of the vasodilation and enhanced circulation that occur with raised tissue temperature and the increase in inflammation caused by increased metabolic rate.

Assess
- Measure limb girth in the area to be treated and compare this with the contralateral side.
- Palpate for pitting or brawny edema.
- Check for other signs of inflammation, including heat, redness, and pain.

Heat should not be applied with the area in a dependent position if edema is present. Heat may be applied with caution with the area elevated if edema is present and is thought to be a result of impaired venous circulation.

Cardiac Insufficiency
Heat can cause both local and generalized vasodilation, which can contribute to increased cardiac demand. Because this may not be well tolerated by patients with cardiac insufficiency, such patients should be monitored closely if heat is applied, particularly if the heat is applied to a large area.

Ask the Patient
- Do you have any problems with your heart?

Assess
- In patients with heart problems, check heart rate and blood pressure before, during, and after intervention.

A slight decrease in blood pressure and an increase in heart rate are normal consensual responses to the application of heat. Heat treatment should be discontinued in a patient with cardiac insufficiency if the patient's heart rate falls or the patient complains of feeling faint.

Metal in the Area
Metal has a higher thermal conductivity and higher specific heat than body tissue and therefore may become very hot with the application of conductive heating modalities. For this reason, jewelry should be removed before the application of superficial heating modalities and caution should be applied when there is metal, such as staples or bullet fragments, in the superficial tissues of the area being treated.

Ask the Patient
- Do you have any metal in you in this area such as staples or bullet fragments?
- Can you remove your jewelry in the area to be heated?

If there is metal present that cannot easily be removed, apply heat with caution. Milder heat should be used at a lower temperature or intensity or with more insulation, and the area should be checked frequently during treatment for any signs of burning.

Assess
- Inspect skin for scars that may cover metal.

Over an Open Wound
Paraffin should not be used over an open wound because it may contaminate the wound and is difficult to remove. All other forms of thermotherapy should be applied over open wounds with caution because the loss of epidermis reduces the insulation of the subcutaneous tissues. If forms of thermotherapy other than paraffin are used in the area of an open wound, they should be applied at a lower temperature or intensity or with more insulation than would be used when treating areas with intact skin. One should also check frequently during treatment for any signs of burning. When applying a heating agent with the goal of increasing circulation and accelerating the healing of an open wound, hydrotherapy with clean, warm water may be applied directly to the wound, or other superficial heating agents may be applied close to but not directly over the wound to provide a therapeutic effect while reducing the risk of cross-contamination and burns.

Over Areas Where Topical Counterirritants Have Recently Been Applied
Topical counterirritants are ointments or creams that cause a sensation of heat when applied to the skin. These preparations generally contain substances such as menthol that stimulate the sensation of heat by causing a mild inflammatory reaction in the skin. These preparations also cause local superficial vasodilation. If a thermal agent is applied to an area that is already vasodilated as the result of application of a topical counterirritant, the vessels in the area may not be able to vasodilate further to dissipate the heat from the thermal agent, and a burn may result.

Ask the Patient
- Have you applied any cream or ointment to this area today? If so, what type?

If the patient has recently applied a topical counterirritant to an area, a superficial heating agent should not be applied. The patient should be told not to use this type of preparation before future treatment sessions and not to apply a superficial heating agent at home after using this type of preparation.

Demyelinated Nerves
Conditions that are associated with demyelination of peripheral nerves include carpal tunnel syndrome and ulnar nerve entrapment. Apply heat with caution to areas with demyelinated nerves as superficial heat, including fluidotherapy, heat lamp, and water bath, has been shown to cause conduction block when applied to peripheral nerves.[109-111]

Ask the Patient
- Do you have carpal tunnel syndrome or ulnar nerve entrapment?

If the patient has a peripheral demyelinating condition, heat should be applied with caution to affected areas.

ADVERSE EFFECTS OF THERMOTHERAPY

BURNS

Excessive heating can cause **protein denaturation** and cell death. These effects may occur when heat is applied for too long, when the heating agent is too hot, or if heat is applied to a patient who does not have the appropriate protective vasodilation response to increased tissue temperature. The effects of heat on cell viability are exploited in the medical treatment of malignancies, in which heat is applied with the goal of killing the malignant cells; however, in application of heat in rehabilitation, cell death is to be avoided. Because protein begins to denature at 45° C (113° F) and cell death has been observed when cells were maintained at 43° C (109° F) for 60 minutes or at 46° C (115° F) for only $7^1/_2$ minutes, when applying heat in rehabilitation, the duration and tissue temperature should be kept below these levels.[153,154]

Overheating and tissue damage can be avoided by using superficial heating agents that get cooler during their application, by limiting the initial temperature of the agent, or by using insulation between the agent and the patient's skin (Box 6-1). For example, hot packs that are warmed in hot water before being placed on the patient start to cool as soon as they are removed from the hot water and applied and are therefore unlikely to cause burns. In contrast, superficial heating agents, such as plug-in electric hot packs or IR lamps that do not cool with use, are more likely to cause burns. The higher the temperature of a conductive superficial heating agent, the greater the rate of heat transfer to the patient and thus the greater the risk of burns; therefore it is important not to overheat a conductive superficial heating agent and to always use adequate insulation.

To avoid burns, heating agents should be applied in the manner recommended here. They should not be applied for longer periods or at higher temperatures, and the treatment time and temperature of the heating agent should be reduced if the patient has impaired circulation. Heating agents should not be applied where contraindicated, and all patients should be provided with a means of calling for assistance, such as a bell, if the clinician or another staff member is not in the immediate treatment area. During the intervention, the clinician should check to be sure that the patient has not fallen asleep and should instruct the patient to use a timer that rings loudly at the end of the treatment time if the patient uses a superficial heating agent at home.

A superficial heating agent used at home should be the type that cools over time, such as a microwavable hot pack

or a hot water bottle. If an electric heating pad is used by a patient at home, it should be the type that requires the patient to hold down a switch at all times for it to stay on. This safety feature ensures that the heating pad will turn off if the patient falls asleep and stops holding down the switch.

It is recommended that the patient's skin be inspected for burns before initiating treatment because a patient may have been burned previously. The skin should also be inspected during and after thermotherapy. A recent superficial burn will appear red and may have blistering. As the burn heals, the skin will appear pale and scarred.

FAINTING

Occasionally, a patient may feel faint when heat is applied. Fainting, which is a sudden, transient loss of consciousness, is generally the result of inadequate cerebral blood flow and is most commonly caused by peripheral vasodilation and decreased blood pressure, generally in association with a decreased heart rate.[155] Heating an area of the body generally causes vasodilation locally and to a lesser extent, in areas distant from the site of application. This distant, or consensual, response can result in a sufficient decrease in cerebral blood flow to cause a patient to faint during the application of thermotherapy. If a patient feels faint while heat is being applied, lowering the head and raising the feet will bring more blood to the brain to help the patient recover. Heating as small an area as clinically beneficial and removing excessive heavy clothing that insulates the whole body may also help limit this consensual decrease in blood pressure and thus reduce the probability of fainting.

Patients may also feel faint when getting up after thermotherapy. This feeling is caused by the additive hypotensive effects of postural (orthostatic) hypotension and the hypotensive effect of the heat, as described previously. The patient's head should be kept elevated with a pillow during the heat application and can help decrease posttreatment postural hypotension by reducing the extent of positional change at the completion of the intervention. It is also recommended that the patient remain in the position used during the treatment for a few minutes after the thermal agent is removed to allow blood pressure to normalize before rising.

BLEEDING

The vasodilation and increased blood flow caused by increasing tissue temperature may cause or aggravate bleeding in areas of acute trauma or in patients with hemophilia. The vasodilation may also cause reopening of any recent vascular lesion.

SKIN AND EYE DAMAGE FROM INFRARED IRRADIATION

IR radiation can produce adverse effects that are not produced by other superficial thermal agents. These include permanent damage to the eyes and permanent changes in skin pigmentation. Injury to the eyes, including corneal burning and retinal and lenticular damage, is considered to be the most likely and most severe hazard of IR radia-

BOX 6-1	How to Avoid Tissue Damage When Using Thermal Agents

- Use superficial heating agents that get cooler during their application (e.g., hot pack, hot water bottle)
- Limit the initial temperature of the agent
- Use enough insulation between the agent and the patient's skin
- Provide a means for the patient to call you

APPLICATION TECHNIQUE 6-6   GENERAL SUPERFICIAL THERMOTHERAPY

1. Evaluate the patient problem and set the goals of treatment.
2. Determine if thermotherapy is the most appropriate intervention.
3. Determine that thermotherapy is not contraindicated for this patient or this condition.

   Inspect the treatment area for open wounds and rashes and assess sensation. Check the patient's chart for any record of previous adverse responses to heat or for any disease that may predispose the patient to an adverse response. Ask the appropriate questions of the patient, as described in the preceding sections on contraindications and precautions.
4. Select the appropriate superficial heating agent according to the body part to be treated and the desired response.

   When applying superficial heat, select an agent that best fits the location and size of the area to be treated, is easily applied in the desired position, allows the desired amount of motion during application, is available, and is reasonably priced. Choose an agent that will conform to the area being treated so that it maintains good contact with the body. If edema is present, an agent that can be applied with the area elevated should be used. When applying thermotherapy with the goal of increasing ROM, it can be beneficial to allow active or passive motion while the treatment is being applied. Any of the heating agents described can be applied in the

clinic; only hot packs and paraffin may be applied by patients at home.
5. Explain to the patient the procedure and the reason for applying thermotherapy, and describe the sensations the patient can expect to feel.

   During the application of thermotherapy the patient should feel a sensation of mild warmth.
6. Apply the appropriate superficial heating agent:

   Select from the following list (see applications for each superficial heating agent on the next pages):
   - Hot packs
   - Paraffin
   - Fluidotherapy
   - IR lamp
   - Whirlpool or contrast bath
7. Inspect the treated area and assess the outcome of treatment.

   After completing thermotherapy with any of these agents, reevaluate the patient, checking particularly for progress toward the set goals of the intervention and for any adverse effects of the intervention. Remeasure quantifiable subjective complaints and objective impairments and disabilities.
8. Document the intervention.

---

tion application.[151] Prolonged exposure to IR radiation may also cause epidermal hyperplasia.[156]

Ⓠ Clinical Pearl

The patient should feel a sensation of mild warmth when a heating agent is applied.

Depending on the agent and the amount of insulation, the warmth may not be felt for the first few minutes of treatment. The patient should not feel excessively hot or feel any sensation of increased pain or burning. If the patient reports any of these sensations, discontinue the treatment or reduce the intensity of the heat.

HOT PACKS

Commercially available hot packs are usually made of bentonite, a hydrophilic silicate gel, covered with canvas. Bentonite is used for this application because it can hold a large quantity of water for the efficient delivery of heat. These types of hot packs are made in various sizes and shapes designed to fit different areas of the body (Fig. 6-21). They are stored in hot water kept at about 70° to 75° C (158° to 167° F) inside a purpose-designed, thermostatically controlled water cabinet (Fig. 6-22) that stays on at all times. This type of hot pack initially takes 2 hours to heat and 30 minutes to reheat between each use.

Although bentonite-filled moist hot packs are generally recommended for clinical use, a variety of other types of hot or warm packs are available. These include chemical heating pads that are activated by mixing and contact of their contents with air and electric plug-in heating pads.

Chemical heating pads are made from a variety of materials that when exposed to air by opening their

package or breaking open an inner sealed bag or when mechanically agitated, warm up and maintain a therapeutic temperature range for 1 to 8 hours. Different chemicals are activated by different means, heat to slightly different temperatures, have different specific heats, and maintain their temperature for different amounts of time. Although most chemical packs cannot be reused, some can, and although none produce moist heat directly, most can be wrapped in a moist towel or cover to produce moist heat.

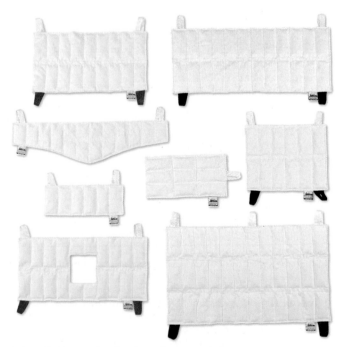

FIG 6-21 Hot packs of various shapes and sizes. *Courtesy Chattanooga Group, Hixson, TN.*

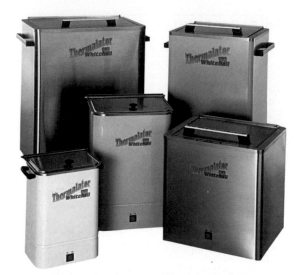

FIG 6-22 Thermostatically controlled hot pack containers. *Courtesy Whitehall Manufacturing, City of Industry, CA.*

These chemical packs also come in a variety of shapes and sizes for application to different body areas, and some are designed to be placed in a wrap allowing them to be worn during activity. Recent studies have found that the low level prolonged heating produced by wearing this type of heating pad during activity can reduce low back and wrist pain and the sensation of stiffness and increase flexibility[132,134,139,140] and may reduce acute low back pain more effectively than ibuprofen or acetaminophen.[158]

Electric plug-in heating pads are not recommended for clinical use because they do not cool during application and therefore may more easily burn a patient. If patients are using an electric plug-in heating pad at home, advise them to use a pad that requires the "on" switch to be held down for the pad to heat, to use only the medium or low settings, to limit application at the medium setting to 20 minutes, and to discontinue use if any sensation of pain, overheating, or burning occurs. Patients should also be advised to inspect their skin for any signs of burns directly after the use of a hot pack and for the following 24 hours.

APPLICATION TECHNIQUE 6-7   HOT PACKS

Equipment Required

- Hot packs in a variety of sizes and shapes appropriate for different areas of the body
- Specialized heating unit
- Towels
- Hot pack covers (optional)
- Timer
- Bell

Procedure

1. Remove clothing and jewelry from the area to be treated and inspect the area.
2. Wrap the hot pack in six to eight layers of dry towels. Hot pack covers, which come in various sizes to match the hot packs, can substitute for two to three layers of towels (Fig. 6-23). More layers should be used if the towels or hot pack covers are old and have become thin or if the patient complains of feeling too warm during treatment. The towels can be preheated to achieve more uniform heating throughout the treatment period. More layers of towels should be used if the body part is on top of the hot pack than if the hot pack is placed over the body part. When the body part is on top of the pack, the towels are compressed, reducing insulation of the body, and the underlying table provides more insulation to the pack, causing it to cool more slowly.[157] If the patient complains of not feeling enough heat, fewer layers of towels may be used for the next treatment session; however, towels should not be removed during heating with hot packs because the increased skin temperature may decrease the patient's thermal sensitivity and the ability to judge the tissue's heat tolerance accurately and safely.
3. Apply the wrapped hot pack to the treatment area and secure it well (Fig. 6-24).

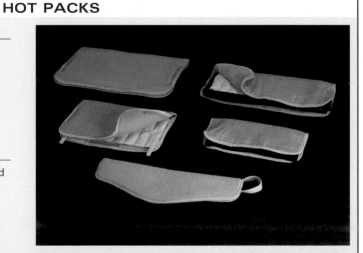

FIG 6-23 Hot pack covers. *Courtesy Whitehall Manufacturing, City of Industry, CA.*

4. Provide the patient with a bell or other means to call for assistance while the hot pack is on and instruct the patient to call immediately if he or she experiences any increase in discomfort. If the patient feels too hot, extra towels should be placed between the hot pack and the patient. If the patient does not feel hot enough, fewer layers of towels should be used at the next treatment session.
5. After 5 minutes, check the patient's report and inspect the area being treated for excessive redness, blistering, or other signs of burning. Discontinue thermotherapy in the presence of signs of burning. If there are any signs of burning, brief application of a cold pack or an ice pack is recommended to curtail the inflammatory response.

APPLICATION TECHNIQUE 6-7	**HOT PACKS**—*cont'd*

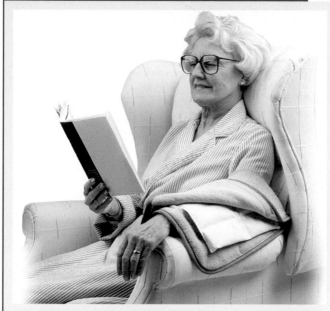

FIG 6-24 Application of a hot pack. *Courtesy Chattanooga Group, Hixson, TN.*

6. After 20 minutes, remove the hot pack and inspect the treatment area. It is normal for the area to appear slightly red and to feel warm to the touch.

Advantages

- Easy to use.
- Inexpensive materials (packs and towels).
- Short use of clinician's time.
- Low level of skill needed for application.
- Can be used to cover moderate to large areas.
- Safe because packs start cooling on removal from the water cabinet.
- Readily available for patient purchase and home use.

Disadvantages

- Hot pack must be moved to observe the treatment area during treatment.
- Patient may not tolerate the weight of the hot pack.
- Pack may not be able to maintain good contact with small or contoured areas.
- Active motion not practical during treatment.
- Moderately expensive equipment (heated water cabinet).

PARAFFIN

Warm, melted paraffin can be used for thermotherapy. For this application, the paraffin is mixed with mineral oil in a 6:1 or 7:1 ratio of paraffin to oil to reduce the melting temperature of the paraffin from 54° C (129° F) to between 45° and 50° C (113° to 122° F). Paraffin can safely be applied directly to the skin at this temperature because of its low specific heat and thermal conductivity. To minimize heat loss, insulating mitts should be applied to the hands or feet (Fig. 6-25). For this application, the paraffin is heated and stored in a thermostatically controlled container that generally can heat the paraffin to 52°-57° C

(126°-134° F).[159] Such containers are available in small portable sizes for home or clinic use and in larger sizes designed primarily for clinic use (Fig. 6-26) The manufacturer's usage and safety instructions for proper setting and adjustment of these devices and selection of the appropriate paraffin wax product should be followed because some units are preset to the correct temperature for a specific product. Paraffin is usually used for heating the distal extremities because it can maintain good contact with these irregularly contoured areas. Paraffin may also be applied to more proximal areas, such as the elbows and knees, or even the low back, by using the paint method described in Application Technique 6-8.

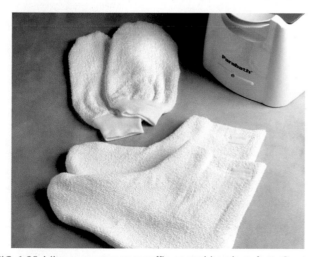

FIG 6-25 Mitts to wear over paraffin-coated hands or feet. *Courtesy The Hygenic Corporation, Akron, OH.*

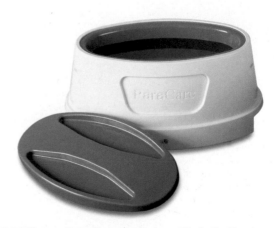

FIG 6-26 Thermostatically controlled paraffin bath. *Courtesy Keitzer Manufacturing, Rolla, MO.*

APPLICATION TECHNIQUE 6-8   PARAFFIN

Equipment Required

- Paraffin
- Mineral oil (or commercially available premixed paraffin intended for this application)
- Thermostatically controlled container
- Plastic bags or paper
- Towels or mitts

Procedure

There are three different methods by which paraffin is commonly applied: dip-wrap, dip-immersion, and paint. The dip-wrap and dip-immersion methods can only be used for treating the distal extremities. The paint method can be used for any area of the body. For all three methods, do the following:

1. Remove all jewelry from the area to be treated and inspect the area.
2. Thoroughly wash and dry the area to be treated to minimize contamination of the paraffin.

For the dip-wrap method (for the wrist and hand):

3. With fingers apart, dip the hand into the paraffin as far as possible and remove (Fig. 6-27). Advise the patient to avoid moving the fingers during the treatment because this will crack the paraffin coating. Also, advise the patient to avoid touching the sides or bottom of the tank because these may be hotter than the paraffin.
4. Wait briefly for the layer of paraffin to harden and become opaque.
5. Redip the hand, keeping the fingers apart. Repeat steps 3 through 5 six to ten times.
6. Wrap the patient's hand in a plastic bag, wax paper, or treatment-table paper and then in a towel or toweling mitt. The plastic bag or paper prevents the towel from sticking to the paraffin, and the toweling acts as insulation to slow the cooling of the paraffin. Caution the patient not to move the hand during dipping or during the rest period because this may crack the coating of paraffin, allowing air to penetrate and the paraffin to cool more rapidly.
7. Elevate the extremity.

8. Leave the paraffin in place for 10 to 15 minutes or until it cools.
9. When the intervention is completed, peel the paraffin off the hand and discard it (Fig. 6-28).

For the dip-immersion method:

3. With fingers apart, dip the hand into the paraffin and remove.
4. Wait 5 to 15 seconds for the layer of paraffin to harden and become opaque.
5. Redip the hand, keeping the fingers apart.
6. Allow the hand to remain in the paraffin for up to 20 minutes and then remove it.

The temperature of the paraffin should be at the lower end of the range for this method of application because the hand cools less during treatment than with the dip-wrap method. The heater should be turned off during the treatment so that the sides and bottom of the tank do not become too hot.

For the paint method:

3. Paint a layer of paraffin onto the treatment area with a brush.
4. Wait for the layer of paraffin to become opaque.
5. Paint on another layer of paraffin no larger than the first layer. Repeat steps 3 through 5 six to ten times.
6. Cover the area with plastic or paper and then with toweling. As with the dip-immersion method, the plastic or paper is used to prevent the towel from sticking to the paraffin and the toweling acts as insulation to slow down the cooling of the paraffin. Caution the patient not to move the area during treatment as this may crack the coating of paraffin, allowing air to penetrate and the treatment area to cool more rapidly.
7. Leave the paraffin in place for 20 minutes or until it cools.
8. When the intervention is completed, peel off the paraffin and discard it.

For all methods:

When the intervention is complete, inspect the treatment area for any signs of adverse effects and document the intervention.

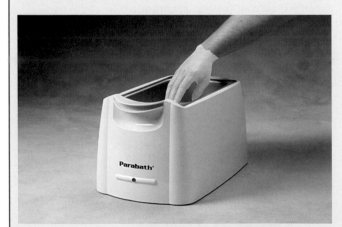

FIG 6-27 Application of paraffin by the dip-wrap method. *Courtesy The Hygenic Corporation, Akron, OH.*

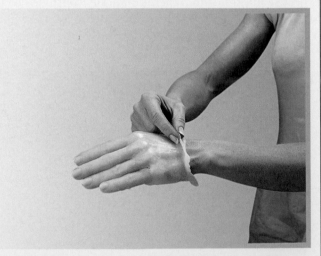

FIG 6-28 Removing paraffin from a patient's hand. *Courtesy HoMedics Inc, Commerce Township, MI.*

APPLICATION TECHNIQUE 6-8 | PARAFFIN—*cont'd*

In most clinics the paraffin bath is left plugged in and on at all times. In this circumstance, it can be used by a number of patients, one after another, and maintain its goal temperature. If the unit is unplugged or turned off and the paraffin is allowed to cool, be sure that the paraffin has returned to between 52° and 57° C (126° and 134° F) before it is used again for treatment. Caution should be used for the first 5 hours after turning a unit on as some units take up to 5 hours to heat the wax and during this heating period parts of the wax may be hotter than the recommended therapeutic temperature range. This could result in burning. Always follow manufacturer's instructions to ensure safe use.

Advantages

- Maintains good contact with highly contoured areas.
- Easy to use.

- Inexpensive.
- Body part can be elevated if using the dip-wrap method.
- Oil lubricates and conditions the skin.
- Can be used by patient at home.

Disadvantages

- Messy and time-consuming to apply.
- Cannot be used over an open skin lesion as it may contaminate the lesion.
- Risk of cross-contamination if the paraffin is reused.
- Part in dependent position for dip-immersion method.

FLUIDOTHERAPY

Fluidotherapy is a dry heating agent that transfers heat by convection.[160] It consists of a cabinet containing finely ground cellulose particles made from corn cobs (Fig. 6-29). Heated air is circulated through the particles, suspending and moving them so that they act like a liquid. The patient extends a body part into the cabinet, where it floats, as if in water. There are also portals in the cabinet that allow the therapist to access the patient's body part while it is being heated. Fluidotherapy units come in a variety of sizes suitable for treating different body parts. Both the temperature and the amount of particle agitation can be controlled by the clinician (Fig. 6-30).

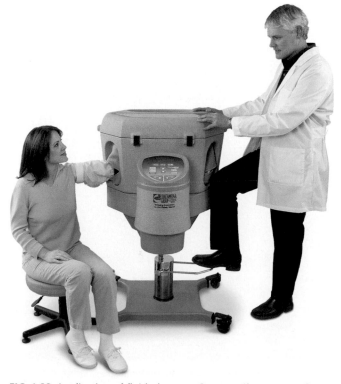

FIG 6-29 Application of fluidotherapy. *Courtesy Chattanooga Group, Hixson, TN.*

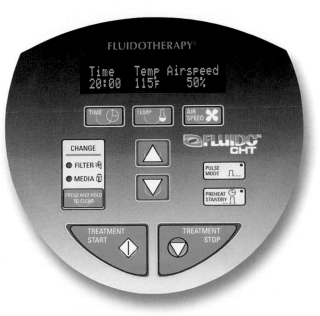

FIG 6-30 Fluidotherapy controls. *Courtesy Chattanooga Group, Hixson, TN.*

APPLICATION TECHNIQUE 6-9	FLUIDOTHERAPY

Equipment Required

- Fluidotherapy unit of appropriate size and shape for areas to be treated

Procedure

1. Remove all jewelry and clothing from the area to be treated and inspect the area.
2. Cover any open wounds with a plastic barrier to prevent the cellulose particles from becoming lodged in the wound.
3. Extend the body part to be treated through the portal of the unit (see Fig. 6-29).
4. Secure the sleeve to prevent particles from escaping from the cabinet.
5. Set the temperature at 38° to 48°C (100° to 118° F).
6. Adjust the degree of agitation to achieve patient comfort.
7. The patient may move or exercise during the intervention.
8. Treat for 20 minutes.

Advantages

- Patient can move during the intervention to work on gaining AROM.
- Minimal pressure applied to the area being treated.
- Temperature well-controlled and constant throughout intervention.
- Easy to administer.

Disadvantages

- Expensive equipment
- Limb must be in dependent position in some units, increasing the risk of edema formation.
- The constant heat source may result in overheating.
- If the corn cob particles spill onto a smooth floor, they will make the floor slippery.

INFRARED LAMPS

IR lamps emit electromagnetic radiation within the frequency range that gives rise to heat when absorbed by matter (Fig. 6-31). IR radiation has a wavelength of 770 nm to 10^6 nm, lying between visible light and microwaves on the electromagnetic spectrum (see Fig. 12-1) and is emitted by many sources that emit visible light or UV radiation such as the sun. IR radiation is divided into three bands with different wavelength ranges: IR-A, with wavelengths of 770 to 1400 nm; IR-B, with wavelengths of 1400 to 3000 nm; and IR-C, with wavelengths of 3000 to 10^6 nm. The IR sources used in rehabilitation include sunlight, IR lamps, IR light-emitting diodes (LEDs), supraluminous diodes (SLDs), and low-intensity lasers. IR lamps currently available for clinical use all emit IR-A, generally with mixed wavelengths of approximately 780 to 1500 nm with a peak intensity at around 1000 nm.

The tissue temperature increase produced by IR radiation is directly proportional to the amount of radiation that penetrates the tissue. This is related to the power and wavelength of the radiation, the distance of the radiation source from the tissue, the **angle of incidence** of the radiation to the tissue, and the absorption coefficient of the tissue. Higher-power IR will deliver more radiation to the skin. Most lamps deliver IR radiation with power in the range of 50 to 1500 watts. Most of the IR radiation produced by today's lamps (780 to 1500 nm wavelength) is absorbed within the first few millimeters of human tissue. It has been shown that at least 50% of IR radiation of 1200 nm wavelength penetrates beyond 0.8 mm and is therefore able to pass through the skin to interact with subcutaneous capillaries and cutaneous nerve endings.[161] Human skin allows maximum penetration of radiation with a wavelength of 1200 nm while being virtually opaque to IR radiation with a wavelength of 2000 nm or greater.[151]

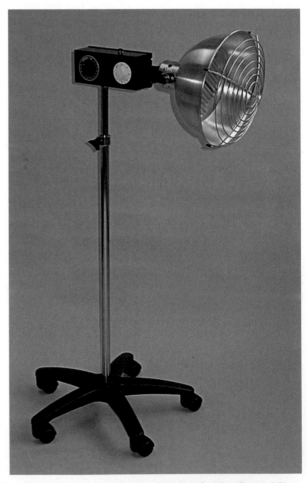

FIG 6-31 Infrared lamp. *Courtesy Brandt Industries, Bronx, NY.*

The amount of energy reaching the patient from an IR radiation source is also related to the distance between the source and the tissue. As the distance of the source from the target increases, the intensity of radiation reaching the target changes in proportion to the inverse square of the distance. For example, if the source is moved from a position 5 cm from the target to a position 10 cm from the target, increasing by a factor of 2, the intensity of radiation reaching the target will fall to one-fourth of its prior level. The amount of energy reaching the target is also related to the angle of incidence of the radiation. As the angle of incidence of the radiation changes, the intensity of the energy reaching the target changes in proportion to the cosine of the angle of incidence of the radiation. For example, if the angle of incidence changes from 0 degrees (i.e., perpendicular to the surface of the skin), with a cosine of 1, to 45 degrees, with a cosine of $\frac{1}{\sqrt{2}}$, the intensity of radiation will fall by a factor of $\frac{1}{\sqrt{2}}$. Thus the intensity reaching the skin is greatest when the radiation source is close to the patient's skin and the radiation beam is perpendicular to the skin surface, and as the distance or the angle of incidence increases, the intensity of the radiation reaching the skin will diminish.

IR radiation is absorbed most by tissues with high IR absorption coefficients. IR absorption coefficients are primarily affected by color, with darker tissue and skin absorbing more radiation than lighter tissue and skin. Therefore, with the same radiation and lamp positioning, dark skin will absorb more IR and therefore increase more in temperature than light skin.

A number of authors have provided formulae for calculating the exact amount of heat being delivered to a patient by IR radiation[149,162] or methodologies for measuring the exact tissue temperature increase;[150] however, in clinical practice, as with other thermal agents, the sensory report of the patient is usually used to gauge the skin temperature. The amount of heat transfer is adjusted by changing the power output of the lamp and/or the distance of the lamp from the patient so that the patient feels a comfortable level of warmth.

Although the clinical use of IR lamps for heating superficial tissues was popular during the 1940s and 1950s, this practice has waned in recent years. This fall in popularity appears to be the result of changes in practice style preferences and concern about overheating patients if they are placed or move too close to the lamp rather than any evidence of excessive adverse effects or lack of therapeutic efficacy. Recent studies continue to show that IR produces expected effects of heat, including reducing pain in patients with chronic low back pain[163] and increasing joint flexibility and thus the increase in ROM produced by stretching in joints with contractures.[143] Most of the current use and literature regarding the use of IR in therapy relates to low-intensity IR lasers with nonthermal effects as discussed in detail in Chapter 12.

APPLICATION TECHNIQUE 6-10 INFRARED LAMPS

Equipment Required

- IR lamp
- IR opaque goggles
- Tape measure to measure distance of treatment area from IR source
- Towels

Procedure

1. Remove clothing and jewelry from the area to be treated and inspect the area. Drape the patient for modesty, leaving the area to be treated uncovered.
2. Put IR opaque goggles on the patient and the therapist if there is a possibility of IR irradiation of the eyes.
3. Allow the IR lamp to warm up for 5 to 10 minutes so it will reach a stable level of output.[149]
4. Position the patient with the surface of the area to be treated perpendicular to the IR beam and about 45 to 60 cm away from the source. Remember that the intensity of the IR radiation reaching the skin decreases, with an inverse square relationship, as the distance from the source increases, and in proportion to the cosine of the angle of incidence of the beam. Adjust the distance from the source and wattage of the lamp output so that the patient feels a comfortable level of warmth. Measure and record the distance of the lamp from the target tissue.
5. Provide the patient with a means to call for assistance, and instruct the patient to call if discomfort occurs.
6. Instruct the patient to avoid moving closer to or farther from the lamp and to avoid touching the lamp since movement toward or away from the lamp will alter the amount of energy reaching the patient.

7. Set the lamp to treat for 15 to 30 minutes. Generally, treatment times of about 15 minutes are used for subacute conditions and up to 30 minutes for chronic conditions. Most lamps have a timer that automatically shuts off the lamp when the treatment time has elapsed.
8. Monitor the patient's response during treatment. It may be necessary to move the lamp farther away if the patient becomes too warm. Be cautious in moving the lamp closer if the patient reports not feeling warm enough as the patient may have accommodated to the sensation and may not judge the heat level accurately once warm.
9. When the intervention is completed, turn off the lamp and dry any perspiration from the treated area.

Advantages

- Does not require contact of the medium with the patient, which reduces the risk of infection and the possible discomfort of the weight of a hot pack and also avoids the problem of poor contact when treating highly contoured areas.
- The area being treated can be observed throughout the intervention.

Disadvantages

- Infrared radiation is not easily localized to a specific treatment area.
- It is difficult to ensure consistent heating in all treatment areas because the amount of heat transfer is affected by the distance of the skin from the radiation source and the angle of the beam with the skin, both of which vary with tissue contours and may be inconsistent between treatment sessions.

OTHER MEANS OF APPLYING THERMOTHERAPY

Superficial heat may also be applied by immersion in a warm whirlpool or a contrast bath, as described in detail in Chapter 9.

DOCUMENTATION

The following should be documented:
- Area of the body treated
- Type of heating agent used
- Treatment parameters, including:
  - Temperature or power of the agent
  - Number and type of insulation layers used
  - Distance of the agent from the patient
  - Patient's position or activity, if these can be varied with the agent used
  - Treatment duration
  - Response to the intervention

Documentation is typically written in the SOAP note format. The following examples only summarize the modality component of intervention and are not intended to represent a comprehensive plan of care.

EXAMPLES

When applying a hot pack (HP) to low back pain (LBP), document the following:

S: Pt reports LBP that worsens with prolonged sitting.
O: Pretreatment: LBP 7/10. Sitting tolerance 30 min.
Intervention: HP low back, 20 min, pt prone, six layers of towels.
Posttreatment: LBP 4/10.
A: Pain decreased from 7/10 to 4/10.
P: Continue use of HP as above before stretching and back exercises. Recheck sitting tolerance at the beginning of next visit.

When applying paraffin to the R hand, document the following:

S: Pt reports R hand stiffness especially with finger extension.
O: Pretreatment: Proximal interphalangeal (PIP) extension limited to −10 degrees. Unable to tie shoelaces without assistance.
Intervention: Paraffin R hand, 50° C (122° F), 10 min, dip-wrap, seven dips.
Posttreatment: PIP extension −5 degrees after active and passive stretching. Able to tie shoelaces without assistance.
A: Decreased joint stiffness and improved ROM and function.
P: Continue use of paraffin as above to R hand before stretching and mobilization.

When applying fluidotherapy to the L leg, ankle, and foot, document the following:

S: Pt reports L ankle stiffness.
O: Pretreatment: Ankle dorsiflexion zero degrees.
Intervention: Fluidotherapy L LE, 42° C (108° F), 20 min. Ankle AROM during heating.
Posttreatment: Ankle dorsiflexion 5 degrees.
A: Ankle dorsiflexion increased from neutral to 5 degrees.
P: Discontinue fluidotherapy. Progress to active and PROM and gait activities in weight-bearing position.

When applying IR radiation to the R forearm, document the following:

S: Pt reports R forearm pain with writing.
O: Pretreatment: Pain with motion associated with writing.
Intervention: IR R forearm, 1000 nm peak wavelength, 100 W at 50 cm for 20 min.
Posttreatment: Mild sensation of warmth at forearm; pain with writing decreased 50%.
A: Tolerated well. Decreased pain with writing.
P: Continue IR as above 2x per week before stretching.

CLINICAL CASE STUDIES

The following case studies summarize the concepts of superficial heat discussed in this chapter. Based on the scenarios presented, an evaluation of the clinical findings and goals of the intervention are proposed. These are followed by a discussion of the factors to be considered in the selection of superficial thermotherapy as the indicated treatment modality and in the selection of the ideal thermotherapy agent to promote progress toward the set goals.

CASE STUDY 6-4

Osteoarthritis of the Hands
Examination
History

MP is a 75-year-old woman referred for therapy with a diagnosis of osteoarthritis of the hands and an order to evaluate and treat with a focus on developing a home program. MP complains of stiffness and aching in all her finger joints, causing difficulties in gripping cooking utensils and performing other household tasks and pain with writing. She reports that these symptoms have gradually worsened over the last 10 years and have become much more severe in the last month since she stopped taking ibuprofen due to gastric side effects.

Tests and Measures

The examination reveals stiffness and restricted flexion PROM of the proximal interphalangeal (PIP) joints of fingers 2 to 5 to approximately 90 degrees and mild ulnar drift at the carpometacarpal (CMC) joints bilaterally. The joints are not warm or edematous, and sensation is intact in both hands.

Is this an acute or chronic condition? What must you consider before using heat in a patient with an inflammatory condition? What types of thermotherapy would be appropriate for this patient? Which type would not be appropriate?

Evaluation, Diagnosis, Prognosis, and Goals
Evaluation and Goals

ICF Level	Current Status	Goals
Body structure and function	Restricted finger ROM	Increase finger ROM
	Pain, stiffness and swelling of the finger joints	Decrease pain Reduce joint stiffness
	Abnormal ulnar drift of the CMC joints of the hands	Prevent further symptoms from developing
Activity	Gripping action difficult	Increase ability to grip
Participation	Difficulty with cooking, household tasks, writing	Optimize patient's ability to cook, do household tasks, and write

Diagnosis
Preferred Practice Pattern 4D: Impaired joint mobility, motor function, muscle performance, and ROM associated with connective tissue dysfunction

Prognosis/Plan of Care
Given the chronic, progressive nature of osteoarthritis, the intervention should focus on maintaining the patient's status, optimizing her function, and slowing progression of her disabilities. Superficial heating agents can increase the extensibility of superficial soft tissue and are therefore indicated for the treatment of joint stiffness and restricted ROM. Superficial heating agents can also reduce joint-related pain. Thermotherapy is not contraindicated for this patient at this time because, although she has a diagnosis of osteoarthritis, which is an inflammatory disease, her hands do not show signs of acute inflammation such as increased temperature or edema of the finger joints. Her hands also have intact sensation. Caution should be used, however, since at the age of 75 years she may have impaired circulation or impaired thermal regulation. Therefore the intensity of the thermal agent should be at the lower end of the range typically used.

Intervention
It is proposed that superficial heat be applied to the wrists, hands, and fingers of both hands. Paraffin, fluidotherapy, or water are appropriate thermal agents for heating these areas; however, a hot pack is not appropriate because it would not provide good contact with these highly contoured areas. Paraffin has the additional advantage of allowing elevation while heat is being applied, thus reducing the risk of edema formation. It is also inexpensive and safe enough to be used at home; however, it has the disadvantage of not allowing motion during application. Therefore, for optimal benefit, if paraffin is used to treat this patient, she should perform active ROM exercises directly after removing the paraffin

from her hands. Fluidotherapy and water have the advantage of allowing motion during their application; however, fluidotherapy is generally too expensive and cumbersome for use at home or in many clinics, and water immersion may result in edema formation because the patient's hands must be in a dependent position while being heated. Given these advantages and disadvantages, warm water soaks together with exercise would be most appropriate if the patient does not develop edema with this intervention, and paraffin followed by exercise would be most appropriate if the patient develops edema with soaking in warm water. If paraffin is used, it should be applied using the dip-wrap method rather than the dip-immersion method because the former allows elevation of the hand and results in less intense and prolonged heating. Therefore it is less likely to result in edema formation and is safer for the older patient who may have impaired circulation or thermal regulation.

Documentation
S: Pt reports bilateral hand pain (7/10) and stiffness.

O: Pretreatment: PIP PROM approximately 90 degrees in fingers 2-5. Stiffness and pain with motion. Mild ulnar drift at bilateral CMC joints.

Intervention: Paraffin to bilateral hands, 50° (108° F), 10 min, dip-wrap, seven dips. ROM exercises after removing paraffin.

Posttreatment: PIP PROM 110 degrees in fingers 2 to 5. Pain (4/10) and decreased subjective stiffness. No visible edema

A: Increased ROM, decreased pain and stiffness without development of edema in response to paraffin.

P: Continue paraffin application as above once daily at home before ROM exercises.

CASE STUDY 6-5

Low Back Pain
Examination
History
KB is a 45-year-old man with mild low back pain. Two months ago he fell 10 feet from a ladder and sustained severe soft tissue bruising; however, there was no evidence of a fracture or disc damage with this trauma. KB was referred for physical therapy 1 month ago with the diagnosis of a lumbar strain and with an order to optimize function to return to work. KB is currently participating in an active exercise program to work on spinal flexibility and stabilization, but he often feels stiff when starting to exercise. He has not returned to his job as a carpenter because of low back pain that is aggravated by forward bending and low back stiffness that is most intense during the first few hours of the day and that prevents him from lifting. He has also not returned to playing baseball with his children because he is scared that this will aggravate his back pain. KB reports that his pain is often worse at night when he lies still making it

Continued

difficult to fall asleep and that it is alleviated to some degree by taking a hot shower. He had been making good progress, with increasing lumbar ROM, strength, and endurance, until the last 2 weeks, when his progress reached a plateau.

Tests and Measures

Palpation reveal spasms of the lumbar paravertebral muscles, and KF is found to have 50% restriction of active forward-bending ROM, and 30% restriction of sidebending bilaterally, with reports of pulling of the low back at the end of the range and pain at a 7/10 level with bending. Other objective measures, including active backward bending, passive joint mobility, and lower extremity strength and sensation, are within normal limits.

How may thermotherapy help this patient? What types of thermotherapy would be appropriate for this patient? Which type would not be appropriate? What types of activities should be combined with thermotherapy to help the patient achieve his goals?

Evaluation, Diagnosis, Prognosis, and Goals
Evaluation and Goals

ICF Level	Current Status	Goals
Body structure and function	Restricted trunk ROM in forward and sidebending Low back pain Paravertebral muscle spasms	Normalize lumbar forward and sidebending ROM Control low back pain Resolve paravertebral muscle spasms
Activity	Inability to bend forward to lift Difficulty falling asleep	Return lifting ability to prior baseline Able to fall asleep within 15 minutes of going to bed
Participation	Inability to work as a carpenter or play baseball	Return to work Return to recreational sports

Diagnosis

Preferred Practice Pattern 4F: Impaired joint mobility, motor function, muscle performance, ROM, and reflex integrity associated with spinal disorders.

Prognosis/Plan of Care

Two months after a soft tissue injury, KB's rehabilitation program should generally focus on active participation in a program of stretching and strengthening; however, applying a physical agent before active exercise may improve performance and accelerate progress. Thermotherapy may be indicated for this patient because it can reduce pain, stiffness, and soft tissue shortening and because this patient has reported that a hot shower, which provides superficial heating, helps to alleviate his symptoms. There are also no contraindications to the use of thermotherapy for this patient.

Intervention

A deep or superficial heating agent would be appropriate for providing thermotherapy to this patient. A deep-heating agent would be ideal because it could directly increase the temperature of both the superficial tissues and the muscles of the low back; however, a superficial heating agent would generally be used because diathermy, which can provide deep heating to large areas, is not available in most clinical settings (see Chapter 14) and ultrasound can only provide deep heating to small areas (see Chapter 7). Superficial heating could be provided to the low back using an IR lamp or a hot pack. A hot pack is most likely to be used because IR lamps are also not available in most clinical settings.

A hot pack could be applied with the patient in a supine, prone, side-lying, or sitting position. More insulating towels may be needed in the supine or sitting position than in the prone or side-lying position because of compression of the towels and the insulating effect of the supporting surface. Treatment with any superficial heating agent would generally be applied for 20 to 30 minutes. Also, to optimize the benefit of increased soft tissue extensibility, active or passive stretching should be performed immediately after the application of the thermal agent.

Documentation

S: Pt reports low back stiffness and pain with forward bending.

O: Pretreatment: LBP 4/10. Lumbar paravertebral muscle spasms. 30% restriction of active forward-bending ROM. 30% restriction of bilateral sidebending.

Intervention: HP low back, 20 min, pt prone, six layers of towels.

Post-treatment: LBP 2/10, decreased paravertebral muscle spasms. 20% restriction of forward-bending and minimal restriction of sidebending.

A: Pt tolerated HP well, with decreased pain and increased ROM.

P: Continue use of HP as above twice daily before stretching and back exercises.

CASE STUDY 6-6

Ulcer caused by Arterial Insufficiency
Examination
History

BD is a 72-year-old woman with a 10-year history of non–insulin-dependent diabetes mellitus and a full-thickness ulcer on her lateral right ankle caused by arterial insufficiency. The ulcer has been present for 6 months and has been treated only with daily dressing changes. BD has poor arterial circulation in her distal lower extremities, but her physician has determined that she is not a candidate for lower extremity bypass surgery. She lives alone at home and is independent in all activities of daily living; however, her walking is limited to approximately 500 feet because of calf pain. Because of this, she has limited her participation in family activities such as taking her grandchildren to the park. BD has been referred to physical therapy for evaluation and treatment of her ulcer.

Tests and Measures

The patient is alert and oriented. Sensation is impaired distal to the patient's knees and is intact proximal to the knees. There is a 2-cm diameter, full-thickness ulcer on the right lateral ankle.

What concerns would you have about the use of thermotherapy in this patient? On what part(s) of the body would you consider applying thermotherapy in this patient?

Evaluation, Diagnosis, Prognosis, and Goals
Evaluation and Goals

ICF Level	Current Status	Goals
Body structure and function	Loss of skin and underlying soft tissue on right lateral ankle Reduced sensation in bilateral distal lower extremities	Decrease wound size Close wound
Activity	Walking is limited to 500 feet Daily dressing changes	Increase walking tolerance to 1 block Decrease the need for dressing changes to 1-2 times per week and thus reduced the risk of infection associated with open wounds
Participation	Decreased participation in family activities, such as taking her grandchildren to the park	Patient able to take her grandchildren to the park Participation in family activities not limited by calf pain

Diagnosis

Preferred Practice Pattern 7D: Impaired integumentary integrity associated with full-thickness skin involvement and scar formation

Prognosis/Plan of Care

Thermotherapy may help achieve some of the proposed goals of treatment because it can improve circulation and thus facilitate tissue healing. Superficial heating agents can increase circulation both in the area to which the heat is applied and distally. Increasing tissue temperature can also increase oxygen-hemoglobin dissociation, increasing the availability of oxygen for tissue healing. Because the application of thermotherapy directly to the distal lower extremities of this patient is contraindicated due to her impaired sensation in these areas, proximal application of thermotherapy to the patient's low back or thighs may be used in an attempt to increase the circulation to her distal lower extremities without excessive risk.

Intervention

Thermotherapy using a deep or superficial heating agent would be appropriate for this patient. As with Case Study 6-2, deep heating would be ideal since this would affect both deep and superficial tissue temperatures; however, a superficial heating agent is more likely to be used because of greater availability. A hot pack or an IR lamp could be used to heat this patient's low back or thighs and should be applied for about 20 minutes. Extra towels should be used during the first treatment because this patient's poor circulation puts her at increased risk for burns.

Documentation

S: Pt reports ulcer on R lateral ankle present for 6 months and walking limited to 500 feet by calf pain.

O: Pretreatment: Full-thickness ulcer right lateral ankle, 1 cm × 1 cm. Decreased sensation from ankle distally bilaterally.

Intervention: HP bilateral thighs, 20 min, pt sitting, 8 layers of towels.

Posttreatment: Skin in area of heat application intact without blistering or burns. Pt reports very mild warmth felt with this application.

A: Pt tolerated treatment without discomfort.

P: Continue application of HP to thighs, with 6 towels at next treatment, in conjunction with appropriate direct wound care.

CHOOSING BETWEEN CRYOTHERAPY AND THERMOTHERAPY

Because some of the effects and clinical indications for the use of cryotherapy and thermotherapy are the same and others are different, there are some situations in which either may be used and others in which only one or the other would be appropriate. Table 6-3 provides a summary of the effects of cryotherapy and thermotherapy to assist the clinician in choosing between these options. Although both heat and cold can decrease pain and muscle spasm, their effects on blood flow, edema formation, nerve conduction velocity, tissue metabolism, and collagen extensibility are the opposite. Cryotherapy decreases these effects, and thermotherapy increases them.

Effect	Cryotherapy	Thermotherapy
TABLE 6-3 Effects of Cryotherapy and Thermotherapy		
Pain	Decrease	Decrease
Muscle spasm	Decrease	Decrease
Blood flow	Decrease	Increase
Edema formation	Decrease	Increase
Nerve conduction velocity	Decrease	Increase
Metabolic rate	Decrease	Increase
Collagen extensibility	Decrease	Increase
Joint stiffness	Increase	Decrease
Spasticity	Decrease	No effect

CHAPTER REVIEW

1. Thermal agents transfer heat to or from patients by conduction, convection, conversion, or radiation.
2. Cryotherapy is the transfer of heat from a patient by use of a cooling agent. Cryotherapy has been shown to decrease blood flow, decrease nerve conduction velocity, increase pain threshold, alter muscle strength, decrease enzymatic activity rate, temporarily decrease spasticity, and facilitate muscle contraction. These effects of cryotherapy are used clinically to control inflammation, pain, edema, and muscle spasm; to reduce spasticity temporarily; and to facilitate muscle contraction. Examples of physical agents used for cryotherapy include ice pack, cold pack, ice massage, and vapocoolant spray.
3. Thermotherapy is the transfer of heat to a patient with a heating agent. Thermotherapy has been shown to increase blood flow, increase nerve conduction velocity, increase pain threshold, alter muscle strength, and increase enzymatic activity rate. These effects of thermotherapy are used clinically to control pain, increase soft tissue extensibility, and accelerate healing. Examples of physical agents used for thermotherapy include hot pack, paraffin, fluidotherapy, and IR lamp.
4. Thermal agents should not be applied in situations in which they may aggravate an existing pathology, such as a malignancy, or may cause damage, such as frostbite or burns.
5. The reader is referred to the Evolve web site for further exercises and links to resources and references.

ADDITIONAL RESOURCES *evolve*

Web Sites

Chattanooga Group: Chattanooga produces a number of physical agents, including cold packs and cooling units, hot packs and warming units, paraffin, and fluidotherapy. The web site may be searched by body part or by product category. Product specifications are available online. www.chattgroup.com

Game Ready: Information on cold compression units along with some discussion of the science behind the product and some references. www.gameready.com

Gebauer Company: Information on vapocoolant spray products, videos on application, and a list of references. www.gebauer.com

Whitehall Manufacturing: Whitehall produces hospital and therapy products, including cold packs and cooling units, moist heat therapy packs and warming units, and paraffin. The web site includes product photographs, as well as sheets outlining the specifications for all products. www.whitehallmfg.com

GLOSSARY *evolve*

General Terms

Angle of incidence: The angle at which a beam (e.g., from an infrared lamp) contacts the skin

Conduction: Heat transfer resulting from energy exchange by direct collision between molecules of two materials at different temperature. Heat is transferred by conduction when the materials are in contact with each other.

Convection: Heat transfer through direct contact of a circulating medium with a material of a different temperature.

Conversion: Heat transfer by the conversion of a nonthermal form of energy, such as mechanical, electrical, or chemical energy, into heat.

Radiation: Transfer of energy from one material to another without the need for direct contact or an intervening medium.

Specific heat: The amount of energy required to raise the temperature of a given weight of a material by a given number of degrees, usually expressed in $J/gm/^\circ C$.

Thermal conductivity: The rate at which a material transfers heat by conduction, usually expressed in $(cal/sec)/(cm^2 \times ^\circ C/cm)$.

Cryotherapy

Cold-induced vasodilation (CIVD): The dilation of blood vessels that occurs after cold is applied for a prolonged time or after tissue temperature reaches less than 10 degrees Celsius. Also known as the hunting response.

Contrast bath: Alternating immersion in hot and cold water.

Controlled cold compression: Alternate pumping of cold water and air into a sleeve wrapped around a patient's limb, used most commonly to control pain and edema immediately after surgery.

Cryokinetics: A technique that combines the use of cold and exercise.

Cryostretch: The application of a cooling agent before stretching.

Cryotherapy: The therapeutic use of cold.

Delayed-onset muscle soreness (DOMS): Soreness that often occurs 24 to 72 hours after eccentric exercise or unaccustomed training levels. DOMS is probably caused by inflammation as result of tiny muscle tears.

Edema: Swelling resulting from accumulation of fluid in the interstitial space.

Quick icing: The rapid application of ice as a stimulus to elicit desired motor patterns in patients with reduced muscle tone or impaired muscle control.

RICE: An acronym for rest, ice, compression, and elevation. RICE is used to decrease edema formation and inflammation after an acute injury.

Spasticity: Muscle hypertonicity and increased deep tendon reflexes.

Vapocoolant spray A liquid that evaporates quickly when sprayed on the skin, causing quick superficial cooling of the skin.

Vasoconstriction A decrease in blood vessel diameter. Cold generally causes vasoconstriction.

Thermotherapy

Diathermy: The application of shortwave or microwave electromagnetic energy to produce heat within tissues, particularly deep tissues.

Fluidotherapy: A dry heating agent that transfers heat by convection. It consists of a cabinet containing finely ground particles of cellulose through which heated air is circulated.

Hubbard tank: A large, stainless steel whirlpool designed for immersion of the entire body that is used primarily for the treatment of patients with extensive burn wounds.

Infrared (IR) lamp: A lamp that emits electromagnetic radiation in the infrared range (wavelength approximately 750 nm to 1300 nm). IR radiation of sufficient intensity can cause an increase in superficial tissue temperature.

Paraffin: A waxy substance that can be warmed and used to coat the extremities for thermotherapy.

Protein denaturation: The breakdown of proteins that permanently alters their biological activity and which can be caused by excessive heat.

Thermotherapy: The therapeutic application of heat.

Ultrasound: Sound with a frequency greater than 20,000 cycles per second that has thermal and nonthermal effects when applied to the body.

Vasodilation: An increase in blood vessel diameter. Heat generally causes vasodilation.

REFERENCES *evolve*

1. Darlas Y, Solassol A, Clouard R, et al: Ultrasonotherapie: calcul del thermogenese, *Ann Readapt Med Phys* 32:181-192, 1989.
2. Coakley WT: Biophysical effects of ultrasound at therapeutic intensities, *Physiotherapy* 64(4):166-168, 1978.
3. Martin SS, Spindler KP, Tarter JW, et al: Cryotherapy: an effective modality for decreasing intraarticular temperature after knee arthroscopy, *Am J Sports Med* 29(3):288-291, 2000.
4. Warren TA, McCarty EC, Richardson AL, et al: Intra-articular knee temperature changes: ice versus cryotherapy device, *Am J Sports Med* 32(2):441-445, 2004.
5. Weston M, Taber C, Casagranda L, et al: Changes in local blood volume during cold gel pack application to traumatized ankles, *J Orthop Sport Phys Ther* 19(4):197-199, 1994.
6. Karunakara RG, Lephart SM, Pincivero DM: Changes in forearm blood flow during single and intermittent cold application, *J Orthop Sports Phys Ther* 29(3):177-180, 1999.
7. Wolf SL: Contralateral upper extremity cooling from a specific cold stimulus, *Phys Ther* 51:158-165, 1971.
8. Palmieri RM, Garrison JC, Leonard JL, et al: Peripheral ankle cooling and core body temperature, *J Athl Train* 41(2):185-188, 2006.
9. Lewis T: Observations upon the reactions of the vessels of the human skin to cold, *Heart* 15:177-208, 1930.
10. Clark RS, Hellon RF, Lind AR: Vascular reactions of the human forearm to cold, *Clin Sci* 17(1):165-179, 1958.
11. Fox R, Wyatt H: Cold-induced vasodilation in various areas of the body surface in man, *J Physiol* 162(1):289-297, 1962.
12. Keating WR: The effect of general chilling on the vasodilation response to cold, *J Physiol* 139(3):497-507, 1957.
13. Taber C, Countryman K, Fahrenbruch J, et al: Measurement of reactive vasodilation during cold gel pack application to nontraumatized ankles, *Phys Ther* 72(4):294-299, 1992.
14. Keating WR: *Survival in cold water*, Oxford, 1978, Blackwell.
15. Comroe JH Jr: *The lung: clinical physiology and pulmonary function tests*, ed 2, Chicago, 1962, Year Book Medical Publishers.
16. Lee JM, Warren MP, Mason SM: Effects of ice on nerve conduction velocity, *Physiotherapy* 64:2-6, 1978.
17. Zankel HT: Effect of physical agents on motor conduction velocity of the ulnar nerve, *Arch Phys Med Rehabil* 47:787-792, 1966.
18. Douglas WW, Malcolm JL: The effect of localized cooling on cat nerves, *J Physiol* 130:53-54, 1955.
19. Bassett FH, Kirkpatrick JS, Engelhardt DL, et al: Cryotherapy induced nerve injury, *Am J Sport Med* 22:516-528, 1992.
20. Ernst E, Fialka V: Ice freezes pain? A review of the clinical effectiveness of analgesic cold therapy, *J Pain Symptom Mgmt* 9(1):56-59, 1994.
21. McMaster WC, Liddie S: Cryotherapy influence on posttraumatic limb edema, *Clin Orthop Relat Res* 150:283-287, 1980.
22. McGown HL: Effects of cold application on maximal isometric contraction, *Phys Ther* 47:185-192, 1967.
23. Oliver RA, Johnson DJ, Wheelhouse WW, et al: Isometric muscle contraction response during recovery from reduced intramuscular temperature, *Arch Phys Med Rehabil* 60:126-129, 1979.
24. Johnson J, Leider FE: Influence of cold bath on maximum handgrip strength, *Percept Mot Skills* 44:323-325, 1977.
25. Davies CTM, Young K: Effect of temperature on the contractile properties and muscle power of triceps surae in humans, *J Appl Physiol* 55:191-195, 1983.
26. Knuttsson E, Mattsson E: Effects of local cooling on monosynaptic reflexes in man, *Scand J Rehabil Med* 52:166-168, 1969.
27. Knuttsson E: Topical cryotherapy in spasticity, *Scand J Rehabil Med* 2:159-162, 1970.
28. Hartvikksen K: Ice therapy in spasticity, *Acta Neurol Scand* 38:79-83, 1962.
29. Miglietta O: Electromyographic characteristics of clonus and influence of cold, *Arch Phys Med Rehabil* 45:502-503, 1964.
30. Miglietta O: Action of cold on spasticity, *Am J Phys Med* 52:198-205, 1973.
31. Price R, Lehmann JF, Boswell-Bassette S, et al: Influence of cryotherapy on spasticity at the human ankle, *Arch Phys Med Rehabil* 74:300-304, 1993.
32. Wolf SL, Letbetter WD: Effect of skin cooling on spontaneous EMG activity in triceps surae of the decerebrate cat, *Brain Res* 91:151-155, 1975.
33. Harris ED, McCroskery PA: The influence of temperature and fibril stability on degradation of cartilage collagen by rheumatoid synovial collagenase, *N Engl J Med* 290:1-6, 1974.
34. Hocutt JE, Jaffe R, Rylander CR, et al: Cryotherapy in ankle sprains, *Am J Sports Med* 10(5):316-319, 1982.
35. Ogilvie-Harris DJ, Gilbart M: Treatment modalities for soft tissue injuries of the ankle: a critical review, *Clin J Sport Med* 5:175-186, 1995. Retrieved from Database of Abstracts of Reviews of Effectiveness [DARE] on November 13, 2006.
36. Schaser KD, Stove JF, Melcher I, et al: Local cooling restores microcirculatory hemodynamics after closed soft-tissue trauma in rats, *J Trauma* 61(3):642-649, 2006.
37. Deal DN, Tipton J, Rosencrance E, et al: Ice reduces edema. A study of microvascular permeability in rats, *J Bone Joint Surg* 84A:1573-1578, 2002.
38. Ohkoshi Y, Ohkoshi M, Nagasaki S: The effect of cryotherapy on intraarticular temperature and postoperative care after anterior cruciate ligament reconstruction, *Am J Sports Med* 27(3):357-362, 1999.
39. Osbahr DC, Cawley PW, Speer KP: The effect of continuous cryotherapy on glenohumeral joint and subacromial space

temperatures in the postoperative shoulder, *Arthroscopy* 18(7): 748-754, 2002.

40. Saito N, Horiuchi H, Kobayashi S, et al: Continuous local cooling for pain relief following total hip arthroplasty, *J Arthro* 19(3):334-337, 2004.

41. Singh H, Osbahr DC, Holovacs TF, et al: The efficacy of continuous cryotherapy on the postoperative shoulder: a prospective, randomized investigation, *J Shoulder & Elbow Surgery*, 10(6):522-525, 2001.

42. Meeusen R, Lievens P: The use of cryotherapy in sport injuries, *Sports Med* 3:398-414, 1986.

43. Friden J, Sjostrom M, Ekblom B: A morphological study of delayed onset muscle soreness, *Experientia* 37:506-507, 1981.

44. Jones D, Newhan D, Round J, et al: Experimental human muscle damage: morphological changes in relation to other indices of damage, *J Physiol* 375:435-448, 1986.

45. Brosseau L, Yonge KA, Robinson V, et al: Thermotherapy for treatment of osteoarthritis, *Cochrane Database Syst Rev* 4: CD004522, 2003.

46. Robinson V, Brosseau L, Casimiro L, et al: Thermotherapy for treating rheumatoid arthritis, *Cochrane Database Syst Rev* 2: CD002826, 2002.

47. Hirvonen HE, Mikkelsson MK, Kautiainen, et al: Effectiveness of different cryotherapies on pain and disease activity in active rheumatoid arthritis. A randomised single blinded controlled trial, *Clin Exp Rheumatol* 24(3):295-301, 2006.

48. Cote DJ, Prentice WE, Hooker DN, et al: Comparison of three treatment procedures for minimizing ankle sprain swelling, *Phys Ther* 68(7):1072-1076, 1988.

49. Wilkerson GB: Treatment of inversion ankle sprain through synchronous application of focal compression and cold, *Athl Train* 26:220-225, 1991.

50. Quillen WS, Roullier LH: Initial management of acute ankle sprains with rapid pulsed pneumatic compression and cold, *J Orthop Sports Phys Ther* 4:39-43, 1982.

51. Boris M, Wiedorf S, Lasinski B, et al: Lymphedema reduction by noninvasive complex lymphedema therapy, *Oncology* 8(9):95-106, 1994.

52. Beenakker EA, Oparina TI, Hartgring A, et al: Cooling garment treatment in MS: clinical improvement and decrease in leukocyte NO production, *Neurology* 57(5):892-894, 2001.

53. Capello E, Gardella M, Leandri M, et al: Lowering body temperature with a cooling suit as symptomatic treatment for thermosensitive multiple sclerosis patients, *Ital J Neurol Sci* 16(8):533-539, 1995.

54. Schwid SR, NASA/MS Cooling Study Group: A randomized controlled study of the acute and chronic effects of cooling therapy for MS, *Neurology* 60(12):1955-1960, 2003.

55. Feys P, Helsen W, Liu X, et al: Effects of peripheral cooling on intention tremor in multiple sclerosis, *J Neurol Neurosurg Psychiatry* 76(3):373-379, 2005 Mar.

56. Umphred DA: *Neurological rehabilitation*, St. Louis, 1985, Mosby.

57. Selbach H: The principles of relaxation oscillation as a special instance of the law of initial value in cybernetic functions, *Ann NY Acad Sci* 98:1221-1228, 1962.

58. Gelhorn E: *Principles of autonomic-somatic integration: physiological basis and psychological and clinical implications*, Minneapolis, 1967, University of Minnesota Press.

59. Knight KL: *Cryotherapy: theory, technique, physiology*, Chattanooga, TN, 1985, Chattanooga Corp.

60. Hayden CA: Cryokinetics in an early treatment program, *J Am Phys Ther Assoc* 44:990, 1964.

61. Bugaj R: The cooling, analgesic, and rewarming effects of ice massage on localized skin, *Phys Ther* 55(1):11-19, 1975.

62. Prentice WE: An electromyographic analysis of the effectiveness of heat or cold and stretching for inducing relaxation in injured muscle, *J Orthop Sports Phys Ther* 3:133-137, 1982.

63. Lin Y: Effects of thermal therapy in improving the passive range of knee motion: comparison of cold and superficial heat applications, *Clin Rehabil* 17:618-623, 2003.

64. Marino FE: Methods, advantages, and limitations of body cooling for exercise performance, *Br J Sports Med* 36(2):89-94, 2002.

65. Day MJ: Hypersensitive response to ice massage: report of a case, *Phys Ther* 54:592-593, 1974.

66. Parker JT, Small NC, Davis DG: Cold-induced nerve palsy, *Athl Train* 18:76-77, 1983.

67. Green GA, Zachazewski JE, Jordan SE: Peroneal nerve palsy induced by cryotherapy, *Phys Sport Med* 17(9):63-70, 1989.

68. Lundgren C, Murren A, Zederfeldt B: Effect of cold vasoconstriction on wound healing in the rabbit, *Acta Chir Scand* 118:1, 1959.

69. Boyer JT, Fraser JRE, Doyle AE: The hemodynamic effects of cold immersion, *Clin Sci* 19:539-543, 1980.

70. Covington DB, Bassett FH: When cryotherapy injures, *Phys Sport Med* 21(3):78-93, 1993.

71. Kanlayanaphotporn R, Janwantanakul P: Comparison of skin surface temperature during the application of various cryotherapy modalities, *Arch Phys Med Rehabil* 86(7):1411-1415, 2005.

72. Chesterton LS, Foster NE, Ross L: Skin temperature response to cryotherapy, *Arch Phys Med Rehabil* 83(4):543-549, 2002.

73. Enwemeka CS, Allen C, Avila P, et al: Soft tissue thermodynamics before, during, and after cold pack therapy, *Med Sci Sports Exerc* 34(1):45-50, 2002.

74. Myrer WJ, Myrer KA, Measom GJ, et al: Muscle temperature is affected by overlying adipose when cryotherapy is administered, *J Athl Train* 36(1):32-36, 2001.

75. Bender AL, Kramer EE, Brucker JB, et al: Local ice-bag application and triceps surae muscle temperature during treadmill walking, *J Athl Train* 40(4):271-275, 2005.

76. Myer JW, Measom G, Fellingham GW: Temperature changes in the human leg during and after two methods of cryotherapy, *J Athl Train* 33(1):25-29, 1998.

77. Knight KL: *Cryotherapy in sport injury management*, Champaign, IL, 1995, Human Kinetics.

78. Metzman L, Gamble JG, Rinsky LA: Effectiveness of ice packs in reducing skin temperature under casts, *Clin Orthop* 330:217-221, 1996.

79. Farry PJ, Prentice NG: Ice treatment of injured ligaments: an experimental model, *NZ Med J* 9:12-14, 1980.

80. Krumhansl BR: Ice lollies for ice massage, *Phys Ther* 49(10):1098, 1969.

81. Knobloch K, Grasemann R, Jagodzinski N, et al: Changes of Achilles midportion tendon microcirculation after repetitive simultaneous cryotherapy and compression using a Cryo/Cuff, *Am J Sports Med* 34:1953-1959, 2006.

82. Schroder D, Passler HH: Combination of cold and compression after knee surgery: a prospective randomized study, *Knee Surg Sports Traumatol Arthro* 2(3):158-165, 1994.

83. Webb JM, Williams D, Ivory JP, et al: The use of cold compression dressings after total knee replacement: a randomized controlled trial, *Orthopedics* 21(1):59-61, 1998.

84. Travel J: Temporomandibular joint pain referred from muscles of the head and neck, *J Prosthetic Dent* 10(4):745-763, 1960.

85. Rubin D: Myofascial trigger point syndromes: an approach to management, *Arch Phys Med Rehabil* 62:107-110, 1981.

86. Simons DG, Travell JG: Myofascial origins of low back pain. I. Principles of diagnosis and treatment, *Postgrad Med* 73(2):70-77, 1983.

87. Travell JG, Simons DG: *Myofascial pain and dysfunction: the trigger point manual*, Baltimore, 1983, Williams & Wilkins.

88. Travell JG: Myofascial trigger points: clinical view. In Bonica JJ, Albe-Fessard D, eds: *Advances in pain research and therapy*, New York, 1976, Raven Press.

89. Simons DG: Myofascial pain syndrome due to trigger points, *Int Rehabil Med Assoc Monogr* 1, 1987.

90. *Gebauer's spray and stretch indications and usage*, The Gebauer Company, Cleveland, OH. http://www.gebauerco.com/Default. asp?strAction=SAS_IndicationsAndUse. Accessed February 6, 2007.

91. Scarcella JB, Cohn BT: The effect of cold therapy on the postoperative course of total hip and total knee arthroplasty patients, *Am J Orthop* 24(11):847-852, 1955.

92. Bickford RH, Duff RS: Influence of ultrasonic irradiation on temperature and blood flow in human skeletal muscle, *Circ Res* 1:534-538, 1953.

93. Imamura M, Biro S, Kihara T et al: Repeated thermal therapy improves impaired vascular endothelial function in patients with coronary risk factors, *J Am Coll Cardiol* 38(4):1083-1088, Oct 2001.

94. Cider A, Svealv BG, Tang MS, et al: Immersion in warm water induces improvement in cardiac function in patients with chronic heart failure, *Eur J Heart Fail* 8(3):308-313, 2006.

95. Kihara T, Biro S, Imamura M, et al: Repeated sauna treatment improves vascular endothelial and cardiac function in patients with chronic heart failure, *J Am Coll Cardiol* 39(5):754-759, 2002.

96. Gong B, Asimakis GK, Chen Z, et al: Whole-body hyperthermia induces up-regulation of vascular endothelial growth factor accompanied by neovascularization in cardiac tissue, *Life Sci* 79(19):1781-178, 2006.

97. Crockford GW, Hellon RF, Parkhouse J: Thermal vasomotor response in human skin mediated by local mechanisms, *J Physiol* 161:10-15, 1962.

98. Kellogg DL Jr, Liu Y, Kosiba IF, et al: Role of nitric oxide in the vascular effects of local warming of the skin in humans, *J Appl Physiol* 86(4):1185-1190, 1999.

99. Minson CT, Berry LT, Joyner MJ: Nitric oxide and neurally mediated regulation of skin blood flow during local heating, *J Appl Physiol* 91(4):1619-1626, 2001.

100. Fox HH, Hilton SM: Bradykinin formation in human skin as a factor in heat vasodilation, *J Physiol* 142:219, 1958.

101. Kellogg DL Jr, Liu Y, McAllister K, et al: Bradykinin does not mediate cutaneous active vasodilation during heat stress in humans, *J Appl Physiol* 93:1215-1221, 2002.

102. Guyton AC: *Textbook of medical physiology*, ed 8, Philadelphia, 1991, WB Saunders.

103. Abramson DI: Indirect vasodilation in thermotherapy, *Arch Phys Med Rehabil* 46:412-415, 1965.

104. Wessman MS, Kottke FJ: The effect of indirect heating on peripheral blood flow, pulse rate, blood pressure and temperature, *Arch Phys Med Rehabil* 48:567-576, 1967.

105. Wyper DJ, McNiven DR: Effects of some physiotherapeutic agents on skeletal muscle blood flow, *Physiotherapy* 62:83-85, 1976.

106. Crockford GW, Hellon RF: Vascular responses in human skin to infra-red radiation, *J Physiol* 149:424-426, 1959.

107. Currier DP, Kramer JF: Sensory nerve conduction: heating effects of ultrasound and infrared radiation, *Physiother Canada* 34:241-246, 1982.

108. Halle JS, Scoville CR, Greathouse DG: Ultrasound effect on the conduction latency of the superficial radial nerve in man, *Phys Ther* 61:345-350, 1981.

109. Kelly R, Beehn C, Hansford A, et al: Effect of fluidotherapy on superficial radial nerve conduction and skin temperature, *J Orthop Sports Phys Ther* 35(1):16-23, 2005.

110. Tilki HE, Stalberg E, Coskun M, et al: Effect of heating on nerve conduction in carpal tunnel syndrome, *J Clin Neurophysiol* 21(6):451-456, 2004.

111. Rutkove SB, Geffroy MA, Lichtenstein SH: Heat-sensitive conduction block in ulnar neuropathy at the elbow, *Clin Neurophysiol*, 112(2):280-285, 2001.

112. Rasminsky M: The effect of temperature on conduction in demyelinated single nerve fibers, *Arch Neurol* 28:287-292, 1973.

113. Lehmann JF, DeLateur BJ: Therapeutic heat. In Lehmann JF (ed): *Therapeutic heat and cold*, ed 4, Baltimore, 1990, Williams & Wilkins.

114. Rennie GA, Michlovitz SL: Biophysical principles of heating and superficial heating agents. In Michlovitz SL, ed: *Thermal agents in rehabilitation*, Philadelphia, 1996, FA Davis.

115. Fountain FP, Gersten JW, Senger O: Decrease in muscle spasm produced by ultrasound, hot packs and IR, *Arch Phys Med Rehabil* 41:293-299, 1960.

116. Fischer M, Schafer SS: Temperature effects on the discharge frequency of primary and secondary endings of isolated cat muscle spindles recorded under a ramp-and-hold stretch, *Brain Res* 840(1-2):1-15, 1999.

117. Lehmann JF, Brunner GD, Stow RW: Pain threshold measurements after therapeutic application of ultrasound, microwaves and infrared, *Arch Phys Med Rehabil* 39:560-565, 1958.

118. Benson TB, Copp EP: The effects of therapeutic forms of heat and ice on the pain threshold of the normal shoulder, *Rheumatol Rehabil* 13:10-104, 1974.

119. Chastain PB: The effect of deep heat on isometric strength, *Phys Ther* 58:543-546, 1978.

120. Wickstrom R, Polk C: Effect of whirlpool on the strength and endurance of the quadriceps muscle in trained male adolescents, *Am J Phys Med* 40:91-95, 1961.

121. Edwards R, Harris R, Hultman E, et al: Energy metabolism during isometric exercise at different temperatures of m. quadriceps femoris in man, *Acta Physiol* Scand 80:17-18, 1970.

122. Miller MW, Ziskin MC: Biological consequences of hyperthermia, *Ultrasound Med Biol* 15(8):707-722, 1989.

123. Barcroft J, King W: The effect of temperature on the dissociation curve of blood, *J Physiol* 39:374-384, 1909.

124. Lentell G, Hetherington T, Eagan J, et al: The use of thermal agents to influence the effectiveness of low-load prolonged stretch, *J Orthop Sport Phys Ther* 16(5):200-207, 1992.

125. Warren C, Lehmann J, Koblanski J: Elongation of rat tail tendon: effect of load and temperature, *Arch Phys Med Rehabil* 52:465-474, 484, 1971.

126. Warren C, Lehmann J, Koblanski J: Heat and stretch procedures: an evaluation using rat tail tendon, *Arch Phys Med Rehabil* 57:122-126, 1976.

127. Gersten JW: Effect of ultrasound on tendon extensibility, *Am J Phys Med* 34:362-369, 1955.

128. Lehmann J, Masock A, Warren C, et al: Effect of therapeutic temperatures on tendon extensibility, *Arch Phys Med Rehabil* 51:481-487, 1970.

129. Kramer JF: Ultrasound: evaluation of its mechanical and thermal effects, *Arch Phys Med Rehabil* 65:223-227, 1984.

130. Steilan J, Habot B: Improvement of pain and disability in elderly patients with degenerative osteoarthritis of the knee treated with narrow band light therapy, *J Am Geriatr Soc* 40(1):23-26, 1992.

131. Magness J, Garrett T, Erickson D: Swelling of the upper extremity during whirlpool baths, *Arch Phys Med Rehabil* 51:297-299, 1970.

132. French SD, Cameron M, Walker BF, et al: Superficial heat or cold for low back pain, *Cochrane Database Syst Rev* 1:CD004750, 2006.

133. Nadler SF, Steiner DJ, Erasala GN, et al: Continuous low-level heatwrap therapy for treating acute nonspecific low back pain, *Arch Phys Med Rehabil* 84:329-334, 2003.

134. Nadler SF, Steiner DJ, Petty SR, et al: Overnight use of continuous low-level heatwrap therapy for relief of low back pain, *Arch Phys Med Rehabil* 8:335-342, 2003.

135. Nuhr M, Hoerauf K, Bertalanffy A, et al: Active warming during emergency transport relieves acute low back pain, *Spine* 29:1499-1503, 2004.

136. Mayer JM, Ralph L, Look M, et al: Treating acute low back pain with continuous low-level heat wrap therapy and/or exercise: a randomized controlled trial, *Spine J* 5:395-403, 2005.

137. Bertalanffy P, Kober A, Andel H, et al: Active warming as emergency interventional care for the treatment of pelvic pain, *BJOG* 113(9):1031-1034, 2006.

138. Kober A, Dobrovits M, Djavan B, et al: Local active warming: an effective treatment for pain, anxiety and nausea caused by renal colic, *J Urol* 170(3):741-744, 2003.

139. Mayer JM, Mooney V, Matheson LN, et al: Continuous low-level heat wrap therapy for the prevention and early phase treatment of delayed-onset muscle soreness of the low back: a randomized controlled trial, *Arch Phys Med Rehabil* 87(10):1310-1357, 2006.

140. Michlovitz S, Hun L, Erasala GN, et al: Continuous low-level heat wrap therapy is effective for treating wrist pain, *Arch Phys Med Rehabil* 85(9):1409-1416, 2004.

141. Loten C, Stokes B, Worsley D, et al: A randomised controlled trial of hot water (45 degrees C) immersion versus ice packs for pain relief in bluebottle stings, *Med J Aust* 184(7):329-333, 2006.

142. Knight CA, Rutledge CR, Cox ME, et al: Effect of superficial heat, deep heat, and active exercise warm-up on the extensibility of the plantar flexors, *Phys Ther* 81(6):1206-1214, 2001.

143. Usuba M, Miyanaga Y, Miyakawa S, et al: Effect of heat in increasing the range of knee motion after the development of a joint contracture: an experiment with an animal model, *Arch Phys Med Rehabil* 87(2):247-253, 2006.

144. Robertson VJ, Ward AR, Jung P: The effect of heat on tissue extensibility: a comparison of deep and superficial heating, *Arch Phys Med Rehabil* 86(4):819-825, 2005.

145. Wright V, Johns R: Physical factors concerned with the stiffness of normal and diseased joints, *Johns Hopkins Hosp Bull* 106:215-229, 1960.
146. Kik JA, Kersley GD: Heat and cold in the physical treatment of rheumatoid arthritis of the knee, *Ann Phys Med* 9:270-274, 1968.
147. Blacklung L, Tiselius P: Objective measurement of joint stiffness in rheumatoid arthritis, *Acta Rheum Scand* 13:275, 1967.
148. Johns R, Wright V: Relative importance of various tissues in joint stiffness, *J Appl Physiol* 17:824-828, 1962.
149. Orenberg EK, Noodleman FR, Koperski JA, et al: Comparison of heat delivery systems for hyperthermia treatment of psoriasis, *Int J Hypertherm* 2(3):231-241, 1986.
150. Westerhof W, Siddiqui AH, Cormane RH, et al: Infra-red hyperthermia and psoriasis, *Arch Dermatol Res* 279:209-210, 1987.
151. Moss C, Ellis R, Murray W, et al: *Infrared radiation, nonionising radiation protection*, ed 2, Geneva, 1989, World Health Organization.
152. Schmidt KL: Heat, cold and inflammation, *Rheumatology* 38:391-404, 1979.
153. Sapareto SA, Dewey WC: Thermal dose determination in cancer therapy, *Int J Radiol Oncol Biol Phys* 10:787-800, 1984.
154. Hornback NB: *Hyperthermia and cancer*, Boca Raton, FL, 1984, CRC Press.
155. Ganong WF: *Review of medical physiology*, ed 13, Norwalk, CT, 1987, Appleton & Lange.
156. Kligman LH: Intensification of ultraviolet-induced dermal damage by infra-red radiation, *Arch Dermatol Res* 272:229-238, 1982.
157. Enwemeka CS, Booth CK, Fisher SL, et al: Decay time of temperature of hot packs in two application positions, *Phys Ther* 76(5):S96, 1996.
158. Nadler SF, Steiner DJ, Erasala GN: Continuous low-level heat wrap therapy provides more efficacy than ibuprofen and acetaminophen for acute low back pain, *Spine* 27(10):1012-1017, 2002.
159. *Parabath paraffin heat therapy owner's guide*, Akron, OH, 2004, The Hygenic Corporation.
160. Borrell RM, Henley ES, Purvis H, et al: Fluidotherapy: evaluation of a new heat modality, *Arch Phys Med Rehabil* 58:69-71, 1977.
161. Hardy JD: Spectral transmittance and reflectance of excised human skin, *J Appl Physiol* 9:257-264, 1956.
162. Selkins KM, Emery AF: Thermal science for physical medicine. In Lehmann JF (ed): *Therapeutic heat and cold*, ed 3, Baltimore, 1982, Williams & Wilkins.
163. Gale GD, Rothbart PJ, Li Y: Infrared therapy for chronic low back pain: a randomized, controlled trial, *Pain Res Mgmt* 11(3):193-196, 2006.

Ultrasound

INTRODUCTION

TERMINOLOGY

It is recommended that the first-time reader and student carefully review the glossary at the end of this chapter before reading the rest of the chapter because much of the terminology used to describe ultrasound is unique to this area.

HISTORY

Methods to generate and detect **ultrasound** first became available in the United States in the 19th century; however, the first large-scale application of ultrasound was for sound navigation and ranging (SONAR) during World War II. With SONAR, a short pulse of ultrasound is sent from a submarine through the water, and a detector picks up the echo of the signal. Because the time required for the echo to reach the detector is proportional to the distance of the detector from a reflecting surface, the duration of this period can be used to calculate the distance to objects under the water such as other submarines or rocks. This pulse-echo technology has since been adapted for medical imaging applications, for "viewing" a fetus or other internal masses. Early SONAR devices used high-intensity ultrasound for ease of detection; however, it was found that these devices can heat and thus damage underwater life. Although this fact limited the **intensity** of ultrasound appropriate for SONAR, it led to the development of clinical ultrasound devices specifically intended for heating biological tissue. Ultrasound was found to heat tissue with a high collagen content, such as tendons, ligaments, or fascia, and for the past 50 years or more, has been widely used clinically for this purpose.

> **© Clinical Pearl**
>
> Ultrasound heats tissue with a high collagen content such as tendons, ligaments, joint capsules, and fascia.

More recently, ultrasound has been found to have nonthermal effects, and, over the past 20 years, therapeutic applications of these effects have been developed. Low-intensity **pulsed ultrasound**, which produces only nonthermal effects, has been shown to facilitate tissue healing, modify inflammation, and enhance transdermal drug delivery.

ULTRASOUND DEFINITION

Ultrasound is a type of sound, and all forms of sound consist of waves that transmit energy by alternately compressing and rarefying material (Fig. 7-1). Ultrasound is sound with a **frequency** greater than 20,000 cycles per second (hertz [Hz]). This definition is based on the limits of normal human hearing. Humans can hear sound with a frequency of 16 to 20,000 Hz; sound with a frequency greater than this is known as ultrasound. Generally, therapeutic ultrasound has a frequency between 0.7 and 3.3 megahertz (MHz) to maximize energy absorption at a depth of 2 to 5 cm of soft tissue.

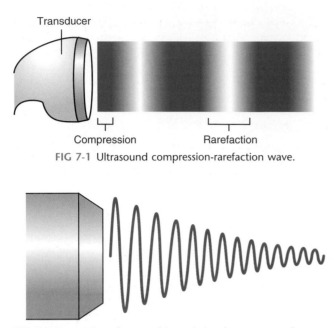

Transducer

Compression   Rarefaction

FIG 7-1 Ultrasound compression-rarefaction wave.

FIG 7-2 Decreasing ultrasound intensity as the wave travels through tissue.

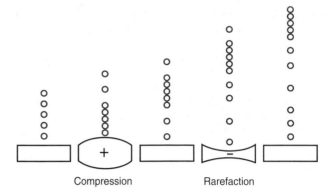

Compression   Rarefaction

FIG 7-3 Ultrasound production by piezoelectric crystal.

TABLE 7-1	Attenuation of 1 MHz Ultrasound	
Tissue	Attenuation (dB/cm)	%/cm
Blood	0.12	3
Fat	0.61	13
Nerve	0.88	0
Muscle	1.2	24
Blood vessels	1.7	32
Skin	2.7	39
Tendon	4.9	59
Cartilage	5.0	68
Bone	13.9	96

Audible sound and ultrasound have many similar properties. For example, as ultrasound travels through material, it gradually decreases in intensity as a result of **attenuation** in the same way that the sound we hear becomes quieter as we move farther from its source (Fig. 7-2). Ultrasound waves cause a slight circular motion of material as they are transmitted, but they do not carry the material along with the wave. Similarly, when someone speaks, the audible sound waves of the voice reach across the room, but the air in front of the speaker's mouth is agitated only slightly, not moved across the room.

Ultrasound has a variety of physical effects that can be classified as thermal or nonthermal. Increasing tissue temperature is its thermal effect. **Acoustic streaming**, **microstreaming**, and **cavitation**, which may alter cell membrane permeability, are its nonthermal effects. This chapter describes the physical properties of ultrasound and its effects on the body to derive guidelines for the optimal clinical application of therapeutic ultrasound.

In brief, ultrasound is a high-frequency sound wave that can be described by its intensity, frequency, **duty cycle**, **effective radiating area** (ERA), and **beam nonuniformity ratio** (BNR). It enters the body and is attenuated in the tissue by absorption, **reflection**, and **refraction**. Attenuation is greatest in tissues with a high collagen content and with the use of high ultrasound frequencies. Attenuation is the result of absorption, reflection, and refraction, with absorption accounting for about one-half of attenuation. Attenuation coefficients are tissue- and frequency-specific. They are higher for tissues with a higher collagen content and increase in proportion to the frequency of the ultrasound (Table 7-1).

Continuous ultrasound is generally used to produce thermal effects, whereas pulsed ultrasound is used for nonthermal effects. Both the thermal and nonthermal effects

of ultrasound can be used to accelerate the achievement of treatment goals when ultrasound is applied to the appropriate pathology at the appropriate time.

GENERATION OF ULTRASOUND

Ultrasound is generated by applying a high-frequency alternating electrical current to the crystal in the **transducer** of an ultrasound unit. The crystal is made of a material with **piezoelectric** properties causing it to respond to the alternating current by expanding and contracting at the same frequency at which the current changes polarity. When the crystal expands, it compresses the material in front of it, and when it contracts, it rarefies the material in front of it. This alternating **compression-rarefaction** is the ultrasound wave (Fig. 7-3).

The property of piezoelectricity, or the ability to generate electricity in response to a mechanical force or to change shape in response to an electrical current, was first discovered by Paul-Jacques and Pierre Currie in the 1880s. A variety of materials are piezoelectric, including bone, natural quartz, synthetic plumbium zirconium titanate (PZT), and barium titanate. At this time, ultrasound transducers are usually made of PZT because this is the least costly and most efficient piezoelectric material readily available.

To obtain a pure single frequency of ultrasound from a piezoelectric crystal, a single frequency of alternating current must be applied to it and the crystal must be the appropriate thickness to resonate with this frequency.

Resonance occurs when the ultrasound frequency and the crystal thickness conform to the following formula:

$$f = \frac{c}{2t}$$

where f is frequency, c is the speed of sound in the material, and t is the thickness of the crystal. Thus thinner, more fragile crystals are generally used to generate higher frequencies of ultrasound. These crystals should be handled with care.

Multifrequency transducers use a single crystal of a thickness optimized for only one of the frequencies. The crystal is made to vibrate at other frequencies by application of those frequencies of alternating electrical currents; however, this is associated with decreased efficiency, variability in the output frequency, reduction of the ERA, and increased BNR.[1] Recently, composite materials have been developed to deliver multiple frequencies of ultrasound more accurately and efficiently.[2]

Pulsed ultrasound is produced when the high-frequency alternating electrical current is delivered to the transducer for only a limited proportion of the treatment time, as determined by the selected duty cycle.

EFFECTS OF ULTRASOUND

Ultrasound has a variety of biophysical effects. It can increase the temperature of deep and superficial tissues and has a range of nonthermal effects. Traditionally, these effects have been considered separately, although to some degree both occur with all applications of ultrasound. Continuous ultrasound has the most effect on tissue temperature; however, nonthermal effects can also occur with the use of continuous ultrasound. Additionally, although pulsed ultrasound as typically applied clinically, with a duty cycle of 20% and a low **spatial average temporal average (SATA) intensity**, produces minimal sustained changes in tissue temperature, it can have a small brief heating effect during the on time of a pulse. A recent study found that continuous ultrasound with an intensity of 0.5 W/cm^2 produced the same temperature increase in the human gastrocnemius muscle at 2 cm depth as pulsed ultrasound with a duty cycle of 50% and an intensity of 1 W/cm^2, both at 3 MHz frequency applied for 10 minutes.[3] In this study the SATA intensity was the same for the continuous and pulsed applications and the 50% duty cycle provided much less time between pulses for cooling than would occur with a 20% duty cycle. Similar comparisons of heating with equal SATA intensity for continuous and 20% duty cycle pulsed ultrasound have not been reported. Although a number of studies have demonstrated the biophysical effects of ultrasound, the degree to which the findings can be extrapolated from the experimental conditions to specific clinical applications is still uncertain and requires further study.[4]

THERMAL EFFECTS
Tissues Affected

The earliest studies demonstrating that ultrasound can increase tissue temperature were published by Harvey in 1930.[5] The thermal effects of ultrasound, including accel-

eration of metabolic rate, reduction or control of pain and muscle spasm, alteration of nerve conduction velocity, increased circulation, and increased soft tissue extensibility, are the same as those obtained with other heating modalities, as described in Chapter 6, except that the structures heated are different.[6-8] Ultrasound reaches more deeply and heats smaller areas than most superficial heating agents.

> **Clinical Pearl**
>
> Ultrasound heats smaller, deeper areas than most superficial heating agents.

Ultrasound also heats tissues with high ultrasound **absorption coefficients** more than those with low absorption coefficients. Tissues with high absorption coefficients are generally those with a high collagen content, while tissues with low absorption coefficients generally have a high water content. Thus ultrasound is particularly well-suited to heating tendons, ligaments, joint capsules, and fascia while not overheating the overlying fat. Ultrasound is generally not the ideal physical agent for heating muscles tissue because muscle has a relatively low absorption coefficient; also, most muscles are much larger than the available ultrasound transducers. However, ultrasound can be very effective for heating small areas of scar tissue in muscle that will likely absorb more ultrasound because of their increased collagen content.

Factors Affecting the Amount of Temperature Increase

The increase in tissue temperature produced by the absorption of ultrasound varies according to the tissue to which the ultrasound is applied, as well as with the frequency, average intensity, and duration of the ultrasound application. The speed with which the ultrasound transducer is moved does not affect the increase in tissue temperature produced. A recent study found that moving the ultrasound transducer at 2 to 3, 4 to 5, or 7 to 8 cm/s while applying 1 MHz frequency, 100% continuous duty cycle, 1.5 W/cm^2 intensity ultrasound for 10 minutes, within an area twice the size of the transducer head, produced the same temperature elevations.[9]

The rate of tissue heating by ultrasound is proportional to the tissue's absorption coefficient at the applied ultrasound frequency.[10] Tissue absorption coefficients increase with increased collagen content and in proportion to the ultrasound frequency. Thus higher temperatures are achieved in tissues with a high collagen content and with the application of higher-frequency ultrasound. When the absorption coefficient is high, the temperature increase is distributed in a smaller volume of more superficial tissue than when the absorption coefficient is low because changing the absorption coefficient alters the heat distribution but does not change the total amount of energy being delivered (Fig. 7-4).

With 3 MHz ultrasound, as compared to 1 MHz ultrasound, and in tissues with higher collagen content, the depth of penetration is lower, although the maximum temperature achieved is higher. One MHz frequency ultrasound is considered best for heating tissues up to 5 cm

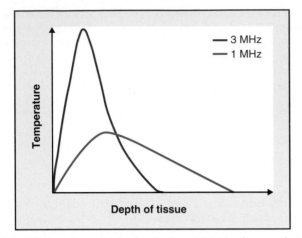

FIG 7-4 Temperature distribution for 1 and 3 MHz ultrasound at the same intensity.

deep, and 3 MHz frequency is considered best for heating tissues only 1 to 2 cm deep. However, a recent study found that 3 MHz frequency ultrasound at an intensity of 1.5 W/cm² produced a greater increase in calf muscle temperature at a depth of 2.5 cm than did 1 MHz frequency ultrasound at the same intensity.[11] This finding suggests that 3 MHz ultrasound is effective for slightly deeper heating than was previously thought. Further studies are needed to verify this finding before a change in practice is recommended.

Although theoretical models predict that 3 MHz ultrasound will increase tissue temperature three times more than 1 MHz ultrasound, an in-vivo study in which ultrasound was applied to human calf muscle found an almost fourfold greater temperature increase with 3 MHz ultrasound than with 1 MHz ultrasound applied at 0.5 to 2.0 W/cm²; therefore, clinically, an intensity 3 to 4 times lower should be used when applying 3 MHz ultrasound than when applying 1 MHz ultrasound.[12]

To increase the total amount of energy being delivered to the tissue, the duration of ultrasound application or the average ultrasound intensity must be increased. Studies have shown that, with all other parameters kept the same, higher intensity ultrasound produces greater temperature increases.[12,13] During ultrasound application, tissue temperature change is also affected by factors other than ultrasound **absorption**. Blood circulating through the tissue will cool the tissues, whereas conduction from one warmed area of tissue to another and reflection of ultrasound waves in regions of soft tissue–bone interfaces will heat the tissues.[14]

On average, soft tissue temperature has been shown to increase by approximately 0.2° C per minute in vivo with ultrasound delivered at 1 W/cm² at 1 MHz.[12,15] Nonuniformity of the intensity of ultrasound output, the variety of tissue types with different absorption coefficients in a clinical treatment area, and reflection at tissue boundaries cause the temperature increase within the ultrasound field not to be uniform. The highest temperature is generally produced at soft tissue–bone interfaces where reflection is greatest. Moving the sound head throughout the application helps to equalize the heat distribution and minimize causing excessively hot or cold areas.

The number of unknown variables, including the thickness of each tissue layer, the amount of circulation, the distance to reflecting soft tissue-bone interfaces, and variability among machines,[16] makes it difficult to predict accurately the temperature increase that will be produced clinically when ultrasound is applied to a patient. Thus initial treatment parameters are set according to theoretical and research predictions; however, the patient's report of warmth is used to determine the final ultrasound intensity.

If the ultrasound intensity is too high, the patient will complain of a deep ache from overheating of the periosteum. If this occurs, the ultrasound intensity must be reduced to avoid burning the tissue. If the ultrasound intensity is too low, the patient will not feel any increase in temperature. More specific guidelines for selection of the optimal ultrasound treatment parameters for tissue heating are given later in the section on application technique. Because the patient's report is used to determine the maximum safe ultrasound intensity, it is recommended that thermal-level ultrasound not be applied to patients who are unable to feel or report discomfort caused by overheating.

Applying Other Physical Agents in Conjunction with Ultrasound

Various physical agents can be applied together with, before, or after the application of ultrasound. Applying a hot pack before ultrasound treatment has been shown to increase the temperature of only the superficial 1 to 2 mm of skin and subcutaneous tissue while not affecting the temperature of deeper tissue layers.[17] Heating (39° C [102° F]) or cooling (18° C [64° F]) the conduction medium may decrease the rate of heating with ultrasound with the fastest rate of heating occurring with slightly warm (25° C [77° F]) conduction gel.[18] Applying ultrasound in cold water cools the superficial skin by conduction and convection, thereby reducing the increase in superficial tissue temperature produced by ultrasound. Applying ice before the application of ultrasound also reduces the temperature increase produced by ultrasound in the deeper tissues.[19] Ice, or any other thermal agent, should be applied with caution before the application of ultrasound because the loss of sensation that may be caused by these agents can reduce the accuracy of the patient's feedback regarding deep tissue temperature. Although many clinicians apply ultrasound in conjunction with electrical stimulation, with the goal of combining the benefits of both modalities, there is little published research at this time evaluating the efficacy of this combination of interventions and one study found that adding ultrasound to electrical stimulation, exercise, or superficial heat provided no additional benefit when managing soft tissue disorders of the shoulder.[20] In general, one should analyze the effects of each physical agent independently when considering applying a combination of agents either concurrently or in sequence.

NONTHERMAL EFFECTS

Ultrasound has a variety of effects on biological processes that are thought to be unrelated to any increase in tissue temperature. These effects are the result of the mechanical events produced by ultrasound, including cavitation, microstreaming, and acoustic streaming. When ultrasound is delivered in a pulsed mode, with a 20% or lower duty cycle, the heat generated during the on time of the cycle is dispersed during the off time, resulting in no measurable net increase in temperature. Thus pulsed ultrasound with a 20% duty cycle has generally been used to apply and study the nonthermal effects of ultrasound. Some recent studies have also used low intensities of continuous ultrasound to study these effects.[21]

Ultrasound with a low average intensity has been shown to increase intracellular calcium levels[22] and increase skin and cell membrane permeability.[23] It has also been shown to promote the normal function of a variety of cell types. Ultrasound increases mast cell degranulation and their release of chemotactic factor and histamine.[24] Ultrasound also promotes macrophage responsiveness[25] and increases the rate of protein synthesis by fibroblasts[26] and tendon cells.[27] Additionally, studies have found that low-intensity ultrasound increases nitric oxide synthesis in endothelial cells[28,29] and increases blood flow when applied to fractures in dogs[30] and to ischemic muscle in rats.[31] Furthermore, low intensity ultrasound has been found to stimulate proteoglycan synthesis by chondrocytes (cartilage cells).[32-35] These effects have been demonstrated using ultrasound at intensities and duty cycles that did not produce any measurable increase in temperature and are therefore considered to be nonthermal effects. They have been attributed to cavitation, acoustic streaming, and microstreaming.[25,36] The greatest changes in intracellular calcium levels have been reported to occur in response to 20% pulsed ultrasound at intensities of 0.5 to 0.75 W/cm^2.[22]

Because the cellular level and vascular processes demonstrated to occur in response to low-intensity ultrasound are essential components of tissue healing, they are thought to underlie the enhanced recovery found to occur in response to the application of ultrasound to people with a variety of pathologies. For example, increasing intracellular calcium can alter the enzymatic activity of cells and stimulate their synthesis and secretion of proteins, including proteoglycans,[37] because calcium ions act as chemical signals (second messengers) to cells. Vasodilation from increased nitric oxide and the resulting increased blood flow may further enhance healing by increasing the delivery of essential nutrients to the area.

The fact that ultrasound can affect macrophage responsiveness explains in part why ultrasound is particularly effective during the inflammatory phase of repair, when the macrophage is the dominant cell type. Pulsed ultrasound has been shown to have a significantly greater effect on membrane permeability than continuous ultrasound delivered at the same SATA intensity.[23]

CLINICAL APPLICATIONS OF ULTRASOUND

Ultrasound is commonly used as a component of the treatment of a wide variety of pathologies. These applications take advantage of the thermal and the nonthermal effects of ultrasound. The thermal effects are used primarily before stretching shortened soft tissue and for the reduction of pain. The nonthermal effects are used primarily for altering membrane permeability to accelerate tissue healing. Although much of the research on the nonthermal effects of ultrasound has been done using in vitro models, ultrasound at nonthermal levels has been found in a number of studies to facilitate the healing of dermal ulcers, surgical skin incisions, tendon injuries, and bone fractures in both humans and animals. Ultrasound has also been shown to enhance transdermal drug penetration, probably via both thermal and nonthermal mechanisms. This mode of transdermal drug delivery is known as **phonophoresis**. Ultrasound may also assist in the resorption of calcium deposits.

A summary of the research on the use of ultrasound for these applications follows. Gaps in current research do not allow one to conclude with certainty that ultrasound can consistently produce the clinical effects described. Although there is evidence to support these recommended clinical applications, most systematic reviews of the randomized controlled studies of the clinical effects of ultrasound found that there were insufficient studies to clearly demonstrate that ultrasound is more effective than placebo.[38-40] Many studies were limited by poor design and by the fact that the ultrasound doses varied considerably without a clear rationale. Further well-controlled studies using appropriate ultrasound doses are needed to determine with greater certainty the clinical efficacy of therapeutic ultrasound and the optimal treatment parameters to use for most clinical applications. An exception is low-intensity pulsed ultrasound for healing fractures treated nonoperatively where there is strong, high-quality, evidence that ultrasound can promote fracture healing.[41]

SOFT TISSUE SHORTENING

Soft tissue shortening can be the result of immobilization, inactivity, or scarring and can cause joint range of motion (ROM) restrictions, pain, and functional limitations. Shortening of the joint capsule, surrounding tendons, or ligaments is frequently responsible for such adverse consequences, and stretching of these tissues can help them regain their normal length and thereby reverse the adverse consequences of soft tissue shortening. Increasing the temperature of soft tissue temporarily increases its extensibility, increasing the length gained for the same force of stretch while also reducing the risk of tissue damage.[42,43] The increase in soft tissue length is also maintained more effectively if the stretching force is applied while the tissue temperature is elevated. This increased ease of stretching is thought to be the result of altered viscoelasticity of collagen and alteration of the collagen matrix.

Because ultrasound can penetrate to the depth of most joint capsules, tendons, and ligaments and these tissues have high ultrasound absorption coefficients, ultrasound can be an effective physical agent for heating these tissues before stretching. The deep heating produced by 1 MHz continuous ultrasound at 1.0 to 2.5 W/cm^2 has been shown to be more effective at increasing hip joint ROM in human patients than the superficial heating produced by infrared radiation when applied in conjunction with exercise.[44] In contrast, a study using rats found that both ultrasound and infrared radiation combined with stretching increased ROM more than stretching alone after the development of a joint contracture.[45] The similarity in the effectiveness of ultrasound and infrared (IR) radiation on rats is likely because these animals are so small that, in contrast to the human hip, the low depth of penetration of IR radiation was sufficient to affect joint mobility. One MHz continuous ultrasound at 1.5 W/cm^2 applied to the triceps surae combined with static dorsiflexion stretching has also been shown to be more effective than static stretching alone at increasing dorsiflexion ROM.[46] However, 1.25 W/cm^2 intensity MHz frequency continuous ultrasound applied to normally functioning medial collateral ligaments during a static stretch produced no greater increase in valgus displacement than stretching alone.[48] This may be because of the limited stretching of a normally functioning medial collateral ligament that is possible without tearing. The increased ROM observed in some studies in humans is attributed to increased extensibility of deep and superficial soft tissues resulting from heating by ultrasound.

These studies indicate that continuous ultrasound of sufficient intensity and duration to increase tissue temperature can increase soft tissue extensibility, thereby combatting soft tissue shortening and increasing joint ROM when applied in conjunction with stretching. The treatment parameters most likely to be effective for this application are 1 or 3 MHz frequency, depending on the tissue depth, at 0.5 to 1.0 W/cm^2 intensity when 3 MHz frequency is used and at 1.5 to 2.5 W/cm^2 intensity when 1 MHz frequency is used, applied for 5 to 10 minutes. For optimal effect, it is recommended that stretching be applied during heating by ultrasound and maintained for 5 to 10 minutes after ultrasound application while the tissue is cooling (Fig. 7-5).

PAIN CONTROL

Ultrasound may control pain by altering its transmission or perception or by modifying the underlying condition causing the pain. These effects may be the result of stimulation of the cutaneous thermal receptors or increased soft tissue extensibility caused by increased tissue temperature, the result of changes in nerve conduction caused by increased tissue temperature or nonthermal effects of ultrasound, or the result of modulation of inflammation caused by nonthermal effects of ultrasound. Animal studies by one researcher have also demonstrated that pulsed ultrasound decreases the number of nitric oxide synthase producing neurons in rats with induced inflammatory arthritis.[49,50] The author hypothesized that ultra-

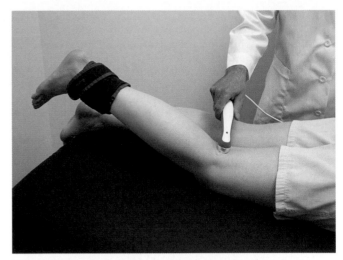

FIG 7-5 Ultrasound being applied to the posterior knee in conjunction with an extension stretching force.

sound may therefore decrease pain in inflammatory conditions by affecting neuronal pain signals.

Studies have shown that ultrasound can be more effective in controlling pain than placebo ultrasound or treatment with other thermal agents, and that the addition of ultrasound to an exercise program can further improve pain relief.[51-54] Continuous ultrasound at 0.5 to 2.0 W/cm^2 intensity and 1.5 MHz frequency has also been reported to be more effective than superficial heating with paraffin or IR radiation or deep heating with shortwave diathermy for relieving the pain from soft tissue injuries when applied within 48 hours of injury.[51] People treated with ultrasound had less pain, tenderness on pressure, erythema, restricted ROM, and swelling than those treated with the other thermal agents. Also, more subjects in the ultrasound-treated group were symptom-free 2 weeks after injury than subjects who received the other interventions.

Continuous ultrasound applied 3 times a week for 4 weeks at 1.0 to 2.0 W/cm^2 for 10 minutes to the low backs of patients with recent onset of pain caused by prolapsed discs and nerve root compression between L4 and S2 has also been shown to result in significantly faster relief of pain and return of ROM than placebo ultrasound or no intervention.[52] The authors discuss the concern that ultrasound at the intensity used may aggravate an acute disc rupture and state that this did not occur because so little ultrasound was able to reach the disc through the overlying bone. Continuous ultrasound applied at 1.5 W/cm^2 for 3 to 5 minutes for 10 treatments over a 3-week period followed by exercise has been found to be more effective than exercise alone in relieving pain and increasing ROM in patients with shoulder pain.[53] Also, at the 3-month follow-up, significantly more patients who received ultrasound treatment reported no pain than those who received exercise alone. A systematic review of two studies on therapeutic ultrasound for patients with rheumatoid arthritis found that ultrasound alone used on the hand increased grip strength and somewhat reduced the number of painful joints, increased wrist dorsiflexion, decreased the number of swollen joints, and decreased morning stiffness.[54]

The studies cited here indicate that continuous ultrasound may be effective for reducing pain. The treatment parameters found to be effective for this application are 1 or 3 MHz frequency, depending on the tissue depth, and 0.5 to 3.0 W/cm² intensity, for 3 to 10 minutes.

DERMAL ULCERS

Some studies have shown that ultrasound accelerates the healing of vascular and pressure ulcers; however, others have failed to demonstrate any beneficial effects with this application. Recent systematic reviews of the randomized controlled trials on the treatment of venous ulcers and pressure ulcers with therapeutic ultrasound concluded that there is no good evidence of a benefit of ultrasound therapy in these types of dermal ulcers.[40,55,56]

An early study by Dyson and Suckling found that the addition of ultrasound treatment to conventional wound care procedures resulted in significantly greater reduction in the area of lower extremity varicose ulcers.[57] Ultrasound was applied pulsed at 20% duty cycle, at 1.0 W/cm² intensity, 3 MHz frequency, for 5 to 10 minutes to the intact skin around the border of 13 lower extremity varicose ulcers 3 times a week for 4 weeks. Sham ultrasound was applied, in a double-blind manner, to 12 other ulcers to serve as a control. At 28 days the treated ulcers were approximately 30% reduced in size, whereas the sham-treated ulcers were not significantly smaller than their initial size. Using a similar procedure, McDiarmid and colleagues found that infected pressure ulcers healed significantly more quickly with the application of ultrasound than with sham treatment, whereas clean wounds did not.[58] The ultrasound was applied pulsed at a 20% duty cycle, 0.8 W/cm² intensity, 3 MHz frequency, for 5 to 10 minutes 3 times a week.

In contrast, three later studies failed to demonstrate improved healing of venous ulcers with ultrasound,[59-61] and a recent study in rats found no evidence of enhanced regeneration of injured gastrocnemius muscles in response to nonthermal ultrasound (3 MHz frequency, 0.1 W/cm² intensity, continuous duty cycle, for 5 minutes daily) applied alone or in conjunction with exercise alone.[62] One MHz ultrasound was used in the first two of these studies, and it is possible that this lower frequency may have altered the effectiveness of the intervention. In the third study, 3 MHz pulsed ultrasound was used; however, 0.1% chlorhexidine, a cytotoxic agent, was used to cleanse some of the wounds. The addition of this cleanser to the intervention may have obscured the benefits of the ultrasound. In the more recent study, the ultrasound intensity may have been too low to produce an effect.

Overall, the studies published so far indicate that pulsed ultrasound may facilitate wound healing but good evidence of this effect is lacking. The treatment parameters that have been found to be effective for this application are 20% duty cycle, 0.8 to 1.0 W/cm² intensity, 3 MHz frequency, for 5 to 10 minutes. Further well-controlled studies with this range of ultrasound dosing are needed to ascertain the effectiveness of this intervention. Ultrasound can be applied to a dermal ulcer either by applying transmission gel to the intact skin around the wound perimeter and treating only over this area (Fig. 7-6A), or the wound can be treated directly by covering it with an ultrasound

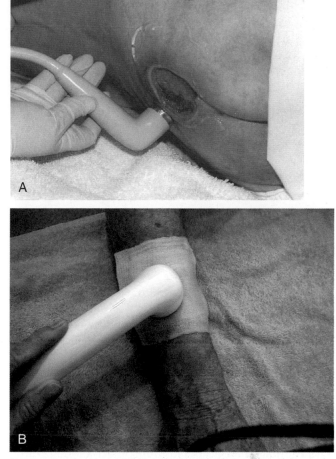

FIG 7-6 A, Ultrasound treatment of a wound: periwound application technique. **B,** Ultrasound being used to treat a venous stasis ulcer. *Courtesy Jim Staicer, Beverly Manor Convalescent Hospital, Fresno, CA.*

coupling sheet (Fig. 7-6B) or by placing it and the ultrasound transducer in water (Fig. 7-7).

Traditionally, megahertz frequency ultrasound has been used to promote wound healing, and the device has contact with the wound or periwound area. In June 2004, a noncontact kilohertz ultrasound device was cleared by the Food and Drug Administration (FDA) for wound cleaning and maintenance debridement and, in May 2005, this device was cleared for use for wound healing. This device applies 40 kHz frequency, 0.1 W/cm² to 0.5 W/cm² intensity ultrasound when held 5 to 15 mm from the wound. The device uses a saline mist as a coupling medium to deliver the ultrasound energy to the tissue. It is held perpendicular to the wound, and multiple vertical and horizontal passes are made over the wound during a treatment. The treatment duration depends on the area of the wound. A wound that is less than 10 cm² is treated for 3 minutes, a wound that is 10 cm² to 19 cm² is treated for 4 minutes, and the time increases by 1 minute for each further 10 cm² increment.[63] Although few published studies have examined the effects of this type of kilohertz ultrasound application, two small randomized controlled trials have been published. One of these trials examined applying this device for 4 minutes to chronic diabetic foot ulcers.[64] This

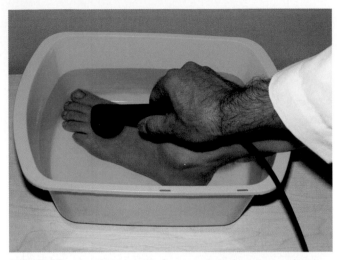

FIG 7-7 Ultrasound treatment of a wound: underwater application technique.

intervention increased the healing rate of the wounds after 12 weeks of treatment 3 times weekly as compared to a sham intervention. In a nonrandomized study, the same authors found that applying this intervention to chronic lower extremity wounds of various etiologies resulted in a decreased time to healing (8 weeks) when compared to standard wound care alone (18 weeks) and that the wounds that eventually healed had evidence of healing at 4 weeks after the start of the ultrasound therapy.[63] A randomized controlled trial by a different group of researchers found that 63% of patients treated with the standard of care plus noncontact kilohertz ultrasound achieved greater than 50% wound healing at 12 weeks, whereas 29% of those treated with the standard of care alone achieved the same results.[65] The patients in this study all had nonhealing leg and foot ulcers associated with chronic critical limb ischemia.[66]

SURGICAL SKIN INCISIONS

The effect of ultrasound on the healing of surgical skin incisions has been studied in both animal and human subjects and has been clearly demonstrated to be beneficial. 0.75 or 3 MHz frequency ultrasound applied at 0.5 W/cm^2, pulsed 20%, for 5 minutes daily to full-thickness skin lesions in adult rats has been shown to accelerate the evolution of **angiogenesis**, a vital component of early wound healing.[67] Noncontact kilohertz ultrasound therapy has also been shown to enhance angiogenesis and collagen deposition in a diabetic mouse model.[61] Angiogenesis is the development of new blood vessels at an injury site that serves to reestablish circulation and thus limit ischemic necrosis and facilitate repair. It is proposed that ultrasound may accelerate the development of angiogenesis by altering cell membrane permeability, particularly to calcium ions, and by stimulating angiogenic factor synthesis and release by macrophages.[53]

Byl and associates reported that low-dose and high-dose ultrasound can increase the breaking strength of incisional wounds in pigs when applied for 1 week and that low-dose ultrasound increases wound breaking strength only in the second week.[68,69] The low dose was 0.5 W/cm^2,

pulsed 20%, 1 MHz, and the high dose was 1.5 W/cm^2, continuous, 1 MHz. Both were applied for 5 minutes daily, starting 1 day after the incision. A more recent study found that pulsed ultrasound at frequencies of 3 MHz or 0.75 kHz reduced the incidence of skin flap necrosis and that 1 W/cm^2 20% duty cycle was more effective than 0.5 W/cm^2, 20% duty cycle.[70]

Ultrasound has also been reported to be beneficial in the treatment of gynecological surgical wounds and episiotomies in humans.[71,72] Ultrasound applied on the first and second postoperative days at 0.5 W/cm^2, 20% duty cycle, 1 MHz for 3 minutes has been reported to reduce pain and accelerate hematoma resolution after these procedures. Treatment with ultrasound has also been found to relieve the pain from episiotomy scars when applied months or years after the procedure. Fieldhouse reported successful treatment of painful, thickened scars with ultrasound at 0.5 to 0.8 W/cm^2, for 5 minutes, 3 times a week for 6 to 16 weeks, at 15 months to 4 years after episiotomy.[72] Earlier intervention was recommended for earlier relief of symptoms.

The preceding studies indicate that ultrasound can accelerate the healing of surgical incisions, relieve the pain associated with these procedures, and facilitate development of stronger repair tissue. The treatment parameters found to be most effective were 0.5 to 0.8 W/cm^2 intensity, pulsed 20% for 3 to 5 minutes, 3 to 5 times a week.

TENDON AND LIGAMENT INJURIES

Ultrasound has been reported to assist in the healing of tendons and ligaments after surgical incision and repair and to be of benefit in tendon inflammation (tendinitis). However, although some studies with both animal and human subjects have reported treatment success, others have failed to support these findings.

Binder and colleagues reported significantly enhanced recovery in patients with lateral epicondylitis treated with ultrasound compared with those treated with sham ultrasound.[73] The ultrasound was applied pulsed with a 20% duty cycle, 1.0 to 2.0 W/cm^2 intensity, 1 MHz frequency, for 5 to 10 minutes for 12 treatments over a 4- to 6-week period. In addition, Ebenbichler and coworkers reported greater resolution of calcium deposits, greater decreases in pain, and greater improvements in the quality of life in patients with calcific tendinitis of the shoulder treated with ultrasound compared with those treated with sham ultrasound.[74] For this study, ultrasound was applied for 24 15-minute sessions with a frequency of 0.89 MHz and an intensity 2.5 W/cm^2 pulsed mode 1 : 4 (sic.).

In contrast to the positive findings of these studies, Lundeberg and colleagues reported no significant difference in the healing of lateral epicondylitis between ultrasound-treated groups and sham ultrasound-treated groups using either continuous or pulsed ultrasound,[75,76] and a more recent randomized controlled trial found that very low-intensity pulsed ultrasound (1.5 MHz, 0.15 W/cm^2 for 20 minutes daily) using a home treatment device intended to promote fracture healing was equivalent to placebo in reducing pain in lateral epicondylitis.[77] Downing and Weinstein also failed to demonstrate any benefit of continuous ultrasound at 10% lower intensity than patient discomfort in the treatment of subacromial symptoms.[78]

The differences in outcomes between the above studies may be due to the use of different treatment parameters and the application of ultrasound at different stages of healing. Because applying ultrasound with parameters that would increase tissue temperature may aggravate acute inflammation and because conversely, pulsed ultrasound may be ineffective in the chronic, late stage of recovery if the tissue requires heating to promote more effective stretching or increased circulation, applying ultrasound with the same parameters to all patients may obscure any treatment effect.

It is recommended that ultrasound be applied in a pulsed mode at a low intensity (0.5 to 1.0 W/cm^2) during the acute phase of tendon inflammation to minimize the risk of aggravating the condition and to accelerate recovery and, that continuous ultrasound at a high enough intensity to increase tissue temperature be applied in combination with stretching to assist in the resolution of chronic tendinitis if the problem is accompanied by soft tissue shortening because of scarring.

◎ Clinical Pearl

Ultrasound should be applied in a pulsed mode at low intensity for acute tendinitis and in a continuous mode at higher intensity along with stretching for chronic tendinitis.

Studies on the effect of ultrasound on tendon healing after surgical incision and repair have yielded more consistently positive results than those on tendonitis, with almost all studies showing improved tendon healing after surgical incision despite the use of a wide range of ultrasound parameters including different intensities (0.5 to 2.5 W/cm^2), modes (pulsed or continuous), and treatment durations (3 to 10 minutes).

Ultrasound at 0.5 or 1.0 W/cm^2, continuous, 1 MHz applied daily for the first 9 postoperative days was found to enhance the breaking strength of cut and sutured Achilles tendons in rabbits.[79,80] The strength of the ultrasound-treated tendons was greater than that of sham-treated controls, and the strength of those treated with 0.5 W/cm^2 intensity ultrasound was greater than that of those treated at 1.0 W/cm^2. Similar benefits were reported from the application of 1.5 W/cm^2, continuous, 1 MHz ultrasound for 3 to 4 minutes starting 1 day postoperatively (daily for the first 8 days and every other day thereafter for up to 3 weeks) to repaired Achilles tendons in rats.[81,82] A more recent study found that both 1 W/cm^2 and 2 W/cm^2 applications of continuous 1 MHz ultrasound applied for 4 minutes daily resulted in improvements in transected rat Achilles tendon tensile strength after 30 days when compared to controls[83] and that the higher intensity of 2 W/cm^2 produced better results than an intensity of 1 W/cm.[2,84] In addition, high-dose pulsed ultrasound (2.5 W/cm^2 and 20% duty cycle for 5 minutes 3 times per week) was found to improve tensile strength and stiffness in rats with Achilles tendon hemitenotomies without surgical repair.[85] One study comparing 1 MHz

pulsed and continuous ultrasound of 0.5 W/cm^2 (SATA) applied for 5 minutes, over a period of 14 consecutive days to transected rat Achilles tendons found that pulsed ultrasound resulted in a faster rate of healing than did continuous ultrasound.[86] Another study comparing the effects of low-intensity pulsed ultrasound and low-level laser therapy in the healing of traumatized rat tendons found that both interventions were associated with increased tendon breaking strength compared to controls at 21 days and that the two together provided no additional benefit.[87] The ultrasound was applied continuously at an intensity of 0.5 W/cm^2 and a frequency of 1 MHz for 5 minutes daily.

In contrast to most studies which have found ultrasound to improve tendon healing, one published study suggested that ultrasound may impair tendon healing. In this study, there appeared to be reduced strength and healing in surgically repaired flexor profundus tendons in 7 rabbits after treatment with pulsed ultrasound at 0.8 W/cm^2, 1 MHz, for 5 minutes daily for 6 weeks as compared to placebo-treated controls.[88] However, the authors of this study questioned the meaning of their findings because the strength of the tendons in both the treated and untreated groups was more than 10 times lower than has been reported in other studies for normal flexor tendon healing in rabbits.[89] Although immobilization was attempted throughout the postinjury period, technical difficulties in maintaining cast fixation and thus apposition of the tendon ends may have resulted in gap formation and poor strength in all subjects. The small sample size and poor reporting of the data also call into question the validity of this study. Furthermore, adverse effects of ultrasound on tendon healing have not been reported in other research.

Overall, research supports the early use of ultrasound for facilitation of tendon healing after rupture with surgical repair. The ultrasound doses found to be effective for this application are 0.5 to 2.5 W/cm^2 intensity, pulsed or continuous, 1 or 3 MHz frequency for 3 to 5 minutes. Although high-intensity ultrasound has been found to promote tendon healing, the lower end of the range is recommended to minimize the risk of any potentially adverse effect from heating acutely inflamed tissue postoperatively.

Some animal studies show that ruptured ligaments may also benefit from low intensity ultrasound while healing. Sparrow and colleagues found that ultrasound applied to transected medial collateral ligaments of rabbits every other day for 6 weeks resulted in an increased proportion of type I collagen and improved biomechanics (ability to resist greater loads and absorb more energy) when compared to ligaments treated with sham ultrasound.[89] In this study, researchers used continuous ultrasound with an intensity of 0.3 W/cm^2 at a frequency of 1 MHz for 10 minutes. Warden and colleagues examined the effect of ultrasound (1 MHz frequency, 0.5 W/cm^2 intensity, pulsed at 20% duty cycle, for 20 minutes 5 days a week) and a nonsteroidal antiinflammatory drug (NSAID) on ligament healing at 2, 4, and 12 weeks and found that low intensity pulsed ultrasound alone accelerated ligament healing, whereas an NSAID alone delayed ligament healing.[91]

When used together, the effect of the NSAID cancelled the positive effect of the ultrasound. Another study found that pulsed ultrasound within the first few days of ligament injury in rats increased the number of inflammatory mediators, thus worsening inflammation in the early stages of healing but possibly accelerating the overall course of the inflammatory and healing process.[92]

Based on the few available studies specifically related to ligament healing and findings related to healing of other soft tissues, it is recommended that low-dose (0.5 to 1.0 W/cm²) pulsed ultrasound be used for this application.

RESORPTION OF CALCIUM DEPOSITS

Ultrasound may facilitate the resorption of calcium deposits. Two published case studies, a randomized controlled trial and a prospective study, have reported functional recovery, pain resolution, and elimination of a calcific deposit in the shoulder after application of ultrasound; however, the mechanisms of this effect are unknown.[74,93-95] Although the mechanism underlying calcific deposits resorption is not known, the decrease in pain and improvements in function may be a result of the reduction in inflammation produced by ultrasound.

BONE FRACTURES

Early texts recommended that ultrasound not be applied over unhealed fractures.[96,97] This recommendation was probably given because applying high-dose continuous ultrasound over an unhealed fracture causes pain. However, numerous studies over the last 25 or more years have demonstrated that low-dose ultrasound can reduce the fracture healing time in animals and humans. Therefore the use of low-dose ultrasound to accelerate fracture healing is now recommended.

The stimulation of bone growth by physical means has been investigated for many years. At the beginning of the 18th century, it was observed that small direct currents acting at the periosteum induced bone formation, and in 1957, Fukada and Yasuda proposed that the piezoelectricity of bone was the mechanism behind this observed phenomenon.[98] In 1983, Duarte proposed that ultrasound may be a safe, noninvasive, and effective means to stimulate bone growth, also theoretically linked to the piezoelectric property of bone.[99] He applied very low-intensity ultrasound, delivered pulsed with a 0.5% duty cycle at approximately 10 W/cm² **spatial average temporal peak** (SATP) intensity, at either 4.93 or 1.65 MHz frequency to 23 rabbit fibulae that were osteomized and 22 femurs with drilled holes. Treatment was applied for 15 minutes per day, starting 1 day postoperatively, for 4 to 18 days. All animals received bilateral osteotomies and were treated with ultrasound unilaterally so that the contralateral extremity could serve as a control. The treated bones were found to develop callus and trabeculae more rapidly than the untreated bones (Fig. 7-8).

A similar study with a larger sample size (139) also reported acceleration of bone healing with ultrasound.[100] The ultrasound was delivered pulsed with a 20% duty cycle, 0.15 W/cm² SATP intensity, 1.5 MHz frequency. Treatment was applied for 20 minutes daily, starting 1 day

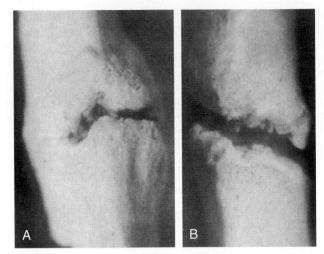

FIG 7-8 Fracture healing 17 days postoperatively. **A,** with, and **B,** without ultrasound application. *From Duarte LR: The stimulation of bone growth by ultrasound,* Arch Orthop Trauma Surg 101:153-159, 1983.

postoperatively, for 14 to 28 days. Biomechanical healing was accelerated by a factor of 1.7, with treated fractures being as strong as intact bone in 17 days compared with 28 days for the control fractures. These parameters, with a purpose-made device in which the parameters cannot be changed, have been used for most studies on the effects of ultrasound on fracture healing in animals and humans since 1990.

In recent years, the amount of research in ultrasound and bone healing has greatly increased. Therefore, this discussion focuses primarily on randomized, placebo-controlled trials in humans and a few key animal studies. Malizos and colleagues' excellent review of this literature summarizes the findings of these studies.[101] Four double-blind, placebo-controlled studies demonstrated acceleration of fracture healing in human subjects with the application of ultrasound, whereas one found no effect. All used the ultrasound signal and treatment durations described previously. One study reported accelerated healing of Colles' and tibial diaphyseal fractures by a factor of 1.5 (as demonstrated by radiography),[102] another reported acceleration of tibial fracture healing by a factor of 1.3 for clinical healing and a factor of 1.6 for overall clinical and radiographic healing,[103] and a third reported accelerated healing of distal radial fractures.[104] A fourth study found that nonunion scaphoid fractures treated with bone grafts healed 38 days sooner with ultrasound than without.[105] A fifth trial compared the effect of active and sham ultrasound on bone healing after placement of a bioabsorbable screw in lateral malleolar fractures and found that radiographs and computed tomography (CT) scans showed no significant difference between the two groups.[106] However, the sample size for this study was small (22 fractures).

One study on fracture healing used the type of ultrasound device typically used by physical therapists and other clinicians in the clinical setting. In this study the ultrasound was 1 MHz frequency, 0.5 W/cm² intensity, and 20% duty cycle. Rats with bilateral femur fractures were treated with active ultrasound on one leg and inactive ultrasound on the other leg starting 1 day after fracture for 5 days a week, 20 minutes a day. At 40 days, the fractures treated with ultrasound had increased bone mineral content at the fracture site, a resulting increase in bone size, and 81% greater mechanical strength than placebo-treated fractures.[107]

Although the use of ultrasound for recent fractures has the most robust body of evidence, some animal studies, human case studies, and one human randomized controlled trial report increased rates of healing in established nonunion fractures. One randomized placebo-controlled trial in humans found that ultrasound accelerated the healing of scaphoid nonunion fractures.[105] A case series of nonunion fractures (fractures that had not healed after an average of 61 weeks) in humans found that 1.5 MHz frequency, 0.15 W/cm^2 intensity, 20% duty cycle ultrasound applied by the patients at home for 20 minutes daily resulted in 86% of the fractures healing in an average of 22 weeks.[108] A similar self-paired control study with the same protocol as the previous study found that 85% of nonunion fractures treated with ultrasound healed after treatment for an average of 168 days,[109] and an animal study using the same treatment protocol found that 50% of nonunion fractures healed with 6 weeks of treatment compared to no healing in the untreated controls.[110]

A device specifically designed for the application of ultrasound for fracture healing was cleared by the FDA in 1994 for home use. In 2000, the FDA expanded its clearance to include the treatment of nonunion fractures with this device. This device has fixed preset treatment parameters of 1.5 MHz frequency, 0.15 W/cm^2 SATP intensity, 20% duty cycle, and a treatment duration of 20 minutes (Fig. 7-9). This device is available by prescription only.

The most recent studies have examined the application of ultrasound to a fracture via a metal pin inserted in the bone approximately 1 cm from the fracture or with implanted transducers. This procedure is known as transosseous ultrasound application. The same ultrasound parameters were used as in the studies discussed previously. The studies of transosseous ultrasound application have shown decreased time to fracture healing, increased bone mineral density, and improved lateral bending strength in the healing fracture.[111-113]

Current research supports the use of very low-dose ultrasound for facilitation of fracture healing. The parameters found to be effective are 1.5 MHz frequency, 0.15 W/cm^2 intensity, 20% duty cycle, for 15 to 20 minutes daily.

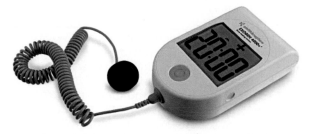

FIG 7-9 Ultrasound device for home use for fracture healing. *Courtesy Exogen, Piscataway, NJ.*

CARPAL TUNNEL SYNDROME

Continuous ultrasound has generally not been recommended for the treatment of carpal tunnel syndrome because of the risk of adversely impacting nerve conduction velocity by overheating.[114,115] However, one study found that pulsed ultrasound produced significantly greater improvement in subjective complaints ($p < 0.001$, paired t test), hand grip and finger pinch strength, and electromyographic variables (motor distal latency $p < 0.001$, paired t test; sensory antidromic nerve conduction velocity $p < 0.001$, paired t test) than sham ultrasound treatment.[116] These benefits were sustained at 6 months follow-up. The ultrasound was applied for 20 sessions at 1 MHz frequency, 1.0 W/cm^2 intensity, pulsed mode 1 : 4, for 15 minutes per session. Another randomized, placebo-controlled trial found clinical improvements in both ultrasound and diclofenac-treated patients with mild to moderate carpal tunnel syndrome.[117] Continuous ultrasound with an intensity of 0.5 W/cm^2 was applied to the palmar carpal tunnel for 10 minutes 5 days a week for 4 weeks. Only the ultrasound-treated group had electrophysiological changes (increased sensory nerve action potential amplitude), but the implications of these results are uncertain. The proposed mechanisms for a potential benefit of ultrasound to patients with carpal tunnel syndrome are the anti-inflammatory and tissue stimulating effects of this intervention.

PHONOPHORESIS

Phonophoresis is the application of ultrasound in conjunction with a topical drug preparation as the ultrasound transmission medium. The ultrasound is intended to enhance delivery of the drug through the skin, thereby delivering the drug for local or systemic effects. Transcutaneous drug delivery has a number of advantages over oral drug administration. It provides a higher initial drug concentration at the delivery site,[118] avoids gastric irritation, and avoids first-pass metabolism by the liver. Transcutaneous delivery also avoids the pain, trauma, and infection risk associated with injection and allows delivery to a larger area than is readily achieved by injection.

The first report of the use of ultrasound to enhance drug delivery across the skin was published in 1954.[119] This was followed by a series of studies by Griffin and colleagues evaluating the location and depth of hydrocortisone delivery and the effects of varying ultrasound parameters on hydrocortisone phonophoresis.[120-123] The authors of these initial studies proposed that ultrasound enhanced drug delivery by exerting pressure on the drug to drive it through the skin. However, because ultrasound exerts only a few grams of force, it is now thought that ultrasound increases transdermal drug penetration by increasing the permeability of the stratum corneum through cavitation.[124] This theory is supported by the observation that ultrasound can enhance drug penetration even when the ultrasound is applied before the drug is put on the skin.[125]

The stratum corneum is the superficial cornified layer of the skin that acts as a protective barrier, preventing foreign materials from entering the body through the skin

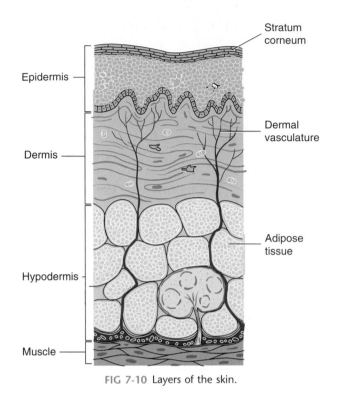

Epidermis —
Dermis —
Hypodermis -
Muscle —

Stratum corneum
Dermal vasculature
Adipose tissue

FIG 7-10 Layers of the skin.

(Fig. 7-10). Ultrasound may change stratum corneum permeability by both thermal and nonthermal mechanisms. It has been proposed that ultrasound alters the skin porous pathways by enlarging the skin effective pore radii and by creating more pores or making the pores less tortuous.[126] Drug diffusion across the stratum corneum depends on both diffusion and partition coefficients. One study demonstrated ultrasound enhancement of diffusion coefficients of a variety of solutes by up to 15-fold. Ultrasound, however, did not significantly enhance partition coefficients.[127] Laboratory research shows that combining ultrasound with surfactants or other materials can increase skin permeability in phonophoresis, although these surfactants may damage the skin.[128] One study concluded that the synergistic effect of ultrasound and sodium lauryl sulfate in increasing skin permeability may be a result of changes in pH in the stratum corneum induced by sodium lauryl sulfate.[129]

When the permeability of the stratum corneum is increased, a drug will diffuse across it because of the difference in concentration on either side of the skin. Once a drug diffuses across the stratum corneum, it is initially more concentrated at the delivery site and is then distributed throughout the body by the vascular circulation; therefore therapists should be aware that drugs delivered by phonophoresis do become systemic and the contraindications for systemic delivery of these drugs also apply to this mode of delivery.

◎ Clinical Pearl

Drugs delivered by phonophoresis become systemic.

Because six phonophoresis treatments with the corticosteroid dexamethasone have been shown not to cause an increase in urinary free cortisol, which is a measure of adrenal suppression, a course of six treatments is considered safe for patients who do not have other contraindications for corticosteroid treatment.[130] It is recommended that a drug not be delivered by phonophoresis if the patient is already receiving a drug of the same type by another route of administration because this increases the risk of adverse effects. For example, if a patient with rheumatoid arthritis or asthma is taking corticosteroids by mouth, hydrocortisone or dexamethasone should not be given by phonophoresis.

Ultrasound frequency is the parameter that has been researched most in the application of phonophoresis. Currently, the understanding is that lower frequency ultrasound, at around 20 to 100 kHz (i.e., much lower than typically used in therapy) results in the greatest increase in skin permeability.[131] Mitragotri and colleagues compared enhancement ratios (ratio of phonophoretic and passive permeabilities across the skin) induced by 1 MHz ultrasound and 20 kHz ultrasound for butanol, corticosterone, salicylic acid, and sucrose in human cadaver skin.[132] They found that low frequency ultrasound induced up to 1,000-fold higher enhancement than 1 MHz ultrasound. A more recent study found that 20 kHz, but not 10 MHz, ultrasound resulted in significantly increased permeation of mannitol and glucose through porcine skin.[133]

In recent years, there has been a wealth of research on the use of phonophoresis to deliver insulin[131] and other drugs that can only be given by injection and that are not typically administered by rehabilitation professionals. Unfortunately, this approach to drug delivery is hampered by difficulties with precise dose control.[134] Ultrasound is also being explored as a method for monitoring blood glucose levels.[135] Most of the recent research on phonophoresis uses low frequency ultrasound, of 100 kHz or lower frequency.[136] In contrast, rehabilitation professionals usually use ultrasound devices that operate in the 1 to 3 MHz frequency range and use phonophoresis primarily for local delivery of corticosteroid and NSAIDs to treat tissue inflammation associated with conditions such as tendinitis or bursitis. Therefore the discussion that follows focuses on the application of megahertz frequency ultrasound to enhance the delivery of antiinflammatory medications. For a more complete review of the principles and research of phonophoresis, consult the literature reviews by Byl and Tachibana.[136,137]

In the 1960s and 1970s, Griffin and colleagues found that with the application of hydrocortisone phonophoresis to pigs, more hydrocortisone was deposited in nerve than in muscle.[120] They also reported that the highest ultrasound frequency they used, 3.6 MHz, was most effective and that a low intensity (0.1 W/cm^2) for a long duration (51 minutes) or a high intensity (3.0 W/cm^2) for a short duration (5 minutes) resulted in the most hydrocortisone delivery.[121-123] Around the same time, Kleinkort and Wood compared the efficacy of different drug concentrations used for phonophoresis and found that 10% hydrocortisone was more effective than 1% hydrocortisone in relieving pain associated with tendinitis or bursitis.[139] However, a later study comparing the ability of different media customarily used for phonophoresis to transmit ultrasound found that the hydrocortisone preparations most commonly used for this application do not transmit ultrasound effectively.[140] This discovery called into question the mechanism of hydrocortisone phonophoresis because when a poorly transmitting medium is used, very little ultrasound is able to reach the tissue. It has been proposed that the enhanced hydrocortisone penetration reported by Griffin and colleagues may have been caused by heating of the skin by conduction from the warm sound head rather than being a direct effect of the ultrasound.[140] Since then, one study found that hydrocortisone gel applied with 1.0 MHz continuous ultrasound at intensity of 1 W/cm^2 for 7 minutes did not increase intramuscular cortisol levels when compared with controls receiving ultrasound only.[141]

However, studies using media that transmit ultrasound effectively have demonstrated enhanced transdermal penetration of drugs other than hydrocortisone using phonophoresis. For example, 1 MHz pulsed or continuous ultrasound has been shown to increase transdermal penetration of mannitol and inulin in rats and guinea pigs, increasing the output of radiolabeled mannitol and inulin in the urine of the ultrasound-treated animals by 5- to 20-fold for 1 to 2 hours after treatment compared with controls.[142] Urinary output was used as a measure of the systemic uptake of these drugs. Phonophoresis for the delivery of NSAIDs in human subjects has been found to produce mixed results. Unfortunately, most of the studies in this area are poorly designed (with no placebo-treated subjects), limiting their interpretation.[143,144] One well-designed randomized controlled trial found greater concentrations of ketoprofen in local synovial tissue with the application of ultrasound than without ultrasound and higher level with pulsed ultrasound than with continuous ultrasound (both at 1 MHz frequency, 1.5 W/cm^2 intensity delivered for 5 minutes).[145]

An in vitro comparison of the penetration of ibuprofen through human skin with ultrasound or with equal heating using a conductive heater demonstrated that the enhancement of transdermal drug penetration by ultrasound was not only the result of the thermal effects of ultrasound.[146] Drug penetration was increased with the application of both conductive heating and ultrasound; however, the increase produced by ultrasound was significantly greater than that produced by conductive heating alone.

The research at this time supports the use of ultrasound for facilitation of transdermal drug penetration. The treatment parameters most likely to be effective are pulsed 20% duty cycle, to avoid heating of any inflammatory condition, at 0.5 to 0.75 W/cm^2 intensity, for 5 to 10 minutes. The drug preparation used should also transmit ultrasound effectively.

CONTRAINDICATIONS AND PRECAUTIONS FOR THE USE OF ULTRASOUND

Although ultrasound is a relatively safe intervention, it must be applied with care to avoid harming the patient. Ultrasound with the range of parameters available on clinical devices may not be used by patients to treat themselves. It must be used by, or under the supervision of, a licensed practitioner.

Even when ultrasound is not contraindicated, if the patient's condition is worsening or not improving within 2 to 3 treatments, reevaluate the treatment approach and consider changing the intervention or referring the patient to a physician for reevaluation.

CONTRAINDICATIONS FOR THE USE OF ULTRASOUND

CONTRAINDICATIONS

for the Use of Ultrasound

- Malignant tumor
- Pregnancy
- Central nervous system (CNS) tissue
- Joint cement
- Plastic components
- Pacemaker
- Thrombophlebitis
- Eyes
- Reproductive organs

Malignant Tumor

Although there are no research data concerning the effects of applying therapeutic ultrasound to malignant tumors in humans, the application of continuous ultrasound at 1.0 W/cm^2, 1 MHz, for 5 minutes for 10 treatments over a period of 2 weeks to mice with malignant subcutaneous tumors has been shown to produce significantly larger and heavier tumors compared to those of untreated controls.[147] The treated mice also developed more lymph node metastases. Because this study indicates that therapeutic ultrasound may increase the rate of tumor growth or metastasis, it is recommended that therapeutic ultrasound not be applied to malignant tumors in humans. Caution should also be used when treating a patient who has a history of a malignant tumor or tumors because it can be difficult to ascertain whether any small tumors remain. It is therefore recommended that the therapist consult with the referring physician before applying ultrasound to a patient with a history of malignancy within the last 5 years.

One should note that ultrasound is used as a component of the treatment of certain types of malignant tumors; however, the devices used for this application allow a number of ultrasound beams to be directed at the tumor in order to achieve a temperature within the range of 42° to 43° C [108° to 109° F].[148-150] Some malignant tumors decrease in size or are eradicated when heated to within this narrow range, whereas healthy tissue is left undamaged. Because the therapeutic ultrasound devices generally available to physical therapists do not allow such precise determination and control of tissue temperature and because primary treatment of malignancy is outside the scope of practice of rehabilitation professionals, therapeutic ultrasound devices intended for rehabilitation applications should not be used for treatment of malignancy.

Ask the Patient

- Have you ever had cancer? Do you have cancer now?
- Do you have fevers, chills, sweats, or night pain?
- Do you have pain at rest?
- Have you had recent unexplained weight loss?

If the patient has cancer at this time, ultrasound should not be used. If the patient has a history of cancer or signs of cancer such as fevers, chills, sweats, night pain, pain at rest, or recent unexplained weight loss, the therapist should consult with the referring physician in order to rule out the presence of malignancy before applying ultrasound.

Pregnancy

Maternal hyperthermia has been associated with fetal abnormalities, including growth retardation, microphthalmia, exencephaly, microencephaly, neural tube defects, and myelodysplasia.[151,152] There is also a published report documenting a case of sacral agenesis, microcephaly, and developmental delay in a child whose mother was treated 18 times with low-intensity pulsed ultrasound for a left psoas bursitis between days 6 and 29 of gestation.[153] It is therefore recommended that therapeutic ultrasound not be applied at any level in areas where it may reach a developing fetus. This includes the abdomen, low back, and pelvis.

The diagnostic ultrasound frequently used during pregnancy to assess the position and development of the fetus and placenta has been shown to be safe and without adverse consequences for the fetus or the mother.[154,155]

Ask the Patient

- Are you pregnant, might you be pregnant, or are you trying to become pregnant?

The patient may not know if she is pregnant, particularly in the first few days or weeks after conception; however, because damage may occur at any time during fetal development, ultrasound should not be applied in any area where the beam may reach the fetus of a patient who is or might be pregnant.

A recent study found that high-frequency (6.7 MHz), low-intensity (1.95 mW/cm^2) ultrasound applied for 30 minutes or longer to the abdomen of pregnant mice impaired neuronal migration in the brain.[156] The ultrasound was applied during the equivalent of the third trimester of pregnancy. The frequency of ultrasound used in this study was much higher than the frequencies used in rehabilitation (1 to 3 MHz) and higher than frequencies used for viewing the human fetus and for other diagnostic procedures (3.5 to 5 MHz). The length of time the ultrasound was applied was also longer than the typical therapeutic session. Nonetheless, this study supports the recommendation that ultrasound exposure should be limited to areas away from the pregnant uterus and that treatment should not exceed the recommended duration.

Central Nervous System Tissue

There is concern that ultrasound may damage CNS tissue. However, because CNS tissue is usually covered by bone,

both in the spinal cord and in the brain, this is rarely a problem. The spinal cord may be exposed if the patient has had a laminectomy above the L2 level. In such cases, ultrasound should not be applied over or near the area of the laminectomy.

Methylmethacrylate Cement or Plastic

Methylmethacrylate cement and plastic are materials used for fixation or as components of prosthetic joints. Because these materials are rapidly heated by ultrasound,[157] it is generally recommended that ultrasound not be applied over a cemented prosthesis or in areas where plastic components are used. Although very little ultrasound is able to reach to the depth of most prosthetic joints, it is still recommended that the clinician err on the side of caution and not use this modality in areas where plastic or cement may be present. Ultrasound may be used over areas with metal implants, such as screws, plates, or all-metal joint replacements, because metal is not rapidly heated by ultrasound and ultrasound has been shown not to loosen screws or plates.[158]

Ask the Patient

- Do you have a joint replacement in this area?
- Was cement used to hold it in place?
- Does it have plastic components?

If the patient has a joint replacement, ultrasound should not be applied in the area of the prosthesis until the therapist has determined that neither cement nor plastic was used.

Pacemaker

Because ultrasound may heat a pacemaker or interfere with its electrical circuitry, ultrasound should not be applied in the area of a pacemaker. Ultrasound may be applied to other areas in patients with pacemakers.

Ask the Patient

- Do you have a pacemaker?

Thrombophlebitis

Because ultrasound may dislodge or cause partial disintegration of a thrombus, which could then result in obstruction of the circulation to vital organs, ultrasound should not be applied over or near an area where a thrombus is or may be present.

Ask the Patient

- Do you have a blood clot in this area?

Eyes

It is recommended that ultrasound not be applied over the eyes because cavitation in the ocular fluid may damage the eyes.

Reproductive Organs

Because ultrasound at the levels used for rehabilitation may affect gamete development, it is recommended that it not be applied in the areas of the male or female reproductive organs.

PRECAUTIONS FOR THE USE OF ULTRASOUND

> ## PRECAUTIONS
> ### for the Use of Ultrasound
>
> • Acute inflammation
> • Epiphyseal plates
> • Fractures
> • Breast implants

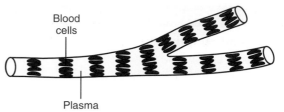

FIG 7-11 Banding of blood cells and plasma due to standing waves.

Acute Inflammation

Because heat can exacerbate acute inflammation, causing increased bleeding, pain, and swelling, impairing healing and delaying functional recovery, ultrasound at sufficient intensity to produce heat should be applied with caution in areas of acute inflammation.

Epiphyseal Plates

The literature regarding the application of ultrasound over epiphyseal plates is controversial. Although one study reported that ultrasound applied at greater than 3.0 W/cm^2 may damage epiphyseal plates,[159] Lehmann states that it is safe to apply ultrasound over epiphyseal plates as long as there is no pain.[6] Also, a recent study reported no change in bone growth in skeletally immature rats with ultrasound applied at the low levels used for fracture healing.[160] At this time, it is recommended that high-dose ultrasound not be applied over growing epiphyseal plates.

Because the age of epiphyseal closure varies, radiographic evaluation rather than age should be used to determine if epiphyseal closure is complete.

Fracture

Although low-dose ultrasound has been shown to accelerate fracture healing, the application of high-intensity ultrasound over a fracture generally causes pain. There is also concern that high-level ultrasound may impair fracture healing. Therefore only low-dose ultrasound, as described in the section on fracture healing, should be applied over the area of a fracture.

Breast Implants

Because heat may increase the pressure inside a breast implant and cause it to rupture, high-dose ultrasound should not be applied over breast implants.

ADVERSE EFFECTS OF ULTRASOUND

In general, ultrasound has rarely been reported to produce adverse effects.[161] However, a variety of adverse effects can occur if ultrasound is applied incorrectly or when contraindicated. The most common adverse effect is a burn, which may occur when high-intensity, continuous ultrasound is applied, particularly if a stationary application technique is used. The risk of burns is further increased in areas with impaired circulation or sensation and with superficial bone. To minimize the risk of burning a patient, always move the ultrasound head and do not apply thermal-level ultrasound to areas with impaired circulation or sensation. Reduce the ultrasound intensity in areas with superficial bone or if the patient complains of any increase in discomfort with the application of ultrasound.

Ultrasound **standing waves** can cause blood cell stasis because of collections of gas bubbles and plasma at antinodes and collection of cells at nodes[162,163] (Fig. 7-11). This is accompanied by damage to the endothelial lining of the blood vessels. These effects have been demonstrated with ultrasound of 1 to 5 MHz frequency, with intensity as low as 0.5 W/cm^2 and as short an exposure as 0.1 second. Although the stasis is reversed when ultrasound application stops, the endothelial damage remains. Therefore, to prevent the adverse effects of standing waves, it is recommended that the ultrasound transducer be moved throughout treatment application.

Another concern is the possibility of cross-contamination and infection of patients. One study found that 27% of ultrasound transducer heads and 28% of ultrasound transmission gels taken from various physiotherapy practices were contaminated with bacteria.[164] The transducer heads were generally contaminated with bacteria normally found on the skin, and cleaning with 70% alcohol significantly reduced the level of contamination. However, the gels were heavily contaminated with opportunistic and potentially pathogenic organisms, including *Staphylococcus aureus*.

APPLICATION TECHNIQUE 7-1   **ULTRASOUND**

Equipment Required

- Ultrasound unit
- Gel, water, or other transmission medium
- Antimicrobial agent
- Towel

Procedure

1. Evaluate the patient's clinical findings and set the goals of treatment.
2. Determine if ultrasound is the most appropriate intervention.
3. Determine that ultrasound is not contraindicated for the patient or the condition. Check with the patient and check the patient's chart for contraindications or precautions regarding the application of ultrasound.
4. Apply an ultrasound transmission medium to the area to be treated. Apply enough medium to eliminate any air between the sound head and the treatment area. Select a medium that transmits ultrasound well, does not stain, is not allergenic, is not rapidly absorbed by the skin, and is inexpensive. Gels or lotions meeting these criteria have been specifically formulated for use with ultrasound. Or, for the application of ultrasound under water, place the area to be treated in a container of water (see Fig. 7-21).
5. Select a sound head with an ERA approximately half the size of the treatment area.
6. Select the optimal treatment parameters, including ultrasound frequency, intensity, duty cycle, and duration; the appropriate size of the treatment area; and the appropriate number and frequency of treatments. Parameters are generally determined by whether the intended effect is thermal or nonthermal. See next section for a general discussion of parameters. Detailed information on parameters for specific conditions is included in previous section.
7. Before treatment of any area with a risk of cross-infection, swab the sound head with 0.5% alcoholic chlorhexidine, or use the antimicrobial approved for this use in the facility.[71]
8. Place the sound head on the treatment area.
9. Turn on the ultrasound machine.
10. Move the sound head within the treatment area. The sound head is moved in order to optimize the uniformity of ultrasound intensity delivered to the tissues and to minimize the risk of standing wave formation.[162,163] See p. 194 for a detailed description of how to move the sound head.
11. When the intervention is completed, remove the conduction medium from the sound head and the patient and reassess for any changes in status.
12. Document the intervention.

APPLICATION TECHNIQUE

This section provides guidelines for the sequence of procedures required for the safe and effective application of therapeutic ultrasound.

ULTRASOUND TREATMENT PARAMETERS

Specific recommendations for different clinical applications are given in the previous sections concerning the specific clinical conditions. General guidelines for treatment parameters follow.

Frequency

The frequency is selected according to the depth of tissue to be treated. For tissue up to 5 cm deep, 1 MHz is used, and 3 MHz is used for tissue 1 to 2 cm deep. The depth of penetration is lower in tissues with a high collagen content and in areas of increased reflection.

Duty Cycle

The duty cycle is selected according to the treatment goal. When the goal is to increase tissue temperature, a 100% (continuous) duty cycle should be used.[47] When applying ultrasound where only the nonthermal effects without tissue heating are desired, pulsed ultrasound with a 20% or lower duty cycle should be used. Although the nonthermal effects of ultrasound are produced by continuous ultrasound, it is thought that they are not optimized with application at this level.[15] Almost all published studies on the effects of pulsed ultrasound have used a duty cycle of 20%.

Intensity

Intensity is selected according to the treatment goal. When the goal is to increase tissue temperature, the patient should feel some warmth within 2 to 3 minutes of initiat-

ing ultrasound application and should not feel increased discomfort at any time during the treatment. When using 1 MHz frequency ultrasound, an intensity of 1.5 to 2.0 W/cm^2 will generally produce this effect. When using 3 MHz frequency, an intensity of about 0.5 W/cm^2 is generally sufficient. A lower intensity is effective at the higher frequency because the energy is absorbed in a smaller, more superficial volume of tissue, resulting in a greater temperature increase with the same ultrasound intensity. The intensity is adjusted up or down from these levels according to the patient's report. The intensity is increased if there is no sensation of warmth within 2 to 3 minutes and decreased immediately if there is any complaint of discomfort. If there is superficial bone in the treatment area, a slightly lower intensity will be sufficient to produce comfortable heating because the ultrasound reflected by the bone will cause a greater increase in temperature.

When applying ultrasound for nonthermal effects, successful treatment outcomes have been documented for most applications using an intensity of 0.5 to 1.0 W/cm^2 SATP (0.1 to 0.2 W/cm^2 SATA), with as low as 0.15 W/cm^2 SATP (0.03 W/cm^2 SATA) sufficient for facilitation of bone healing.

Duration

The treatment duration is selected according to the treatment goal, the size of the area to be treated, and the ERA of the sound head. For most thermal or nonthermal applications, ultrasound should be applied for 5 to 10 minutes for each treatment area that is twice the ERA of the transducer. For example, when treating an area 20 cm^2 with a sound head that has an ERA of 10 cm^2, the treatment duration should be 5 to 10 minutes. When treating an area of 40 cm^2 with the same 10 cm^2, the treatment duration should be extended to between 10 and 20 minutes.

When the goal of treatment is to increase tissue temperature, the treatment duration should also be adjusted according to the frequency and intensity of the ultrasound. For example, if the goal is to increase tissue temperature by 3° C (37° F) and thus reach the minimal therapeutic level of 40° C (104° F) and if 1 MHz ultrasound at an intensity of 1.5 W/cm^2 is applied to an area twice the ERA of the transducer, the treatment duration must be at least 9 minutes, whereas if the intensity is increased to 2 W/cm^2, the treatment duration need be only 8 minutes.[8] If 3 MHz ultrasound is used at an intensity of 0.5 W/cm^2, the treatment duration must be at least 10 minutes to achieve the same temperature level.

In general, treatment duration should be increased when lower intensities or lower frequencies of ultrasound are used, when treating areas larger than twice the ERA of the transducer, or when higher tissue temperatures are desired. Treatment duration should be decreased when higher intensities or frequencies of ultrasound are used, when treating areas smaller than twice the ERA of the transducer, or when lower tissue temperatures are desired.

When ultrasound is used to facilitate bone healing, longer treatment times of 15 to 20 minutes are recommended.

Area to be Treated

The size of area that can be treated with ultrasound depends on the ERA of the transducer and the duration of treatment. As explained in the previous discussion of duration of treatment, a treatment area equal to twice the ERA of the sound head can be treated in 5 to 10 minutes. Smaller areas can be treated in proportionately shorter times; however, it is impractical to treat areas less than 1$\frac{1}{2}$ times the ERA of the sound head and still keep the sound head moving within the area. Larger areas can be treated in proportionately longer times; however, ultrasound should not be used to treat areas larger than four times the ERA of the transducer, such as the whole low back, because this requires excessively long treatment durations and, when heating is desired, results in some areas being heated while other previously heated areas are already cooling (Figs. 7-12 and 7-13).

Number and Frequency of Treatments

The recommended number of treatments depends on the goals of treatment and the patient's response. If the patient is making progress at an appropriate rate toward the established goals for this intervention, the treatment should be continued. If the patient is not progressing appropriately, the intervention should be modified, either by changing the ultrasound parameters or by selecting a different intervention. In most cases, an effect should be detectable within 1 to 3 treatments. For problems in which progress is commonly slow, such as chronic wounds, or in which progress is hard to detect, such as with fractures, treatment may need to be continued for a longer period. The frequency of treatments depends on the level of ultrasound being used and the stage of healing. Thermal-level ultrasound is usually applied only during the subacute or chronic phase of healing, when treatment 3 times a week

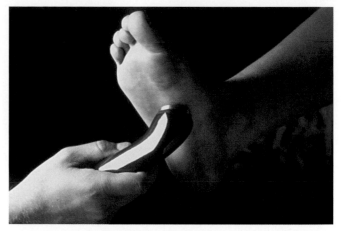

FIG 7-12 Ultrasound application to the foot. *Courtesy Mettler Electronics, Anaheim, CA.*

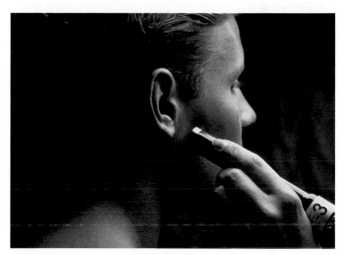

FIG 7-13 Ultrasound application to the temporomandibular joint (TMJ) area. *Courtesy Mettler Electronics, Anaheim, CA.*

is recommended; ultrasound at nonthermal levels may be applied at earlier stages, when treatment may be as frequent as daily. These frequencies of treatment are based on current clinical standards of practice because there are no published studies at this time comparing the efficacy of different treatment frequencies.

Sequence of Treatment

In most cases, ultrasound may be applied before or after other interventions; however, when using ultrasound to heat tissue, it should not be applied after any intervention that may impair sensation, such as ice. Also, when thermal-level ultrasound is used to increase collagen extensibility in order to maximize the increase in length produced with stretching, the ultrasound must be applied directly before, and if possible during, the application of the stretching force. The clinician should not wait or apply another intervention between applying the ultrasound and stretching because the tissue starts to cool as soon as the ultrasound application ends.

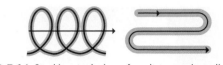

FIG 7-14 Stroking technique for ultrasound application.

Moving the Sound Head

The sound head is moved at approximately 4 cm/sec, quickly enough to maintain motion and slowly enough to maintain contact with the skin. If the sound head is kept stationary or moved too slowly, the area of tissue under the center of the transducer, where the intensity is greatest, will receive much more ultrasound than the areas under the edges of the transducer. With continuous ultrasound, this can result in overheating and burning of the tissues at the center of the field, and with pulsed ultrasound, this can reduce the efficacy of the intervention. A stationary sound head should not be used when applying either continuous or pulsed ultrasound. If the sound head is moved too quickly, the therapist may not be able to maintain good contact of the sound head with the skin and thus the ultrasound will not be able to enter the tissue.

The sound head should be moved in a manner that causes the center of the head to change position so that all parts of the treatment area receive similar exposure. Strokes overlapping by half the ERA of the sound head are recommended (Fig. 7-14). The clinician should keep within the predetermined treatment area of one and a half to four times the ERA only.

The surface of the sound head is kept in constant parallel contact with the skin to ensure that the ultrasound is transmitted to the tissues. Poor contact will impede the transmission of ultrasound because much of it will be absorbed by intervening air or reflected at the air-tissue interface. To promote more effective intervention, some clinical ultrasound units are equipped with a transmission sensor that gives a signal when contact is poor.

DOCUMENTATION

The following should be documented:
- Area of the body treated
- Ultrasound frequency
- Ultrasound intensity
- Ultrasound duty cycle
- Treatment duration
- Whether the ultrasound was delivered under water
- Patient's response to the intervention

Documentation is typically written in the SOAP note (Subjective, Objective, Assessment, Plan) format. The following examples only summarize the modality component of the intervention and are not intended to represent a comprehensive plan of care.

EXAMPLES

When applying ultrasound (US) to the left lateral knee (L lat knee) over the lateral collateral ligament (LCL) to facilitate tissue healing, document the following:

S: Pt reports L lat knee pain with turning has decreased from frequent 8/10 to occasional 5/10 since last week after therapy treatment.

O: Intervention: US L lat knee, LCL, 0.5 W/cm^2, pulsed 20%, 3 MHz, 5 min.

A: Pt tolerated treatment well, with decreased knee pain since ultrasound initiated.

P: Reassess pain level next treatment; if pain resolved then discontinue US.

When applying ultrasound to the R inferior (inf) anterior (ant) shoulder capsule, document the following:

S: Pt notes slowly improving R shoulder ROM and is now able to use R UE when combing her hair since last treatment.

O: Pretreatment: R shoulder active abduction ROM 120 degrees, passive abduction ROM 135 degrees.

Intervention: US R inf ant shoulder, 2.0 W/cm^2, continuous, 1 MHz, 5 min, followed by joint mobility inf glide grade IV.

Posttreatment: R shoulder passive abduction 150 degrees.

P: Continue US as above followed by mobilization and ROM to R shoulder.

CLINICAL CASE STUDIES

The following case studies summarize the concepts of applying therapeutic ultrasound as discussed in this chapter. Based on the scenarios presented, an evaluation of the clinical findings and goals of treatment are proposed. These are followed by a discussion of factors to be considered in the selection of ultrasound as the indicated intervention modality and in selection of the ideal treatment parameters to promote progress toward the goals (Fig. 7-15).

CASE STUDY 7-1

Soft Tissue Shortening
Examination
History

TR is a 60-year-old man, 3 months after open-reduction and internal-fixation of a right hip fracture with placement of a plate and screws. He has been referred to

CLINICAL CASE STUDIES—*cont'd*

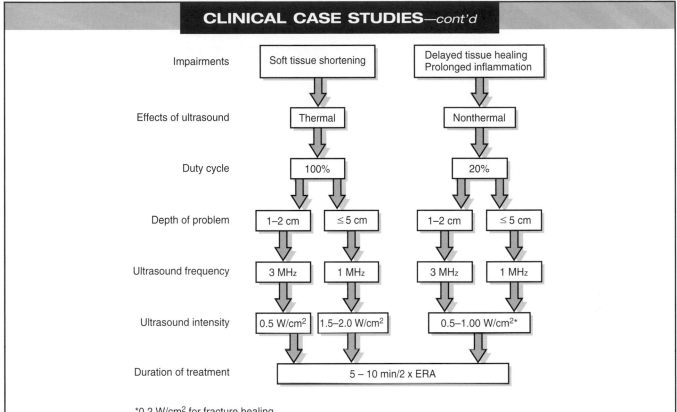

FIG 7-15 Decision-making chart for ultrasound treatment parameters. *ERA,* Effective radiating area.

*0.2 W/cm² for fracture healing

physical therapy for gait training with the restriction of limiting weight bearing to his tolerance. TR reports intermittent dull pain in the right anterior groin that is aggravated by standing or walking without an assistive device and by lying prone. His pain is eased when he sits or lies on his side. Since the hip fracture he has walked only up to approximately 50 feet, maintaining partial weight bearing on his right lower extremity by using bilateral crutches and by flexing his right hip and knee throughout the gait cycle. He has not been able to return to work due to his restricted ambulation. Before the hip fracture, TR walked 2 miles a day at his job without an assistive device and without pain.

Tests and Measures

The patient has decreased right hip passive ROM (PROM) in extension (–20 degrees) and abduction (10 degrees right versus 40 degrees left), with tightness of the anteromedial hip capsule and guarding and spasms of the hip adductor and flexor muscles. All other measures are within normal limits.

What problems would ultrasound address in this patient? What effect will the plate and screws have on ultrasound application? What ultrasound parameters would you use for this patient?

Evaluation, Diagnosis, Prognosis, and Goals
Evaluation and Goals

ICF Level	Current Status	Goals
Body structure and function	Right hip pain	Resolve hip pain
	Shortening of right anteromedial hip capsule and reduced hip PROM	Normalize the length of the right hip capsule and right hip PROM
Activity	Limited ambulation	Return to 2 miles of ambulation per day without an assistive device
Participation	Unable to work	Full return to work

Diagnosis

Preferred Practice Pattern 4I: Impaired joint mobility, muscle performance, and ROM associated with bony or soft tissue surgery.

Prognosis/Plan of Care

Therapeutic ultrasound is an indicated intervention for pain and for shortened deep soft tissue with a high collagen content. A superficial heating agent would not be appropriate because the heat will not penetrate to the

Continued

CLINICAL CASE STUDIES—*cont'd*

hip capsule, and diathermy would not be appropriate because the presence of metal contraindicates diathermy application. Therapeutic ultrasound can reach deep tissues and is not contraindicated in the presence of metal plates and screws. The presence of malignancy should be ruled out, and the patient's sensation in the anterior hip should be assessed prior to initiating treatment. Ultrasound should not be used if the hip fracture was associated with a malignancy. Thermal-level ultrasound should not be used if sensation in the treatment area is not intact.

Intervention

It is proposed that ultrasound be applied over the area of greatest soft tissue shortening, the right anterior groin. A frequency of 1 MHz to reach the depth of the hip joint capsule, a continuous duty cycle to increase tissue temperature and thereby increase soft tissue extensibility, and an intensity of 1.5 to 2.0 W/cm^2, adjusting as necessary so that the patient feels a sensation of mild warmth after 2 to 3 minutes of ultrasound application to produce an adequate increase in the temperature of the hip capsule are recommended. Because the treatment area will probably be in the range of 20 cm^2, a large sound head with an ERA of 10 cm^2 should be used. Given this relationship of sound head ERA to treatment area, ultrasound should be applied for approximately 10 minutes to raise the temperature of the hip capsule to within the therapeutic range of 40° to 45° C. It is essential that the shortened soft tissues be stretched immediately after the ultrasound application and ideally during the ultrasound application as well. Treatment would generally be applied 2 or 3 times per week, consistent with present practice patterns, and should be continued as long as progress is being made toward the treatment goals.

Documentation

S: Pt reports dull pain in R groin and difficulty walking 3 months after hip fx repair.

O: Pretreatment: Decreased R hip PROM in extension (−20 degrees) and abduction (10 degrees R versus 40 degrees L). Tight anteromedial hip capsule. Guarding and spasms in hip adductors and flexors.

Intervention: US to R anterior groin ×10 minutes with stretching during and after. Sound head ERA 10 cm^2. Frequency 1 MHz, continuous duty cycle, intensity 1.5 W/cm^2.

Posttreatment: R hip PROM extension (−10 degrees) and abduction (20 degrees), decreased guarding and spasms in R hip adductors and flexors.

A: Pt tolerated treatment well, with a sensation of mild warmth and improved ROM, and with good increase in ROM.

P: Continue US 2-3 times weekly as above as long as progress continues.

CASE STUDY 7-2

Tendon Healing
Examination
History

BJ is an 18-year-old female college student. She sustained a complete rupture of her left Achilles tendon 6 weeks ago while playing basketball, and the tendon was surgically repaired 2 weeks later. She has been referred for physical therapy to attain a pain-free return to sports as rapidly as possible. She reports mild discomfort at the surgical incision site that increases with walking. Her leg was in a cast, and BJ ambulated without weight bearing on the left, using bilateral axillary crutches, for 4 weeks postoperatively. The cast was removed yesterday, and she has been instructed to walk, bearing weight as tolerated, wearing a heeled "boot." She has been instructed to avoid running or jumping for 6 more weeks.

Tests and Measures

The patient has restricted passive dorsiflexion ROM of −15 degrees on the left compared with +10 degrees on the right. There is also mild swelling, tenderness, and redness in the area of the surgical repair and atrophy of the calf muscles on the left. All other measures are within normal limits.

What do tenderness, swelling, and erythema indicate? How will ultrasound help this patient? What studies should be performed before using ultrasound on this patient?

Evaluation, Diagnosis, Prognosis, and Goals
Evaluation and Goals

ICF Level	Current Status	Goals
Body structure and function	Restricted left dorsiflexion PROM Tenderness, swelling, and erythema at site of surgical repair Atrophy of left calf muscles	Resolve inflammation and limit scar tissue formation Maximize tendon strength in shortest time possible In the longer term, normalize left ankle ROM, normalize left calf size and strength
Activity	Limited ambulation	Return to normal ambulation
Participation	Unable to participate in sports	Return to sports in 2 months

Diagnosis

Preferred Practice Pattern 4I: Impaired joint mobility, motor function, muscle performance, and ROM associated with bony or soft tissue surgery.

Prognosis/Plan of Care

Therapeutic ultrasound may be used at this time for facilitation of tendon repair in order to promote the development of greater strength in the repaired tendon. Therapeutic ultrasound may also promote completion of the inflammation stage of tissue healing and progression to the proliferation and remodeling stages. As the signs of inflammation resolve, ultrasound may be used to increase the temperature of the tendon to facilitate stretching and recovery of normal ankle ROM; however, ultrasound will not promote the recovery of muscle mass or strength.

Because ultrasound should be used with caution over unclosed epiphyseal plates and this patient is of an age where epiphyseal closure may or may not be complete, radiographic studies of skeletal maturity should be performed before applying ultrasound. If the studies indicate that the epiphyseal plates are closed, ultrasound may be applied in the usual manner. If they indicate that the epiphyseal plates are not closed, thermal-level ultrasound should not be used; however, most authors agree that low-level, pulsed ultrasound may be used.

Intervention

It is proposed that ultrasound be applied over the area of the tendon repair. A frequency of 3 MHz is selected to maximize absorption in the Achilles tendon, which is a superficial structure. For the initial treatment, a 20% pulsed duty cycle is used to avoid increasing the tissue temperature, thereby potentially aggravating the inflammatory reaction, and an intensity of 0.5 W/cm² is selected, consistent with the studies demonstrating improved tendon repair with ultrasound. When the signs of inflammation have resolved and the goal of treatment with ultrasound is to increase dorsiflexion ROM, the duty cycle should be increased to 100%, and the intensity may be increased to between 0.5 and 0.75 W/cm² to heat the tendon before stretching. Because the treatment area will probably be in the range of 5 cm², a small sound head with an ERA of 2 to 3 cm² should be used. Given this relationship of sound head ERA to treatment area, ultrasound should be applied for 5 to 10 minutes. Treatment would generally be applied 3 to 5 times per week, depending on the availability of resources and the importance of a rapid functional recovery. In studies demonstrating enhanced tendon healing with the application of therapeutic ultrasound, the ultrasound was applied daily; however, treatment 3 times per week is more consistent with present practice patterns. Because of the contouring of this area and its accessibility, treatment may be applied under water.

Documentation

S: Pt reports L ankle swelling, tenderness, and decreased ROM 4 weeks after Achilles tendon repair.

O: Pretreatment: L ankle dorsiflexion PROM −15 degrees. Mild swelling, tenderness, erythema over surgical repair site. L calf muscle atrophy (midcalf girth 37 cm L, 42 cm R).

Intervention: US applied to left Achilles tendon underwater ×5 minutes. Sound head ERA 2 cm². Frequency 3 MHz, 20% pulsed duty cycle, intensity 0.5 W/cm².

Posttreatment: Decreased tenderness over surgical site.

A: Pt tolerated treatment well.

P: Continue treatment as above 5× weekly for 2 weeks. Initiate stretching when cleared by MD. Consider use of continuous ultrasound to promote tendon stretching at that time.

Wound Healing
Examination
History

JG is an 80-year-old woman with a 10 cm² stage IV infected pressure ulcer over her left greater trochanter. She is bedridden, minimally responsive, and completely dependent on others for feeding and bed mobility as the result of three strokes over the past 5 years. She developed the present ulcer 6 months ago after suffering a loss of appetite because of an upper respiratory infection. JG is turned every 2 hours, avoiding left sidelying, has been placed on systemic antibiotics, and is receiving conventional wound care; however, her wound has not improved in the last month. She has been referred to physical therapy with the hope that the addition of other interventions may promote tissue healing.

Tests and Measures

The patient is not responsive to questions. There is a 3 × 3.5 cm stage IV pressure ulcer with purulent drainage over her left greater trochanter.

Is this an acute or chronic wound? Why is ultrasound a good choice for intervention? Does this patient have any contraindications for the use of ultrasound?

Evaluation, Diagnosis, Prognosis, and Goals
Evaluation and Goals

ICF Level	Current Status	Goals
Body structure and function	Soft tissue ulceration and infection Delayed tissue healing	Resolution of wound infection Decrease wound size Wound closure Prevention of reulceration
Activity	Decreased strength Limited mobility	Increase strength and mobility
Participation	Dependent on others for moving and eating	Decrease dependence on others for activities of daily living (ADLs)

Continued

Diagnosis

Preferred Practice Pattern 7E: Impaired integumentary integrity associated with skin involvement extending into fascia, muscle, or bone and scar formation

Prognosis/Plan of Care

Therapeutic ultrasound has been shown in some studies to facilitate the healing of chronic wounds, including those with infection. Because conventional modes of treatment have failed to promote any improvement in wound status over the last month, it is appropriate to consider the addition of adjunctive treatments, such as ultrasound, to the treatment regimen at this time. The use of ultrasound is not contraindicated in this patient, although thermal-level ultrasound should not be used because the patient is minimally responsive and would therefore not be able to report excessive heating by the ultrasound.

Intervention

In most studies demonstrating improved healing with the application of ultrasound to chronic wounds, ultrasound was applied to the periwound area alone; therefore it is recommended that treatment of this patient should focus on the area of intact periwound skin using a gel conduction medium. A frequency of 3 MHz is selected in accordance with research findings regarding the use of ultrasound for wound healing and to maximize absorption in the superficial tissues surrounding the wound. A 20% pulsed duty cycle is used to produce the nonthermal effects of ultrasound while avoiding increasing tissue temperature. An intensity of 0.5 to 1.0 W/cm^2 is selected, consistent with the studies demonstrating improved wound healing with ultrasound. Because the treatment area is in the range of 10 cm^2, a medium-sized sound head with an ERA of approximately 5 cm^2 should be used. Given this relationship of sound head ERA to treatment area, ultrasound should be applied for 5 to 10 minutes, and the treatment should be provided 3 to 5 times per week, depending on the availability of resources. Treatment with ultrasound should be continued until the wound closes or progress plateaus. One can expect approximately a 30% reduction in wound size per month. It is important to note that standard wound care procedures should be continued when ultrasound is added to the treatment regimen for a chronic wound.

Documentation

S: Minimally responsive pt with nonhealing (6 months) pressure ulcer.

O: Pretreatment: 3 × 3.5 cm stage IV ulcer with purulent drainage over L greater trochanter.

Intervention: US to periwound area with gel transmission medium ×5 minutes. Sound head ERA 5 cm^2. Frequency 3 MHz, 20% pulsed duty cycle, intensity 0.5 W/cm^2.

Posttreatment: Same as before treatment.

A: Pt appeared to be comfortable during US application.

P: Apply US as above 5× weekly until wound closes or stops healing. Monitor wound size. Continue standard wound care. Coordinate pressure relief with nursing staff.

CHAPTER REVIEW

1. Ultrasound is sound with a frequency greater than that audible by the human ear. It is a mechanical compression-rarefaction wave that travels through tissue, producing both thermal and nonthermal effects.

2. The thermal effects of ultrasound can produce increases in the temperature of deep tissue with a high collagen content and thus increase the tissue's extensibility or control pain.

3. The nonthermal effects of ultrasound can alter cell membrane permeability and thus facilitate tissue healing and transdermal drug penetration. Therapeutic ultrasound may also facilitate calcium resorption.

4. To achieve these treatment outcomes, the appropriate frequency, intensity, duty cycle, and duration of ultrasound must be selected and applied.

5. Ultrasound should not be applied in situations where it may aggravate an existing pathology, such as a malignancy, or when it may cause tissue damage, such as a burn.

6. When evaluating an ultrasound device for clinical application, one should consider the appropriateness of the available frequencies, pulsed duty cycles, sizes of sound heads, and BNRs to the types of problems expected to be treated with the device.

7. The reader is referred to the Evolve web site for further exercises and links to resources and references.

ADDITIONAL RESOURCES *evolve*

Web Sites

Chattanooga Group: Chattanooga produces many physical agents, including ultrasound. Photographs of ultrasound units and heads, user manuals, product specifications, and contact information are available on the web site.
www.chattgroup.com

Mettler Electronics: Mettler produces ultrasound, diathermy, and electrical stimulation devices. The web site contains product pictures, brochures, and specifications.
www.mettlerelectronics.com

GLOSSARY *evolve*

General

Absorption: Conversion of the mechanical energy of ultrasound into heat. The amount of absorption that occurs in a tissue type at a specific frequency is expressed by its absorption coefficient, which is determined by measuring the rate of temperature rise in a homogeneous tissue model exposed to an ultrasound field of known intensity. Absorption coefficients are tissue- and frequency-specific. They are highest for tissues with the highest collagen content and increase in proportion to the ultrasound frequency.

Absorption coefficient: The degree to which a material absorbs ultrasound. Note that absorption coefficients are different for different materials and ultrasound frequencies.

Absorption Coefficients in Decibels/Centimeters at 1 and 3 MHz

Tissue	1 MHz	3 MHz
Blood	0.025	0.084
Fat	0.14	0.42
Nerve	0.2	0.6
Muscle (parallel)	0.28	0.84
Muscle (perpendicular)	0.76	2.28
Blood vessels	0.4	1.2
Skin	0.62	1.86
Tendon	1.12	3.36
Cartilage	1.16	3.48
Bone	3.22	

Acoustic streaming: The steady, circular flow of cellular fluids induced by ultrasound. This flow is larger in scale than with microstreaming and is thought to alter cellular activity by transporting material from one part of the ultrasound field to another.[47]

Angiogenesis: The development of new blood vessels at an injury site.

Attenuation: The decrease in ultrasound intensity as ultrasound travels through tissue.

Beam nonuniformity ratio (BNR): The ratio of the spatial peak intensity to the spatial average intensity (Fig. 7-16). For most units this is usually between 5:1 and 6:1, although it can be as low as 2:1. The FDA requires that the maximum BNR for an ultrasound transducer be specified on the device.

Using a transducer with a maximum BNR of 5:1, when the spatial average intensity is set at 1 W/cm², the

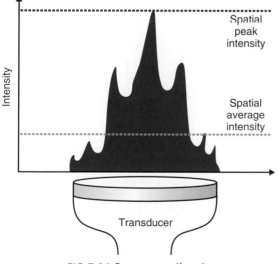

FIG 7-16 Beam nonuniformity.

spatial peak intensity within the field could be as high as 5 W/cm².

Using a transducer with a maximum BNR of 6:1, when the spatial average intensity is set at 1.5 W/cm², the spatial peak intensity within the field could be as high as 9 W/cm².

Cavitation: The formation, growth, and pulsation of gas-filled bubbles caused by ultrasound. During the compression phase of an ultrasound wave, bubbles present in the tissue are made smaller, and during the rarefaction phase, they expand. Cavitation may be stable or unstable (transient). With stable cavitation, the bubbles oscillate in size throughout many cycles but do not burst. With unstable cavitation, the bubbles grow over a number of cycles and then suddenly implode (Fig. 7-17). This implosion produces large, brief, local pressure and temperature increases and causes free radical formation. Stable cavitation has been proposed as a mechanism for the nonthermal therapeutic effects of ultrasound, while unstable cavitation is thought not to occur at the intensities of ultrasound used therapeutically.[165]

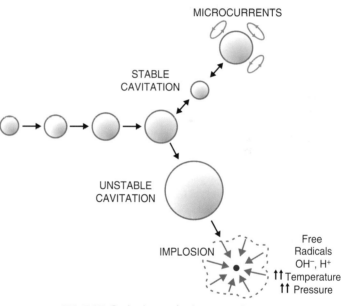

FIG 7-17 Cavitation and microstreaming.

Compression: Increase in density of a material as ultrasound waves pass through it.

Half depth: The depth of tissue at which the ultrasound intensity is half its initial intensity.

Half-Depths in Millimeters at 1 and 3 MHz

Tissue	1 MHz	3 MHz
Water	11,5000	3833
Fat	50	16.5
Muscle (parallel)	24.6	8
Muscle (perpendicular)	9	3
Skin	11.1	4
Tendon	6.2	2
Cartilage	6	2
Bone	2.1	0

Microstreaming: Microscale eddying that takes place near any small, vibrating object. Microstreaming occurs around the gas bubbles set into oscillation by cavitation.[47]

Near field/far field: The ultrasound beam delivered from a transducer initially converges and then diverges (Fig. 7-18). The near field, also known as the Fresnel zone, is the convergent region, and the far field, also known as the Fraunhofer zone, is the divergent region. In the near field, there is interference of the ultrasound beam, causing variations in ultrasound intensity. In the far field, there is little interference, resulting in a more uniform distribution of ultrasound intensity. The length of the near field is dependent on the ultrasound frequency and the ERA of the transducer and can be calculated from the following formula:

$$\text{Length of near field} = \frac{\text{Radius of transducer}^2}{\text{Wavelength of ultrasound}}$$

In most human tissue the majority of the ultrasound intensity is attenuated within the first 2 to 5 cm of tissue depth, which, for transducers of most frequencies and sizes, lies within the near field.

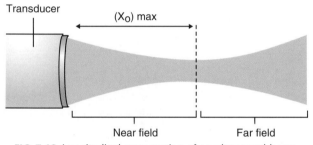

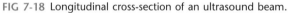

FIG 7-18 Longitudinal cross-section of an ultrasound beam.

Length of the Near Field for Different Frequencies of Ultrasound and Different Areas (ERA) of Ultrasound Transducers

Ultrasound Frequency (MHz)	ERA (cm²)	Length of Near Field (cm)
1	5	11
3	5	33
1	1	2.1
3	1	6.3

Phonophoresis: The application of ultrasound with a topical drug in order to facilitate transdermal drug delivery.

Piezoelectric: The property of being able to generate electricity in response to a mechanical force, or being able to change shape in response to an electrical current (as in an ultrasound transducer).

Rarefaction: Decrease in density of a material as ultrasound waves pass through it.

Reflection: The redirection of an incident beam away from a surface at an angle equal and opposite to the angle of incidence (Fig. 7-19). Ultrasound is reflected at tissue interfaces, with most reflection occurring where

there is the greatest difference between the acoustic impedance of adjacent tissues. In the body, most reflection, about 35%, occurs at soft tissue-bone interfaces. There is 100% reflection of ultrasound at the air-skin interface and only 0.1% reflection at the transmission medium–skin interface. There is no reflection at the transmission medium–sound head interface. A transmission medium that eliminates the air between the sound head and the body is used in order to avoid an air-skin interface with high reflection.

Refraction: The redirection of a wave at an interface (see Fig. 7-19). When refraction occurs, the ultrasound wave enters the tissue at one angle and continues through the tissue at a different angle.

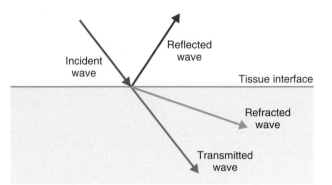

FIG 7-19 Ultrasound reflection and refraction.

Standing Wave: Intensity maxima and minima at fixed positions one-half wavelength apart. Standing waves occur when the ultrasound transducer and a reflecting surface are an exact multiple of wavelengths apart, allowing the reflected wave to superimpose on the incident wave entering the tissue (Fig. 7-20). Standing waves can be avoided by moving the sound head throughout the treatment.

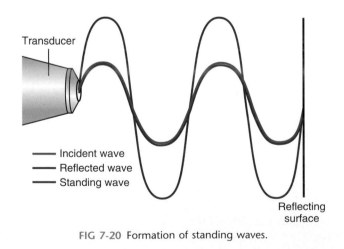

FIG 7-20 Formation of standing waves.

◎ Clinical Pearl

Avoid standing waves by moving the sound head throughout treatment.

Transducer: Also called sound head; a crystal that converts electrical energy into sound. This term is also used to describe the part of an ultrasound unit that contains the crystal.

Ultrasound: Sound with a frequency greater than 20,000 cycles per second that, when applied to the body, has thermal and nonthermal effects (Fig 7-21).

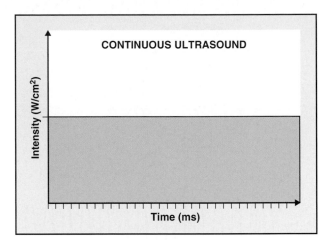

FIG 7-22 Continuous ultrasound.

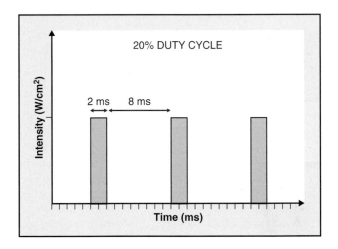

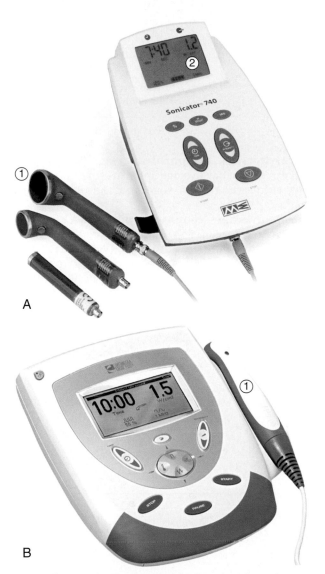

FIG 7-21 Ultrasound units: *1,* transducer; *2,* power/intensity indicator. *A, Courtesy Mettler Electronics, Anaheim, CA; B, courtesy Chattanooga Group, Hixson, TN.*

Treatment Parameters

Continuous ultrasound: Continuous delivery of ultrasound throughout the treatment period (Fig. 7-22).

Duty cycle: The proportion of the total treatment time that the ultrasound is on. This can be expressed either as a percentage or a ratio: 20% or 1:5 duty cycle, is on 20% of the time and off 80% of the time and generally delivered 2 ms on, 8 ms off (Fig. 7-23); 100% duty cycle is on 100% of the time and is the same as continuous ultrasound.

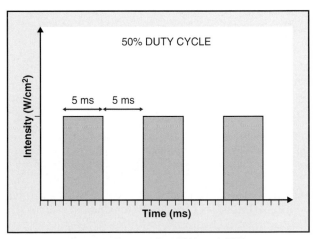

FIG 7-23 Duty cycles: 20% and 50%.

Effective radiating area (ERA): The area of the transducer from which the ultrasound energy radiates (Fig. 7-24). Because the crystal does not vibrate uniformly, the ERA is always smaller than the area of the treatment head.

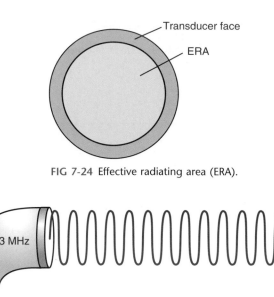

FIG 7-24 Effective radiating area (ERA).

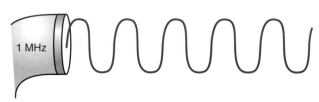

FIG 7-25 Ultrasound frequencies: 1 and 3 MHz.

Frequency: The number of compression-rarefaction cycles per unit of time, expressed in cycles per second, or hertz (Hz) (Fig. 7-25). Therapeutic ultrasound is usually in the frequency range of 1 to 3 million cycles per second (i.e., 1 to 3 MHz). Increasing the frequency of ultrasound causes a decrease in its depth of penetration and concentration of the ultrasound energy in the superficial tissues (Fig. 7-26).

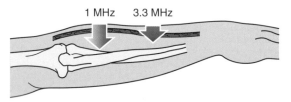

FIG 7-26 Frequency controls the depth of penetration of ultrasound; 1 MHz ultrasound penetrates approximately 3 times as far as 3.3 MHz ultrasound. *Courtesy Mettler Electronics, Anaheim, CA.*

Intensity: The power per unit area of the sound head, expressed in watts per centimeter squared (W/cm²) The World Health Organization limits the average intensity output by therapeutic ultrasound units to 3 W/cm².[166]

Power: The amount of acoustic energy per unit time, expressed in watts (W).

Pulsed ultrasound: Intermittent delivery of ultrasound during the treatment period. Delivery of ultrasound is pulsed on and off throughout the treatment period. Pulsing the ultrasound minimizes its thermal effects (Fig. 7-27).

Spatial average intensity: The average intensity of the ultrasound output over the area of the transducer.

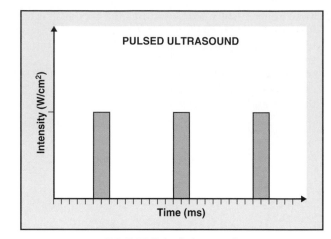

FIG 7-27 Pulsed ultrasound.

Spatial average temporal average (SATA) intensity: The spatial average intensity of the ultrasound averaged over the on time and the off time of the pulse.

Spatial average temporal peak (SATP) intensity: The spatial average intensity of the ultrasound during the on time of the pulse (Fig. 7-28). This is a measure of the amount of energy delivered to the tissue. SATA units are frequently used in the nonclinical literature on ultrasound. Note that clinical ultrasound units generally display the SATP intensity when pulsed ultrasound is applied. In this chapter, all intensities are expressed as SATP, followed by the duty cycle, unless stated otherwise. Note that SATA is equal to SATP for continuous ultrasound:

$$SATP \times duty\ cycle = SATA$$

$$1\ W/cm^2\ SATP\ at\ 20\%\ duty\ cycle = 1 \times 0.2 = 0.2\ W/cm^2\ SATA$$

$$1\ W/cm^2\ SATP\ at\ 100\%\ duty\ cycle = 1 \times 1 = 1\ W/cm^2\ SATA$$

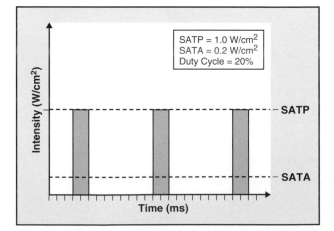

FIG 7-28 Spatial average temporal peak (SATP) and spatial average temporal average (SATA) intensity.

Spatial peak intensity: The peak intensity of the ultrasound output over the area of the transducer. The intensity is usually greatest in the center of the beam and lowest at the edges of the beam.

REFERENCES *evolve*

1. Pye SD, Milford C: The performance of ultrasound physiotherapy machines in Lothian Region, Scotland, 1992, *Ultrasound Med Biol* 20(4):347-359, 1994.
2. Chapelon JY, Cathignol D, Cain C, et al: New piezoelectric transducers for therapeutic ultrasound, *Ultrasound Med Biol* 26(1):153-159, 2000.
3. Gallo JA, Draper DO, Brody LT, Fellingham GW: A comparison of human muscle temperature increases during 3-MHz continuous and pulsed ultrasound with equivalent temporal average intensities, *J Orthop Sports Phys Ther* 34(7):395-401, 2004.
4. Baker KG, Robertson VJ, Duck FA: A review of therapeutic ultrasound: biophysical effects, *Phys Ther* 81(7):1351-1358, 2001.
5. Harvey EN: Biological aspects of ultrasonic waves: a general survey, *Biol Bull* 59:306-325, 1930.
6. Lehmann JF: *Ultrasound therapy in therapeutic heat and cold*, ed 4, Baltimore, 1990, Williams & Wilkins.
7. Lehmann JF, DeLateur BJ, Stonebridge JB, et al: Therapeutic temperature distribution produced by ultrasound as modified by dosage and volume of tissue exposed, *Arch Phys Med Rehabil* 48:662-666, 1967.
8. Lehmann JF, DeLateur BJ, Warren G, et al: Bone and soft tissue heating produced by ultrasound, *Arch Phys Med Rehabil* 48:397-401, 1967.
9. Weaver SL, Demchak TJ, Stone MB, et al: Effect of transducer velocity on intramuscular temperature during a 1-MHz ultrasound treatment, *J Orthop Sports Phys Ther* 36(5):320-325, 2006.
10. Nyborg WN, Ziskin MC: Biological effects of ultrasound, *Clin Diagn Ultrasound* 16:24, 1985.
11. Hayes BT, Merrick MA, Sandrey MA, et al: Three-MHz ultrasound heats deeper into the tissues than originally theorized, *J Athl Train* 39(3):230-234, 2004.
12. Draper DO, Castel JC, Castel D: Rate of temperature increase in human muscle during 1 MHz and 3 MHz continuous ultrasound, *J Orthop Sport Phys Ther* 22(4):142-150, 1995.
13. Levine D, Mills DL, Mynatt T: Effects of 3.3-MHz ultrasound on caudal thigh muscle temperature in dogs, *Vet Surg* 30(2):170-174, 2001.
14. Darlas Y, Solasson A, Clouard R, et al: Ultrasonotherapie: calcul de la thermogenese, *Ann Readaptation Med Phys* 32:181-192, 1989.
15. TerHaar G: Basic physics of therapeutic ultrasound, *Physiotherapy* 64(4):100-103, 1978.
16. Merrick MA, Bernard KD, Devor ST, et al: Identical 3-MHz ultrasound treatments with different devices produce different intramuscular temperatures, *J Orthop Sports Phys Ther* 33(7):379-385, 2003.
17. Lehmann JF, Stonebridge JB, DeLateur BJ, et al: Temperatures in human thighs after hot pack treatment followed by ultrasound, *Arch Phys Med Rehabil* 59:472-475, 1978.
18. Oshikoya CA, Shultz SJ, Mistry D, et al: Effect of coupling medium temperature on rate of intramuscular temperature rise using continuous ultrasound, *J Athl Train* 35(4):417-421, 2000.
19. Draper DO, Schulties S, Sorvisto P, et al: Temperature changes in deep muscle of humans during ice and ultrasound therapies: an in vivo study, *J Orthop Sport Phys Ther* 21(3):153-157, 1995.
20. Kurtais Gursel Y, Ulus Y, Bilgic A, et al: Adding ultrasound in the management of soft tissue disorders of the shoulder: a randomized placebo-controlled trial, *Phys Ther* 84(4):336-343, 2004.
21. Harle J, Salih V, Mayia F, et al: Effects of ultrasound on the growth and function of bone and periodontal ligament cells in vitro, *Ultrasound Med Biol* 27(4):579-586, 2001.
22. Mortimer AJ, Dyson M: The effect of therapeutic ultrasound on calcium uptake in fibroblasts, *Ultrasound Med Biol* 14(6):499-506, 1988.
23. Dinno MA, Crum LA, Wu J: The effect of therapeutic ultrasound on electrophysiological parameters of frog skin, *Ultrasound Med Biol* 15(5):461-470, 1989.
24. Fyfe MC, Chahl LA: Mast cell degranulation: a possible mechanism of action of therapeutic ultrasound, *Ultrasound Med Biol* 8(suppl 1):62, 1982.
25. Young SR, Dyson M: Macrophage responsiveness to therapeutic ultrasound, *Ultrasound Med Biol* 16(8):809-816, 1990.
26. Harvey W, Dyson M, Pond JB, et al: The stimulation of protein synthesis in human fibroblasts by therapeutic ultrasound, *Rheumatol Rehabil* 14:237, 1975.
27. Tsai WC, Pang JH, Hsu CC, et al: Ultrasound stimulation of types I and III collagen expression of tendon cell and upregulation of transforming growth factor beta, *J Orthop Res* 24(6):1310-1316, 2006.
28. Altland OD, Dalecki D, Suchkova VN, et al: Low-intensity ultrasound increases endothelial cell nitric oxide synthase activity and nitric oxide synthesis, *J Thromb Haem* 2(4):637-643, 2004.
29. Hsu SH, Huang TB: Bioeffect of ultrasound on endothelial cells in vitro, *Biomol Eng* 21(3-5):99-104, 2004.
30. Rawool NM, Goldberg BB, Forsberg F, et al: Power Doppler assessment of vascular changes during fracture treatment with low-intensity ultrasound, *J Ultrasound Med* 22(2):145-153, 2003.
31. Barzelai S, Sharabani-Yosef O, Holbova R, et al: Low-intensity ultrasound induces angiogenesis in rat hind-limb ischemia, *Ultrasound Med Biol* 32(1):139-145, 2006.
32. Kopakkala-Tani M, Karjalainen HM, Karjalainen T, et al: Ultrasound stimulates proteoglycan synthesis in bovine primary chondrocytes, *Biorheology* 43(3-4):271-282, 2006.
33. Miyamoto K, An HS, Sah RL, et al: Exposure to pulsed low intensity ultrasound stimulates extracellular matrix metabolism of bovine intervertebral disc cells cultured in alginate beads, *Spine* 30(21):2398-2405, 2005.
34. Choi BH, Woo JI, Min BH, et al: Low-intensity ultrasound stimulates the viability and matrix gene expression of human articular chondrocytes in alginate bead culture, *J Biomed Materials Res Part A* 79(4):858-864, 2006.
35. Min BH, Woo JI, Cho HS: Effects of low-intensity ultrasound (LIUS) stimulation on human cartilage explants, *Scand J Rheumatol* 35(4):305-311, 2006.
36. Dinno MA, Al-Karmi AM, Stoltz DA, et al: Effect of free radical scavengers on changes in ion conductance during exposure to therapeutic ultrasound, *Membr Biochem* 10(4):237-247, 1993.
37. Parvizi J, Parpura V, Greenleaf JF, et al: Calcium signaling is required for ultrasound-stimulated aggrecan synthesis by rat chondrocytes, *J Orthop Res* 20(1):51-57, 2002.
38. Robertson VJ, Baker KG: A review of therapeutic ultrasound: effectiveness studies, *Phys Ther* 81(7):1339-1350, 2001.
39. van der Windt DAWM, van der Heijden GJMG, van der Berg SG, et al: Ultrasound therapy for musculoskeletal disorders: a systematic review, *Pain* 81:257-271, 1999.
40. Baba-Akbari SA, Flemming K, Cullum NA, et al: Therapeutic ultrasound for pressure ulcers, *Cochrane Database Syst Rev* 3: CD001275, 2006.
41. Busse JW, Bhandari M, Kulkarni AV, et al: The effect of low-intensity pulsed ultrasound therapy on time to fracture healing: a meta-analysis. *Canadian Med Assoc J* 166(4):437-441, 2002.
42. Warren CG, Lehmann JF, Koblanski JN: Elongation of rat tail tendon: effect of load and temperature, *Arch Phys Med* 52:465, 1971.
43. Lehmann JF, Masock AJ, Warren CG, et al: Effects of therapeutic temperatures on tendon extensibility, *Arch Phys Med* 51:481, 1970.
44. Lehmann JF: Clinical evaluation of a new approach in the treatment of contracture associated with hip fracture after internal fixation, *Arch Phys Med Rehabil* 42:95, 1961.
45. Usuba M, Miyanaga Y, Miyakawa S, et al: Effect of heat in increasing the range of knee motion after the development of a joint contracture: an experiment with an animal model, *Arch Phys Med Rehabil* 87(2):247-253, 2006.
46. Wessling KC, DeVane DA, Hylton CR: Effects of static stretch versus static stretch and ultrasound combined on triceps surae

muscle extensibility in healthy women, *Phys Ther* 67(5):674-679, 1987.

47. Kramer JF: Ultrasound: Evaluation of its mechanical and thermal effects, *Arch Phys Med Rehabil* 65:223-227, 1984.

48. Reed BV, Ashikaga T, Fleming BC, et al: Effects of ultrasound and stretch on knee ligament extensibility, *J Orthop Sports Phys Ther* 30:341-347, 2000.

49. Hsieh YL: Reduction in induced pain by ultrasound may be caused by altered expression of spinal neuronal nitric oxide synthase-producing neurons, *Arch Phys Med Rehabil* 86(7):1311-1317, 2005.

50. Hsieh YL: Effects of ultrasound and diclofenac phonophoresis on inflammatory pain relief: suppression of inducible nitric oxide synthase in arthritic rats, *Phys Ther* 86(1):39-49, 2006.

51. Middlemast S, Chatterjee DS: Comparison of ultrasound and thermotherapy for soft tissue injuries, *Physiotherapy* 64(11):331-332, 1978.

52. Nwuge VCB: Ultrasound in treatment of back pain resulting from prolapsed disc, *Arch Phys Med Rehabil* 64:88-89, 1983.

53. Munting E: Ultrasonic therapy for painful shoulders, *Physiotherapy* 64(6):180-181, 1978.

54. Robinson V, Brosseau L, Casimiro L, et al: Thermotherapy for treating rheumatoid arthritis. *Cochrane Database Syst Rev* 2: CD002826, 2002.

55. Flemming K, Cullum N: Therapeutic ultrasound for venous leg ulcers, *Cochrane Database Syst Rev* 4:CD001180, 2000.

56. Flemming K, Cullum H: Therapeutic ultrasound for pressure sores, *Cochrane Database Syst Rev* 4: CD001275, 2000.

57. Dyson M, Suckling J: Stimulation of tissue repair by ultrasound: survey of the mechanisms involved, *Physiotherapy* 63:105-108, 1978.

58. McDiarmid T, Burns PN, Lewith GT, et al: Ultrasound and the treatment of pressure sores, *Physiotherapy* 71(2):66-70, 1985.

59. Lundeberg T, Nordstrom F, Brodda-Jansen G, et al: Pulsed ultrasound does not improve healing of venous ulcers, *Scand J Rehabil Med* 22:195-197, 1990.

60. Eriksson SV, Lundeberg T, Malm M: A placebo-controlled trial of ultrasound therapy in chronic leg ulceration, *Scand J Rehabil Med* 23:211-213, 1991.

61. TerRiet G, Kessels AGH, Knipschild P: A randomized clinical trial of ultrasound in the treatment of pressure ulcers, *Phys Ther* 76(12):1301-1312, 1996.

62. Markert CD, Merrick MA, Kirby TE, et al: Nonthermal ultrasound and exercise in skeletal muscle regeneration, *Arch Phys Med Rehabil* 86(7):1304-1310, 2005.

63. Ennis WJ, Valdes W, Gainer M, et al: Evaluation of clinical effectiveness of MIST ultrasound therapy for the healing of chronic wounds, *Adv Skin Wound Care* 19(8):437-446, 2006.

64. Ennis WJ, Foreman P, Mozen N, et al: Ultrasound therapy for recalcitrant diabetic foot ulcers: results of a randomized, double-blind, controlled, multicenter study, *Ostomy Wound Manage* 51(8):24-39, 2005.

65. Kavros SJ, Miller JL, Hanna SW: Treatment of ischemic wounds with noncontact, low-frequency ultrasound: The Mayo Clinic experience, 2004-2006, *Adv Skin Wound Care* 20(4):221-226, 2007.

66. Thawer HA, Houghton PE: Effects of ultrasound delivered through a mist of saline to wounds in mice with diabetes mellitus, *J Wound Care* 13(5):171-176, 2004.

67. Young SR, Dyson M: The effect of therapeutic ultrasound on angiogenesis, *Ultrasound Med Biol* 16(3):261-269, 1990.

68. Byl NN, McKenzie AL, West JM, et al: Low dose ultrasound effects on wound healing: a controlled study with Yucatan pigs, *Arch Phys Med Rehabil* 73:656-664, 1992.

69. Byl NN, McKenzie AL, Wong T, et al: Incisional wound healing: a controlled study of low dose and high dose ultrasound, *J Orthop Sport Phys Ther* 18(5):619-628, 1993.

70. Emsen IM: The effect of ultrasound on flap survival: an experimental study in rats, *Burns* 33(3):369-371, 2007.

71. Ferguson HN: Ultrasound in the treatment of surgical wounds, *Physiotherapy* 67(2):43, 1981.

72. Fieldhouse C: Ultrasound for relief of painful episiotomy scars, *Physiotherapy* 65(7):217, 1979.

73. Binder A, Hodge G, Greenwood AM, et al: Is therapeutic ultrasound effective in treating soft tissue lesions? *Br Med J* 290:512-514, 1985.

74. Ebenbichler GR, Erdogmus CB, Resch KL, et al: Ultrasound therapy for calcific tendinitis of the shoulder, *N Engl J Med* 340:1533-1538, 1999.

75. Lundeberg T, Abrahamsson P, Haker E: A comparative study of continuous ultrasound, placebo ultrasound and rest in epicondylalgia, *Scand J Rehab Med* 20:99-101, 1988.

76. Haker E, Lundeberg T: Pulsed ultrasound treatment in lateral epicondylitis, *Scand J Rehab Med* 23:115-118, 1991.

77. D'Vaz AP, Ostor AJ, Speed CA et al: Pulsed low-intensity ultrasound therapy for chronic lateral epicondylitis: a randomized controlled trial, *Rheumatology* 45(5):566-570, 2006.

78. Downing DS, Weinstein A: Ultrasound therapy of subacromial bursitis: a double blind trial, *Phys Ther* 66(2):194-199, 1986.

79. Enwemeka CS: The effects of therapeutic ultrasound on tendon healing, *Am J Phys Med Rehabil* 6:283-287, 1989.

80. Enwemeka CS, Rodriguez O, Mendosa S: The biomechanical effects of low intensity ultrasound on healing tendons, *Ultrasound Med Biol* 16(8):801-807, 1990.

81. Frieder SJ, Weisberg B, Fleming B, et al: A pilot study: the therapeutic effect of ultrasound following partial rupture of Achilles tendons in male rats, *L Orthop Sport Phys Ther* 10:39-46, 1988.

82. Jackson BA, Schwane JA, Starcher BC: Effect of ultrasound therapy on the repair of Achilles tendon injuries in rats, *Med Sci Sport Exerc* 23(2):171-176, 1991.

83. Ng CO, Ng GY, See EK, Leung MC: Therapeutic ultrasound improves strength of Achilles tendon repair in rats, *Ultrasound Med Biol* 29(10):1501-1506, 2003.

84. Ng GY, Ng CO, See EK: Comparison of therapeutic ultrasound and exercises for augmenting tendon healing in rats, *Ultrasound Med Biol* 30(11):1539-1543, 2004.

85. Yeung CK, Guo X, Ng YF: Pulsed ultrasound treatment accelerates the repair of Achilles tendon rupture in rats, *J Orthop Res* 24(2):193-201, 2006.

86. da Cunha A, Parizotto NA, Vidal Bde C: The effect of therapeutic ultrasound on repair of the Achilles tendon (tendo calcaneus) of the rat, *Ultrasound Med Biol* 27(12):1691-1696, 2001.

87. Demir H, Menku P, Kirnap M, et al: Comparison of the effects of laser, ultrasound, and combined laser + ultrasound treatments in experimental tendon healing, *Lasers Surg Med* 35(1):84-89, 2004.

88. Roberts M, Rutherford JH, Harris D: The effect of ultrasound on flexor tendon repairs in rabbits, *Hand* 14(1):17-20, 1982.

89. Turner SM, Powell ES, Ng CS: The effect of ultrasound on healing of repaired cockerel tendon: is collagen cross-linkage a factor? *J Hand Surg* 14B(4):428-433, 1989.

90. Sparrow KJ, Finucane SD, Owen JR, et al: The effects of low-intensity ultrasound on medial collateral ligament healing in the rabbit model, *Am J Sports Med* 33(7):1048-1056, 2005.

91. Warden SJ, Avin GA, Beck EM, et al: Low-intensity pulsed ultrasound accelerates and a nonsteroidal anti-inflammatory drug delays knee ligament healing, *Am J Sports Med* 34:1094-1102, 2006.

92. Leung MC, Ng GY, Yip KK: Effect of ultrasound on acute inflammation of transected medial collateral ligaments, *Arch Phys Med Rehabil* 85(6):963-966, 2004.

93. Cline PD: Radiographic follow-up of ultrasound therapy in calcific bursitis, *Phys Ther* 43:16, 1963.

94. Gorkiewicz R: Ultrasound for subacromial bursitis: a case report, *Phys Ther* 64(1):46-47, 1984.

95. Rahman MH, Khan SZ, Ramiz MS: Effect of therapeutic ultrasound on calcific supraspinatus tendinitis, *Mymensigh Med J* 16(1):33-35, 2007.

96. Griffin J, Karselis T: *Physical agents for physical therapists*, Springfield, IL, 1982, Charles C Thomas.

97. Hecox B, Mehreteab TA, Weisberg J: *Physical agents: a comprehensive text for physical therapists*, East Norwalk, CT, 1994, Appleton & Lange.

98. Fukada E, Yasuda I: On the piezoelectric effect of bone, *J Phys Soc Jap* 12:10, 1957.

99. Duarte LR: The stimulation of bone growth by ultrasound, *Archiv Orthop Trauma Surg* 101:153-159, 1983.

100. Pilla AA, Mont MA, Nasser PR, et al: Non-invasive low-intensity ultrasound accelerates bone healing in the rabbit, *J Orthop Trauma* 4(3):246-253, 1990.

101. Malizos KN, Hantes ME, Protopappas V, et al: Low-intensity pulsed ultrasound for bone healing: an overview, *Injury* 37 (suppl 1):S56-62, 2006.

102. Kristiansen T, Pilla AA, Siffert RS, et al: A multicenter study of Colles' fracture healing by noninvasive low intensity ultrasound. Presented at the 57th meeting of the American Association of Orthopedic Surgeons, New Orleans, February 1990.

103. Heckman JD, Ryaby JP, McCabe J, et al: Acceleration of tibial fracture healing by non-invasive, low-intensity pulsed ultrasound, *J Bone Joint Surg* 76A(1):26-34, 1994.

104. Kristiansen TK, Ryaby JP, McCabe J, et al: Accelerated healing of distal radial fractures with the use of specific, low-intensity ultrasound. A multicenter, prospective, randomized, double-blind, placebo-controlled study. *J Bone Joint Surg* 79A(7):961-973, 1997.

105. Ricardo M: The effect of ultrasound on the healing of muscle-pediculated bone graft in scaphoid non-union, *Int Orthop* 30(2):123-127, 2006.

106. Handolin L, Kiljunen V, Arnala I, et al: Effect of ultrasound therapy on bone healing of lateral malleolar fractures of the ankle joint fixed with bioabsorbable screws, *J Orthop Sci* 10(4):391-395, 2005.

107. Warden SJ, Fuchs RK, Kessler CK, et al: Ultrasound produced by a conventional therapeutic ultrasound unit accelerates fracture repair, *Phys Ther* 86(8):1118-1127, 2006.

108. Nolte PA, van der Krans A, Patka P, et al: Low-intensity pulsed ultrasound in the treatment of nonunions, *J Trauma* 51(4):693-703, 2001.

109. Gebauer D, Mayr E, Orthner E, et al: Low-intensity pulsed ultrasound: effects on nonunions, *Ultrasound Med Biol* 31(10):1391-1402, 2005.

110. Takikawa A, Matsui N, Kokubu T, et al: Low-intensity pulsed ultrasound initiates bone healing in rat nonunion fracture model, *J Ultrasound Med* 20(3):197-205, 2001.

111. Hantes ME, Mavrodontidis AN, Zalavras CG, et al: Low-intensity transosseous ultrasound accelerates osteotomy healing in a sheep fracture model. *J Bone Joint Surg* 86A(10):2275-2282, 2004.

112. Protopappas VC, Baga DA, Fotiadis PG, et al: An ultrasound wearable system for the monitoring and acceleration of fracture healing in long bones, *IEEE Trans Biomed Eng* 52(9):1597-1608, 2005.

113. Malizos KN, Papachristos AA, Protopappas VC, et al: Transosseous application of low-intensity ultrasound for the enhancement and monitoring of fracture healing process in a sheep osteotomy model, *Bone* 38(4):530-539, 2006.

114. Herrick JF: Temperatures produced in tissues by ultrasound: experimental study using various technics, *J Acoust Soc Am* 25:12-16, 1953.

115. Oztas O, Turan B, Bora I, et al: Ultrasound therapy effect in carpal tunnel syndrome, *Arch Phys Med Rehabil* 79(12):1540-1544, 1988.

116. Ebenbichler GR, Resch KL, Nicolakis P, et al: Ultrasound treatment for treating the carpal tunnel syndrome: randomised "sham" controlled trial, *BMJ* 316:731-735, 1988.

117. Piravej K, Boonhong J: Effect of ultrasound thermotherapy in mild to moderate carpal tunnel syndrome, *J Med Assoc Thailand,* 87 (suppl 2):S100-106, 2004.

118. McNeill SC, Potts RO, Francoer ML: Local enhanced topical drug delivery (LETD) of drugs: does it truly exist? *Pharm Res* 9:1422-1427, 1992.

119. Fellinger K, Schmid J: *Klinik und Therapie des Chronischen Gelenkheumatismus*, Vienna, 1954, Maudrich.

120. Griffin JE, Touchstone JC: Ultrasonic movement of cortisol into pig tissues. I. Movement into skeletal muscle, *Am J Phys Med* 42:77-85, 1963.

121. Griffin JE, Touchstone JC, Liu ACY: Ultrasonic movement of cortisol into pig tissues. II: Movement into paravertebral nerve, *Am J Phys Med* 44:20-25, 1965.

122. Griffin JE, Touchstone JC: Low intensity phonophoresis of cortisol in swine, *Phys Ther* 48:1336-1344, 1968.

123. Griffin JE, Touchstone JC: Effects of ultrasonic frequency on phonophoresis of cortisol into swine tissues, *Am J Phys Med* 51:62-78, 1972.

124. Mitragotri S, Farrell J, Tang H, et al: Determination of threshold energy dose for ultrasound-induced transdermal drug transport, *J Control Release* 63(1-2):41-52, 2000.

125. Bommannan D, Okuyama H, Stauffer P, et al: Sonophoresis. I. The use of high frequency ultrasound to enhance transdermal drug delivery, *Pharm Res* 9:559-564, 1992.

126. Tang H, Mitragotri S, Blankschtein D, et al: Theoretical description of transdermal transport of hydrophilic permeants: application to low-frequency sonophoresis, *J Pharm Sci* 90(5):545-568, 2001.

127. Mitragotri S: Effect of therapeutic ultrasound on partition and diffusion coefficients in human stratum corneum, *J Control Release* 71(1):23-29, 2001.

128. Nokhodchi A, Shokri J, Dashbolaghi A, et al: The enhancement effect of surfactants on the penetration of lorazepam through rat skin, *Int J Pharm* 250(2):359-369, 2003.

129. Lavon I, Grossman N, Kost J: The nature of ultrasound-SLS synergism during enhanced transdermal transport, *J Control Release* 107(3):484-494, 2005.

130. Franklin ME, Smith ST, Chenier TC, et al: Effect of phonophoresis with dexamethasone on adrenal function, *J Orthop Sport Phys Ther* 22(3):103-107, 1995.

131. Mitragotri S, Kost J: Low-frequency sonophoresis: a review, *Adv Drug Deliv Rev* 56(5):589-601, 2004.

132. Mitragotri S, Blankschtein D, Langer R: Transdermal drug delivery using low-frequency sonophoresis, *Pharm Res* 13(3):411-420, 1996.

133. Merino G, Kalia YN, Delgado-Charro MB, et al: Frequency and thermal effects on the enhancement of transdermal transport by sonophoresis, *J Control Release* 88(1):85-94, 2003.

134. Smith NB, Lee S, Malone E, et al: Ultrasound-mediated transdermal transport of insulin in vitro through human skin using novel transducer designs, *Ultrasound Med Biol* 29(2):311-317, 2003.

135. Chuang H, Taylor E, Davison TW: Clinical evaluation of a continuous minimally invasive glucose flux sensor placed over ultrasonically permeated skin, *Diabetes Technol Ther* 6(1):21-30, 2004.

136. Merino G, Kalia YN, Guy RH: Ultrasound-enhanced transdermal transport, *J Pharm Sci* 92(6):1125-1137, 2003.

137. Byl NN: The use of ultrasound as an enhancer for transcutaneous drug delivery: phonophoresis, *Phys Ther* 75(6):539-553, 1995.

138. Tachibana K, Tachibana S: The use of ultrasound for drug delivery, *Echocardiography* 18(4):323-328, 2001.

139. Kleinkort JA, Wood AF: Phonophoresis with 1% versus 10% hydrocortisone, *Phys Ther* 55:1320-1324, 1975.

140. Cameron MH, Monroe LG: Relative transmission of ultrasound by media customarily used for phonophoresis, *Phys Ther* 72:142-148, 1992.

141. Kuntz AR, Griffiths CM, Rankin JM, et al: Cortisol concentrations in human skeletal muscle tissue after phonophoresis with 10% hydrocortisone gel, *J Athl Train* 41(3):321-324, 2006.

142. Levy D, Kost J, Meshulam Y, et al: Effect of ultrasound on transdermal drug delivery to rats and guinea pigs, *J Clin Invest* 83:2074-2078, 1989.

143. Kozanoglu E, Basaran S, Guzel R, et al: Short term efficacy of ibuprofen phonophoresis versus continuous ultrasound therapy in knee osteoarthritis, *Swiss Med Weekly* 133(23-24):333-338, 2003.

144. Bakurt F, Ozcan A, Algun C: Comparison of effects of phonophoresis and iontophoresis of naproxen in the treatment of lateral epicondylitis, *Clin Rehab* 17(1):96-100, 2003.

145. Cagnie B, Vinck E, Rimbaut S, et al: Phonophoresis versus topical application of ketoprofen: comparison between tissue and plasma levels, *Phys Ther* 83(8):707-712, 2003.

146. Brucks R, Nanavaty M, Jung D, et al: The effect of ultrasound on the in vitro penetration of ibuprofen through human epidermis, *Pharm Res* 6(8):697-701, 1989.

147. Sicard-Rosenbaum L, Lord D, Danoff JV, et al: Effects of continuous therapeutic ultrasound on growth and metastasis of subcutaneous murine tumors, *Phys Ther* 75(1):3-11, 1995.

148. Marmor JB, Pounds D, Hahn GM: Treating spontaneous tumors in dogs and cats by ultrasound-induced hyperthermia, *Int J Radiat Oncol Biol Phys* 4:967-973, 1978.

149. Marmor JB, Hilerio FB, Hahn GM: Tumor eradication and cell survival after localized hyperthermia induced by ultrasound, *Cancer Res* 39:2166-2171, 1979.

150. Smachlo K, Fridd CW, Child SZ, et al: Ultrasonic treatment of tumors. I Absence of metastases following treatment of a hamster fibrosarcoma, *Ultrasound Med Biol* 5:45-49, 1979.

151. Shista K: Neural tube defects and maternal hyperthermia in early pregnancy: epidemiology in a human embryo population, *Am J Med Genet* 12:281-288, 1982.

152. Kalter H, Warkany J: Congenital malformations: etiological factors and their role in prevention, *N Engl J Med* 308:424-431, 1983.

153. McLeod DR, Fowlow SB: Multiple malformations and exposure to therapeutic ultrasound during organogenesis, *Am J Med Genet* 34:317-319, 1989.

154. Carstensen EL, Gates AH: The effects of pulsed ultrasound on the fetus, *J Ultrasound Med* 3:145-147, 1984.

155. National Council of Radiation Protection and Measurements: *Biological effects of ultrasound: mechanisms and clinical implications*, NCRP Report No. 74. Bethesda, MD, 1983, The Council.

156. Ang ES Jr, Gluncic V, Duque A, et al: Prenatal exposure to ultrasound waves impacts neuronal migration in mice, *Proc National Acad Sci USA* 103(34):12903-12910, 2006.

157. Normand H, Darlas Y, Solassol A, et al: Etude experimentale de l'effet thermique des ultrasons sur le materiel prothetique, *Ann Readaptation Med Phys* 32:193-201, 1989.

158. Skoubo-Kristensen E, Sommer J: Ultrasound influence on internal fixation with rigid plate in dogs, *Arch Phys Med Rehabil* 63:371-373, 1982.

159. Deforest RE, Herrick JF, Janes JM: Effects of ultrasound on growing bone: an experimental study, *Arch Phys Med Rehab* 34:21, 1953.

160. Spadaro JA, Skarulis T, Albanese SA: Effect of pulsed ultrasound on bone growth in rats. Proceedings of the 14th Annual Meeting of the Society for Physical Regulation in Biology and Medicine, Washington DC, 1994.

161. Nyborg WL: Biological effects of ultrasound: development of safety guidelines. II. General review, *Ultrasound Med Biol* 27(3):301-333, 2001.

162. Dyson M, Pond JB, Woodward B, et al: The production of blood cell stasis and endothelial damage in blood vessels of chick embryos treated with ultrasound in a stationary wave field, *Ultrasound Med Biol* 63:133-138, 1974.

163. TerHaar GR, Dyson M, Smith SP: Ultrastructural changes in the mouse uterus brought about by ultrasonic irradiation at therapeutic intensities in standing wave fields, *Ultrasound Med Biol* 5:167-179, 1979.

164. Schabrun S, Chipchase L, Rickard H: Are therapeutic ultrasound units a potential vector for nosocomial infection? *Physiother Res Int* 11(2):61-71, 2006.

165. Goodman CE, Al-Karmi AM, Joyce JM, et al: The biological effects of therapeutic ultrasound: frequency dependence. Proceedings of the 14th annual meeting of the Society for Physical Regulation in Biology and Medicine, Washington DC, 1994.

166. Hill CR, Ter Haar G: *Ultrasound and non-ionizing radiation protection*, Copenhagen, 1981, World Health Organization.

Chapter 8

Electrical Currents

Sara Shapiro

TERMINOLOGY

The terminology used to describe electrical stimulation is complex and can be confusing. Clinicians, manufacturers, researchers, educators, and engineers often use different words to denote the same feature or parameter and there are many different parameters that need to be identified. In an attempt to standardize the terminology used to describe therapeutic electrical currents, in 1986 the Clinical Electrophysiology Section of the American Physical Therapy Association (APTA) published a guide to electrical stimulation terminology that included recommended standard terminology and definitions. A second edition of this guide was published in 2000.[1] This guide has helped promote more consistent use of terms describing therapeutic electric currents. However, this terminology is not consistently adhered to. This chapter uses the terminology and definitions provided in the APTA guide; however, because a variety of terms are in use, alternative commonly used terms are also noted in the glossary. In this chapter, we particularly recommend that the reader become familiar with the terms listed at the end of the chapter in the glossary of useful terms and concepts before reading the text.

INTRODUCTION AND HISTORY

An **electrical current** is a flow of charged particles. The charged particles may be electrons or ions. Electrical currents have been applied to biological systems to change physiological processes since at least 46 CE, when it was recorded that the electric discharge from torpedo fish was used to alleviate pain.[2,3]

In the late 18th and early 19th centuries there was a revival of interest in medical applications of electrical currents. In 1791, Galvani first recorded producing muscle contractions by touching metal to a frog's muscle. He called this effect "animal electricity." A few years later, when Volta constructed the precursor to the battery, Galvani used the current put out by this device to produce muscle contractions. He named the current "Galvanic current." In an attempt to understand the mechanisms by which electrical currents cause muscle contractions, Duchenne mapped out the locations on the skin where electrical stimulation most effectively caused specific muscles to contract. He called these locations "motor points."[4] During the 1830s, Faraday discovered that bidirectional electrical currents could be induced by a moving magnet. He called this current "Faradic current." Faradic current can be used to produce muscle contractions. In 1905, Lapicque developed the "law of excitation" relating the intensity and duration of a stimulus to whether it would produce a muscle contraction. Lapicque introduced the concept of the strength-duration curve, which is described later in this chapter.

The use of electrical currents for controlling pain is derived from the **gate control theory** of pain perception developed by Melzack and Wall in the 1960s. A more complete description of the historical development of electrical stimulation can be found in Sidney Licht's *Electrodiagnosis and Electromyography*.[5]

Today, electrical stimulation has a wide range of clinical applications in rehabilitation. These include muscle strengthening and reeducation,[6,7] pain control,[8,9] facilitating the healing of recalcitrant wounds,[9] resolving edema and inflammatory reactions after injury or surgery,[11] and enhancing transdermal drug delivery.[12,13]

Many professionals, including physical therapists, occupational therapists, physicians, and chiropractors, find electrical stimulation to be a valuable and effective component of their therapeutic armamentarium. In an ongoing effort to provide evidence-based treatment, researchers have evaluated the efficacy of electrical stimulation for its common clinical applications. The proliferation of more sophisticated machines has also increased interest in the use of electrical stimulation as an adjunct to rehabilitation interventions. These machines have multiple waveforms, allow a wide variety of parameter selection, may include computer-generated images of body parts and electrode placement for specific diagnoses, and may be integrated into bracing devices to facilitate functional use. The availability of small, patient-friendly units that can be used at home has also enhanced the effectiveness of electrical stimulation by allowing ongoing treatment between clinic visits.

Electrical stimulation can be applied to the body in a variety of ways. The electricity may be delivered by a stimulator implanted in the body, as occurs with a cardiac pacemaker, or an external stimulator can be used to deliver current to implanted or external, surface, transcutaneous electrodes. This chapter describes only the application of electrical stimulation by external stimulators that deliver current transcutaneously via surface electrodes applied to the skin.

EFFECTS OF ELECTRICAL CURRENTS

NERVE DEPOLARIZATION

For most applications, electrical currents exert their physiological effects by depolarizing nerve membranes and thereby producing action potentials, the message unit of the nervous system. Electrical currents with sufficient amplitude and that last for a sufficient length of time will cause enough of a change in nerve membrane potential to generate an action potential. Once that action potential is propagated along the axon, the human body responds to it in the same way as it does to action potentials that are initiated by physiological stimuli.

> ### ◎ Clinical Pearl
>
> Most of the clinical effects of electrical currents are the result of the current stimulating the production of action potentials in nerves.

An **action potential** (AP) is the basic unit of nerve communication. When a nerve is at rest, without physiological or electrical stimulation, the inside is more negatively charged than the outside by 60 to 90 mV. This is known as the **resting membrane potential** (Fig. 8-1).

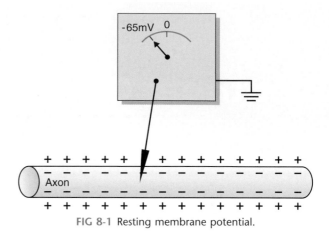

FIG 8-1 Resting membrane potential.

The resting membrane potential is maintained by most of the sodium ions being outside the cell and most of the potassium ions being inside the cell. When a sufficient stimulus is applied, sodium channels in the cell membrane open rapidly, whereas the potassium channels open slowly. Because of the high extracellular concentration of sodium, sodium ions rush into the cell through the open channels. This makes the inside of the cell more positively charged, reversing the membrane potential. When the membrane potential reaches +30 mV, the permeability to sodium decreases and potassium channels rapidly open, increasing the permeability to potassium. Because there is a high intracellular concentration of potassium ions, potassium ions then flow out of the cell, returning the membrane polarization to its resting state of –60 to –90 mV. This sequential **depolarization** and repolarization of the cell membrane caused by the changing flow of ions across the cell membrane is the AP (Fig. 8-2).

While the nerve is depolarized, no additional APs can be generated. During this time, the nerve cannot be further excited, however strong a stimulus is applied. This period is known as the **absolute refractory period**. After depolarization, before returning to the resting potential, there is a brief period of membrane hyperpolarization. During this period, a greater stimulus than usual is required to produce another AP. This period of hyperpolarization is known as the **relative refractory period**.

Strength-Duration Curve

The amount of electrical current required to produce an AP in a specific type of nerve varies and can be represented by the nerve's strength-duration curve (Fig. 8-3). The strength-duration curve for a nerve is a graphic representation of the minimum combination of current strength (**amplitude**) and **pulse duration** needed to depolarize that nerve. This interplay of amplitude and pulse duration is the basis for the specificity of the effect of electrical stimulation. In general, lower-current amplitudes and shorter pulse durations can depolarize sensory nerves, whereas higher amplitude or longer pulses are needed to depolarize motor nerves. Even higher amplitudes and longer pulses are needed to depolarize pain-transmitting C fibers.

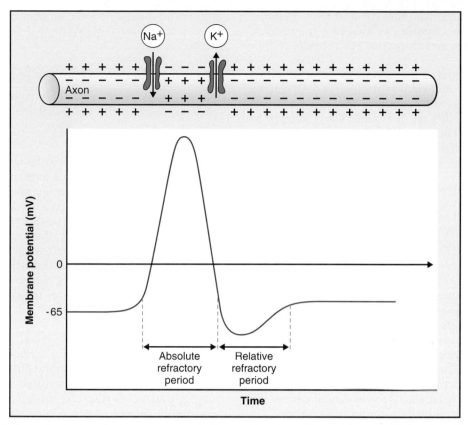

FIG 8-2 An action potential is the basic unit of nerve communication and is achieved by rapid sequential depolarization and repolarization in response to stimulation. Note that depolarization starts when the Na+ gate opens and Na+ flows into the cell, causing a rapid change from the normal resting membrane potential to a more positively charged state. Sequential repolarization occurs as permeability to sodium decreases, causing the K+ channels to open and K+ to flow out of the cell, returning the membrane polarization to its resting state.

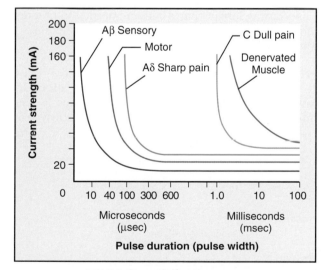

FIG 8-3 Strength-duration curve.

ⓒ Clinical Pearl

Short pulses and low-current amplitudes are used for sensory stimulation, and longer pulses and higher amplitudes are used for motor stimulation.

Thus short pulses, generally less than 80 μs (80×10^{-6} seconds) in duration, are used to produce sensory stimulation only, whereas longer pulses, 150 to 350 μs in duration, are used to produce muscle contractions. Most but not all portable electrical stimulation units intended to be used to produce muscle contractions have a fixed pulse duration of 200 to 300 μs. The larger clinical units usually allow adjustment and selection of the pulse duration. When stimulating contractions of smaller muscles and muscles in younger children and in the frail elderly, shorter pulses, of 125 to 250 μs pulse duration range, may be effective, more comfortable and better tolerated than longer duration pulses. By keeping pulse durations well below 1 ms (10^{-3} seconds) at all times, pain is minimized because C fibers are not depolarized. Much longer pulses, of more than 10 ms, are required to produce contractions of denervated muscle where the stimulus directly depolarizes the muscle cell rather than the motor nerve. This type of stimulation is generally uncomfortable because it also stimulates pain transmitting A-delta and C fibers if they are present.

When the current amplitude and pulse duration fall below the curve for a particular nerve type, the stimulation is considered to be subthreshold and no response will occur. For any type of tissue, the minimum current amplitude, with a very long pulse duration, required to produce an action potential is called **rheobase**. The minimum duration it takes to stimulate that tissue at twice rheobase intensity is known as **chronaxie**. Rheobase is a measure of current amplitude, and chronaxie is a measure of time (duration).

Increasing the current amplitude or pulse duration beyond that which is sufficient to stimulate an AP will not change the AP in any way. Neither a larger nor a longer AP occurs. All nerve APs are the same. They occur in an all-or-none fashion. The same AP occurs with any stimulus above threshold, and no AP will occur with any stimulus below threshold level.

> ◎ **Clinical Pearl**
>
> An action potential occurs in a nerve when its threshold is reached. Further increasing the current amplitude or pulse duration does not make the action potential larger or longer.

In addition to sufficient current amplitude and pulse duration, the current amplitude must rise quickly for an AP to be triggered. If the current rises too slowly, the nerve will accommodate to the stimulus. **Accommodation** is the process of a nerve gradually becoming less responsive to stimulation; a stimulus of sufficient amplitude and duration that usually produces a response no longer does so. Accommodation occurs with a slow rate of current rise because of the prolonged subthreshold stimulation.

Once an AP is generated, it triggers an AP in the adjacent area of the nerve membrane. This process is called **propagation** or conduction of the AP along the neuron. In general, with physiological stimulation, AP propagation occurs in only one direction. With electrically stimulated APs, propagation occurs in both directions from the site of stimulation; however, only those APs transmitted in the usual physiological direction have an effect.

The speed at which an AP travels depends on the diameter of the nerve along which it travels and whether the nerve is myelinated. The greater the diameter of the nerve the faster the AP will travel. For example, large-diameter myelinated A-alpha motor nerves conduct at between 60 and 120 m/sec, whereas smaller-diameter myelinated A-gamma and A-delta nerves conduct at only 12 to 30 m/sec. APs also travel faster in myelinated nerves than in unmyelinated nerves.

> ◎ **Clinical Pearl**
>
> Action potentials travel faster in large-diameter myelinated nerves than in small-diameter or unmyelinated nerves.

Myelin is a fatty sheath that wraps around certain axons. The sheath has small gaps in it that are called **nodes of Ranvier**. APs propagate along myelinated nerve fibers by jumping from one node to the next node—a process called **saltatory conduction** (Fig. 8-4). Saltatory conduction accelerates the conduction of action potentials along a nerve. For example, unmyelinated C-fibers that transmit slow pain and temperature sensations conduct at only 0.5 to 2 m/sec, which is much slower than the 12 to 30 m/sec conduction speed of similar diameter myelinated A-delta nerves.[14]

MUSCLE DEPOLARIZATION

In the late 1800s, it was found that denervated muscles do not contract in response to the pulses of electricity that produce contractions in innervated muscles. Innervated muscles contract in response to short pulses of electricity because the current causes depolarization of their motor nerves. This is known as **neuromuscular electrical stimulation** (NMES). Denervated muscles only contract in response to pulses of electricity lasting 10 ms or longer.

> ◎ **Clinical Pearl**
>
> Pulses lasting longer than 10 ms are needed to produce contractions in denervated muscle, and this requires a stimulator designed for this purpose.

These longer-duration pulses depolarize the muscle cell membrane directly. This is known as **electrical muscle stimulation** (EMS). Denervated muscle membrane does not accommodate. Therefore, a slowly rising

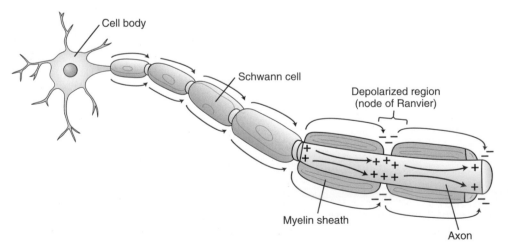

FIG 8-4 Saltatory conduction along a myelinated nerve.

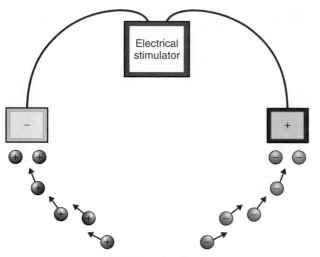

FIG 8-5 Ionic effects.

stimulus can be used to produce contractions in denervated muscle.[15]

IONIC EFFECTS OF ELECTRICAL CURRENTS

Most electrical currents used therapeutically have balanced biphasic waveforms that leave no **charge** in the tissue and thus have no ionic effects. In contrast, **direct current** (DC), pulsed monophasic currents, and unbalanced biphasic waveforms, which are used occasionally for electrical stimulation, do leave a net charge in the tissue. This charge can produce ionic effects. The negative electrode (**cathode**) attracts positively charged ions and repels negatively charged ions while the positive electrode (**anode**) attracts negatively charged ions and repels positively charged ions (Fig. 8-5).

These ionic effects can be exploited therapeutically. For example, DC can be used to repel ionized drug molecules and may thus provide a force to increase transdermal drug penetration. This application of electrotherapy is known as **iontophoresis**. The ionic effects of electricity are also exploited for the treatment of inflammatory states, to facilitate tissue healing, and to reduce the formation of edema, as described in detail later.

CLINICAL APPLICATIONS OF ELECTRICAL CURRENTS

MUSCLE CONTRACTION

Innervated Muscle

When APs are propagated along motor nerves the muscle fibers innervated by those nerves become depolarized and contract. The muscle contraction produced by electrically stimulated APs is similar to that produced by physiological generation of APs; however, there are some important differences between these contractions.

The primary difference between electrically stimulated muscle contractions and physiologically initiated muscle contractions is the order of recruitment of motor units. With electrical stimulation, nerve fibers with the largest diameter axons, which innervate the larger fast-twitch

type II muscle fibers, are activated first and those with a smaller axonal diameter are recruited later.[16,17] In contrast, with physiological contractions, the smaller nerve fibers, and thus the smaller, slow-twitch type I muscle fibers are activated before larger nerve and muscle fibers. The large, fast-twitch muscle fibers, which contract preferentially in response to electrical stimulation, fatigue rapidly and atrophy rapidly with disuse, whereas the smaller, slow-twitch muscle fibers, preferentially recruited physiologically, are more fatigue- and atrophy-resistant (Fig. 8-6). One clinical implication of this difference is that electrically stimulated contractions can be very effective at specifically strengthening those muscle fibers weakened by disuse. However, patients should perform both electrically stimulated and physiological contractions, if possible, to optimize the functional integration of strength gains produced by stimulation. In addition, because stimulated contractions are more fatiguing than physiological contractions, long rest times should be provided between contractions (Fig. 8-7).

> **ⓒ Clinical Pearl**
>
> When using electrical currents to stimulate muscle contractions, patients should also perform physiological contractions, and long rest times should be provided between contractions.

Another difference between electrically stimulated contractions and physiologically initiated contractions is the smoothness of the onset of the contraction. Physiological contractions usually gradually increase in force in a smoothly graded manner. The force is regulated by physiological control of motor unit recruitment and the rate of motor unit activation. The contraction is kept smooth by asynchronous recruitment of motor units. In contrast, electrically stimulated contractions generally have a rapid, and often jerky, onset because all motor units of a given size fire simultaneously when the stimulus reaches motor threshold.

> **ⓒ Clinical Pearl**
>
> Physiological muscle contractions usually have a smooth onset, whereas electrically stimulated muscle contractions have a rapid and jerky onset.

Electrical stimulation is thought to strengthen muscles by two mechanisms: overload and specificity.[18] According to the **overload principle**, the greater the load placed on a muscle and the higher force contraction it produces, the more strength that muscle will gain. This principle applies to contractions produced by electrical stimulation and to those produced by physiological exercise.[19] With physiological exercise, the load can be progressively increased by increasing the resistance, as with weights. With electrically stimulated contractions, the force is increased primarily by increasing the total amount of current, which is limited by patient tolerance and fatigue. In healthy human subjects, combining electrical stimulation with a voluntary exercise regimen has been shown to produce no greater strengthening than either intervention

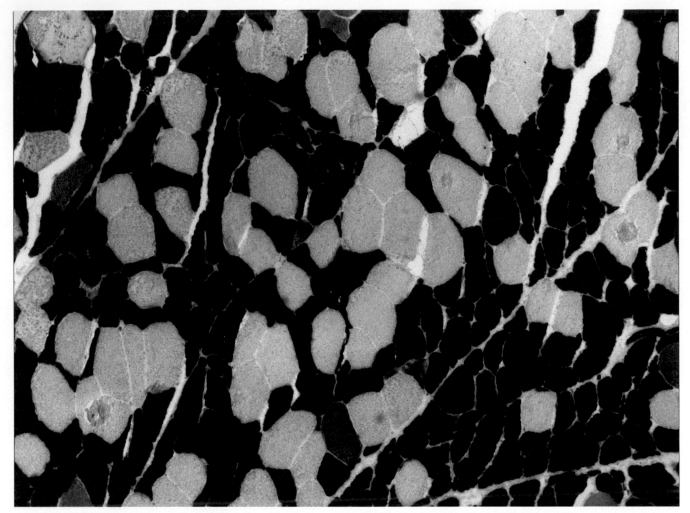

FIG 8-6 Type II muscle fiber atrophy from disuse. In this fresh frozen muscle biopsy, the dark brown/black fibers are the atrophic type II fibers, and the light beige fibers are normal-sized type I fibers. *Courtesy Sakir Gultekin, MD, Oregon Health & Science University, Portland, OR.*

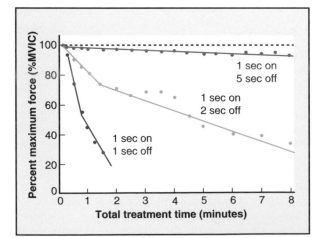

FIG 8-7 The effect of changing the on:off ratio on the force of contraction produced. Note that stronger contractions are produced when longer off times are used. *Adapted from Benton LA, Baker LL, Bowman BR, et al: Functional electrical stimulation: a practical clinical guide, Downey, CA, 1981, Rancho Los Amigos Hospital.*

alone, if the same force of contraction is produced.[20] In addition, in healthy subjects, the gains in muscle strength are similar for electrically stimulated contractions and exercise when the same amount of force is produced.[21] However, in subjects with weakness after surgery, adding electrical stimulation to physiological exercise has been shown to amplify and accelerate strength gains.[22]

According to the specificity theory, because electrical stimulation causes larger fast-twitch type II muscle fibers, which produce a greater level of force, to contract before smaller slow-twitch type I muscle fibers, electrical stimulation should have more effect on type II muscle fibers than on type I muscle fibers. This theory is supported by the findings that in weak patients with reduced muscle strength, or in those with specific muscle weakness after surgery, in whom there is generally primarily type II fiber atrophy, early use of electrical stimulation can result in a more rapid functional recovery and greater strength gains than exercise alone.[22-28] Research supports the clinical observation that after joint surgery, the strength of the muscles supporting the joint is highly related to functional performance after surgery.[29] Although electrical stimulation appears to accelerate postoperative recovery of strength by 12 weeks after surgery, the strength of patients who exercise is not significantly different from that of patients who also receive electrical stimulation.[30]

Electrical stimulation of muscle contractions can accelerate and improve patient rehabilitation by increasing muscle strength and endurance.[31] This can enhance the quality of motor recruitment and carry over to improved performance of functional activities. To produce strength gains in healthy muscle, the force of the stimulated contraction needs to be at least 50% of the maximum voluntary isometric contraction (MVIC) force, although the greatest strength gains will be achieved with the maximally tolerated force of contraction. To produce strength gains in injured patients, the stimulated contractions may have a force of as little as 10% of the MVIC, although stronger contractions will be more effective if they are tolerated. To optimize gains in endurance, more prolonged periods of stimulation with more lower-force contractions will be more effective.[14,32]

◎ Clinical Pearl

To increase strength, higher force contractions should be used. To increase endurance, prolonged stimulation with more lower-force contractions should be used.

Electrical stimulation has traditionally been used to increase strength and function in patients with orthopedic problems and intact peripheral and central nervous systems (CNS). However, electrical stimulation can also be used to increase strength and improve control in patients with CNS damage, such as from stroke or cerebral palsy, as long as the peripheral motor nerves are intact. For example, NMES of the lower extremity in patients with hemiplegia due to stroke has been shown to improve voluntary recruitment of motor units and gait, increase ankle-dorsiflexion torque, reduce agonist:antagonist cocontraction, and increase the probability of returning home, as compared to traditional treatment without electrical stimulation or with placebo.[33,34] Several studies have also reported an improvement in gait in children with cerebral palsy when NMES of the lower extremities has been included in their treatment regimen and an improvement in upper extremity function when NMES of the upper extremities has been included.[35-38] This effect may be a direct result of muscle strengthening but may also be influenced by the increased general excitability of the motor neuron pool produced by motor level electrical stimulation enhancing descending control of muscle recruitment. The sensory input always produced by motor level stimulation may also provide a cue for the patient to initiate a movement or activate a muscle group.[39] NMES may also be integrated into the performance of functional activities by stimulating contractions at the time during an activity when the muscle should contract. An example of this is stimulating the anterior tibialis muscle to produce dorsiflexion during the swing phase of gait. This is known as **functional electrical stimulation** (FES). Patterned sensory-level stimulation, using an intermittent sensory stimulus, with an on:off time but without stimulation of

muscle contractions, may also enhance motor control, likely by promoting reciprocal inhibition of antagonist muscles.[40-42]

Studies concerning the use of NMES in patients with spasticity have primarily focused on stimulating the antagonist muscles. However, stimulating the agonist and the antagonist sequentially, with brief rest periods after each contraction, may be more effective since this more closely mimics normal motor activity. For example, individuals without CNS dysfunction flex and extend the elbow by firing the biceps and triceps sequentially, with a brief latency period between activation of these muscle groups. In contrast, individuals with CNS dysfunction maintain some ongoing motor activity of both agonist and antagonist throughout the movement, and the latency period between contractions is absent.

Electrically stimulated muscle contractions can also support or assist with joint positioning, functioning like an orthosis. For example, Baker and colleagues reported that an aggressive program of electrically stimulated contraction of the muscles surrounding the shoulder over a 6-week period reduced shoulder subluxation in patients with hemiplegia caused by stroke more effectively than facilitation programs, slings, or sitting support.[43] A smaller study in patients with hemiplegia caused by stroke demonstrated that subjects who received NMES had slightly reduced shoulder subluxation whereas glenohumeral separation increased in the control group even though the affected arm was supported at all times.[44] A recent study also found that a home-based sensory and motor level electrical stimulation program resulted in improvements in arm function, voluntary movement, and muscle tone in patients after stroke.[45]

Electrical stimulation can be used to strengthen and improve the function of muscles throughout the body. Although traditionally used primarily for strengthening limb muscles, there is growing interest and clinical application of electrical stimulation for the treatment of swallowing difficulties (dysphagia), particularly in patients with dysphagia resulting from stroke.[46] This intervention involves applying electrodes to the neck and stimulating contractions in the muscles responsible for swallowing. Several studies have found this intervention to be more effective than other approaches used to treat dysphagia of various etiologies.[47-50] In addition, a metaanalysis examining the evidence on electrical stimulation for swallowing, in which 7 out of a total of 81 published studies met inclusion criteria, concluded that, from the small amount of high-quality data available, there was a small but significant summary effect-size supporting the use of electrical stimulation to improve swallowing.[51] One study found that this application of electrical stimulation only produced clinically relevant results in patients with mild to moderate dysphagia and not in those with severe dysphagia.[52]

Another use of electrically stimulated muscle contractions is for the treatment of urinary incontinence associated with pelvic floor dysfunction.[53,54] Electrical stimulation for this purpose has been applied transcutaneously, percutaneously, and via intravaginal probes.[55,56] Most reports have focused on urinary incontinence in women, although some review protocols for men. In 1996, the Agency for Health Care Policy and Research (AHCPR) Guidelines on urinary incontinence stated that pelvic floor electrical stimulation has been shown to decrease incontinence in women with stress urinary incontinence and may be useful for urge and mixed incontinence.[57]

Additionally, studies have shown that electrically stimulated muscle contraction can promote blood flow in healthy individuals and in patients with poor circulation.[58-61] This increase in circulation can accelerate tissue healing and has been demonstrated to help reduce the risk of deep venous thrombosis formation.[60-63] Some studies suggest that sensory-level electrical stimulation may also augment peripheral blood flow, but this effect has been found to occur only in patients and not in healthy individuals.[58,59,64-66]

Denervated Muscle

When a muscle becomes denervated by nerve injury or disease, it no longer contracts physiologically nor can a contraction be produced by the usual electrical stimulus used for NMES. However, if the electrical current lasts for more than 10 ms, the denervated muscle will contract. Usually a continuous DC is applied for a number of seconds to produce contractions in denervated muscle. The duration of stimulation is controlled directly by the clinician depressing a manually controlled switch on a DC stimulator. To produce a graded contraction in a denervated muscle, the current amplitude can be gradually increased to reach full amplitude over a number of seconds.

Denervation causes muscle to atrophy and fibrose. The entire muscle and the individual muscle fibers become smaller, and fibrous tissue forms between the muscle fibers. It has been suggested that ongoing electrical stimulation of denervated muscles may retard, or even reverse, this atrophy and fibrosis[67-69]; however, studies have not found maintained improvement in the final functional outcome of denervated muscles or improvement in enervation as a result of this intervention.[70-72] In addition, there is conflicting evidence about the effects of electrical stimulation on motor nerve regeneration. Studies in rats have found that electrically stimulated contractions of denervated muscles may retard motor nerve sprouting and muscle reinnervation,[73] whereas pulsed electrical stimulation of denervated muscles in rats and rabbits has been found to accelerate nerve healing and increase muscle strength.[74,75] At this time, most do not recommend stimulation of contractions in denervated muscles with DC. Although DC electrical stimulation has traditionally been used for treatment of Bell's palsy (facial paralysis resulting from damage to the seventh cranial nerve), evidence indicates that this treatment is no more effective than placebo.[76,77] Some studies have shown improved clinical recovery in patients with chronic facial palsy in response to long-term sensory-level electrical stimulation.[78,79]

Parameters for Electrical Stimulation of Contractions in Innervated Muscles

Electrode Placement. When electrical stimulation is applied to produce a muscle contraction, one electrode

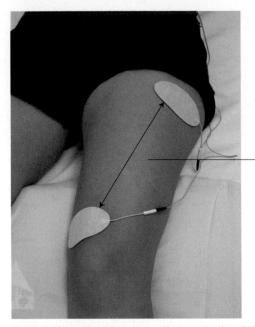

FIG 8-8 Electrodes placed over the proximal and distal ends of the quadriceps muscles for maximum efficacy.

Electrode configuration (approximately parallel to fiber direction)

should be placed over the **motor point** for the muscle and the other electrode should be placed on the muscle to be stimulated so that the two electrodes are aligned parallel to the direction of the muscle fibers allowing the current to travel parallel to the direction of the muscle fibers (Fig. 8-8). The electrodes should be at least 2-inches apart to avoid them becoming too close (less than 1-inch apart) when the muscle changes shape during a contraction, potentially moving the electrodes close together. The motor point is the place where an electrical stimulus will produce the greatest contraction with the least amount of electricity and is the area of skin over which the motor nerve enters the muscle. Charts of motor points are available; however, because most motor points are over the middle of the muscle belly, it is generally easy and effective to place electrodes over the middle of the muscle belly.

Waveform. A pulsed biphasic waveform or **Russian protocol** should be used when electrical stimulation is used to produce muscle contractions. The pulsed biphasic waveform is available on most devices and is effective for this application. The Russian protocol, which is available on select units, may produce greater and faster strength gains.

Pulse Duration. When using electrical stimulation to produce a muscle contraction in an innervated muscle, the pulse duration should be between 150 and 350 μs to stimulate motor nerves (see Fig. 8-3). Most units with an adjustable pulse duration allow a maximum duration of 300 μs, and many units intended to be used only for stimulation of muscle contractions have a fixed pulse duration of around 300 μs. If the pulse duration is adjustable, most patients find shorter pulse durations more comfortable when stimulating smaller muscles and longer pulse durations more comfortable when stimulating larger muscles. In addition, for similar applications, smaller people and children also often find shorter pulse durations to be more comfortable, and as effective, as longer pulse durations. It is important to remember that as the pulse duration is shortened a greater amplitude will be required to achieve the same strength of contraction produced by a longer pulse duration.

> ### ⊚ Clinical Pearl
>
> As the pulse duration is shortened a greater amplitude will be needed to achieve the same strength of contraction produced by a longer pulse duration.

Selection of the ideal combination of pulse duration and current amplitude should be based on patient comfort and achievement of the desired outcome.

Frequency. Pulse **frequency** determines the type of response or muscle contraction that the electrical stimulation will produce. When a low frequency of less than approximately 30 pps is used to stimulate a motor nerve, each pulse will produce a separate muscle twitch contraction (Fig. 8-9). As the frequency increases, the twitches will occur more closely together, eventually summating to produce a smooth tetanic contraction. This requires approximately 35 to 50 pps. Increasing the frequency beyond 50 to 80 pps may produce greater muscle strengthening but will also result in more rapid fatigue during stimulation.[14,80,81] Therefore, clinically, a frequency of between 35 and 50 pps is generally recommended and may be increased to a maximum of 80 pps if needed for comfort.

On:Off Time. When used to produce muscle contractions, an **on:off time** must be set to allow the muscles to contract and then relax during the treatment. The relaxation time is needed to limit fatigue.

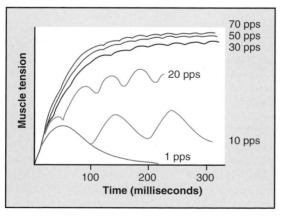

FIG 8-9 Effect of stimulus frequency on the type of muscle contraction produced. Note that a frequency of at least 30 pps is needed to produce a sustained contraction.

When electrical stimulation is used for muscle strengthening, the recommended on time is in the range of 6 to 10 seconds and the recommended off time is in the range of 50 to 120 seconds, with an initial on:off ratio of 1:5. The long off time is required to minimize muscle fatigue. With subsequent treatments, as the patient gets stronger, the on:off ratio may be decreased to 1:4 or even 1:3. When the goal of electrical stimulation is to relieve a muscle spasm, the on:off ratio is set at 1:1, with both the on and off times set between 2 and 5 seconds, to produce muscle fatigue and relax the spasm. When the treatment is intended to pump out edema, the on:off ratio is also set at 1:1 with both the on and off times set between 2 and 5 seconds.

Ramp Time. A ramp time may be needed when a muscle contraction is stimulated. The ramp time allows for a gradual increase and decrease of force rather than a sudden increase when switching from off time to on time and a sudden decrease when switching from on time to off time. When stimulation is used to facilitate repetitive exercise and when on times are in the range of 6 to 10 seconds, a **ramp up/ramp down time** of 1 to 4 seconds is recommended. However, for some activities, shorter or longer ramp times are indicated. For example, when electrical stimulation is used for gait training, where the muscles should contract and then relax rapidly, a ramp time should not be used. In contrast, when stimulating contraction of the antagonist to a spastic muscle in a patient with stroke, a long ramp time of 4 to 8 seconds may be necessary to avoid a rapid stretch of the agonist and thus increased spasticity.

Current Amplitude. When using electrical stimulation for muscle strengthening, the current amplitude is adjusted according to the strength of contraction desired. When the goal is to strengthen muscles in people without injury, the amplitude of the current must be high enough to produce a contraction that is at least 50% of MVIC strength. However, during recovery from injury or surgery, such as anterior cruciate ligament reconstruction, a current amplitude that produces contractions of a strength equal to or greater than 10% of the MVIC of the uninjured limb has been shown to increase strength and accelerate functional recovery more than a control intervention of strengthening without stimulation.[82]

When electrical stimulation is used for motor reeducation, the goal of treatment is functional movement that may not require maximum strength. Electrical stimulation can assist with functional recovery by providing sensory input, proprioceptive feedback of normal motion, and increased muscle strength. In this circumstance the lowest current amplitude to produce the desired functional movement is probably the best. Initially, this may require strong motor-level stimulation that makes the muscles move by stimulating the motor nerves. As the patient progresses and regains voluntary control, a lower amplitude sensory-level stimulus may be sufficient to cue the patient to move appropriately. Ideally, the patient will learn over time

TABLE 8-1	Recommended Parameter Settings for Electrically Stimulated Muscle Contractions						
Parameter Settings/ Treatment Goal	Pulse Frequency	Pulse Duration	Amplitude	On:Off Times and Ratio	Ramp Time	Treatment Time	Times per Day
Muscle strengthening	35-80 pps	150-200 µs for small muscles, 200-350 µs for large muscles	To >10% of MVIC in injured, >50% MVIC in uninjured	6-10 sec on, 50-120 sec off, ratio of 1:5, initially. May reduce the off time with repeated treatments	At least 2 sec	10-20 min to produce 10-20 repetitions	Every 2-3 hours when awake
Muscle reeducation	35-50 pps	150-200 µs for small muscles, 200-350 µs for large muscles.	Sufficient for functional activity	Depends on functional activity	At least 2 sec	Depends on functional activity	NA
Muscle spasm reduction	35-50 pps	150-200 µs for small muscles, 200-350 µs for large muscles	To visible contraction	2-5 sec on: 2-5 sec off. Equal on:off times	At least 1 sec	10-30 min	Every 2-3 hours until spasm relieved
Edema reduction using muscle pump	35-50 pps	150-200 µs for small muscles, 200-350 µs for large muscles	To visible contraction	2-5 sec on: 2-5 sec off. Equal on:off times	At least 1 sec	30 min	Twice a day

MVIC, Maximum voluntary isometric contraction; *NA*, not applicable.

to perform the movement without the need for stimulation.

When electrical stimulation is used to reduce muscle spasms, the current amplitude need only be sufficient to produce a visible contraction.

Treatment Time. When using electrical stimulation for muscle strengthening, it is generally recommended that the treatment should last long enough to allow for 10 to 20 contractions. This will usually take 10 to 20 minutes. This treatment session should be repeated multiple times throughout the day if the patient has an electrical stimulation device available for home use. When treating in the clinic, electrical stimulation is generally applied once each visit for 10 to 20 minutes.

When electrical stimulation is used for muscle reeducation, the treatment time will vary based on the functional activity being addressed but is generally no more than 20 minutes at a single session, or less if a patient shows signs of inattentiveness or fatigue (Table 8-1).

PAIN MODULATION

A substantial body of research demonstrates that electrical stimulation can modulate pain.[83-88] Melzack and Wall first proposed that electrical stimulation may reduce the sensa-

tion of pain by interfering with its transmission at the spinal cord level.[8] This approach to pain control is known as the gate control theory of pain and is described in detail in Chapter 3.

Noxious stimuli are transmitted from the periphery along small myelinated A-delta nerves and small unmyelinated C nerve fibers. According to the gate control theory, activation of nonnociceptor A-beta nerve fibers can inhibit transmission of noxious stimuli from the spinal cord to the brain. Electrical stimulation, when applied with appropriate parameters, can selectively activate A-beta nerves. Because pain perception is determined by the relative activity of A-delta and C fibers compared with A-beta fibers, when greater A-beta activity is produced by electrical stimulation, pain perception is decreased.[89]

A-beta nerves can be activated by both short- and long-duration electrical current pulses.[90] However, short duration pulses, lasting between 50 and 80 µs and with a current amplitude that produces a comfortable level of sensation, selectively activate these nerves without activating motor nerves. Pulse frequencies of 100 to 150 pps are generally found to be most comfortable for this application. This application of electrical stimulation is known as conventional or high-rate **transcutaneous electrical nerve stimulation** (TENS).

Because the primary pain-modulating effects of **conventional TENS**, as produced by gating, last only while the stimulation is being applied, this type of TENS should be applied when the patient has pain and may be used for up to 24 hours a day if necessary. Conventional TENS can also interrupt the pain-spasm-pain cycle, thereby resulting in some reduction of pain after the stimulation stops. The pain is reduced directly by the electrical stimulation, and this indirectly reduces muscle spasms, further reducing pain unless the muscle spasm recurs.

The stimulus used for conventional TENS is generally modulated to limit adaptation. **Adaptation** is a decrease in the frequency of action potentials, and a decrease in the subjective sensation of stimulation, when electrical stimulation is applied, if there are no changes in the applied stimulus. Adaptation is a known property of sensory receptors caused by decreased excitability of the nerve membrane with repeated stimulation. Modulation of any of the stimulation parameters, including frequency, pulse duration, or current amplitude, is likely to be equally effective in helping to prevent adaptation to stimulation.

It is also proposed that electrical stimulation may control pain by stimulating the production and release of endorphins and enkephalins. These substances, known as endogenous opioids, act in a manner similar to morphine and are known to modulate pain perception. They modulate pain by binding to opiate receptors in the brain and other areas and acting as neurotransmitters and neuromodulators.[91] They also activate descending inhibitory pathways that involve nonopioid (serotonin) systems. It has been shown that endorphin and enkephalin levels are increased after the application of certain types of electrical stimulation.[92]

Repetitive stimulation of motor or nociceptive A-delta nerves to produce repetitive muscle contractions or brief sharp pain can stimulate endogenous opioid production and release. To achieve this, longer pulse durations and higher current amplitudes than used for conventional TENS are required because motor nerves, and possibly A-delta nerves, must be depolarized. Lower frequencies of 2 to 10 pps are usually used for this application to minimize the risk of muscle soreness. This application of electrical stimulation is known as **low rate** or **acupuncture-like TENS.** Low rate TENS will usually control pain for 4 to 5 hours after a 20- to 30-minute treatment. It is effective for this amount of time because the half-life of the endogenous opioids released is approximately 4½ hours. Low rate TENS should not be applied for more than 45 minutes at a time because prolonging the repetitive muscle contraction produced by the stimulus can result in delayed-onset muscle soreness.

Stimulation with **pulsed current** with frequencies of less than 10 pps has been found to most effectively increase

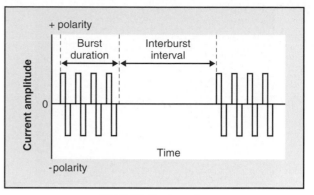

FIG 8-10 Burst mode.

endorphin and enkephalin levels,[93] and naloxone, a mu-opioid receptor blocker, blocks the analgesia produced by low rate TENS (4 pps) but not that produced by conventional high rate TENS (100 pps), whereas naltrindole, a delta opioid receptor blocker, blocks only the analgesia produced by high rate TENS.[94] In a more recent study, investigators looked specifically for difference in effects between high and low rate TENS on experimental inflammatory edema and pain. They found that both interventions reduced the hyperalgesia but not the edema; however, the effect of the low rate TENS lasted longer. Naltrexone-treated animals showed a complete reversal of analgesia in by low but not high rate TENS, again confirming the participation of endogenous opioids on low rate TENS associated analgesia.[95]

Another form of TENS used for pain modulation is known as **burst mode TENS**. This mode of TENS is thought to work by the same mechanisms as low rate TENS but may be more effective or better tolerated in some individuals. For burst mode TENS, the stimulation is delivered in bursts, or packages, composed of a number of pulses each (Fig. 8-10).

Electrical stimulation may also control pain when the electrodes are placed on acupuncture points. This method of application is thought to stimulate energy flow along acupuncture meridians that connect acupuncture points in the body.[96,97] The application of TENS over acupuncture points has been shown to decrease chronic neck pain when applied with exercise.[98] Recent studies have also investigated electroacupuncture, which involves the application of an electrical stimulus to acupuncture needles inserted into the body at the appropriate points.[99,100] This application requires special training and licensure that allows the clinician to place needles through the patient's skin.

Although most applications of TENS use a pulsed biphasic waveform, **interferential current** may also be used to control pain, likely by the same mechanisms. Interferential current has been shown to reduce pain and swelling, increase range of motion (ROM) after knee surgery,[101] and relieve pain related to chronic inflammatory conditions such as osteoarthritis and psoriatic arthritis.[102,103] Interferential current was found in one study to produce a longer duration of pain relief than pulsed biphasic current.[104]

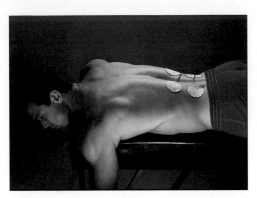

FIG 8-11 Electrodes placed over the low back for electrical stimulation treatment to control low back pain. *Courtesy Mettler Electronics, Anaheim, CA.*

Parameters for Electrical Stimulation for Pain Modulation

Electrode Placement. When electrical stimulation is applied for pain control, a variety of electrode placements can be effective.[105] If two channels, and thus four electrodes are used, the electrodes can be placed to surround the area of pain. The two channels can be placed so that they intersect, allowing the current to cross at the area of pain (Fig. 8-11) or they may be placed parallel, either horizontally or vertically. The two channels must intersect if an interferential current is desired. If one channel and thus two electrodes are used, placement around the painful area is also most common. Placement over trigger points or acupuncture points, which are generally areas of decreased skin **resistance**, has also been reported to be effective.[80] When the electrodes cannot be placed near or over the painful area, for example, if the area is in a cast or local application of the electrodes is not tolerated, the electrodes can be placed proximal to the site of pain along the pathway of the sensory nerves supplying the area.[105] For all applications the electrodes should be at least 1-inch apart.

Waveform. A pulsed biphasic waveform or an interferential current are recommended when electrical stimulation is used to modulate pain. The pulsed biphasic waveform requires only two electrodes and is therefore quicker to set up, but the interferential current may be more comfortable, affect a larger area, and provide a longer-lasting effect.

Pulse Duration. Most clinical units with biphasic waveforms intended to be used for pain control and most portable units intended for use for pain control (usually called TENS units) allow the clinician to adjust the pulse duration. When using a biphasic waveform for conventional TENS, the pulse duration should be between 50 and 80 μs to depolarize only the A-beta sensory nerves. When applying low rate TENS, the pulse duration should be between 200 and 300 μs to depolarize the motor nerves and possibly the A-delta nerves.

When using interferential current for pain control, one cannot select the pulse duration. Interferential current is composed of **alternating current** (AC) where the **wavelength**, which is equivalent to the pulse duration of a pulsed waveform, changes inversely with the carrier frequency. If the carrier frequency is higher, the wavelength is shorter, and if the carrier frequency is lower, the wavelength is longer.

$$\text{Wavelength} = \frac{1}{\text{carrier frequency}}$$

When the carrier frequency is 2,500 Hz, the wavelength is 400 μs, when the carrier frequency is 4,000 Hz, the wavelength is 250 μs, and when the carrier frequency is 5,000 Hz, the wavelength is 200 μs. Most units have a fixed carrier frequency of 4,000 or 5,000 Hz.

Frequency. Selection of pulse frequency for pain control depends both on the selected mode (high rate, conventional, or low rate) and the waveform and parameter options available on the unit being used. With high rate TENS, the pulse frequency is set between 100 to 150 pps, and with low rate, the pulse frequency is set below 10 pps. TENS units that have burst mode available are generally preset by the manufacturer to provide 10 or fewer bursts each second, with the pulses within the burst being at 100 to 150 pps, thereby attempting to combine the effects of high rate and low rate TENS.

On:Off Time. Electrical stimulation is delivered continuously throughout the treatment time with no off time when applied for pain control.

Current Amplitude. To control pain with electrical stimulation, the treatment should be as comfortable as possible. For high rate TENS, it is generally recommended that the amplitude be set to produce a gentle sensation only, generally perceived as tingling or vibration. However, some recommend a strong or maximally tolerated level of sensory stimulation for this application. It is likely that different individuals respond best to different levels of sensory stimulation and that the ideal for a particular individual will need to be determined by the patient and the clinician. For low rate and burst TENS to be effective, the amplitude must be sufficient to produce a visible contraction.

Treatment Time. When using electrical stimulation for pain control using high rate TENS, a patient may wear a home unit at all times as needed to relieve pain. The low rate or burst mode TENS modes should be applied for a maximum of 20 to 45 minutes every 4 hours. Low rate and burst mode TENS should not be used for longer periods because the muscle contractions they produce can cause delayed-onset muscle soreness if the stimulation is applied for prolonged periods (Table 8-2).

TABLE 8-2	Recommended Parameter Settings for Electrical Stimulation for Pain Control					
Parameter Settings	Pulse Frequency (or Beat Frequency for Interferential)	Pulse Duration	Amplitude	Modulation (Frequency, Duration, or Amplitude)	Treatment Time	Possible Mechanism of Action
Conventional (high rate)	100-150 pps	50-80 µs	To produce tingling	Use if available	May be worn 24 hours, as needed for pain control	Gating at the spinal cord
Acupuncture-like (low rate)	2-10 pps	200-300 µs	To visible contraction	None	20-30 min	Endorphin release
Burst mode	Generally preset in unit at 10 bursts	Generally preset and may have max of 100-300 µs	To visible contraction	Is generally not possible in burst mode	20-30 min	Endorphin release

TISSUE HEALING

A number of studies have demonstrated that electrical stimulation can enhance tissue healing.[10,11,106-108] In 2002, the Centers for Medicare and Medicaid Services in the United States approved payment for electrical stimulation for the treatment of chronic lower extremity ulcers that have not responded to standard wound treatment.[109] Kloth's 2005 review of studies of electrical currents for wound healing *in-vitro*, and *in-vivo* in human and animal models, found that overall, electrical stimulation aids wound healing, particularly when applied in conjunction with standard wound care.[106] Kloth proposes several mechanisms for this effect, including increased protein synthesis and cell migration, antibacterial effects, increased blood flow, and improved tissue oxygenation.

Similarly, in 1999, Gardner, Frantz, and Schmidt's metaanalysis of studies on the effects of electrical stimulation on chronic wound healing found that electrical stimulation was associated with faster healing in the majority of clinical trials.[110] They evaluated four different types of electrical currents for this application: low-intensity DC (LIDC), high-voltage pulsed current (HVPC), AC, and TENS (i.e., sensory-level pulsed biphasic current). For all types of electrical current, electrical stimulation was associated with faster wound healing. Although the usual control treatment in the clinical trials varied, the treatment of the control samples in at least 10 of the studies appeared to be standardized. Moist dressings were used on the majority of controls, and whirlpool was used in a few cases. A number of the control subjects were treated with an electrical stimulation placebo. Fifteen studies were included in the final metaanalysis. The most common measure used to report change was percentage healing per week. The net effect of electrical stimulation across all studies evaluated was 13% increased healing per week, which represents a 144% increase over the control rate of healing. When wounds were categorized by type, it was found that electrical stimulation was most effective for accelerating the healing of pressure ulcers. The proposed mechanisms by which electrical stimulation promotes

tissue healing include attraction of appropriate cell types to the area, activation of these cells by altering cell membrane function, modification of endogenous electrical potential of the tissue in concert with healing potentials, reduction of edema, enhancement of antimicrobial activity, and promotion of circulation.

Specific cells, including neutrophils, macrophages, lymphocytes and fibroblasts, can be attracted to an injured healing area by an electrical charge because the cells themselves carry a charge.[111,112] This process of attraction is known as **galvanotaxis**. Activated neutrophils, which are present when a wound is infected or inflamed, are attracted to the negative pole, whereas inactive neutrophils move toward the positive pole. Macrophages and epidermal cells are also attracted to the positive pole, whereas lymphocytes, platelets, mast cells, keratinocytes, and fibroblasts are attracted to the negative pole. It is generally recommended that to attract the most appropriate cell types, the negative electrode be used for treatment of infected or inflamed wounds and the positive electrode be used if there is necrosis without inflammation and when the wound is in the proliferative stage of healing.[113]

> **◎ Clinical Pearl**
>
> In general, the negative electrode should be used to promote healing of inflamed or infected wounds and the positive electrode should be used to promote healing of wounds with no inflammation.

Not only can electrical stimulation attract cells to an injury site, but it has also been shown to enhance fibroblast replication and increase the synthesis of DNA and collagen by fibroblasts.[114,115] Fibroblasts, and the collagen they produce, are essential for the proliferation phase of tissue healing. The proposed mechanism of enhanced cell function is that the electrical current pulse triggers calcium channels in the fibroblast cell membrane to open. The open channels allow calcium to flow into the cells, increasing intracellular calcium levels to induce exposure of additional insulin receptors on the cell surface. Insulin can then bind to the exposed receptors, stimulating the fibroblasts to synthesize collagen and DNA.[116] This sequence of events is voltage dependent, with a maximum calcium influx and protein and DNA synthesis occurring with HVPC with a peak **voltage** in the range of 60 to 90 V. Both higher and lower voltages have less effect. Electrical stimulation can also promote epidermal cell and lymphocyte migration, proliferation, and function.[117]

When skin and cell membranes are intact, they have an electrical charge across them as a result of the action of the sodium/potassium pumps. When tissue is injured, thereby rupturing cell membranes, charged ions leak out of the cells, causing the wound and the adjacent area to become positively charged relative to the surrounding uninjured tissue.[118,119] This has been demonstrated in children with accidental finger amputations where the stump tips were positively charged relative to the uninjured forearm.[120] This electrical potential difference steadily declines over time, returning to normal only after the wound closes. Electrical stimulation may accelerate tissue healing by replicating or enhancing this process.

Electrical stimulation may also promote tissue healing through antimicrobial activity. Monophasic currents, both microampere level DC and HVPC, have been shown to kill bacteria *in-vitro*, whereas ACs have not been found to affect bacterial growth or survival.[106,121-123] However, it is likely that to inhibit bacterial growth, electrical currents must be applied either at much higher voltages or for much longer times than used in the clinical setting.[124-126]

It is also possible that electrical stimulation facilitates tissue healing by increasing circulation during or after the stimulation.[127] However, in general, muscle contraction is required for electrical stimulation to increase circulation, whereas tissue healing has been shown to be enhanced by submotor levels of stimulation.[61,64,65,128] Over the longer term, electrical currents may enhance wound circulation by promoting the growth of new blood vessels.[129]

Parameters for Electrical Stimulation for Tissue Healing

Electrode Placement. For electrical stimulation to promote wound healing, the treatment electrodes may be placed in or around the wound (Fig. 8-12). One treatment electrode is used when stimulation is applied directly in the wound and two or more treatment electrodes may be used when the stimulation is applied to the area around the wound. If stimulation is applied directly to the wound, a single-use electrode constructed by the therapist should be used. This type of electrode is made of saline-soaked gauze placed directly in the wound. Aluminum foil or a single-patient, reusable electrode may be placed over the gauze. The electrode is attached to the lead wire with an alligator clip (Fig. 8-13). If stimulation is applied to the intact tissue around the wound, the usual commercially available electrodes, as described at the end of this chapter, may be used. One large dispersive electrode, of opposite **polarity** to the treatment electrode, should be placed on intact skin close to the wound site.

Waveform. A monophasic waveform, where the electrodes are of consistent opposite polarity, should be used when electrical stimulation is applied to promote tissue healing. HVPC, a monophasic pulsed waveform (Fig. 8-14), was used in most studies showing benefit for this application, although LIDC has also been found to be effective. The parameter recommendations that follow are for the HVPC waveform.

Polarity. The polarity of the electrode on or nearest to the wound is selected according to the type of cells required to advance a particular stage of wound healing and the presence or absence of infection or inflammation in the wound. Negative polarity is generally used during the early inflammatory stage of healing, whereas positive polarity is used later to facilitate epithelial cell migration across the wound bed. Kloth recommends using negative polarity for the first 3 to 7 days of treatment and changing to positive polarity thereafter; however, some researchers recommend using negative polarity for all treatments.[64,65,130]

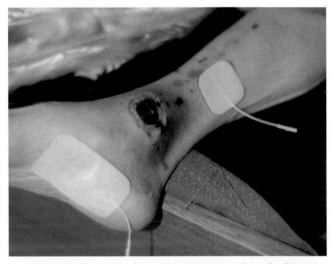

FIG 8-12 Electrode placement to promote tissue healing.

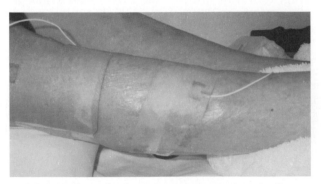

FIG 8-13 Electrode placement to promote tissue healing.

Alternatively, it has been recommended that polarity be switched when wound healing reaches a plateau. Another recommendation is to use negative polarity initially and for 3 days after the wound bed becomes free of necrotic tissue and the drainage becomes serosanguineous and thereafter to use positive polarity.[131,132]

Pulse Duration. The pulse duration recommended when using HVPC to promote wound healing is between 40 and 100 μs. This parameter is generally preset in the device by the manufacturer and cannot be changed by the clinician.

Frequency. Pulse frequency for promoting tissue healing should be in the range of 60 to 125 pps.

On:Off Time. Electrical stimulation is delivered continuously throughout the treatment time when applied for tissue healing.

Current Amplitude. The current amplitude should be sufficient to produce a comfortable sensation without a motor response. If the patient has decreased or altered sensation in the treatment area, the appropriate amplitude can be determined by first applying the electrode to another area with normal intact sensation.

Treatment Time. At this time, the majority of studies recommend treating for at least 5 days each week, with each treatment lasting 45 to 60 minutes (Table 8-3).

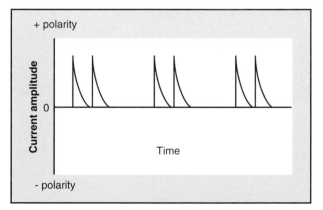

FIG 8-14 High-voltage pulsed current.

EDEMA CONTROL

Edema forms directly after an acute injury and as part of the inflammatory response. An area with this type of edema will appear red and feel warm. The application of electrical stimulation to control this type of edema has been studied extensively by Fish, Mendel, and co-workers.[11,133-137] The application of certain types of electrical stimulation during the inflammatory response can retard the formation of edema, although it does not decrease the amount of edema already present. Negative[137] (but not positive) polarity[136] HVPC below the threshold for motor contraction has been found to retard the formation of edema after acute injury in animal models. HVPC was found to reduce the formation of acute edema by roughly 50% as compared to untreated limbs, an effect similar to that of ibuprofen[138] or cool-water immersion.[139]

A number of theories have been suggested for how HVPC retards edema formation associated with inflammation. It is suggested that the negative charge repels negatively charged serum proteins, essentially blocking their movement out of blood vessels. Another theory is that the current decreases blood flow by reducing microvessel diameter, although cathodal stimulation has not been shown to have an effect on microvessel diameter.[140] Still another suggested mechanism involves a reduction in pore size in the microvessel walls, thereby preventing large plasma protein from leaking through pores[141]. In the normal histamine response to acute trauma, these pores would be enlarged. Prior studies referenced have found that both negative polarity and positive polarity HVPC decrease microvessel permeability, suggesting that some other mechanism possibly underlies the reduced edema formation produced by negative polarity stimulation only.

Electrical stimulation can also reduce edema caused by poor peripheral circulation due to lack of motion.[142] Edema can form in the distal extremities when the area is dependent and there is reduced or absent muscle activity. When the distal muscles can contract, return flow of fluid from the periphery is promoted by contracting muscles compressing the veins and lymphatic vessels. If the muscles do not contract, fluid in the form of edema will accumulate. An area with this type of edema will appear pale and feel cool. Edema of this type can be treated by applying motor-level electrical stimulation to the muscles around

TABLE 8-3	Recommended Parameter Settings for Electrical Stimulation for Tissue Healing					
Parameter Settings/ Goal of Treatment	Waveform	Polarity	Pulse Frequency	Pulse Duration	Amplitude	Treatment Time
Tissue healing: inflammatory phase/infected	HVPC	Negative	60-125 pps	Usually preset for HVPC at 40-100 μs	To produce comfortable tingling	45-60 min
Tissue healing: proliferation phase/clean	HVPC	Positive	60-125 pps	Usually preset for HVPC at 40-100 μs	To produce comfortable tingling	45-60 min

HVPC, High-voltage pulsed current.

the main draining veins. Motor-level electrical stimulation, in conjunction with elevating the legs, has been shown to increase popliteal blood flow in subjects with a history of lower limb surgery or thromboembolism[143] and was found to reduce the increase in foot and ankle volume produced in healthy volunteers after standing motionless for 30 minutes.[141] In contrast, submotor (i.e., sensory level) electrical stimulation (NMES) has, as expected, not been found to be effective for this application.[144] This intervention should be applied in conjunction with elevation and followed by use of a compression garment (see Chapter 11).

Parameters for Electrical Stimulation for Edema Control

When electrical stimulation is used for edema control, the therapist must determine whether the edema is caused by acute inflammation, lack of muscle contraction, or other causes (heart, kidney, or liver failure). Electrical stimulation can be used to treat edema associated with acute inflammation or lack of muscle contraction, but different parameters must be used for these different types of edema. Electrical stimulation should not be used to treat edema with other causes. Patients with edema of other causes should be evaluated by a medical provider.

Electrical Stimulation for Edema Associated with Inflammation

Electrode Placement. For retarding the formation of edema associated with acute inflammation, the negative polarity treatment electrode(s) should be placed directly over the area of edema, with the dispersive electrode more proximal if possible (Fig. 8-15).

Waveform. When using electrical stimulation to inhibit the formation of edema during the acute inflammatory response, HVPC is the recommended waveform.

Pulse Duration. When using HVPC to inhibit the formation of edema associated with acute inflammation, the pulse width of the device will be fixed and in the range of 40 to 100 μs.

Polarity. When using HVPC to inhibit the formation of edema associated with acute inflammation the negative polarity electrode should be placed over the area of edema.

Frequency. When electrical stimulation is used to control the formation of edema associated with inflammation, the pulse frequency is set to 100 to 120 pps.

On:Off Time. Electrical stimulation is delivered continuously throughout the treatment time when used to control edema associated with acute inflammation.

Current Amplitude. When using electrical stimulation to retard the formation of inflammatory edema, the current amplitude should be set to a comfortable sensory level.

Treatment Time. When used to retard the formation of edema associated with inflammation, electrical stimulation is generally applied for 20 to 30 minutes but may be used more than once a day.

Electrical Stimulation for Edema Associated with Lack of Muscle Contraction

Electrode Placement. To reduce edema associated with lack of muscle activity, electrically stimulated contractions of the muscles around the deep veins supplying the area can pump away the excess fluid. For this application, the electrodes should be placed on the muscle around the main veins draining the area in the same way as recommended for muscle contractions (Fig. 8-16).

Waveform. When using electrical stimulation to reduce edema associated with lack of muscle activity, a pulsed biphasic waveform or Russian protocol is recommended.

Pulse Duration. When using a pulsed biphasic waveform to reduce edema associated with lack of muscle activity, the pulse duration should be between 150 and 350 μsec, sufficient to produce a muscle contraction.

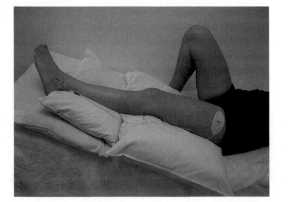

FIG 8-15 Electrode placement to retard acute edema formation at the ankle.

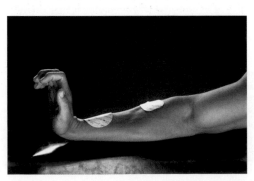

FIG 8-16 Electrode placement to reduce edema in the wrist and hand caused by lack of motion. *Courtesy Mettler Electronics, Anaheim, CA.*

TABLE 8-4	Recommended Parameter Settings for Electrical Stimulation for Edema Control					
Parameter Settings/ Goal of Treatment	**Waveform**	**Polarity**	**Pulse Frequency**	**Pulse Duration**	**Amplitude**	**Treatment Time**
Edema control: For edema associated with inflammation	HVPC	Negative	100-120 pps	Usually preset for HVPC at 40-100 µs	To produce comfortable tingling	20-30 min
Edema control: For edema associated with lack of motion	Biphasic (can use interferential if on:off time available)	NA	35-50 pps, 2-5 sec equal on:off times	150-350 µs	To visible contraction	20-30 min

HPVC, High-voltage pulsed current; *NA*, not applicable.

Frequency. When electrical stimulation is used to control edema associated with lack of muscle contraction, the frequency should be 35 to 50 pps, as used to produce muscle contractions for other purposes.

On:Off Time. An on time of 1 to 2 seconds and an off time of 1 to 2 seconds is recommended to promote muscle pumping when electrical stimulation is used to reduce edema caused by lack of muscle activity.

Current Amplitude. When using electrical stimulation to control edema associated with lack of muscle activity, the amplitude should be sufficient to produce a small, visible muscle contraction.

Treatment Time. When used to control edema associated with lack of muscle activity, electrical stimulation is generally applied for 20 to 30 minutes but may be used more than once a day (Table 8-4).

IONTOPHORESIS

Iontophoresis is the use of low-amplitude DC to facilitate transdermal drug delivery. The use of iontophoresis was first reported in the early 1900s.[145,146] Iontophoresis is based on the principle that like charges repel and that therefore a fixed charge electrode on the skin can drive charged ions of a drug through the skin by "pushing" them away.[147] However, more recent studies suggest that iontophoresis may promote transdermal drug penetration primarily by increasing the permeability of the outermost layer of the skin, the stratum corneum, the main barrier to transdermal drug uptake.[148-150]

The depth of drug delivery with iontophoresis is uncertain. Most studies have demonstrated penetration to a depth of 3 to 20 mm.[151] For example, in comparing iontophoretic delivery with passive delivery of salicylic acid and lidocaine to rats, it was found that both drugs penetrated 3 to 4 mm below the skin when delivered by iontophoresis if the epidermis was intact or by passive delivery if the epidermis was removed.[152] Passive delivery was the application of the drug to the skin without additional enhancement. Penetration was negligible with passive delivery when the epidermis was not removed. The authors of this study concluded that iontophoresis allows salicylic acid and lidocaine to penetrate through the stratum corneum. Another study demonstrated that sodium ethanolamine and lidocaine could be detected up to 2 cm laterally away from the iontophoresis treatment electrode in the intact skin of rats.[153] Declining drug concentration with distance was thought to be a result of clearance from the site of application by the skin's microcirculation, resulting in systemic uptake of the drug.

TABLE 8-5	Current Amplitude and Treatment Duration for Iontophoresis Treatment	
Current Amplitude (mA)	**Treatment Time (min)**	**Dose (mA-min)**
1	40	40
2	20	40
3	13.3	40
4	10	40

For an electrical current to facilitate transdermal drug penetration, the current must be at least sufficient to overcome the combined resistance of the skin and the electrode being used.[154] The amount of electricity used for performing iontophoresis is described according to charge, in milliamp minutes (mA-min). This is the product of the current amplitude, measured in milliamps, and the time, measured in minutes. The number of milliamp minutes depends on the specific electrode being used and is determined by the manufacturer of the electrode. At this time, most manufacturers recommend using 40 mA-min for each iontophoresis treatment, although some recommend up to 80 mA-min. Studies have shown effective drug delivery with a range of 40 to 80 mA-min treatments.[155]

One can use a number of combinations to achieve the currently recommended 40 mA-min dosage level. For example, a 1 mA current for 40 minutes, a 2 mA current for 20 minutes, or a 4 mA current for 10 minutes all give a 40 mA-min treatment (Table 8-5). In practice, one should set the current amplitude to patient comfort and then adjust the time to produce the desired product. Typical treatment current amplitudes used in research studies are between 1.0 mA and 5.0 mA; however, currently available clinical devices only allow a maximum current amplitude of 4.0 mA.[156]

To promote continuous delivery of the ionized drug, a direct current must be used for iontophoresis. Unfortunately, this type of current can also produce undesirable chemical changes under the electrodes. Sodium hydroxide, which is caustic, can form under the negative electrode, causing discomfort, skin irritation, or chemical burns.[157] This is known as the alkaline reaction. Reducing the **current density** by making the negative electrode larger or reducing the current amplitude will help decrease the risk of adverse effects. Hydrochloric acid can form under the positive electrode. This is known as the acidic reaction and is generally less uncomfortable than the alkaline reaction.

To reduce the risk of skin irritation, optimize comfort, and provide prolonged drug delivery, iontophoresis delivery systems that have low voltage output and apply an extremely low current for a much longer period of time have recently been developed. These devices have a battery within the electrodes and deliver between 0.1 and 0.3 mA for a period of 1 to 24 hours, delivering a total dose of approximately 40 to 80 mA-min (Fig. 8-17). The battery activates when the drug is applied to the electrode (also called a patch) and the patch is applied to the skin. The patch can be worn under clothing and requires no machine or external battery. A recent study demonstrated that this type of iontophoresis delivery increases drug retention in the treatment area because it causes less increase in local circulation.[158,159]

Although the low-voltage patches are more comfortable than traditional iontophoresis delivery, their lower voltage and current may reduce drug delivery because of high skin resistance. To address this, a new device combining traditional and low-volt technology has been designed and has recently become available (Hybresis System, Iomed, Salt Lake City, UT). This device has a small rechargeable wireless dose controller that attaches to a patch containing the drug to be delivered (Fig. 8-18). Three minutes of 3 mA current is applied by the clinician using the controller at the beginning of treatment to decrease skin resistance. The controller is then removed and the patch, which then delivers a low level of current, is worn for 1 to 2 hours and turns off automatically after a preset dose of 40, 60, or 80 mA-min has been delivered.

This device may also be used to deliver standard iontophoresis in the clinic or patch-only treatment, without the 3 minutes of 3 mA current at the beginning, for a longer period. Although this device shows promise, it is not yet in wide clinical use and has only undergone limited study.[160]

Many drugs can be delivered by iontophoresis as long as they can be ionized and are stable in solution, are not altered by the application of an electrical current, and their ions are small or moderate in size. Different drugs have been used for the treatment of different pathologies (Table 8-6). At this time the manufacturers of iontophoresis electrodes recommend using iontophoresis only for delivering dexamethasone or lidocaine. However, the use

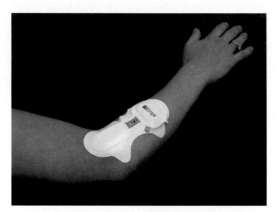

FIG 8-17 24-hour iontophoresis patch.

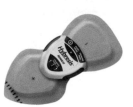

FIG 8-18 Hybrid iontophoresis device. *Courtesy Iomed, Salt Lake City, UT.*

TABLE 8-6	Ions Used Clinically for Iontophoresis, Including Ion Source, Polarity, Recommended Indications, and Concentration				
Ion	**Source**	**Polarity**	**Indications**		**Concentration (%)**
Acetate	Acetic acid	Negative	Calcium deposits		2.5-5
Chloride	NaCl	Negative	Sclerotic		2
Copper	CuSO₄	Positive	Fungal infection		2
Dexamethasone phosphate	DexNa₂PO₃	Negative	Inflammation		0.4
Hyaluronidase	Wydase	Positive	Edema reduction		
Iodine	—	Negative	Scar		5
Lidocaine	Lidocaine 1:50,000 with epinephrine	Positive	Local anesthetic		5
Magnesium	MgSO₄	Positive	Muscle relaxant, vasodilator		
Salicylate	NaSal	Negative	Inflammation, plantar warts		2
Tap water	—	Negative/positive	Hyperhidrosis		
Zinc	ZnO₂	Positive	Dermal ulcers, wounds		

of other substances, such as acetic acid for treatment of calcific tendinitis or heel pain, has been reported.[161] There is also a new iontophoretic delivery system available by physician order only for delivering fentanyl to hospitalized patients.[162]

Dexamethasone is a corticosteroid with antiinflammatory action that is recommended for treatment of inflammatory conditions such as tendonitis or bursitis. Dexamethasone iontophoresis has been found to be more effective than placebo in the treatment of lateral epicondylitis and plantar fasciitis.[163,164] Dexamethasone is delivered by iontophoresis, using a 0.4% solution of dexamethasone sodium phosphate. The negative polarity electrode is used to promote the penetration of the negatively charged dexamethasone phosphate ion through the skin (Fig. 8-19).

Lidocaine is an anesthetic drug. In the past, dexamethasone and lidocaine were delivered together by iontophoresis, with a positive charge being used initially to promote lidocaine delivery and then a negative charge being used to promote dexamethasone delivery.[165] This combined procedure mimicked the combined application of lidocaine and dexamethasone by injection and provided chemical buffering. However, because iontophoresis should not be as painful as an injection, the lidocaine is not needed. Also, newer electrodes are buffered, adding to the safety of the treatment. It is therefore recommended that dexamethasone be delivered alone with the negative electrode only. One randomized controlled trial found that low-dose lidocaine iontophoresis provided effective topical anesthesia for venipuncture and venous cannulation within 10 minutes in adults and children.[166] The manufacturers of iontophoresis electrodes have recommended lidocaine iontophoresis for local anesthesia in children.

There has also been much research exploring the use of iontophoresis to deliver a wide range of other molecules including insulin, leuprolide, calcitonin analogues, cyclosporin, and beta-blockers.[13] There is also a product currently available by prescription that uses reverse iontophoresis to measure a patient's blood sugar level (GlucoWatch Biographer, Animas Technologies, Westchester, PA). In the future, reverse iontophoresis may provide a nonin-vasive way of checking the blood levels of other substances that now require taking a blood sample and analyzing it in a laboratory.[167]

Parameters for the Application of Iontophoresis

Electrode Placement and Size. For iontophoresis the drug delivery electrode is placed over the area of pathology and the dispersive or return electrode is placed a few inches away, at a site of convenience over a large muscle belly (Fig. 8-20). The electrode should be large enough that the current density does not exceed $0.5\,mA/cm^2$ when using the cathode as the delivery electrode and $1.0\,mA/cm^2$ if the anode is used.[64]

Polarity. For iontophoresis the drug delivery electrode should have the same polarity as the polarity of the active ion of the drug to be delivered.

Current Amplitude. For iontophoresis the amplitude should be determined by patient comfort and should be no greater than 4 mA.

Treatment Time. For iontophoresis the treatment time is affected by the current amplitude and should be adjusted to produce a total treatment dose of 40 mA-min, which is achieved by setting the amplitude to patient tolerance and then setting, or having the device select, the treatment time to achieve the desired treatment dose (Table 8-7). It is important to check the patient's skin during this treatment because the DC and the small electrodes used for iontophoresis produce a high current density, increasing the risk of burning the patient.

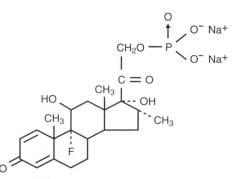

FIG 8-19 The molecular structure of dexamethasone sodium phosphate. Note that the negatively charged dexamethasone phosphate ion is moved across the dermal barrier by iontophoresis using the negatively charged electrode.

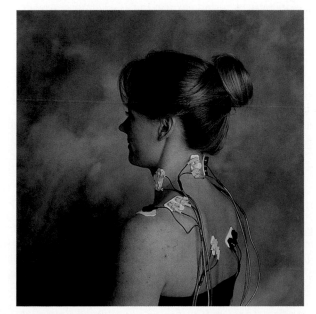

FIG 8-20 Electrode placement for iontophoresis. *Courtesy Iomed, Salt Lake City, UT.*

TABLE 8-7	Recommended Parameter Settings for Electrical Stimulation for Iontophoresis					
Parameter Settings/ Goal of Treatment	Waveform	Pulse Frequency	Pulse Duration	Amplitude	Polarity	Treatment Time
Iontophoresis	DC	NA	NA	To patient tolerance, no greater than 4 mA	Same as drug ion. See Table 8-5	Depends on amplitude, to produce a total of 40 mA-min

DC, Direct current; *NA,* not applicable.

CONTRAINDICATIONS AND PRECAUTIONS FOR THE USE OF ELECTRICAL CURRENTS

The use and application of electrical currents is not without risks. There are widely accepted contraindications and precautions that have been established to ensure the best clinical practice and application of these tools. These contraindications and precautions are presented in the next section.

CONTRAINDICATIONS FOR THE USE OF ELECTRICAL CURRENTS

CONTRAINDICATIONS
for the Use of Electrical Currents

- Demand cardiac pacemaker or unstable arrhythmias
- Placement of electrodes over carotid sinus
- Areas where venous or arterial thrombosis or thrombophlebitis is present
- Pregnancy—over or around the abdomen or low back

Demand Pacemaker or Unstable Arrhythmias

Electrical stimulation devices should not be used on patients with demand cardiac pacemakers because electrical stimulation may interfere with the functioning of this type of pacemaker and could alter the heart rate. Electrical stimulation may also aggravate an unstable arrhythmia that is not treated with a pacemaker.

Ask the Patient
- Do you have a cardiac pacemaker?
- Do you have a history of heart problems or have you been treated for heart problems?
- What type of heart problems?
- How recently has your doctor checked your heart?

If the patient has a pacemaker, electrical stimulation should not be applied. If the patient is unsure of his or her cardiac status or has recently had episodes of cardiac arrhythmias or pain, the therapist should consult with the referring physician to rule out the possibility of cardiac compromise during the use of electrical stimulation as a treatment modality.

Over the Carotid Sinus

Care should be taken to avoid placement of electrodes on the anterior or lateral neck in the areas over the carotid sinuses because stimulation to these areas may induce a rapid fall in blood pressure and heart rate that may cause the patient to faint.

Venous or Arterial Thrombosis or Thrombophlebitis

Stimulation should not be placed over areas of known venous or arterial thrombosis or thrombophlebitis because stimulation may increase circulation, increasing the risk of releasing emboli.

Ask the Patient
- Do you have a blood clot in this area?

Assess
- Check the area for increased swelling, redness, and increased tenderness. If any of these are present, do not apply electrical stimulation until the possibility of a thrombus has been ruled out.

Pelvis, Abdomen, Trunk, and Low Back Area During Pregnancy

The effects of electrical stimulation on the developing fetus and on the pregnant uterus have not been determined. Therefore it is recommended that stimulation electrodes not be placed in any way that the current may reach the fetus. Electrodes should not be applied to the low back, abdomen, or hips (as might be the case for bursitis), where the path of the current might cross the uterus.

Occasionally, electrical stimulation is used for pain control during labor and delivery as an alternative to general anesthesia or a spinal block.[168-170] Electrodes can be placed on the low back or on the anterior lower abdominal region, depending on where the pain is felt. The patient increases the current amplitude during a contraction and turns the amplitude down or off between contractions.

Ask the Patient
- Are you pregnant?
- Could you be pregnant?
- Are you trying to get pregnant?

The patient may not know if she is pregnant, particularly in the first few days or weeks after conception. Because damage may occur early during development, electrical stimulation should not be applied in any area where the current may reach the fetus of a patient who is or might be pregnant.

PRECAUTIONS FOR THE USE OF ELECTRICAL CURRENTS

PRECAUTIONS

for the Use of Electrical Currents

- Cardiac disease
- Patients with impaired mentation or in areas with impaired sensation
- Malignant tumors
- Areas of skin irritation or open wounds
- Iontophoresis after other physical agents

Cardiac Disease

Cardiac disease includes previous myocardial infarction or other specifically known congenital or acquired cardiac abnormalities.

Ask the Patient

- Do you have a known history of cardiac disease?
- Have you had a previous myocardial infarction?
- Have you ever had rheumatic fever as a child or an adult?
- Are you aware of having any cardiac problems at this time?

Assess

- Check for surgical incisions in the thoracic area, both anteriorly and posteriorly.
- Check the patient's resting pulse and respiratory rate before initiating treatment and check for changes in these values during and after applying electrical stimulation.

Impaired Mentation or Impaired Sensation

The patient's sensation and reporting of pain are usually used to limit the intensity of current applied to within safe limits. If the patient cannot report or feel pain, electrical stimulation must be applied with caution and close attention must be paid to any possible adverse effects. In addition, patients with impaired mentation may also be agitated and try to pull off the stimulation electrodes. Electrical stimulation may be used to treat chronic open wounds in areas with decreased sensation by first determining the appropriate current amplitude in an area with intact sensation.

Assess

- Sensation in the area
- Patient orientation and level of alertness
- Patient agitation

Malignant Tumors

Although there is no research concerning the effects of applying electrical stimulation to malignant tumors, because electrical currents can enhance tissue growth, in most cases it is recommended that electrical stimulation not be applied to patients with known or suspected malignant tumors. Electrical stimulation should not be applied to any area of the body of a patient with a malignancy because malignant tumors can metastasize to areas beyond where they are first found or known to be. Occasionally, electrical stimulation is used to control pain in patients with known malignancy. This is done when the improvement in quality of life afforded by this intervention is considered to be greater than the possible risks associated with the treatment.

Ask the Patient

- Have you ever had cancer? Do you have cancer now?
- Do you have fever, sweats, chills, or night pain?
- Do you have pain at rest?
- Have you had recent unexplained weight loss?

Skin Irritation or Open Wounds

Electrodes should not be placed over abraded skin or known open wounds unless the electrical stimulation is being used to treat the wound. Open or damaged skin should be avoided because it has lower **impedance** and less sensation than intact skin, and this may result in too much current being delivered to the area.

Assess

- Inspect the patient's skin carefully before placing electrodes.
- Check for increased redness, swelling, warmth, rashes or broken and abraded areas.

Iontophoresis After Another Physical Agent

It is recommended that iontophoresis not be applied after the application of any physical agent that may alter skin permeability, such as heat, ice, or ultrasound. In addition, heat will cause vasodilation and increased blood flow that can accelerate dispersion of the drug from the treatment area.

ADVERSE EFFECTS OF ELECTRICAL CURRENTS

There are very few potential adverse effects from the clinical application of electrical currents. Careful evaluation of the patient and review of the patient's pertinent medical history and current medical status will minimize the likelihood of any adverse effects. In addition, patients should be monitored throughout the initial treatment with electrical stimulation for any adverse effects of the stimulation. If a patient is provided with an electrical stimulation unit for home use, the patient should be clearly instructed in its use and in early identification of potential adverse effects.

Electrical currents can cause burns. This effect is seen most commonly when a DC or AC (including interferential current) is being applied. DC and AC are always on, unlike pulsed currents, resulting in high total charge delivery and high skin impedance. In addition, the chemical effects produced under DC electrodes can be caustic. If there is not enough conduction medium on an electrode, as can occur with repeated use of self-adhesive electrodes or poorly applied nonadhesive electrodes, the risk of burns also increases because of the increased current density in the areas where there is adequate conduction. The risk of burns can be minimized by using at least 2 × 2-inch electrodes for interferential currents and only using electrodes that adhere well to the skin.

Skin irritation or inflammation may occur in the area where electrical stimulation electrodes are applied because the patient is allergic to the contact surface of the electrode such as the adhesive or foam rubber. If this occurs, a different type of electrode should be tried.

Some patients find electrical stimulation to be painful. In such patients, increasing the current amplitude slowly over a longer period of time may be better tolerated. In patients who find all forms of electrical stimulation painful, other treatment approaches should be used.

APPLICATION TECHNIQUE

This section provides guidelines for the sequence of procedures required for the safe and effective application of therapeutic electrical stimulation.

PATIENT POSITIONING

Patient positioning is dictated by the area to be treated, the goal(s) of the treatment, and the device used. Primary to these three issues are patient comfort and modesty. Upper extremity set-ups require short sleeves or a halter top for women, whereas men may or may not be comfortable with their shirts off. When treating the neck, upper and lower back, or hips, the clinician should ask the patient if they feel protected or covered enough by their clothing or additional sheets or towels the clinician has in place. If in doubt, an additional covering may add to a patient's comfort. For lower extremity set-ups, shorts are generally adequate and allow the patient to perform voluntary exercise with the stimulation in place.

When applying electrical stimulation for muscle strengthening, the limb should be secured to prevent motion through the range, with the joint that the stimulated muscles cross in midrange. This will allow the patient to perform a strong isometric contraction in midrange rather than moving through the range and then applying maximum force at the end of the available ROM. The limb may be secured by placing a barrier to motion in either direction or by using cuff weights to overpower the strength of the muscle. In addition, most treatment tables have positioning straps that can be used to facilitate appropriate and comfortable positioning for the patient, whereas maintaining the joint in a single position to facilitate an isometric contraction.

ELECTRODE TYPE

Many different types of electrodes are available for use with electrical stimulation devices. The electrodes serve as the interface between the patient and the stimulator. They are connected from the machine to the electrodes by cables or lead wires. Surgically implantable electrodes are also available but since these are not placed by therapists they are not discussed further in this book. A number of factors, including electrode material, size and shape, the need for conductive gel, and the tissues to be treated, should be considered when selecting electrodes for electrical stimulation.

The electrodes most commonly used today are disposable and flexible and have a self-adhesive gel coating that serves as the conduction medium (Fig. 8-21). The gel decreases resistance between the electrode and the skin.

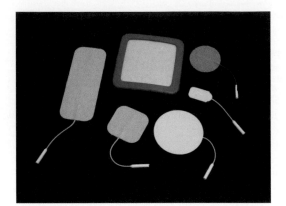

FIG 8-21 Examples of different types of electrodes.

These self-adhesive electrodes may be designed for single use or for multiple uses over a period of 1 month or more. Although many electrodes on the market may appear to be made with similar material and conductive gel, their conductivity, impedance, and comfort may differ. How often an electrode can be used depends on the nature of the gel coating. Once this coating starts to dry out, the current delivery becomes less uniform, causing uneven current density. In areas where the electrode is still able to conduct, the current density will be high, and this can cause the skin under the electrode to burn. Therefore electrodes must be inspected regularly, and dry or discolored ones should be discarded.

More long-lasting electrodes are made of carbon-impregnated silicone rubber (see Fig. 8-21). These electrodes are used with a gel conduction medium or with a sponge soaked in tap water to promote conduction. Because these types of electrodes are not self-adhesive, they must be secured to the patient with tape, elastic straps, or bandages. Carbon rubber electrodes should be cleaned with warm, soapy water and not alcohol.

Selection of electrode size, shape, and type depends on the treatment goals, the area to be treated, and the amount of tissue or muscle bulk targeted. Because current density is inversely proportional to the size of the electrode, larger electrodes are more comfortable than smaller ones. However, large electrodes cannot target small areas.

ELECTRODE PLACEMENT

To ensure even delivery of current, electrodes must lie smoothly against the skin without wrinkles or gaps. Self-adhesive electrodes usually maintain good contact; however, with other types of electrodes, flexible bandaging is generally needed to maintain good electrode-to-skin contact. Electrodes should not be placed directly over bony prominences because the higher resistance of bone and the poor adhesion of electrodes to highly contoured surfaces increases the risk of discomfort and burns and is less likely to produce therapeutic benefits.

> ◎ **Clinical Pearl**
>
> Electrodes should not be placed directly over bony prominences.

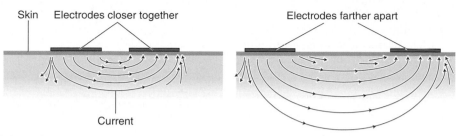

FIG 8-22 The effect of electrode spacing. When the electrodes are closer together, the current travels more superficially. When the electrodes are further apart, the current goes deeper.

The distance or spacing between electrodes affects the depth and course of the current. The closer together electrodes are configured, the more superficially the current travels, and conversely, the greater the distance between them, the deeper the current travels (Fig. 8-22).

The ideal electrode placement should be documented, noting distance or approximation to bony landmarks or anatomical structures, so that follow-up sessions can replicate the placement. Diagrams are often helpful.

> ◎ **Clinical Pearl**
>
> Document electrode placement using diagrams.

GENERAL INSTRUCTIONS FOR ELECTRICAL STIMULATION

APPLICATION TECHNIQUE 8-1	ELECTRICAL STIMULATION

1. Assess the patient and set treatment goals.
2. Determine if electrical stimulation is the most appropriate intervention.
3. Determine that electrical stimulation is not contraindicated for this patient or for the specific diagnosis you are treating. Check with the patient and review the patient's chart for contraindications or precautions regarding the application of electrical stimulation.
4. Select an electrical stimulation unit with the necessary waveform and adjustable parameters for the intervention (muscle contraction, pain modulation, tissue healing, etc).
5. Explain the procedure to the patient, including an explanation of what he/she might expect to experience, and any instructions or directions regarding patient participation with the electrical stimulation.
6. Position the patient appropriately and comfortably for the intervention.
7. Inspect the skin where the stimulation is to be applied for any signs of abrasions or skin irritation. Clean the skin and clip hair if necessary for good adhesion of the electrode to the skin, and thus good current flow. The hair should not be shaved as this can cause skin cuts or abrasions.
8. Check electrodes and lead wires for continuity or signs of excessive wear and replace any of those found faulty or of concern.
9. Apply the electrodes to the area being treated. Use conductive gel if electrodes are not pregelled. Use the appropriate size and number of electrodes to address the problem. For specific information on electrode selection and placement, please see the sections later on these topics.
10. Attach the lead wires to electrodes and to the stimulation unit.
11. Set optimal parameters for treatment including waveform, polarity, frequency, pulse duration, on:off time, ramp up/ramp down, and length of treatment time, as indicated for the goals of the intervention. For specific information on parameter selection for different treatment effects, refer to Tables 8-1 to 8-4 and Table 8-7, and the sections on parameter selection within the clinical application discussions earlier in this chapter.
12. Slowly advance the amplitude until the patient is just able to notice a sensation under the electrodes. If a muscle contraction is needed to achieve the treatment objectives, continue to increase the amplitude until the indicated strength of contraction is produced.
13. Observe the patient's reaction to the stimulation over the first few minutes of the treatment. If the treatment includes muscle contraction, observe the amplitude, direction, and quality of the contraction. The parameters may need to be adjusted or the electrodes may need to be moved slightly if the expected outcome is not achieved.
14. When the treatment is completed, remove the electrodes and inspect the patient's skin for any signs of adverse reaction to the treatment.
15. Document the treatment, including all treatment parameters and the patient's response to the treatment.

DOCUMENTATION

The following should be documented:
- Area of the body treated with electrical stimulation
- Patient positioning
- Stimulation parameters
- Electrode placement
- Treatment duration
- Response to treatment

Documentation is typically written in the SOAP note (Subjective, Objective, Assessment, Plan) format. The following examples only summarize the modality component of treatment and are not intended to represent a comprehensive plan of care.

EXAMPLES

When applying electrical stimulation (ES) to the right (R) knee for quadriceps muscle reeducation after R anterior cruciate ligament (ACL) reconstruction, document the following:

S: Pt reports she is unable to independently perform the quad set exercise she was instructed to do at her last treatment.

O: Pretreatment: Pt unable to perform quad exercises.

Intervention: ES to R quadriceps muscles ×20 min. Electrodes placed over vastus medialis oblique (VMO) muscle and proximal lateral anterior thigh. Biphasic waveform, pulse duration 300 μsec, frequency 50 pps, on : off time 10 sec : 50 sec, ramp up/ramp down: 2 sec/2 sec, amplitude to produce maximum tolerated contraction. Pt instructed to attempt to contract quadriceps muscle with the ES.

Posttreatment: Pt able to perform 4 visible quadriceps contractions independently after ES treatment.

A: Pt tolerated ES with increased ability to contract VMO during exercise.

P: Discontinue ES when pt can perform quad sets ×10 independently as part of home program.

When applying TENS for relief of acute pain in bilateral (B) upper trapezius (trap) and neck because of a motor vehicle accident (MVA), docum.ent the following:

S: Pt reports constant B trap area pain after MVA 10 days ago. He awakens 6-10 × each night from neck pain. Pt denies pain, numbness, or tingling in his upper extremities.

O: Intervention: TENS to B upper trap area ×30 min, 2 channels, 4 electrodes, 2 at level of cervical thoracic junction and 2 at level of proximal-medial scapulae, crossed channels. Biphasic waveform, pulse duration 70 μsec, frequency 120 pps, with amplitude modulation. Pt set amplitude to his comfort.

Posttreatment: After 20 min of treatment, pt notes a 50% decrease in his trap area discomfort. Pt instructed in appropriate application and use; he then correctly demonstrated set up and operation of unit. Given written instruction for independent home use of TENS.

A: Pt tolerated TENS, with decrease in pain.

P: Pt to use TENS independently at home up to 24 hrs/day for pain. Pt to monitor the condition of his skin under the electrodes and discontinue TENS if irritation or redness occurs. Pt to call therapist at clinic if he has any questions or concerns re: independent TENS use.

When applying ES to a full thickness venous ulcer on the left (L) lateral ankle, document the following:

S: Pt alert and oriented ×3. She states she has been keeping her L lower extremity elevated as much as possible because the edema in her L ankle increases with dependent positioning.

O: Intervention: Pt supine with 2 pillows under L leg for elevation. HVPC to L lower extremity ×1 hr. 2 treating electrodes placed periwound, 1 dispersive electrode placed on proximal posterior calf. Frequency 100 pps, negative (−) polarity to treatment area, intensity to sensory level.

Posttreatment: Wound area decreased from 10 × 5 cm on first treatment 3 weeks ago to 8 × 3 cm today.

A: Pt tolerated treatment well. Wound size decreasing.

P: Continue HVPC to L lateral ankle area until wound closes. Change polarity if healing plateaus.

CLINICAL CASE STUDIES

The following case studies demonstrate the concepts of the clinical application of electrical stimulation discussed in this chapter. Based on the scenarios presented, an evaluation of the clinical findings and goals of treatment are proposed. These are followed by a discussion of the factors to be considered in the selection of electrical stimulation as an indicated intervention and in the selection of the ideal electrical stimulation parameters to promote progress toward the set goals of treatment.

CASE STUDY 8-1

Upper Back and Neck Pain
Examination
History

DS is a 28-year-old woman who was referred to physical therapy with a diagnosis of upper back and neck pain. DS complains of gradually increasing neck and upper trapezius pain over the past 6 weeks. She reports her pain is worse at the end of her work day as a supermarket checker. She notes that her pain has become more intense and frequent in the past month. DS states her pain increases with lifting, carrying, and any twisting motion of her neck, and she has had to cut short some of her workdays this month because of her pain. She has been evaluated by a physician, and her cervical spine x-rays were negative. She has no history of cardiac arrhythmias and does not have a pacemaker.

Tests and Measures

The patient states that her neck pain severity is 6/10. Her upper extremity active ROM (AROM) is within normal limits, her strength is 4+/5 bilaterally, and she is limited by neck pain. Her rhomboid and lower trapezius strength are 4−/5 bilaterally. Neck rotation and lateral flexion are 75% of normal, with pain on overpressure bilaterally. Forward flexion is uncomfortable in the final 30% of the range. Extension is within normal limits. On palpation, there are significant nodules in bilateral upper trapezius and trigger points along the medial borders of both scapulae. DS denies numbness or tingling in her upper extremities.

Why is this patient a candidate for electrical stimulation? What else should be included in her treatment program? What other physical agents might be useful?

Evaluation, Diagnosis, Prognosis, and Goals
Evaluation and Goals

ICF Level	Current Status	Goals
Body structure and function	Cervical and upper back pain	Control pain
		Regain normal cervical ROM
	Restricted cervical ROM	Regain normal upper body strength
	Decreased upper body strength	
Activity	Difficulty lifting and carrying	Resume usual ability to lift and carry
Participation	Decreased work hours	Perform all work-related duties and return to regular work hours

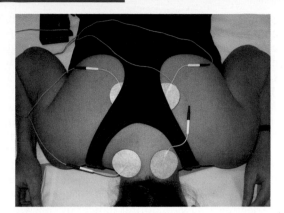

FIG 8-23 Treatment of upper back and neck pain with electrical stimulation.

Diagnosis
Preferred Practice Pattern 4B: Impaired posture.
Prognosis/Plan of Care
This patient does not appear to have a skeletal problem, given her normal x-ray and lack of tingling or numbness. The nodules in her trapezius and the scapular trigger points indicate a muscular cause of her pain. In general, TENS is an indicated treatment for the reduction of pain. Other physical agents, such as ultrasound or ice and heat, may be used in conjunction with electrical stimulation. This patient has no contraindications for the use of electrical stimulation.

Intervention
It is proposed that electrical stimulation be used for the control of pain, with the patient using a unit at home after evaluation and instruction (Fig. 8-23). The following parameters are chosen:

Type	Parameters
Electrode placement	One pair of electrodes upper cervical, one pair lower cervical
Waveform	Pulsed biphasic (or interferential)
Pulse rate	100-150 pps (or 100 bps-150 bps for interferential)
Pulse duration	50-80 μs
Modulation	Yes
Amplitude	Sensory only—to patient comfort
Treatment duration	The patient may wear unit throughout the day for pain control.

The patient will initially feel a gentle humming or buzzing under the electrodes. Once comfortable, patient may switch the unit to modulation mode so there is little or no adaptation to the stimulus. Because the patient will have a home unit, she will be able to receive treatment throughout the day to minimize her pain at all times. DS will be reevaluated for revision of parameters as well as update of her home exercise program weekly, with the frequency of visits decreasing as her problem resolves. Use of the electrical stimulation is generally discontin-

ued at the patient's request upon reaching tolerable resolution of pain.

If the patient is experiencing significant relief while wearing the TENS unit, she may use it at work. The lead wires can be placed under clothing, and the unit can be placed in a pocket or clipped onto a waistband. With present technology, amplitude controls are covered so that they cannot be accidentally moved, increasing or decreasing the current.

Documentation
S: Pt reports bilateral upper back and neck pain that is worse at the end of the day.
O: Pretreatment: Overall neck pain 6/10. UE strength 4+/5 bilaterally, limited by neck pain. Rhomboid and lower trapezius strength are 4−/5 bilaterally. Neck rotation and lateral flexion 75% of normal. Forward flexion uncomfortable in final 30% of range.
Intervention: TENS home unit to bilateral cervical area ×30 min, 4 electrodes, 2 upper and 2 lower cervical. Biphasic waveform, pulse duration 60 μs, frequency 130 pps, with amplitude modulation. Pt set amplitude to her comfort (sensory only).
During treatment: Approximately 50% decreased pain in neck and upper back.
A: Pt tolerated with no adverse effects. Demonstrated independent set-up and use of TENS.
P: Pt to use TENS at home up to 24 hr/day for pain and will discontinue TENS if irritation or redness occurs at the electrode site. Pt instructed in home exercises.

CASE STUDY 8-2

Medial Knee Pain
Examination
History
VP is a 47-year-old female carpet layer who developed right medial knee pain 4 months ago. Arthroscopic surgery revealed a flap tear abrasion of the trochlear surface of the femur, which was then débrided. VP had

Continued

surgery 3 weeks ago and comes to the physical therapy clinic with an order from her surgeon to evaluate and treat. She has had difficulty straightening her right leg and bearing full weight on the right when walking and has been unable to work since surgery.

Tests and Measures

VP states that right knee pain is 8/10. On palpation, there is mild warmth and tenderness of the patient's right knee. The surgical sites are healing well. Girth at the level of the midpatella is 43 cm on the right, 38 cm on the left. The right knee AROM is from 10 to 50 degrees of flexion. VP is ambulating household distances without any assistive device but with her right knee in about 15 to 20 degrees of flexion during stance. She has 4/5 quadriceps strength on the right, within the available ROM.

Why would electrical stimulation be a good choice in this patient? Does she have any contraindications to electrical stimulation? What are some appropriate goals?

Evaluation, Diagnosis, Prognosis, and Goals

Evaluation and Goals

ICF Level	Current Status	Goals
Body structure and function	R knee pain, loss of motion, increased girth	Control pain and edema Improve ROM Increase strength
Activity	Limited and altered ambulation	Return to normal ambulation
Participation	Unable to work	Return to limited, then normal work hours

Diagnosis

Preferred Practice Pattern 4I: Impaired joint mobility, motor function, muscle performance, and ROM associated with bony or soft tissue surgery.

Prognosis/Plan of Care

Electrical stimulation would be an appropriate treatment for this patient because it would help generate a greater level of force than the patient can generate on her own. Electrically stimulated muscle contractions would help increase the patient's lower extremity strength and may assist in eliminating fluid from around her knee, both of which would contribute to functional improvements. This patient has no contraindications for the use of electrical stimulation.

Intervention

Electrical stimulation with either a biphasic square waveform or Russian protocol should be used for this patient (Fig. 8-24). With a square wave the recommended parameters are as follows:

Type	Parameters
Electrode placement	One channel is set up on the quadriceps with one electrode over the VMO and the second electrode at the proximal lateral anterior thigh. Placement may need to be varied slightly, depending on quality of contraction and patient comfort. The second channel is placed on the hamstrings, also using large electrodes for comfort. The stimulation is applied alternately to the quadriceps and hamstrings, with a rest period in between. The channels should not run simultaneously as this would produce a co-contraction of the quads and hamstrings.
Pulse duration	200-350 μs (based on patient comfort, with longer durations used for larger muscles).
Pulse frequency	50-80 pps to achieve a smooth tetanic contraction.
On:off time	10 sec on, 50 sec off to initiate treatment, moving to 10/30 as the patient progresses.
Ramp up/ramp down time	2-3 sec ramp up/2 sec ramp down for comfort.
Amplitude	10%-50% of MVIC muscle contraction, as tolerated. The patient should be encouraged to actively contract with the stimulation if she is able.
Treatment time	Sufficient to produce 10-20 contractions. If available, the patient should use a portable stimulation device at home 3-4 times a day to accelerate her recovery.

Documentation

S: Pt reports R knee pain, increased girth and difficulty walking after R knee surgery.

O: Pretreatment: R knee pain 8/10. R knee girth 43 cm, L knee 38 cm. R knee AROM 10 to 50 degrees of flexion. R knee in about 15 to 20 degrees of flexion during stance when ambulating. R quadriceps strength 4/5.

Intervention: ES with biphasic square waveform, 2 channels, 2 electrodes from 1 channel over VMO, 2 electrodes from second channel over proximal lateral anterior thigh. Apply stimulation simultaneously to both channels. Pulse duration 250 μs, pulse frequency 50 pps, ramp up 3 sec, ramp down 2 sec, amplitude 20% of MVIC muscle contraction. Repeat for 15 contractions.

Posttreatment: Pt able to straighten knee in non–weight-bearing.

A: Pt tolerated ES, with improved quad control.

P: Pt given home device and demonstrated correct use. Pt to use 3-4 times daily at home, along with strengthening exercises.

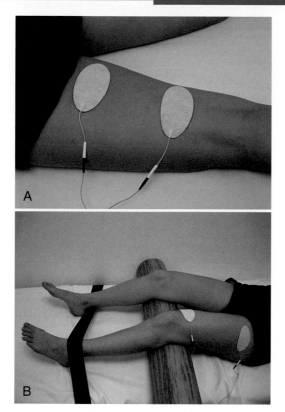

FIG 8-24 **A,** Electrical stimulation to increase hamstring; **B,** quadriceps strength.

CASE STUDY 8-3

Lateral Ankle Sprain
Examination
History

MC is a 23-year-old student. He injured his left ankle during a soccer game at school. He was seen by the attending physician on the field and diagnosed with a grade II lateral ankle sprain. MC's ankle was packed in ice and he was sent to the locker room for immediate physical therapy follow-up. The physician instructed MC to use non–weight-bearing on crutches to rest the injured ankle.

Tests and Measures

Visual inspection shows the patient holding his ankle in a single position with extreme hesitancy in allowing the therapist to move the joint. Gentle passive ROM (PROM) reveals restrictions in all directions. There is minimal AROM. The lateral talofibular joint is tender to touch, with discoloration indicative of internal bleeding along the lateral surface and an inability to view the lateral malleolus because of swelling. The area is warm

to the touch and slightly reddened. The student is otherwise healthy and denies a history of cancer, diabetes, or other significant health problems.

What kind of process is occurring in this patient's ankle? What kind of electrical stimulation would be most useful? What aspects of the patient's injury would electrical stimulation address? What other physical agent may be used along with electrical stimulation?

Evaluation, Diagnosis, Prognosis, and Goals
Evaluation and Goals

ICF Level	Current Status	Goals
Body structure and function	Left ankle pain, edema, and decreased ROM	Control edema and pain Accelerate resolution of the acute inflammatory phase of healing Increase ROM
Activity	Limited ambulation	Increase ambulation
Participation	Unable to play soccer	Return to playing soccer

Diagnosis

Preferred Practice Pattern 4D: Impaired joint mobility, motor function, muscle performance, and ROM associated with connective tissue dysfunction.

Prognosis/Plan of Care

Given the mechanism of injury, there is most likely an active inflammatory process occurring. Electrical stimulation using HVPC would be an appropriate choice of treatment as it has been shown to retard the formation of edema during the inflammatory stage of injury. It is also known to help control pain. There is nothing in the patient's history to indicate a contraindication to using electrical stimulation.

Intervention

Electrical stimulation using HVPC waveform is chosen based on the literature indicating that it is effective at decreasing edema formation after injury (see Fig. 8-15). The following parameters are chosen:

Type	Parameter
Electrode placement	One or two treating electrodes may be used over the swollen, discolored area. (Polarity is negative for treating electrodes.) The larger dispersive electrode is placed proximally over either the calf or the quadriceps. This may be based on comfort or other suspected areas of swelling. Ice may be added over the electrodes to further inhibit the formation of edema.
Pulse duration	Generally fixed at 40-100 μs for HVPC
Pulse frequency	120 pps
Mode	Continuous

Continued

CLINICAL CASE STUDIES—cont'd

Amplitude	Sensory ONLY. Ask the patient to state when a tingling or vibratory sensation just begins to occur. Continue to increase the amplitude until it reaches the maximum tolerable level. If a contraction is seen, decrease the amplitude
Treatment time	30 minutes

Documentation

S: Pt reports severe (9/10) L ankle pain immediately after injuring himself playing soccer.

O: Pretreatment: Pt unable to bear weight. L ankle PROM limited in all directions. Edema and discoloration over lateral L ankle.

Intervention: One treating electrode, negative polarity, place over lateral L ankle; one dispersive electrode on L calf. HVPC at 120 pps, continuous. Amplitude sensory only x30 minutes.

Posttreatment: Pain 5/10. Mildly increased L ankle PROM. Pt unable to bear weight.

A: Pt tolerated ES well, with a decreased pain and increased PROM.

P: Continue treatment 2-3 times daily for 30 minutes. Pt should remain non–weight-bearing and apply ice and elevation to the L ankle.

CHAPTER REVIEW

1. An electrical current is a flow of charged particles.
2. The effects of electrical currents include nerve depolarization, muscle depolarization, and ionic effects.
3. Most uses of electrical stimulation are based on its ability to depolarize nerves to produce action potentials (APs). Once an AP is generated by an electrical current, the body responds to it in the same way as it does to an AP that is generated physiologically. An electrically stimulated AP can affect sensory nerves producing a pleasant or painful sensation, or motor nerves producing a muscle contraction.
4. The sensations produced by electrically stimulated APs in sensory nerves can control pain.
5. The muscle contractions produced by electrically stimulated APs in motor nerves can strengthen muscles, increase muscle endurance, improve function, assist with joint positioning, decrease spasticity, increase circulation, and control pain.
6. The ionic effects of electrical currents can be used to facilitate tissue healing, control the formation of inflammation-related edema, and promote transdermal drug penetration.
7. For each application, the clinician must determine which parameters to use. Parameters include electrode placement, waveform, polarity, current amplitude, pulse duration, pulse frequency, on:off times, ramp time, and treatment time. These are summarized in tables throughout this chapter.
6. Contraindications for electrical stimulation include cardiac pacemaker, placement over carotid sinus, areas of thrombosis, and pregnancy. Precautions include cardiac disease, impaired mentation, impaired sensation, malignant tumor, skin irritation, and the use of iontophoresis after other physical agents.
7. The reader is referred to the Evolve web site for further exercises and links to resources and references.

ADDITIONAL RESOURCES *evolve*

Textbooks

Baker LL, Wederich CL, McNeal DR, et al: *Neuromuscular Electrical Stimulation: A Practical Guide*, ed 4, Downey, CA, 2000, Rancho Los Amigos Research and Educational Institute.

Gersh MR, Wolf SR: *Electrotherapy in Rehabilitation*, ed 2, Philadelphia, 2000, FA Davis.

Kitchen S, ed: *Electrotherapy Evidence-Based Practice*, ed 11, Edinburgh, 2002, Churchill Livingstone.

Nelson RM, Currier DP, Hayes K, eds: *Clinical Electrotherapy*, ed 3, Norwalk, CT, 1999, Appleton & Lange.

Web Sites

Chattanooga Group: Chattanooga produces a number of physical agents, including cold packs and cooling units, hot packs and warming units, paraffin, and fluidotherapy. The web site may be searched by body part or by product category. Product specifications are available online. www.chattgroup.com

Dynatronics Corporation: Dynatronics produces a variety of physical agents, including electrical stimulation devices. www.dynatronics.com

Empi: Empi specializes in noninvasive rehabilitation products, including iontophoresis and electrical stimulation. In addition to product brochures and protocols, the web site lists references. www.empi.com

Iomed: Iomed sells iontophoresis units and patches. The web site includes product brochures, specifications, and instructions. www.iomed.com

Mettler Electronics: Mettler Electronics carries a wide variety of electrical stimulation products. www.mettlerelectronics.com

GLOSSARY *evolve*

General Terms

Acupuncture-like TENS: TENS with long-duration, high-amplitude pulses used to control pain; also called low rate TENS.

Anode: The positive electrode.

Burst mode TENS: TENS using burst mode current.

Conventional TENS: TENS with short duration, low-amplitude pulses used to control pain; also called high rate TENS.

Cathode: The negative electrode.

Charge: One of the basic properties of matter, which either has no charge (is electrically neutral), or may be negatively (–) or positively (+) charged. Charge is noted as Q and is measured in Coulombs (C). Charge is equal to current × time.

$$Q = It$$

Current density: The amount of current delivered per unit area.

Electrical current: The movement or flow of charged particles through a conductor in response to an applied electrical field. Current is noted as I and is measured in amperes (A).

Electrical muscle stimulation (EMS): Application of an electrical current directly to muscle to produce a muscle contraction.

Functional electrical stimulation (FES): Application of an electrical current to produce muscle contractions that are applied during a functional activity. An example of FES is the electrical stimulation of dorsiflexion during the swing phase of gait.

Galvanotaxis: The attraction of cells to an electrical charge.

Gate control theory: A theory of pain control and modulation that states pain is modulated at the spinal cord level by inhibitory effects of nonnoxious afferent input.

Impedance: The total frequency-dependent opposition to current flow. Impedance is noted by Z and is measured in Ohms (Ω). For biological systems, impedance describes the ratio of voltage to current more accurately than resistance because it includes the effects of capacitance and resistance.

Iontophoresis: The transcutaneous delivery of ions into the body for therapeutic purpose using an electrical current.

Low rate TENS: TENS with long duration, high amplitude pulses used to control pain; also called acupuncture-like TENS.

Motor point: The place in a muscle where electrical stimulation will produce the greatest contraction with the least amount of electricity, generally located over the middle of the muscle belly.

Neuromuscular electrical stimulation (NMES): Application of an electrical current to motor nerves to produce contractions of the muscles they innervate.

Ohm's law: A mathematical expression of how voltage, current, and resistance relate where voltage equals current multiplied by resistance.

$$V = IR$$

Overload principle: A principle of strengthening muscle that states the greater the load placed on a muscle and the higher force contraction it produces, the more strength that muscle will gain.

Phase: In pulsed current, the period from when current starts to flow in one direction to when it stops flowing or starts to flow in the other direction. A biphasic pulsed current is made up of two phases; the first phase begins when current starts to flow in one direction and ends when the current starts to flow in the other direction, which is also the beginning of the second phase. The second phase ends when current stops flowing.

Polarity: The charge of an electrode that will be positive (the anode) or negative (the cathode) with a direct or monophasic pulsed current and constantly changing with an alternating or biphasic pulsed current.

Pulse: In pulsed current, the period when current is flowing in any direction.

Resistance: A material's opposition to the flow of electrical current. Resistance is noted as R and is measured in Ohms (Ω).

Transcutaneous electrical nerve stimulation (TENS): The application of electrical current through the skin to modulate pain.

Voltage: The force or pressure of electricity; the difference in electrical energy between two points that produces the electrical force capable of moving charged particles through a conductor between those two points. Voltage is noted as V and is measured in volts (V); also called potential difference.

Waveforms

Alternating current (AC): A continuous bidirectional flow of charged particles (Fig. 8-25). AC has equal ion flow in each direction, and thus no pulse charge remains in the tissues. Most commonly, AC is delivered as a sine wave. With AC, when the frequency increases, the cycle duration decreases and when the frequency decreases, the cycle duration increases (Fig. 8-26).

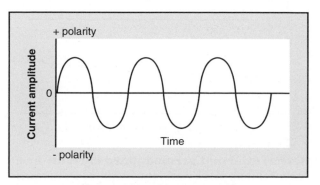

FIG 8-25 Alternating current (AC).

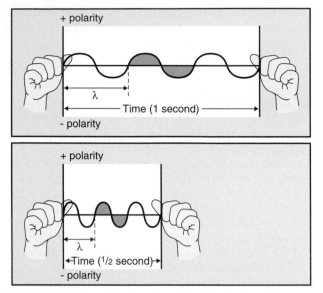

FIG 8-26 Illustration of the inverse relationship between frequency and cycle duration for an alternating current. (λ = Wavelength).

Medium frequency AC: An AC with a frequency between 1000 and 10,000 Hz (1-10 kHz). Most medium frequency currents available on clinical units have a frequency of 2500 to 5000 Hz. Medium frequency AC is rarely used alone therapeutically but two medium frequency ACs of different frequency may be applied together to produce an interferential current (see Interferential current).

Continuous current: A continuous flow of charged particles without interruptions or breaks. A continuous current that goes in one direction only is known as a *direct current* (DC). A continuous current that goes back and forth in two directions is known as an *alternating current* (AC).

Direct current (DC): A continuous unidirectional flow of charged particles. DC is used for iontophoresis and for stimulating contraction of denervated muscle and also occasionally to facilitate wound healing (Fig. 8-27).

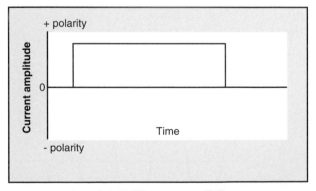

FIG 8-27 Direct current (DC).

Interferential and premodulated current: Interferential current is the waveform produced by the interference of two medium frequency (1000 to 10,000 Hz)

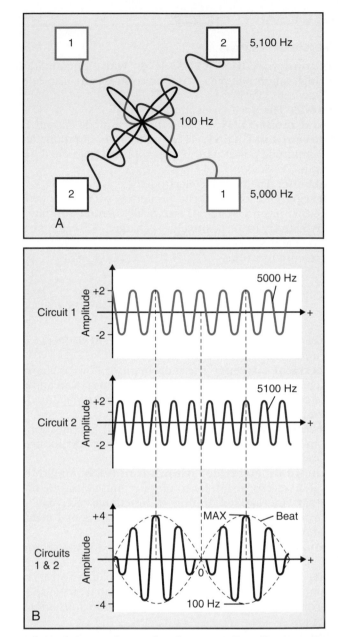

FIG 8-28 **A,** Intersecting medium frequency alternating currents producing an interferential current between two crossed pairs of electrodes. **B,** An alternating current with a frequency of 5000 Hz interfering with an alternating current with a frequency of 5100 Hz to produce an interferential current with a beat frequency of 100 Hz. Modified *from May H-U, Hansjürgens A:* Nemectrodyn Model 7 manual of Nemectron GmbH, *Karlsruhe, Germany, 1984, Nemectron GmbH.*

sinusoidal ACs of slightly different frequencies. These two waveforms are delivered through two sets of electrodes through separate channels in the same stimulator. The electrodes are configured on the skin so that the two ACs intersect (Fig. 8-28, *A*). When the currents intersect, they interfere, producing a higher amplitude when both currents are in the same phase and a lower amplitude when the two currents are in opposite phases. This produces envelopes of pulses known as beats. The beat frequency is equal to the difference between the frequencies of the two original ACs. The frequency of the original AC is called the carrier frequency. For example, when a carrier frequency of 5000 Hz interferes with a current with a frequency of 5100 Hz, a beat frequency of 100 Hz will be produced in the tissue (Fig. 8-28, *B*). Typically, electrical stimulation units that produce interferential stimulation allow the clinician to set the beat frequency and some also allow the clinician to select the carrier frequency.

It is proposed that interferential current is more comfortable than other waveforms because it allows a low-amplitude current to be delivered through the skin, where most discomfort is produced, while delivering a higher current amplitude to deeper tissues. Interferential current also delivers more total current than pulsed waveforms and may stimulate a larger area than other waveforms. However, although a number of studies have found that interferential current can decrease pain associated with inflammation or ischemia in animals and humans,[102,103,171,172] the few studies where biphasic pulsed currents (as typically used for TENS) have been compared with interferential current have not found one to be more effective than the other, although one study found that the effects of interferential current lasted longer.[104,173]

Premodulated current is an alternating current with a medium frequency and sequentially increasing and decreasing current amplitude, produced with a single circuit and only two electrodes. This current has the same form as an interferential current that is produced by the interference of two medium-frequency sinusoidal ACs that requires four electrodes. The advantages of interferential current, including a lower current amplitude being delivered to the skin and a larger area of stimulation, are not reproduced by premodulated current (Fig. 8-29).

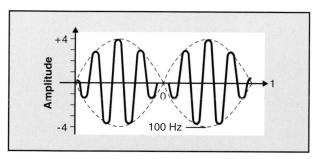

FIG 8-29 Premodulated current.

Pulsed current (pulsatile current): An interrupted flow of charged particles where the current flows in a series of pulses separated by periods when no current flows. The current may flow in one direction only or flow back and forth during each pulse. A series of pulses where the charged particles move only in one direction is known as a monophasic pulsed current. A series of pulses where the charged particles move in one direction and then in the opposite direction is known as a biphasic pulsed current (Fig. 8-30).

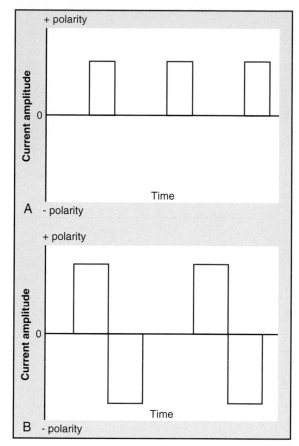

FIG 8-30 **A,** Monophasic; **B,** biphasic pulsed currents.

Monophasic pulsed currents may be used for any clinical application of electrical stimulation but are most commonly used in tissue healing and acute edema management applications. The most commonly encountered monophasic pulsed current in HVPC, also known as pulsed galvanic current). This waveform is made up of pulses composed of a pair of short, exponentially decaying phases, both in the same direction (see Fig 8-14).

A biphasic pulsed current may be symmetrical or asymmetrical, and if asymmetrical, may be balanced or unbalanced (Fig. 8-31). With a symmetrical or a balanced asymmetrical biphasic pulsed current the charge of the phases are equal in amount and opposite in polarity, resulting in a net charge of zero. With an unbalanced asymmetrical biphasic current the charge of the phases are not equal, and there is a net charge. In general, the biphasic pulsed current waveforms available are balanced. Although there is often little clinical difference in the effects of symmetrical and asymmetrical pulsed currents, one study found that subjects found asymmetrical biphasic waveforms to be more comfortable when used to produce contractions of smaller muscle groups, such as the wrist flexors or extensors, and symmetrical biphasic waveforms to be comfortable when used to produce contractions of larger muscle groups, such as the quadriceps.[174]

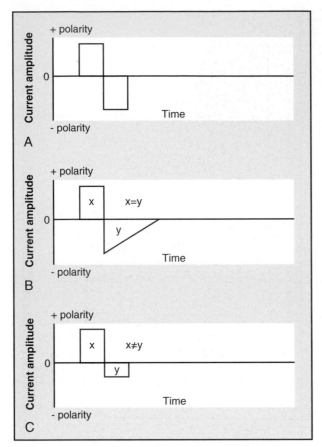

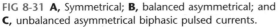

FIG 8-31 **A,** Symmetrical; **B,** balanced asymmetrical; and **C,** unbalanced asymmetrical biphasic pulsed currents.

Russian protocol: The Russian protocol is a waveform with specific parameters intended for quadriceps muscle strengthening. This protocol was developed by Kots who was involved in the training of Russian Olympic athletes.[175] It uses a medium frequency AC with a frequency of 2500 Hz delivered in 50 bursts/second. Each burst is 10 ms long and is separated from the next burst by a 10 ms interburst interval (Fig. 8-32). This type of current is also known as medium-frequency burst AC (MFburstAC), and when this term is used, the frequency of the medium-frequency current or the bursts may be different from the original protocol.

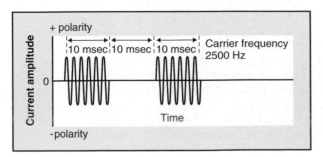

FIG 8-32 Russian protocol.

Time-Dependent Parameters

Frequency: The number of cycles or pulses per second. Frequency is measured in Hertz (Hz) for cycles or pulses per second (pps) for pulses (Fig. 8-33).

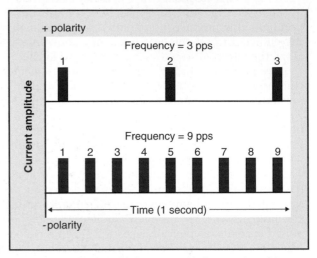

FIG 8-33 Monophasic pulsed current with frequencies of 3 pps and 9 pps.

Interphase interval (intrapulse interval): The time between phases of a pulse (Fig. 8-34).

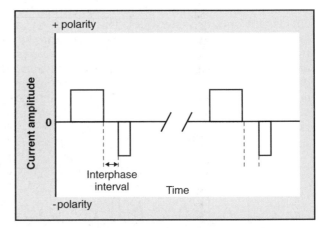

FIG 8-34 Interphase interval for a biphasic pulsed current.

Interpulse interval: The time between pulses (Fig. 8-35).

On:off time: On time is the time during which a train of pulses occurs. Off time is the time between trains of pulses when no current flows. On and off times are usually only used when electrical stimulation is used to produce muscle contractions. During the on time, the muscle contracts, and during the off time it relaxes. The off times are needed to reduce muscle fatigue during the stimulation session. The sequential on and off times also attempt to mimic the voluntary contract and relax phases of normal physiological exercise. The relationship of the on and off time is often expressed as a ratio. For example, if a muscle is stimulated for 10 seconds and then allowed to relax for 50 seconds, this may be written as a 10 : 50 second on : off time or a 1 : 5 on : off ratio (Fig. 8-36).

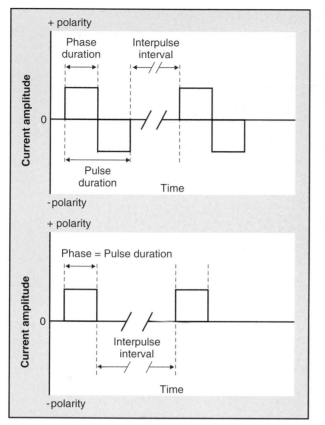

FIG 8-35 Pulse duration, phase duration, and interpulse interval for biphasic and monophasic pulsed currents.

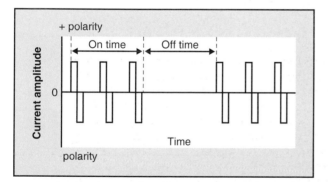

FIG 8-36 On:off times for a biphasic current.

Phase duration: The duration of one phase of a pulse. Phase duration is generally expressed in microseconds ($\mu s = 10^{-6}$ seconds) or milliseconds ($ms = 10^{-3}$ seconds) (see Fig. 8-35).

Pulse duration: The time from the beginning of the first phase of a pulse to the end of the last phase of a pulse. Pulse duration is generally expressed in microseconds ($\mu s = 10^{-6}$ seconds) (see Fig. 8-35).

Ramp up/ramp down time: The ramp up time is the time it takes for the current amplitude to increase from zero, at the end of the off time, to its maximum amplitude during the on time. A current ramps up by having the amplitude of first few pulses of the on time gradually be sequentially higher than the amplitude of the previous pulse. The ramp down time is the time it takes

for the current amplitude to decrease from its maximum amplitude during the on time back to zero (Fig. 8-37). Ramping is used to produce a "soft start," allowing patients to become accustomed to the stimulation as it increases to reach motor threshold. The ramp up time is generally included in the on time while the ramp down time is generally included in the off time. Ramp up and ramp down time are different from rise and decay time. The latter describe the time for the current amplitude to increase and decreased during a phase.

Rise time/decay time: Rise time is the time it takes for the current to increase from zero to its peak during any one phase. Decay time is the time it takes for the current to decrease from its peak level to zero during any one phase (Fig. 8-38). Note that this is different from ramp up/ramp down time described previously.

Wavelength: The duration of 1 cycle of AC. A cycle lasts from the time the current departs from the isoelectric line (zero current amplitude) in one direction and then crosses the isoelectric line in the opposite direction to when it returns to the isoelectric line. The wavelength of alternating current is similar to the pulse duration of pulsed current (Fig. 8-39).

Other Electrical Current Parameters

Amplitude (intensity): The magnitude of current or voltage (Fig. 8-40).

Amplitude modulation: Variation in peak current amplitude over time.

Burst mode: A current composed of series of pulses delivered in groups known as bursts. The burst is generally delivered with a preset frequency and duration. Burst duration is the time from the beginning to the end of the burst. The time between bursts is called the interburst interval (see Fig. 8-10).

Frequency modulation: Variation in the number of pulses or cycles per second delivered.

Modulation: Any pattern of variation in one or more of the stimulation parameters. Modulation is used to limit neural adaptation to an electrical current. Modulation may be cyclic or random (Fig. 8-41).

Phase duration or pulse duration modulation: Variation in the phase or pulse duration.

Scan: Amplitude modulation of an interferential current. Amplitude modulation of an interferential current moves the effective field of stimulation, causing the patient to feel the focus of the stimulation in a different location. This may allow the clinician to target a specific area in soft tissue.

Sweep: The frequency modulation of an interferential current.

Nerves and Electrical Current

Absolute refractory period: The period of time immediately after nerve depolarization when no action potential can be generated.

Accommodation: A transient increase in threshold to nerve excitation.

Action potential (AP): The rapid sequential depolarization and repolarization of a nerve that occurs in response to a stimulus and transmits along the axon.

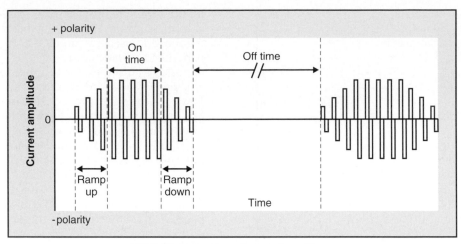

FIG 8-37 Ramp up and ramp down times.

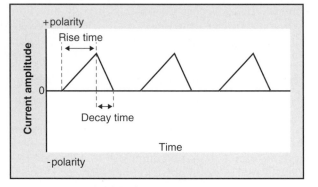

FIG 8-38 Rise and decay times.

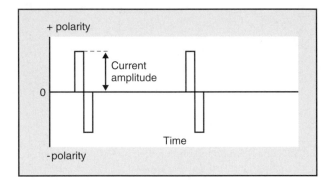

FIG 8-40 Current amplitude.

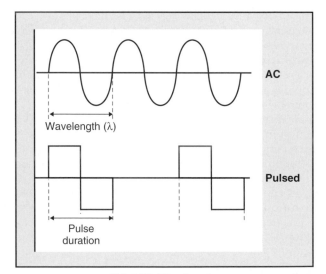

FIG 8-39 Wavelength.

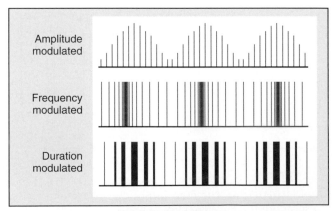

FIG 8-41 Modulation.

Adaptation: A decrease in the frequency of APs and a decrease in the subjective sensation of stimulation that occurs in response to electrical stimulation with unchanging characteristics.

Chronaxie: The minimum duration an electrical current at twice rheobase intensity needs to be applied to produce an AP.

Depolarization: The reversal of the resting potential in excitable cell membranes, where the inside of the cell becomes positive relative to the outside.

Myelin: A fatty tissue that surrounds the axons of neurons, allowing electrical signals to travel more quickly.

Nodes of Ranvier: Small, unmyelinated gaps in the myelin sheath covering myelinated axons.

Propagation: The movement of an AP along a nerve axon; also called conduction.

Relative refractory period: The period after nerve depolarization in which the nerve membrane is hyperpolarized, and a greater stimulus than usual is required to produce an action potential.

Resting membrane potential: The electrical difference between the inside of a neuron and the outside when the neuron is at rest, usually 60 to 90 mV, with the inside being negative relative to the outside.

Rheobase: The minimum current amplitude, with a long pulse duration, required to produce an AP.

Saltatory conduction: The rapid propagation of an electrical signal along a myelinated nerve axon, with the signal appearing to jump from one node of Ranvier to the next (see Fig. 8-4).

REFERENCES evolve

1. American Physical Therapy Association: Clinical electrophysiology. In *Electrotherapeutic terminology in physical therapy*, Alexandria, VA, 2000, APTA.
2. McNeal DR: 2000 years of electrical stimulation. In Hambrecht FT, Reswick JB, eds: *Functional electrical stimulation: applications in neural prostheses*, New York, 1977, Marcel Dekker.
3. Cambridge NA: Electrical apparatus used in medicine before 1900, *Proc Roy Soc Med* 70:635-641, 1977.
4. Duchenne G-B: *A treatise on localized electrization and its applications to pathology and therapeutics*, London, 1871, Hardwicke.
5. Licht S: History of electrodiagnosis. In Licht S, ed: *Electrodiagnosis and electromyography*, ed 3, New Haven, CT, 1971, Elizabeth Licht.
6. Currier DP, Mann R: Muscular strength development by electrical stimulation in healthy individuals, *Phys Ther* 63:915-921, 1983.
7. Kralj A, Acimovic R, Stanic U: Enhancement of hemiplegic patient rehabilitation by means of functional electrical stimulation, *Prosthet Ortho Int* 17(2):107-114, 1993.
8. Melzack R, Wall PD: Pain mechanisms: a new theory, *Science* 150:971-979, 1965.
9. Schuster G, Marsden B: Treatment of pain by transcutaneous electric nerve stimulation in general practice, *J Neurol Orthop Surg* 1:137-1141, 1980.
10. Kloth LC, Feedar JA: Acceleration of wound healing with high voltage, monophasic, pulsed current, *Phys Ther* 68:503-508, 1988.
11. Mendel FC, Wylegala JA, Fish DR: Influence of high voltage pulsed current on edema formation following impact injury in rats, *Phys Ther* 72:668-673, 1992.
12. Kalia YN, Naik A, Garrison J, et al: Iontophoretic drug delivery, *Adv Drug Deliv Rev* 56(5):619-658, 2004.
13. Viscusi ER, Reynolds L, Chung F, et al: Patient-controlled transdermal fentanyl hydrochloride vs intravenous morphine pump for postoperative pain: a randomized controlled trial, *JAMA* 291(11):1333-1341, 2004.
14. Baker LL, Wederich CL, McNeal DR, et al: *Neuromuscular electrical stimulation*, ed 4, Downey, CA, 2000, LAREI.
15. Petrofsky JS, Petrofsky S: A wide-pulse-width electrical stimulator for use on denervated muscles, *J Clin Eng* 17:331-338, 1992.
16. Garnett R, Stephens JA: Changes in the recruitment threshold of motor units produced by cutaneous stimulation in man, *J Physiol* (London) 311:463-473, 1981.
17. Hennings K, Kamavuako EN, Farina D: The recruitment order of electrically activated motor neurons investigated with a novel collision technique, *Clin Neurophysiol* 118(2):283-291, 2007.
18. Delitto A, Snyder-Mackler: Two theories of muscle strength augmentation using percutaneous electrical stimulation, *Phys Ther* 70:158-164, 1990.
19. DeLuca CJ, LeFever RS, McCue MP, et al: Behavior of human motor units in different muscles during linearly varying contractions, *J Physiol* (London) 329:113-128, 1982.
20. Alon G, McCombe SA, Koutsantonis S, et al: Comparison of the effects of electrical stimulation and exercise on abdominal musculature, *J Orthop Sports Phys* Ther 8:567-573, 1987.
21. Wolf SL, Gideon BA, Saar D, et al: The effect of muscle stimulation during resistive training on performance parameters, *Am J Sports Med* 14:18-23, 1986.
22. Delitto A, Rose SJ, McKowen JM, et al: Electric stimulation vs. voluntary exercise in strengthening thigh musculature after anterior cruciate ligament surgery, *Phys Ther* 68:660-663, 1988.
23. Eriksson E, Haggmark T: Comparison of isometric muscle training and electrical stimulation supplementing isometric muscle training in the recovery after major knee ligament surgery, *Am J Sports Med* 7:169-171, 1979.
24. Godfrey CM, Jayawardena H, Quance TA, et al: Comparison of electrostimulation and isometric exercise in strengthening the quadriceps muscle, *Physiother Can* 31:265-267, 1979.
25. Snyder-Mackler L, Delitto A, Bailey S, et al: Quadriceps femoris muscle strength and functional recovery after anterior cruciate ligament reconstruction: a prospective randomized clinical trial of electrical stimulation, *J Bone Joint Surg* 77(8):1166-1173, 1995.
26. Stevens JE, Mizner RL, Snyder-Mackler L: Neuromuscular electrical stimulation for quadriceps muscle strengthening after bilateral total knee arthroplasty: a case series, *J Orthop Sports Phys Ther* 34(1):21-29, 2004.
27. Mizner RL, Petterson SC, Snyder-Mackler L: Quadriceps strength and the time course of functional recovery after total knee arthroplasty, *J Orthop Sports Phys Ther* 35(7):424-436, 2005.
28. Lewek M, Stevens J, Snyder-Mackler L: The use of electrical stimulation to increase quadriceps femoris muscle force in an elderly patient following a total knee arthroplasty, *Phys Ther* 81(9):1565-1571, 2001.
29. Mizner RL, Petterson SC, Snyder-Mackler L: Quadriceps strength and the time course of functional recovery after total knee arthroplasty, *J Orthop Sports Phys Ther* 35(7):424-436, 2005.
30. Morrissey MC, Brewster CE, Shields CL, et al: The effects of electrical stimulation on the quadriceps during postoperative knee immobilization, *Am J Sports Med* 13:40-45, 1985.
31. Trimble MH, Enoka RM: Mechanisms underlying the training effects associated with neuromuscular electrical stimulation, *Phys Ther* 71:273-282, 1991.
32. Alon G, Dar A, Katz-Behiri D, et al: Efficacy of a hybrid upper limb neuromuscular electrical stimulation system in lessening selected impairments and dysfunctions consequent to cerebral damage, *J Neuro Rehab* 12:73-80, 1988.
33. Mahdad M, Baker L: Effect of electrical stimulation on recruitment of motor units in patients with hemiparesis, *Phys Ther* 77:S17-S18, 1977.
34. Yan T, Hui-Chan CW, Li LS: Functional electrical stimulation improves motor recovery of the lower extremity and walking ability of subjects with first acute stroke: a randomized placebo-controlled trial, *Stroke* 36(1):80-85, 2005.
35. Carmick J: Clinical use of neuromuscular electrical stimulation for children with cerebral palsy. I. Lower extremity, *Phys Ther* 73:505-613, 1993.
36. Comeaux P, Patterson N, Rubin M, et al: Effect of neuromuscular electrical stimulation during gait in children with cerebral palsy, *Pediatr Phys Ther* 9:103-109, 1997.
37. Carmick J: Clinical use of neuromuscular electric stimulation for children with cerebral palsy. II. Upper extremity, *Phys Ther* 73:514-527, 1993.
38. Carmick J: Guidelines for application of neuromuscular electric stimulation for children with cerebral palsy, *Pediatr Phys* Ther 9:128-136, 1997.
39. Maenpaa H, Jaakkola R, Sandstrom M, et al: Electrostimulation at sensory level improves function of the upper extremities in children with cerebral palsy, *Dev Med Child Neurol* 46(2):84-90, 2004.
40. Perez MA, Field-Fote EC, Floeter MK: Patterned sensory stimulation induces plasticity in reciprocal 1a inhibition in humans, *J Neurosci* 15:23(6):2014-2018, 2003.
41. Peurala SH, Pitkanen K, Sivenius J, et al: Cutaneous electrical stimulation may enhance sensorimotor recovery in chronic stroke. *Clin Rehabil* 16(7):709-716, 2002.
42. Wu CW, Seo HJ, Cohen LG: Influence of electric somato-sensory stimulation on paretic hand function in chronic stroke, *Arch Phys Med Rehabil* 87(3):351-357, 2006.
43. Baker L, Parker K: Neuromuscular electrical stimulation of the muscles surrounding the shoulder, *Phys Ther* 66:1930-1937, 1986.
44. Faghri PD, Rodgers MM, Glaser RM, et al: The effects of functional electrical stimulation on shoulder subluxation, arm function

recovery, and shoulder pain in hemiplegic stroke patients, *Arch Phys Med Rehabil* 75:73-79, 1994.

45. Sullivan JE, Hedman LD: Effects of home-based sensory and motor amplitude electrical stimulation on arm dysfunction in chronic stroke, *Clin Rehabil* 21(2):142-150, 2007.

46. Crary MA, Carnaby-Mann GD, Faunce A: Electrical stimulation therapy for dysphagia: descriptive results of two surveys, *Dysphagia* 22(3):165-167, 2007.

47. Kiger M, Brown CS, Watkins L: Dysphagia management: an analysis of patient outcomes using VitalStim therapy compared to traditional swallow therapy, *Dysphagia* 21(4):243-253, 2006.

48. Leelamanit V, Limsakul C, Geater A: Synchronized electrical stimulation in treating pharyngeal dysphagia, *Laryngoscope* 112(12): 2204-2210, 2002.

49. Blumenfeld L, Hahn Y, Lepage A, et al: Transcutaneous electrical stimulation versus traditional dysphagia therapy: a nonconcurrent cohort study, *Otolaryngol Head Neck Surg* 135(5):754-757, 2006.

50. Freed ML, Freed L, Chatburn RL, et al: Electrical stimulation for swallowing disorders caused by stroke, *Respir Care* 46(5):466-474, 2001.

51. Carnaby-Mann G, Crary M: Examining the evidence on neuromuscular electrical stimulation for swallowing: a meta-analysis, *Arch Otolaryngol Head Neck Surg* 133:1-8, 2007.

52. Shaw GY, Sechtem PR, Searl J, et al: Transcutaneous neuromuscular electrical stimulations (VitalStim) curative therapy for severe dysphagia: myth or reality? *Ann Otol Rhinol Laryngol* 116(1):36-44, 2007.

53. Siegel SW, Richardson DA, Miller KL, et al: Pelvic floor electrical stimulation for the treatment of urge and mixed urinary incontinence in women, *Urology* 50(6):934-940, 1977.

54. Soomro NA, Khadra MH, Robson W, et al: A crossover randomized trial of transcutaneous electrical nerve stimulation and oxybutynin in patients with detrusor instability, *J Urol* 166(1):146-149, 2001.

55. Govier FE, Litwiller S, Nitti V, et al: Percutaneous neuromodulation for the refractory overactive bladder: results of a multicenter study, *J Urol* 165(4):1193-1198, 2001.

56. van Balken MR, Vandoninck V, Gisolf KW, et al: Posterior tibial nerve stimulation as neuromodulative treatment of lower urinary tract dysfunction, *J Urol* 166(3):914-918, 2001.

57. Agency for Health Care Policy and Research : *Guidelines on urinary incontinence*, US Public Health Service Pub No, March 1992, US Department of Health and Human Services.

58. Walker DC, Currier DP, Threlkeld AJ: Effects of high voltage pulsed electrical stimulation on blood flow, *Phys Ther* 68:481-485, 1988.

59. Indergand HJ, Morgan BJ: Effects of high frequency transcutaneous electrical nerve stimulation on limb blood flow in healthy humans, *Phys Ther* 74:361-367, 1994.

60. Klecker N, Theiss W: Transcutaneous electric muscle stimulation: a "new" possibility for the prevention of thrombosis? *Vasa* 23(1):23-29, 1994.

61. Mohr T, Akers T, Wessman HC: Effect of high voltage stimulation on blood flow in the rat hind limb, *Phys Ther* 67:526-533, 1987.

62. Faghri PD, Van Meerdervort HF, Glaser RM, et al: Electrical stimulation-induced contraction to reduce blood stasis during arthroplasty, *IEEE Trans Rehabil Eng* 5(1):62-69, 1997.

63. Merli GJ, Herbison GJ, Ditunno JF, et al: Deep vein thrombosis: prophylaxis in acute spinal cord injured patients, *Arch Phys Med Rehabil* 69(9):661-664, 1988.

64. Lundeberg TC, Eriksson SV, Malm M: Electrical nerve stimulation improves healing in diabetic ulcers, *Ann Plast Surg* 29:328-331, 1992.

65. Lundeberg T, Kjartansson J, Samuelsson UE: Effect of electric nerve stimulation on healing of ischemic skin flaps, *Lancet* 24:712-714, 1988.

66. Bergslien O, Thereson M, Odemark H: The effects of three electrotherapeutic methods on blood velocities in human peripheral arteries, *Scand J Rehabil Med* 20:29-33, 1988.

67. Kanaya F, Tajima T: Effect of electrostimulation on denervated muscle, *Clin Orthop* 283:296-301, 1992.

68. Mokrush T, Engelhardt A, Eichhorn KF, et al: Effects of long-impulse electrical stimulation on atrophy and fibre type

composition of chronically denervated fast rabbit muscle, *J Neurol* 237(1):29-34, 1990.

69. Dennis RG, Dow DE, Faulkner JA: An implantable device for stimulation of denervated muscles in rats, *Med Eng Phys* 25(3):239-253, 2003.

70. Girlanda P, Dattola R, Vita G, et al: Effect of electrotherapy in denervated muscles in rabbits: an electrophysiological and morphological study, *Exp Neurol* 77:483-491, 1982.

71. Pachter BR, Eberstein A, Goodgold J: Electrical stimulation effect on denervated skeletal myofibers in rats: a light and electron microscopic study, *Arch Phys Med Rehabil* 63:427-430, 1982.

72. Johnston TE, Smith BT, Betz RR, et al: Strengthening of partially denervated knee extensors using percutaneous electric stimulation in a young man with spinal cord injury, *Arch Phys Med Rehabil* 86(5): 1037-1042, 2005.

73. Schimrigk K, McLaughlin J, Gruninger W: The effect of electrical stimulation on the experimentally denervated rat muscle, *Scand J Rehabil Med* 9:55-60, 1977.

74. Nix WA, Hopf HC: Electrical stimulation of regenerating nerve and its effect on motor recovery, *Brain Res* 272:21-25, 1983.

75. Al-Majed AA, Neumann CM, Brushart TM, et al: Brief electrical stimulation promotes the speed and accuracy of motor axonal regeneration, *J Neurosci* 20(7):2602-2608, 2000.

76. Bisschop G, Aaron C, Bence G, et al: Indications and limits of electrotherapy in Bell's palsy. In Portmann M, ed: *Facial nerve*, New York, 1985, Masson.

77. Huizing EH, Mechelse K, Staal A: Treatment of Bell's Palsy. An analysis of the available studies, *Acta Otolaryngol* 92(1-2):115-121, 1981.

78. Farragher D, Kidd G, Tallis R: Eutrophic electrical stimulation for Bell's palsy, *Clin Rehab* 1:265-271, 1987.

79. Targan RS, Alon G, Kay SL: Effect of long-term electrical stimulation on motor recovery and improvement of clinical residuals in patients with unresolved facial nerve palsy, *Otolaryngol-Head Neck Surg* 122:246-252, 2000.

80. Jones DA, Bigland-Ritchie B, Edwards RH: Excitation frequency and muscle fatigue: mechanical responses during voluntary and stimulated contractions, *Exp Neurol* 64(2):401-413, 1979.

81. Selkowitz DM: Improvement in isometric strength of the quadriceps femoris muscle after training with electrical stimulation, *Phys Ther* 65:186-196, 1985.

82. Snyder-Mackler L, Delitto A, Stralka SW, et al: Use of electrical stimulation to enhance recovery of quadriceps femoris muscle force production in patients following anterior cruciate ligament reconstruction, *Phys Ther* 74:901-907, 1994.

83. Chabal C, Fishbain A, Weaver M, et al: Long term transcutaneous electrical nerve stimulation (TENS) use: impact on medication utilization and physical therapy costs, *Clin J Pain* 14(1):66-73, 1988.

84. Forster EL, Kramer JF, Lucy SD, et al: Effect of TENS on pain, medications, and pulmonary function following coronary artery bypass graft surgery, *Chest* 106(5):1343-1348, 1994.

85. Ali J, Yaffe GS, Serrette C: The effect of transcutaneous electric nerve stimulation on postoperative pain and pulmonary function, *Surgery* 89:507-512, 1981.

86. Dawood MY, Ramos J: Transcutaneous electrical nerve stimulation (TENS) for the treatment of primary dysmenorrhea: a randomized crossover comparison with placebo TENS and ibuprofen, *Obstet Gynecol* 75:656-660, 1990.

87. Bertalanffy A, Kober A, Bertalanffy P, et al: Transcutaneous electrical nerve stimulation reduces acute low back pain during emergency transport, *Acad Emerg Med* 12(7): 607-611, 2005.

88. Cheing GL, Luk ML: Transcutaneous electrical nerve stimulation for neuropathic pain, *J Hand Surg* [Br] 30(1): 50-55, 2005.

89. Wall PD: The gate control theory of pain mechanisms: a re-examination and restatement, *Brain* 101:1-18, 1978.

90. Levin MF, Hui-Chan C: Conventional and acupuncture-like transcutaneous electrical nerve stimulation excite similar afferent fibers, *Arch Phys Med Rehabil* 74(1):54-60, 1993.

91. Pert CB, Snyder SH.: Opiate receptor: demonstration in nervous tissue, *Science* 179:1011-1014, 1973.

92. Sjolund BH, Terenius L, Eriksson, M: Increased cerebrospinal fluid levels of endorphins after electroacupuncture, *Acta Physiol Scand* 100:382-384, 1977.

93. Mannheimer JS, Lampe GN, eds: *Clinical transcutaneous electrical nerve stimulation*, Philadelphia, 1984, FA Davis.

94. Kalra A, Urban MO, Sluka KA: Blockade of opioid receptors in rostral ventral medulla prevents antihyperalgesia produced by transcutaneous electrical nerve stimulation (TENS), *J Pharmacol Exp Ther* 298(1):257-263, 2001.

95. Resende MA, Sabino GG, Candido CR, et al: Local transcutaneous electrical stimulation (TENS) effects in experimental edema and pain, *Eur J Pharmacol* 504(3):217-222, 2004.

96. Omura Y: Basic electrical parameters for safe and effective electro-therapeutics [electro-acupuncture, TES, TENMS (or TEMS), TENS and electro-magnetic field stimulation with or without drug field] for pain, neuromuscular skeletal problems, and circulatory disturbances, *Acupunct Electrother Res* 12:201-225, 1987.

97. Debreceni L: Chemical releases associated with acupuncture and electric stimulation: critical reviews, *Phys Rehab Med* 5(3):247-275, 1993.

98. Chiu TT, Hui-Chan CW, Chein G: A randomized clinical trial of TENS and exercise for patients with chronic neck pain, *Clin Rehabil* 19(8):850-860, 2005.

99. Kim HW, Roh DH, Yoon SY, et al: The anti-inflammatory effects of low- and high-frequency electroacupuncture are mediated by peripheral opioids in a mouse air pouch inflammation model, *J Altern Complement Med* 12(1):39-44, 2006 Jan-Feb.

100. Ng MM, Leung MC, Poon DM: The effects of electro-acupuncture and transcutaneous electrical nerve stimulation on patients with painful osteoarthritis knees: a randomized controlled trial with follow-up evaluation, *J Altern Complement Med* 9(5):641-649, 2003.

101. Jarit GJ, Mohr KJ, Waller R, et al: The effects of home interferential therapy on post-operative pain, edema, and range of motion of the knee, *Clin J Sport Med* 13(1):16-20, 2003.

102. Walker UA, Uhl M, Weiner SM, et al: Analgesic and disease modifying effects of interferential current in psoriatic arthritis, *Rheumatol Int* 26(10):904-907, 2006.

103. Defrin R, Ariel E, Peretz C: Segmental noxious versus innocuous electrical stimulation for chronic pain relief and the effect of fading sensation during treatment, *Pain*. 115:152-160, 2005.

104. Cheing GL, Hui-Chan CW: Analgesic effects of transcutaneous electrical nerve stimulation and interferential currents on heat pain in healthy subjects, *J Rehabil Med* 35(1):15-19, 2003.

105. Long DM: Stimulation of the peripheral nervous system for pain control, *Clin Neurosurg* 31:323-343, 1984.

106. Kloth LC: Electrical stimulation for wound healing: a review of evidence from in vitro studies, animal experiments, and clinical trials, *Int J Low Extrem Wounds* 4(1):23-44, 2005.

107. Brown M, Gogia PP, Sinacore DR, et al: High voltage galvanic stimulation on wound healing in guinea pigs: longer term effects, *Arch Phys Med Rehabil* 76:1134-1137, 1995.

108. Kloth LC, Feedar JA: Acceleration of wound healing with high voltage, monophasic, pulsed current, *Phys Ther* 69(8):503-508, 1989.

109. Centers for Medicare and Medicaid Services. Electrostimulation for wounds: decision memorandum (#CAG-00068R). Centers for Medicare and Medicaid Services, 2002. http://www.cms.hhs.gov/mcd/viewdecisionmemo.asp?id=28. Accessed 4/19/07.

110. Gardner S, Frantz R, Schmidt F: Effect of electrical stimulation on chronic wound healing: a meta-analysis, *Wound Repair Regen* 11:495-503, 1999.

111. Fukushima K, Senda N, Inui H, et al: Studies on galvanotaxis of leukocytes. I. Galvanotaxis of human neutrophilic leukocytes and methods of its measurement, *Med J Osaka* 4:195-208, 1953.

112. Erickson CA, Nuccitelli R: Embryonic fibroblast motility and orientation can be influenced by physiological electric fields, *J Cell Biol* 98:296-307, 1984.

113. Kloth LC: Electric stimulation in tissue repair. In Kloth L, Feedar J, eds: *Wound healing alternatives in management*, ed 2, Philadelphia, 1995, FA Davis.

114. Cheng N, Van Hoof H, Bock E, et al: The effects of electric currents on ATP generation, protein synthesis, and membrane transport in rat skin, *Clin Orthop* 171:264-272, 1982.

115. Bourguignon GJ, Bourguignon LYW: Electric stimulation of protein and DNA synthesis in human fibroblasts, *FASEB J* 1:398-402, 1987.

116. Bourguignon GJ, Wenche JY, Bourguignon LYW: Electric stimulation of human fibroblasts causes an increase in Ca 2+ influx and the exposure of additional insulin receptors, *J Cell Physiol* 140:379-385, 1989.

117. Cooper MS, Schliwa M: Electrical and ionic controls of tissue cell locomotion in DC electric fields, *J Neurosci Res* 13:223-244, 1985.

118. Jaffe LF, Vanable JW Jr: Electric fields and wound healing, *Clin Dermatol* 2:34-44, 1984.

119. Borgens RB, Vanable JS, Jaffe LF: Bioelectricity and regeneration: large currents leave the stumps of regenerating newt limbs, *Proc Natl Acad Sci USA* 74:4528-4532, 1977.

120. Illingworth CM, Barker AT: Measurement of electrical currents emerging during the regeneration of amputated finger tips in children, *Clin Phys Physiol Meas* 1:87, 1980.

121. Barranco SD, Spadaro JA, Berger TJ et al: In vitro effect of weak direct current on *Staphylococcus aureus*, *Clin Orthop* 100:250-255, 1974.

122. Ong PC, Laatsch LJ, Kloth LC: Antibacterial effects of a silver electrode carrying microamperage direct current in vitro, *J Clin Electrophysiol* 6:14-18, 1994.

123. Rowley B: Electrical current effects on E. coli growth rates, *Proc Soc Exp Biol Med* 139:929-934, 1972.

124. Kincaid C, Lavoie K: Inhibition of bacterial growth in vitro following stimulation with high voltage, monophasic, pulsed current, *Phys Ther* 69:29-33, 1989.

125. Szuminsky NJ, Albers AC, Unger P, et al: Effect of narrow, pulsed high voltages on bacterial viability, *Phys Ther* 74:660-667, 1994.

126. Rowley BA, McKenna J, Chase GR: The influence of electrical current on an infecting microorganism in wounds, *Ann NY Acad Sci* 238:543-551, 1974.

127. Petrofsky J, Schwab E, Lo T, et al: Effects of electrical stimulation on skin blood flow in controls and in and around Stage III and IV wounds in hairy and non hairy skin, *Med Sci Monit* 11(7):CR309-316, 2005.

128. Sherry JE, Oehrlein KM, Hegge KS, et al: Effect of burst-mode transcutaneous electrical nerve stimulation on peripheral vascular resistance, *Phys Ther* 81(6):1183-1191, 2001.

129. Junger M, Zuder D, Steins A, et al: Treatment of venous ulcers with low frequency pulsed current (Dermapulse): effects on cutaneous microcirculation, *Der Hautartz* (18)879-903, 1997.

130. Griffin JW, Tooms RE, Mendius RE, et al: Efficacy of high voltage pulsed current for healing of pressure ulcers in patients with spinal cord injury, *Phys Ther* 71:433-444, 1991.

131. Unger P, Eddy J, Raimastry S: A controlled study of the effect of high voltage pulsed current (HVPC) on wound healing, *Phys Ther* 71(suppl):S119, 1991.

132. Unger PC: A randomized clinical trial of the effect of HVPC on wound healing, *Phys Ther* 71(suppl):S118, 1991.

133. Bettany JA, Fish DR, Mendel FC: The effect of high voltage pulsed direct current on edema formation following impact injury, *Phys Ther* 70:219-224, 1990.

134. Bettany JA, Fish DR, Mendel FC: The effect of high voltage pulsed direct current on edema formation following hyperflexion injury, *Arch Phys Med Rehabil* 71:677-681, 1990.

135. Bettany JA, Fish DR, Mendel FC: Influence of cathodal high voltage pulsed current on acute edema, *J Clin Electrophysiol* 2:724-733, 1990.

136. Fish DR, Mendel FC, Schultz AM, et al: Effect of anodal high voltage pulsed current on edema formation in frog hind limbs, *Phys Ther* 71(10)724-730, 1991.

137. Taylor K, Mendel FC, Fish DR, et al: Effect of high voltage pulsed current and alternating current on macromolecular leakage in hamster cheek pouch microcirculation, *Phys Ther* 77:1729-1740, 1997.

138. Dolan MG, Grave P, Nakazawa C, et al: Effects of ibuprofen and high-voltage electric stimulation on acute edema after blunt trauma to limbs of rats. *J Athl Train* 40(2):111-115, 2005.

139. Dolan MG, Mychaskiw AM, Mendel FC: Cool-water immersion and high-voltage electric stimulation curb edema formation in rats. *J Athl Train* 38(3):225-230, 2003.

140. Karnes JL, Mendel FC, Fish DR, et al: High voltage pulsed current: its influences on diameters of histamine-dilated arterioles in

hamster cheek pouches, *Arch Phys Med Rehabil* 76:381-386, 1995.

141. Reed BV: Effect of high voltage pulsed electrical stimulation on microvascular permeability to plasma proteins: a possible mechanism in minimizing edema, *Phys Ther* 68:491-495, 1988.

142. Man IO, Lepar GS, Morrissey MC, et al: Effect of neuromuscular electrical stimulation on foot/ankle volume during standing, *Med Sci Sports Exerc* 35(4):630-634, 2003.

143. Morita H, Abe C, Tanaka K, et al: Neuromuscular electrical stimulation and an ottoman-type seat effectively improve popliteal venous flow in a sitting position, *J Physiol Sci* 56(2):183-186, 2006.

144. Man IO, Morrissey MC, Cywinski JK: Effect of neuromuscular electrical stimulation on ankle swelling in the early period after ankle sprain, *Phys Ther* 87(1):53-65, 2007.

145. Leduc S: Introduction of medicinal substances into the depths of tissues by electrical current, *Ann Electrobiol* 3:545, 1900.

146. Leduc S: *Electric ions and their use in medicine*, London, 1908, Rebman.

147. Starkey C: Electrical agents. In *Therapeutic modalities for athletic trainers*, ed 2, Philadelphia, 1999, FA Davis.

148. Chen T, Langer R, Weaver JC: Skin electroporation causes molecular transport across the stratum corneum through localized transport regions, *J Investig Dermatol Symp Proc* 3(2):159-165, 1998.

149. Nimmo WS: Novel delivery systems: electrotransport, *J Pain Symptom Manage* 8:160, 1992.

150. Cullander C: What are the pathways of iontophoretic current flow through mammalian skin? *Adv Drug Del Dev* 9:119, 1992.

151. Glass JM, Stephen RL, Jacobsen SC: The quantity and distribution of radiolabeled dexamethasone delivered to tissue by iontophoresis, *Int J Dermatol* 19:519-525, 1980.

152. Singh J, Roberts MS: Iontophoretic transdermal delivery of salicylic acid and lidocaine to local subcutaneous structures, *J Pharm Sci* 82(2):127-131, 1993.

153. Lai PM, Anissimov YG, Roberts MS: Lateral iontophoretic solute transport in skin, *J Pharm Res* 16(1):46-54, 1999.

154. Bertolucci LE: Introduction of anti-inflammatory drugs by iontophoresis: a double blind study, *J Orthop Sport Phys Ther* 4:103-108, 1982.

155. Delacerda FG: A comparative study of three methods of treatment for shoulder girdle myofascial syndrome, *J Orthop Sport Phys Ther* 4:51-54, 1982.

156. Harris PR: Iontophoresis: Clinical research in musculoskeletal inflammatory conditions, *J Orthop Sports Phys Ther* 4:109-112, 1982.

157. Henley EJ: Transcutaneous drug delivery: iontophoresis and phonophoresis, *Crit Rev Phys Rehabil Med* 2:139-151, 1991.

158. Anderson CR, Morris RL, Boeh SD, et al: Effects of iontophoresis current magnitude and duration on dexamethasone deposition and localized drug retention, *Phys Ther* 83(2):161-170, 2003.

159. Anderson C, Sembrowich W, Morris R: *The mechanism of skin penetration by iontophoresis*, Minneapolis, 2001, Birchpoint Medical Inc.

160. Parkinson TM, Szlek MA, Isaacson JD: Hybresis: the hybridization of traditional with low-voltage iontophoresis, *Drug Delivery Technology* 7(4):54-60, 2007.

161. Japour CJ, Vohra R, Vohra PK, et al: Management of heel pain syndrome with acetic acid iontophoresis, *J Am Pod Med Assoc* 89(5):251-257, 1999.

162. Hartrick CT, Bourne MH, Gargiulo K, et al: Fentanyl iontophoretic transdermal system for acute-pain management after orthopedic surgery: a comparative study with morphine intravenous patient-controlled analgesia, *Reg Anesth Pain Med* 31(6):546-554, 2006.

163. Nirschl RP, Rodin DM, Ochiai DH, et al: DEX-AHE-01-99 Study Group: Iontophoretic administration of dexamethasone sodium phosphate for acute epicondylitis. A randomized, double-blinded, placebo-controlled study, *Am J Sports Med* 31(2):189-195, 2003.

164. Gudeman SD, Eisele SA, Heidt RS Jr, et al: Treatment of plantar fasciitis by iontophoresis of 0.4% dexamethasone. A randomized, double-blind, placebo-controlled study, *Am J Sports Med* 25(3):312-316, 1997.

165. Gangarosa LP, Mahan PE, Ciarlone AE: Pharmacologic management of temporo-mandibular joint disorders and chronic head and neck pain, *Cranio* 2:139-151, 1991.

166. Zempsky WT, Sullivan J, Paulson DM, et al: Evaluation of a low-dose lidocaine iontophoresis system for topical anesthesia in adults and children: a randomized, controlled trial, *Clin Ther* 26(7):1110-1119, 2004 Jul.

167. Leboulanger B, Guy RH, Delgado-Charro MB: Reverse iontophoresis for non-invasive transdermal monitoring, *Physiol Meas* 25(3):R35-50, 2004.

168. Labrecque M, Nouwen A, Bergeron M, et al: A randomized controlled trial of nonpharmacologic approaches for relief of low back pain during labor, *J Fam Pract* 48(4):259-263, 1999.

169. Harrison RF, Woods T, Shore M, et al: Pain relief in labour using transcutaneous electrical nerve stimulation (TENS): A TENS/TENS placebo-controlled study in two parity groups, *Br J Obstet Gynaecol* 93(7):739-746, 1986.

170. Kaplan B, Rabinerson D, Lurie S, et al: Transcutaneous electrical nerve stimulation (TENS) for adjuvant pain-relief during labor and delivery, *Int J Gynaecol Obstet* 60(3):251-255, 1988.

171. Jorge S, Parada CA, Ferreira SH, et al: Interferential therapy produces antinociception during application in various models of inflammatory pain, *Phys Ther* 86(6):800-808, 2006.

172. Johnson MI, Tabasam G: A single-blind placebo-controlled investigation into the analgesic effects of interferential currents on experimentally induced ischaemic pain in healthy subjects, *Clin Physiol Funct Imaging* 22(3):187-196, 2002.

173. Johnson MI, Tabasam G: An investigation into the analgesic effects of interferential currents and transcutaneous electrical nerve stimulation on experimentally induced ischemic pain in otherwise pain-free volunteers, *Phys Ther* 83(3):208-223, 2003.

174. Baker LL, Bowman BR, McNeal DR: Effects of waveform on comfort during neuromuscular electrical stimulation, *Clin Orthop Relat Res* 233:75-85, 1988.

175. Ward AR, Shkuratova N: Russian electrical stimulation: the early experiments, *Phys Ther* 82(10):1019-1030, 2002.

Hydrotherapy

Hydrotherapy, derived from the Greek words hydro and therapeia, meaning "water" and "healing," is the application of water, either internally or externally, for the treatment of physical or psychological dysfunction. This chapter concerns only the external application of water when used as a component of physical rehabilitation. **Hydrotherapy** can be applied externally, either by immersion of the whole body or of parts of the body in water, or without immersion by spraying or pouring water onto the body. The effects and applications of both immersion and nonimmersion hydrotherapy are discussed in this chapter. Although not a form of hydrotherapy, **negative pressure wound therapy** is also discussed in this chapter because it is often used as a component of wound care in conjunction with nonimmersion hydrotherapy.

Bathing in water has been considered healing since the beginning of recorded time and across many cultures, from Hippocrates in the 4th and 5th centuries BCE, who used hot and cold water to treat a variety of diseases, to the Romans at the beginning of the 1st century CE, who constructed therapeutic baths across their empire, to the Japanese, who have used ritual baths from ancient times to the modern day.[1] The therapeutic use of water gained particular popularity in Europe in the late 19th century, with the development of health spas in areas of natural springs, such as Baden-Baden and Bad Ragaz, and shortly thereafter in the United States in similar areas of natural hot springs. At this time, hydrotherapy was used for its effects on both the mind and the body: "It is readily shown that no remedy for lunacy exists which is at all comparable to the bath, owing to its purifying action on the blood."[2] The transition of hydrotherapy from a preventive and recreational role to a curative or rehabilitative role for diseases and their sequelae took place during the polio epidemic of the 1940s and 1950s, when Sister Kenny included activities in water as a component of her treatment of patients recovering from polio. She found that the unique properties of the water environment, including **buoyancy**, **resistance**, and support, allowed these weakened patients to perform a wide range of therapeutic activities with greater ease and safety than was possible on dry land.[3]

Although hydrotherapy has been shown to have wide-ranging therapeutic effects and benefits, its use today continues to be limited in most clinical settings, largely a result of the expenses associated with establishing and maintaining a safe hydrotherapy environment. Hydrotherapy is used today primarily as a component of the treatment of wounds or to provide an enhanced environment for therapeutic exercise. It is also used occasionally to control pain or **edema**. Rehabilitation professionals may also be involved in designing and instructing water exercise programs intended for health maintenance or disease prevention in the community rather than in the clinical setting.

PHYSICAL PROPERTIES OF WATER

Water has a number of unique physical properties that make it well-suited to a variety of rehabilitation applications. These properties include a relatively high **specific heat** and **thermal conductivity** and the ability to provide buoyancy, resistance, and **hydrostatic pressure** to the body.

SPECIFIC HEAT AND THERMAL CONDUCTIVITY

Water can transfer heat by conduction and convection and can therefore be used as a superficial heating or cooling agent. It is particularly effective for this application because it has a high specific heat and thermal conductivity. The specific heat of water is approximately 4 times that of air, and its thermal conductivity is approximately 25 times that of air (Table 9-1). Thus water retains four times as much thermal energy as an equivalent mass of air at the same temperature, and it transfers this thermal energy 25 times faster than air at the same temperature. More details regarding the effects of specific heat and thermal conductivity on heat transfer, and on the principles of heat transfer by conduction and convection, are provided in Chapter 6 in the section on modes of heat transfer.

Clinically, during hydrotherapy, heat is generally transferred from warm water to a patient by placing the patient's limb in a basin or whirlpool filled with warm water. Heat may also be transferred from the patient to cooler water by immersing a limb or part of a limb in a basin or whirlpool filled with cold or ice water. The ability of water to transfer heat rapidly and efficiently is one of the advantages of performing exercises in a swimming pool that is colder than the patient's body temperature because, in such circumstances, immersion in water helps to dissipate the heat generated by the patient through exertion and may also counteract the heat of a hotter climate.

Stationary water transfers heat by conduction; moving water also transfers heat by convection. As explained in detail in Chapter 6, the rate of heat transfer by convection increases as the rate of fluid flow relative to the body increases. Thus heating of a patient's limb in a whirlpool is accelerated with increasing agitation of the water, and cooling of a patient in a cold swimming pool is accelerated as the patient moves more quickly through the water in the pool.

BUOYANCY

Buoyancy is a force experienced as an upward thrust on the body in the opposite direction to the force of gravity. According to Archimedes' principle, when a body is entirely or partially immersed in a fluid at rest, it experiences an upward thrust equal to the weight of the fluid it displaces. The amount of fluid it displaces depends on the density of the immersed body relative to the density of the fluid. If the density of the immersed body is less than the density of the fluid, then it will displace a smaller volume of fluid and will float. Conversely, if the density of the immersed body is greater than the density of the fluid, it will displace a larger volume of fluid and will sink. Because the density of the human body is less than that of water, having a **specific gravity** of about 0.974 compared with that of water, it floats in water (Table 9-2). If the relative density of the body compared with the water is further decreased, either by the addition of salt to the water or by attaching air-filled objects, such as a belt, vest, or arm bands, to the patient, the body will float even higher in the water (Fig. 9-1). This effect is commonly experienced when a person swims in sea water or uses a life jacket.

Exercising in water takes advantage of the buoyancy of the human body in water. Submersion of most of the body decreases stress and compression on weight-bearing joints, muscles, and connective tissue (Fig. 9-2). Submersion may also be used to help raise weakened body parts against gravity or to assist the therapist in supporting the weight of the patient's body during therapeutic activities.

RESISTANCE

The **viscosity** of water provides resistance to the motion of a body in water. This resistance occurs against the direction of the motion of the body and increases in proportion to the relative speed of the body's motion and the frontal area of the body part(s) in contact with the water (Fig. 9-3).[4] In the clinical setting, the relative speed of motion of the body can be increased by having the patient move

TABLE 9-1	Comparison of Specific Heat and Thermal Conductivity of Water and Air	
	Specific Heat (J/gm/° C)	Thermal Conductivity ([Cal/sec]/[cm² × ° C/cm])
Water	4.19	0.0014
Air	1.01	0.000057
Water:Air ratio	4.14	24.56

TABLE 9-2	Specific Gravity of Different Substances
Substance	Specific Gravity
Pure water	1
Salt water	1.024
Ice	0.917
Air	1.21×10^{-3}
Average human body	0.974
Subcutaneous fat	0.85

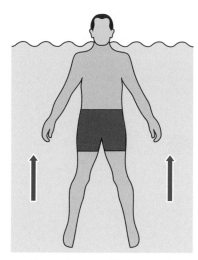

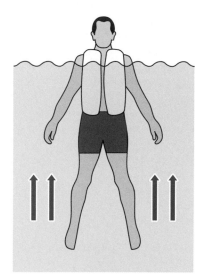

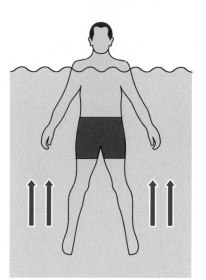

Person in water, floating head above water

Person with air-filled vest in water, floating head and shoulders above water

Person in water, with a high concentration of dissolved salt, floating head and shoulders above water

FIG 9-1 Buoyancy.

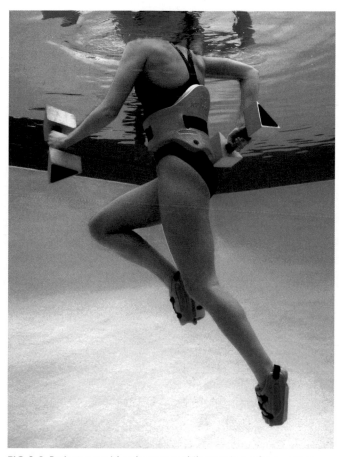

FIG 9-2 Patient exercising in water while wearing a foam vest to increase buoyancy. *Courtesy AquaJogger, Eugene, OR.*

faster in the water or by increasing the speed at which the water moves toward the patient. The frontal area of the body part in contact with the water can be increased by the use of paddles or fins and can be decreased by keeping the limbs more parallel to the direction of movement (Fig. 9-4). The velocity-dependent resistance provided by water makes it a safe and effective strengthening and conditioning medium for many patients. The fact that the resistance of water falls to zero when motion stops provides safety, whereas the fact that the resistance can be readily increased by increasing the speed of motion or the frontal area in contact with the water, makes water a very effective environment for training. The variable resistance and thus **pressure** provided by moving water can also be beneficial for débriding and cleansing wounds.

HYDROSTATIC PRESSURE

Hydrostatic pressure is the pressure exerted by a fluid on a body immersed in the fluid. According to Pascal's law, a fluid exerts equal pressure on all surfaces of a body at rest at a given depth, and this pressure increases in proportion to the depth of the fluid (Fig. 9-5). Water exerts 0.73 mm Hg pressure per centimeter of depth (22.4 mm Hg per foot).[5] Because hydrostatic pressure increases as the depth of immersion increases, the amount of pressure exerted on the distal extremities of an upright immersed patient is greater than that exerted on the more proximal or cranial parts of the body. Thus, for example, when a patient's feet are immersed under 4 feet of water, the pressure exerted by the water will be approximately 88.9 mm Hg, which is slightly greater than normal diastolic blood pressure. This external pressure can have the same effects as the pressure

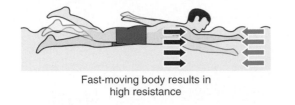

Fast-moving body results in
high resistance

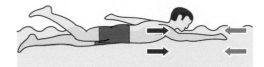

Slow-moving body results in
moderate resistance

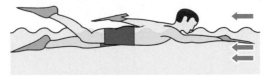

Paddles and fins increase frontal area
and increase resistance

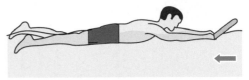

Limbs straight in front decrease frontal
area and decrease resistance

FIG 9-3 Resistance.

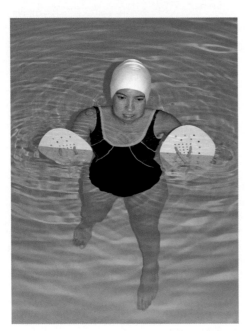

FIG 9-4 Patient exercising in water using hand-held devices to increase the frontal area and thus increase the resistance of the water.

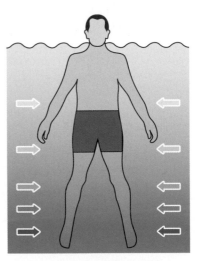

FIG 9-5 Hydrostatic pressure.

exerted by devices intended to produce compression, such as elastic garments or bandages, as described in detail in Chapter 11. Therefore, immersion in water can assist in promoting circulation or alleviating peripheral edema caused by venous or lymphatic insufficiency. However, in contrast to most other devices used to provide external compression, because the limbs must be in a dependent position to maximize the hydrostatic pressure exerted by the water, some of the benefits of the compression produced by immersion are counteracted by the increase in circulatory hydrostatic pressure produced by placing a limb in this position. The increase in venous return that results from increasing external hydrostatic pressure on the limbs may also facilitate cardiovascular function, whereas the support provided by this external pressure may help to brace unstable joints or weak muscles.

It is important to note that because hydrostatic pressure increases with depth of immersion, the physiological and clinical benefits of the hydrostatic pressure of water will vary with patient positioning. The greatest effects will occur with vertical positioning, in which the feet are immersed deep in the water. The effects will be much less pronounced if the patient is swimming or performing other activities in more horizontal positions close to the water surface, in which the limbs are kept at lower depths of immersion. There are also no hydrostatic pressure effects when nonimmersion hydrotherapy techniques are used.

PHYSIOLOGICAL EFFECTS OF HYDROTHERAPY

The physiological effects of water are the result of its physical properties, as described previously. The physiological effects of superficial heating or cooling by warm or cold water are the same as the physiological effects of heating or cooling with other superficial heating or cooling agents and include hemodynamic, neuromuscular, and metabolic changes and modification of soft tissue extensibility. Chapter 6 includes detailed descriptions of the effects of heat and cold. The physiological effects of water that are distinct from those of superficial thermal agents are described in the next section. These effects include cleansing, as well as musculoskeletal, cardiovascular, respiratory, renal, and psychological, changes (Box 9-1).

CLEANSING EFFECTS

Water can be used as a cleanser because it can soften materials and exert pressure. Water is most commonly used for cleansing intact skin; however, in rehabilitation, its cleansing properties are most often used as a component of the treatment of open wounds in which there are exposed areas of subcutaneous tissue and the skin is no longer intact. In this circumstance, the hydrating effects and friction of water are used to soften and remove debris that is lodged in a wound or adhered to the tissue. Water is well-suited to this application because the force it exerts is proportional to its rate of flow and can thus be readily controlled. In addition, water can quickly and easily get into and out of the contoured areas of open wounds. Water is used clinically both as a debriding agent to remove endogenous debris, such as wound **exudate** or **necrotic tissue**, and as a cleanser to remove exogenous waste, such as gravel or adhered dressing materials, and to reduce bacterial burden. The presence of necrotic tissue and contamination by high concentrations or multiple (more than four) types of microorganisms delay wound healing.[6-8]

| **BOX 9-1** | **Physiological Effects of Hydrotherapy** |

Cleansing Effects
- Pressure to remove debris
- Dissolved surfactants and antimicrobials to assist with cleaning

Musculoskeletal Effects
- Decreased weight bearing
- Strengthening
- Effects on bone density loss
- Less fat loss than with other forms of exercise

Cardiovascular Effects
- Increased venous circulation
- Increased cardiac volume
- Increased cardiac output
- Decreased heart rate, systolic blood pressure, and $\dot{V}O_2$ response to exercise

Respiratory Effects
- Decreased vital capacity
- Increased work of breathing
- Decreased exercise-induced asthma

Renal Effects
- Diuresis
- Increased sodium and potassium excretion

Psychological Effects
- Relaxing or invigorating, depending on temperature

Products can be added to water to increase its cleansing power. Such additives are generally antimicrobials or surfactants. Antimicrobials reduce the microbe count in the water and thus on the surface of the wound, whereas surfactants, such as soap or detergent products, reduce surface tension and thereby reduce the adhesion of debris to the tissue. A number of clinical benefits and risks are associated with putting additives in the water used for treating open wounds. These are discussed in detail in the section of this chapter concerning the clinical use of hydrotherapy for wound care.

MUSCULOSKELETAL EFFECTS

The buoyancy of water unloads the weight-bearing anatomical structures and can thus allow patients with load-sensitive joints to perform exercises with less trauma and pain. This effect can help patients with arthritis, ligamentous instability, cartilage breakdown, or other degenerative or traumatic conditions of the articular or periarticular structures of the weight-bearing joints to progress more rapidly with rehabilitation activities. For example, at 75% immersion, weight bearing on the lower extremities is reduced by 75%, thus patients may be able to perform weight-bearing exercises or walk unassisted with a normal gait pattern in a pool, when they can only perform such activities on dry land with the support of crutches.[9]

Buoyancy can also be particularly helpful for obese patients for whom land-based exercise places extreme stresses on the weight-bearing joints. Because such individuals are more buoyant in water than average, having more subcutaneous fat (see Table 9-2), they have greatly reduced joint loading with water-based activities. Therefore water-based exercises may be used to restore fitness in obese patients who have difficulty with other forms of exercise, although paradoxically, exercise in water has been shown to produce less weight and fat loss than exercise of similar intensity and duration on dry land.[10-12] Therefore water-based exercise is recommended for improving the fitness and function of obese patients but is not generally recommended for weight loss.

The velocity-dependent resistance provided by water can also be used to provide a force against which muscles can work to gain or maintain strength. For example, water-based exercises have been shown to result in increased extremity strength in patients with musculoskeletal and neuromuscular diseases, such as fibromyalgia and multiple sclerosis, and to maintain strength in healthy individuals.[13-15] If the direction of water flow is adjusted to be in the same direction as the patient's motion, the resistance of the water can also be used to aid the patient's motion.

The hydrostatic pressure exerted by water has also been shown to increase resting muscle blood flow by 100% to 225% during immersion of the body up to the neck.[16] This is proposed to be the result of reduced peripheral vasoconstriction or increased venous return produced by the external compression provided by the water. This increase in muscular blood flow may improve muscular performance by increasing oxygen availability and accelerating the removal of waste products and may thus promote more effective muscular training.

CARDIOVASCULAR EFFECTS

The cardiovascular benefits of hydrotherapy are primarily a result of the effects of hydrostatic pressure. The hydrostatic pressure exerted on the distal extremities with upright immersion in water displaces venous blood proximally from the extremities and thus enhances venous return by shifting blood from the periphery to the trunk vessels and thence to the thorax and the heart. It has been shown that central venous pressure rises with immersion to the chest and continues to increase until the body is fully immersed.[17,18] With immersion to the neck, central blood volume increases by about 60%, and cardiac volume increases by nearly 30%.[18,19] This increase in cardiac volume results in an increase in right atrial pressure of 14 to 18 mm Hg, to which the heart responds, according to Starling's law, with an increase in the force of cardiac contraction and an increase in stroke volume.[17] This results in approximately 30% increased cardiac output over baseline in response to upright immersion up to the neck (Fig. 9-6).[17]

The increase in cardiac work associated with this increased cardiac output is in contrast to the decrease in heart rate that occurs in response to immersion in water and counters the reduced heart rate and reduced systolic blood pressure that occur when exercise at the same metabolic rate or perceived level of exertion is performed in water rather than on dry land.[18,20-22] The rate of oxygen consumption ($\dot{V}O_2$) is also lower when exercise is performed in water than when exercise at the same level of perceived exertion is performed on dry land, and the maximum rate of oxygen consumption ($\dot{V}O_{2max}$) has been found to be slightly lower with maximal running in water than with maximal running on dry land.[23-25] Because of these reduced physiological responses, exercise in water has often been considered to be less effective for cardiac conditioning than similar exercise on dry land. However, it is important to realize that these reduced physiological responses are accompanied by an increase in stroke volume and cardiac output, which may increase myocardial efficiency. Thus there is a physiological basis for using exercise in water for cardiac conditioning and rehabilitation. Also, a number of studies have shown that cardiovascular training effects, including an increased $\dot{V}O_{2max}$ and a decreased resting heart rate, do occur in healthy individuals in response to water-based exercise programs.[25,26]

In patients with congestive heart failure (CHF), there is a concern that the increase in cardiac volume that occurs during immersion (as result of hydrostatic pressure) may overwhelm the heart's pumping ability. Clinicians should use judgment in the use of hydrotherapy in patients with CHF, although studies have shown that such patients can benefit from hydrotherapy, particularly immersion in warm water.[27,28] When immersed in warm water, subjects with CHF experienced increased early diastolic filling accompanied by a decrease in heart rate, leading to an increase in stroke volume and ejection fraction.[27] These cardiorespiratory responses were similar to those of healthy controls.[28] Additionally, an 8-week warm-water exercise program for patients with CHF resulted in improved exercise capacity and muscle function when compared to a control intervention of similar exercises performed out of the water.[29] Another small study found that home-based warm and cold water immersion of the arms and feet for up to 30 minutes daily for 6 weeks improved quality of life, heart failure–related symptoms and heart rate response to exercise in patients with mild CHF when compared with controls who did not receive this intervention.[30]

Because the heart rate response to exercise is blunted when exercise is performed in water, clinically, the target heart rate is not the ideal guide for water exercise intensity prescription. Therefore, when a patient exercises in water, it is recommended that the level of perceived exertion, rather than the heart rate response, be used as a guide for exercise intensity.

> ◎ **Clinical Pearl**
>
> Perceived exertion rather than heart rate should be used to guide exercise intensity when a patient exercises in water.

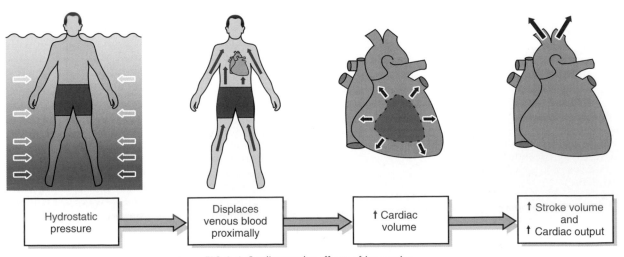

| Hydrostatic pressure | → | Displaces venous blood proximally | → | ↑ Cardiac volume | → | ↑ Stroke volume and ↑ Cardiac output |

FIG 9-6 Cardiovascular effects of immersion.

The reader should also note that the blunting of heart rate and systolic blood pressure in response to exercises that occur with water immersion may be obscured if warm water is used because increasing the body's temperature may elevate the heart rate and reduce the systolic blood pressure.[18,31]

The velocity-dependent resistance to motion provided by water also increases the metabolic rate and energy expenditure, as measured by $\dot{V}O_2$, by approximately a factor of three when an activity is performed at the same speed in water as on dry land.[32] Thus exercise performed in water at one-half to one-third of the speed with which similar exercise is performed on dry land has the same effect on metabolic rate.[33] This altered response can allow individuals with musculoskeletal conditions that limit their speed of movement to perform exercise in water to maintain or improve their cardiovascular fitness.

RESPIRATORY EFFECTS

Immersion of the whole body in water increases the work of breathing because the shift of venous blood from the peripheral to the central circulation increases the circulation in the chest cavity, and the hydrostatic pressure on the chest wall increases the resistance to lung expansion[14] (Fig. 9-7).[17] Immersion in water up to the neck has been shown to decrease expiratory reserve volume by about 50% and to decrease vital capacity by 6% to 12%; these effects, when combined, increase the total work of breathing by about 60%.[34-36] Thus the workload challenge to the respiratory system that occurs when exercise is performed in water can be used to improve the efficiency and strength of the respiratory system. However, because this additional respiratory challenge may overload patients with respiratory or cardiovascular impairments that prevent or limit adaptation to this additional workload, such patients

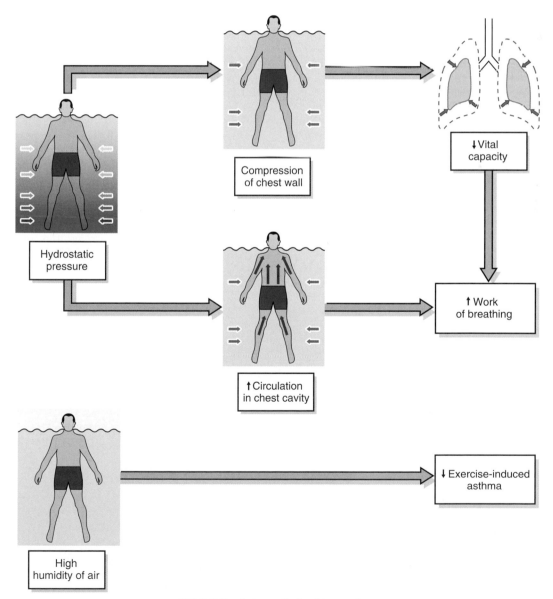

FIG 9-7 Respiratory effects of immersion.

should always be carefully monitored during water-based exercise.[33]

Water-based exercise is also often recommended for patients with exercise-induced asthma because several studies have shown that water-based exercise is less likely to cause asthma in these individuals than exercise on dry land.[37,38] Various properties of water, including the absence of pollen over the water, hydrostatic pressure on the chest, hypoventilation, hypercapnia, peripheral vasoconstriction, and the high humidity of the inspired air in the pool environment, have been proposed as mechanisms for this effect.[39] Although most of these factors have not been studied experimentally, it appears that the high humidity of the air inspired during water exercise, which prevents drying or cooling of the respiratory mucosa, is the most important factor in reducing exercise-induced asthma.

RENAL EFFECTS

Immersion of an individual up to the neck in water has been shown to increase urine production and urinary sodium and potassium excretion (Fig. 9-8).[21,40,41] It is proposed that these effects are the result of increased renal blood flow and decreased antidiuretic hormone (ADH) and aldosterone production.[40,42] Water immersion is thought to cause these circulatory and hormonal changes in response to the redistribution of blood volume and the relative central hypervolemia that result from the hydrostatic pressure that water exerts on the periphery. These renal effects can be taken advantage of in the treatment of patients with hypervolemia, hypertension, or peripheral edema. In patients with chronic kidney disease, low-intensity water exercise twice weekly for 12 weeks was found to improve kidney function, as well as cardiorespiratory function, and decrease blood pressure when compared to no exercise.[43]

PSYCHOLOGICAL EFFECTS

As is well known to those who bathe or exercise in water, water immersion can be invigorating and relaxing. The variations in these psychological effects appear to depend primarily on the temperature of the water. Soaking in warm water is generally relaxing, whereas cold water immersion is found by most people to be invigorating and energizing. Thus the neutral stimulation and support of warm water can be used clinically to provide a comforting and calming environment for overstimulated or agitated patients, and the invigorating effects of cold water can be used to facilitate more active exercise participation by those who are generally less active or responsive.[44] A small study of 18 women in labor found that anxiety decreased after 15 minutes of immersion in 37° C (99° F) water, while anxiety increased in the control group who were not immersed in water.[45] It has been proposed that the clinically observed psychological effects of water immersion may be mediated by a central process within the reticular activating system.[5]

USES OF HYDROTHERAPY

SUPERFICIAL HEATING OR COOLING

Warm or cold water can be used clinically to heat or cool superficial tissues. Warm water and cold water transfer heat primarily by conduction, whereas warm and cold whirlpools transfer heat by conduction and by convection.[46] The effects and clinical applications of heating or cooling superficial tissues with water are the same as those produced when other superficial heating or cooling agents are used. These are described in detail in Chapter 6. However, water has a number of advantages over most other superficial thermal agents. It provides perfect contact with the skin, even in very contoured areas; it does not need to be fastened to the body; and, it allows movement during heating or cooling. Its primary disadvantage is that when it is applied to the extremities only, the distal extremity must be in a dependent position, which may aggravate edema. However, the edema-producing effect of the dependent position is somewhat counteracted during

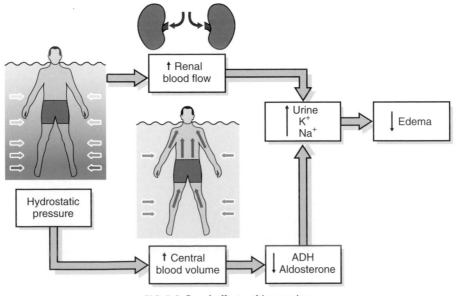

FIG 9-8 Renal effects of immersion.

immersion in water by the compression provided by the hydrostatic pressure of the water.

WATER EXERCISE
Types of Water Exercise

Various types of exercise, including swimming, running with or without a vest or belt, walking, cycle ergometry, and other forms of upright exercise can be performed in water (Fig. 9-9). In general, patients are free to move about the pool while exercising, although they may be tethered to the side, as during in-place water running. The tether may be used to facilitate monitoring of the exercise by the therapist or to increase resistance and allow a wider range of activities, particularly in a small pool. The principles, mechanisms of action, and rationales for performing exercise in water are discussed later in this chapter; however, specific water exercise programs are not covered because they are described in detail in other texts devoted to aquatic therapy.[47]

General Uses of Water Exercise

Exercise in water can be used to increase circulation, muscle strength, joint viscoelasticity, flexibility, and range of motion (ROM); to improve ambulation, coordination, cardiovascular and respiratory conditioning, and psychological well-being; and to decrease pain, muscle spasm, and stiffness. The specific contributions of the unique physical properties of water, including its ability to retain and conduct heat, and its buoyancy, resistance, and hydrostatic pressure in producing these effects, are discussed in detail in the next section.

The ability of water to retain and conduct heat is used clinically when a patient or a part of a patient exercises while immersed in warm water. The combination of heat transfer and exercise is particularly effective in certain cases because increasing the temperature of soft tissue can augment the vasodilation, increased circulation, decreased joint stiffness, increased joint ROM, and enhanced functional abilities that result from exercise.[48,49] The relaxing effects of immersion in warm water may also improve the psychological well-being of the patient during and after water-based exercise.

Because the buoyancy of water decreases the gravitational forces placed on weight-bearing structures, patients with weakened limbs or load-sensitive joints can often perform strengthening, conditioning, and coordination exercises in water that they would not be able to perform on dry land. This can contribute to improved functional mobility and strength.

The resistance provided by water during movement can also serve as a force against which muscles can work to develop strength or when applied in the direction of patient movement, can be used to assist weakened muscles in the production of movement.[50]

Because the hydrostatic pressure provided by immersion in water can facilitate venous return from the extremities, circulation may be enhanced during exercise in water compared to similar exercise performed on dry land. As described previously, the circulatory changes produced by the hydrostatic pressure of water on the extremities during water-based exercise can also facilitate cardiovascular and respiratory conditioning and help to reverse and control the formation of peripheral edema.

Specific Uses of Water Exercise (Box 9-2)

Orthopedic Rehabilitation. The water environment can be used to provide graded weight bearing and patient-controlled resistance to help individuals with spinal or peripheral musculoskeletal dysfunction perform exercises

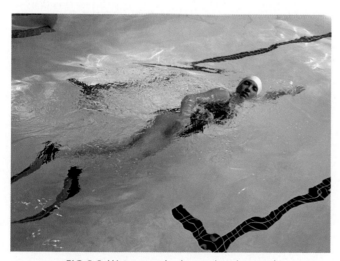

FIG 9-9 Water exercise in a swimming pool.

BOX 9-2   Specific Uses of Water Exercise

Musculoskeletal Problems
- Decreased weight bearing on joints
- Velocity-dependent resistance
- Closed or open chain exercises
- Effects on bone density loss
- Fibromyalgia

Neurological Problems
- Proprioceptive input
- Increased safety
- Improved balance

Cardiac Fitness
- Cardiac conditioning in patients with poor tolerance for land-based exercise

Exercise in Water During Pregnancy
- Decreased weight bearing
- Less elevation of heart rate with exercise
- Decreased risk of maternal hyperthermia

Exercise-Induced Asthma
- Less exercise-induced asthma than with other forms of exercise

Age-Related Deficits
- Improved balance
- Improved strength
- Improved cardiorespiratory fitness
- Improved functional mobility

they would have difficulty performing on dry land.[51,52] This can allow for earlier exercise participation after injury, surgery, or immobilization, and greater exercise participation by patients with load-sensitive conditions such as osteoarthritis or spinal disc displacement.[53] Such exercise participation may also result in earlier recovery of and greater final functional mobility in these individuals.

Several studies have examined the effects of water exercise on people with osteoarthritis. One randomized controlled trial found that both land-based and pool-based strengthening programs resulted in improved physical function in people with osteoarthritis.[54] Similarly, another study comparing land-based and aquatic exercise in people with osteoarthritis found improved knee ROM, thigh girth, and timed 1-mile walk in both groups. However, the aquatic exercise group reported significantly greater reduction in pain levels than the land exercise group.[55] A third study comparing the effects of land exercise, water exercise, and no exercise in adults with arthritis found similar improvements in function in the land and water exercise groups.[56] Yet another study found that a 6-week aquatic physical therapy program resulted in significantly less pain and joint stiffness and greater physical function, quality of life, and hip muscle strength than no program.[57] These benefits persisted 6 weeks after the completion of the hydrotherapy program. Another randomized controlled trial found that exercise in a 34° C (93° F)pool was as effective as electroacupuncture in reducing pain and increasing activity and quality of life in people with osteoarthritis of the hip.[58] Overall, these studies demonstrate that water exercise is as, or more, effective than land-based exercise for improving physical function and reducing pain in people with arthritis.

Weight bearing during aquatic exercise can be graded by varying the depth of water immersion or by the use of flotation devices, such as belts, arm bands, or hand-held floats, with deeper immersion or more flotation devices providing more unloading. Flotation devices also allow greater muscular relaxation in the water by eliminating or reducing the amount of work required by the patient to stay afloat. Therefore the use of such devices is particularly appropriate for the patient who can benefit from both decreased joint loading and decreased muscular activity. For example, patients with load-sensitive spinal conditions, such as disc bulges or herniations or nerve root compression, may benefit from relaxed vertical floating in water, supported by a flotation belt, to allow unloading of the spinal intraarticular structures and relaxation of the paraspinal muscles.

Varying the resistance provided by water during exercise, by altering the speed or direction of the motion of the water or the speed of movement of the patient, can alter the clinical effects of exercise in water. The faster the water moves toward the patient, against the patient's direction of movement, or the faster the patient moves in the water, the greater the resistance against the patient's movement and thus the greater the strengthening or endurance-building effect of the activity. Exercise intensity can thus be graded by modifying the speed of water motion in a pool that allows control of water motion or by altering the speed at which the patient moves while

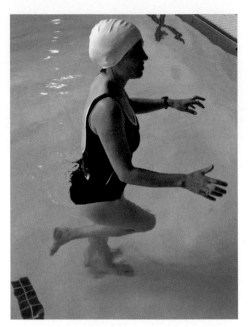

FIG 9-10 Closed-chain exercise in water.

exercising. If the flow of the water can be directed to be in the same direction as the patient's motion rather than against the direction of the patient's motion, the resistance of the water can also be used to assist with motion when muscles are weak allowing strengthening through a greater ROM.

The types of exercises performed in water must be carefully designed and selected to address different conditions and to avoid exacerbating existing problems or causing new ones. The patient can perform either **closed-chain** or **open-chain exercises** in water. Closed-chain exercises can be performed using the bottom of the pool to fix the distal extremity when the patient is in shallow water (Fig. 9-10) or using the side of the pool to fix the distal extremity when the patient is in deeper water. Open-chain exercises can also be performed in either deep or shallow water, depending on the area of the body involved and the type of exercise to be performed (Fig. 9-11). It is important to select the appropriate exercise for a particular problem and to be aware of the changes in biomechanics if an exercise usually performed on dry land is transferred to a water environment.

> **◎ Clinical Pearl**
>
> Changes in biomechanics should be noted when a land-based exercise is performed in the water.

For example, running on dry land is primarily a closed-chain activity, whereas running in deep water using a flotation vest is entirely an open-chain activity. This change may reduce pain from tibiofemoral joint compression by decreasing the weight bearing on this joint but it may increase patellofemoral joint pain by increasing compression at this joint during open-chain knee extension.

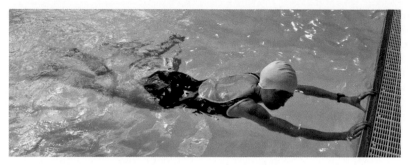

FIG 9-11 Open-chain exercise in water.

When designing rehabilitation programs that involve swimming, it is particularly important to guard against adverse effects of compensatory motions because such motions can cause problems in other areas.[51]

> **Clinical Pearl**
>
> Water rehabilitation programs should be designed so that compensatory motions by the patient do not cause problems in other areas.

For example, if the patient has limited shoulder ROM and increases lumbar or cervical motion to bring the shoulder out of the water during freestyle swimming this may cause problems in these spinal areas. In a similar manner, a patient with hypomobility of the thoracic spine may overuse the shoulder during freestyle or breast stroke swimming and increase subacromial compression of the rotator cuff, causing tendon breakdown.

Because exercise in water results in reduced weight bearing on the bones, it has generally been assumed that exercise in this environment does not assist in maintaining bone density in postmenopausal women. However, a cross-sectional longitudinal study found that exercise in water can slow bone mineral density loss in the lumbar spine in this population,[59] and one randomized controlled trial found that exercise in water can increase calcaneal bone density.[60] However, another cross-sectional prospective study found that bone mineral density in the spine decreased and in the femur remained the same in a group of osteopenic women, although fitness and psychological well-being improved, after a 12-month water exercise program.[61] Water exercise can have a positive impact on the overall health of women with osteoporosis and can be a safe way to exercise for those at high risk of falls, but it may not increase bone density as effectively as weight-bearing exercise.

Several studies have examined the effects of water exercise on people with fibromyalgia. Overall, these studies have found that, among other benefits, water exercise can reduce pain in people with fibromyalgia.[15,62] A randomized controlled trial comparing 15 weeks of deep water running with a land-based exercise program in sedentary women with fibromyalgia found that both groups experienced improved aerobic fitness and reduced pain, but the water exercise group experienced decreased depression sooner than the land exercise group.[63] Another randomized controlled trial found that hydrotherapy resulted in greater total sleep time and less total nap time than a conventional physical therapy program,[64] and an uncontrolled trial noted that improvements in symptom severity, physical function, and social function after completion of a 6-month pool exercise program were still present 6 and 24 months later.[65]

Neurological Rehabilitation. Water-based exercise has been recommended to address the impairments, disabilities, and handicaps resulting from neurological dysfunction because it provides proprioceptive input, weight relief, and a safe environment for movement.[66] The proprioceptive input may be particularly beneficial for patients with central sensory deficits, such as those that can occur after a stroke or traumatic brain injury, and the weight relief can increase ease of movement and reduce the risk of falling to facilitate greater movement exploration, functional activity training, and strengthening in patients with weakness or impaired motor control.[67] It has been proposed that the greater movement exploration and the increased production of movement errors that occur in water-based exercise are responsible for the balance enhancement that has been shown to result from water-based exercise programs.[68] In patients with spasticity after a spinal cord injury, passive ROM combined with water exercise resulted in greater reductions in spasticity and use of antispasmodic medications and greater increases in functional independence than a passive ROM program alone.[69] A small study of patients with brain injury found that water exercise resulted in improved cardiovascular endurance; body composition; muscular strength, endurance, and flexibility; and corresponding improvements in function and ability to perform activities of daily living.[70] These improvements were not seen in the control group, which did not exercise.

Reduced loading as a result of buoyancy and the increased abdominal support from the hydrostatic pressure of water may also provide assistance for breathing in patients with a weak diaphragm, which can occur after a spinal cord injury or with amyotrophic lateral sclerosis (ALS), although this must be balanced against the increased breathing workload produced by the shift of fluids to the central circulation. The decreased patient weight caused by the buoyancy of the patient's body in water and the support provided by the buoyancy and hydrostatic pressure of water may also contribute to patient progress by allowing for easier patient handling by the therapist.

Exercise in water using a variety of specific approaches, such as neurodevelopmental training (NDT) or the Bad Ragaz method, has been recommended for improving function in patients with neurological problems.[71,72] These methods use verbal instructions and tactile cues to guide the patient to practice normal movement progression and sequencing. The challenge of the activities can then be modified by varying the depth of the water or by using the support of one or more flotation devices. These methods are particularly recommended for improving stability and motor control.

Cardiorespiratory Fitness. Because water-based exercise programs have been shown to maintain and increase aerobic conditioning, exercise in water can be used to provide general conditioning for deconditioned patients or for those who wish to increase their cardiovascular fitness.[25,73] This form of exercise can be particularly beneficial for cardiac conditioning in patients with conditions, such as osteoarthritis, postoperative recovery, or joint instability, that are aggravated by joint loading and thus limit land-based exercise. Water exercise has also been found to benefit patients with chronic obstructive pulmonary disease, resulting in improved physical capacity and quality of life[74] and, as mentioned earlier, when closely monitored, patients with congestive heart failure can also benefit from water exercise.

The increased cardiac output resulting from the hydrostatic pressure of water immersion, as described previously, has led some to investigate the effects of exercise in water for cardiac rehabilitation. Two studies of patients with a history of myocardial infarction or ischemic heart disease have demonstrated improvement in heart function of about 30% in patients performing exercise in water for a month.[75,76] Exercise in water has also been shown to reduce the resting heart rate and increase $\dot{V}O_{2max}$, maximum heart rate, and work capacity in healthy older adults and to improve respiratory function in patients with chronic obstructive pulmonary disease.[12,19]

A novel form of water exercise consisting of immersion in water in combination with expiring into water has been found to increase cardiac ejection fraction and to decrease left ventricular end-diastolic and systolic dimensions at rest in patients with emphysema.[77] This exercise also resulted in an increase in the ratio of forced expired volume in 1 second (FEV_1) to forced vital capacity (FVC) ($FEV_1 : FVC$) and a decrease in $PaCO_2$. These results suggest that this type of water exercise may improve both breathing and cardiac function in patients with emphysema.[78]

Exercise in Water During Pregnancy. A number of studies on the effects of exercise in water during pregnancy indicate that this form of exercise may be particularly appropriate for pregnant women.[20,21,79] Exercise in water provides the benefits of unloading the weight-bearing joints, controlling peripheral edema, and causing less elevation of heart rate, blood pressure, and body temperature than similar exercise performed on dry land. Researchers found that pregnant women who participated

in a 1-hour water exercise program three times weekly for 6 weeks had less physical discomfort, greater mobility, and improved body image and health-promoting behaviors than control subjects who did not exercise.[80] The American College of Obstetricians and Gynecologists recommends that women keep their heart rate below 140 beats per minute throughout pregnancy. Thus, given the lower heart rate response to exercise in water, women may be able to perform exercise in water at a higher level of perceived exertion and at a higher metabolic rate than they could on dry land while staying within safe heart rate limits.[20,81] One study also found that on immersion in water, pregnant women had a slight decrease in blood pressure and maintained this until about 10 minutes after exiting the water.[82]

Exercise in water is also thought to pose less risk to the fetus than land-based exercise because it has been shown that the incidence of postexercise fetal tachycardia is lower with this type of exercise than with land-based exercise.[21,79]

Immersion in water, and thus upright exercise or even immersion in an upright position in water, places hydrostatic pressure on the immersed areas and can therefore be used to help reduce peripheral edema in pregnant patients. This effect is the result of improved venous and lymphatic flow and renal-influenced diuresis caused by the hydrostatic pressure of water on the lower extremities. Because hydrostatic pressure increases at increasing depths of water, control of peripheral edema is most marked when the patient exercises in an upright position to produce the greatest pressure on the distal lower extremities.

Exercise-Induced Asthma. Water-based exercise, including swimming, is particularly suited to patients with exercise-induced asthma because the water environment has been found to reduce the incidence of asthma in these individuals compared with land-based exercise.[37,38] Also, a number of studies have shown decreased symptoms of asthma and increased fitness in individuals who have asthma, particularly children, in response to swimming exercise.[83,84]

Age-Related Deficits. While exercise in general can be beneficial to those over 60 years old, water exercise is particularly helpful. Studies of people at least 60 years old find that water exercise programs can increase strength, functional mobility, balance, and quality of life in this population.[85-87] The buoyancy of water helps alleviate age-related aches and pains during exercise and helps support people who have poor balance on land. Working against the resistance of water also helps increase strength in this population.

PAIN CONTROL

Hydrotherapy is often recommended as a treatment for the control of pain. Studies on water exercise in patients with osteoarthritis or fibromyalgia show that, along with other benefits, patients experience decreased pain with

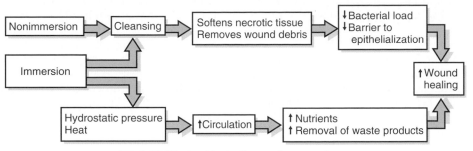

FIG 9-12 Effects of hydrotherapy for wound care.

water exercise.[55,56,58,62] Hydrotherapy is thought to control pain by providing a high level of sensory stimulation to the peripheral mechanoreceptors to gate the transmission of pain sensations at the spinal cord. Such a mechanism is consistent with the reports by many clinicians that forms of hydrotherapy that provide the greatest sensory stimulation, such as **contrast baths**, or water at a high temperature with a high level of agitation, are particularly effective in reducing pain. Cold water may also contribute to the reduction of pain by reducing acute inflammation. Pain control may also result from the decreased weight bearing and increased ease of movement produced by water immersion.

EDEMA CONTROL

Water immersion has been shown to reduce peripheral edema. It is proposed that this effect is caused by the hydrostatic pressure of water and the resulting changes in circulation and renal function. Therefore water immersion has been recommended for the treatment of peripheral edema with a variety of etiologies, including venous or lymphatic insufficiency, renal dysfunction, and postoperative inflammation.[5,88] In addition to the effects of hydrostatic pressure on postoperative edema, the cooling effects of cold water may also contribute to edema reduction by causing vasoconstriction and reducing vascular permeability. Therefore, cold water immersion of a limb, or part of a limb, is frequently used as a component of the treatment of edema that results from recent trauma when other signs of acute inflammation are present. Immersion in warm or hot water is not recommended in such circumstances because heating the area and placing it in a dependent position can increase tissue temperature and intravascular pressure, resulting in increased inflammation and peripheral arterial flow and thus increased rather than decreased edema.[89] In such cases it has been found that the higher the temperature of the water, the greater the amount of edema.[89]

Contrast baths are frequently recommended and clinically used to control edema, with the rationale that the alternating vasodilation and vasoconstriction produced by the alternating immersion in hot and cold water may help to train or condition the smooth muscles of the blood vessels. However, because there are no research data on the efficacy or mechanisms of this effect, it is recommended that clinicians carefully assess the effect of such treatment on the individual patient when considering using this form of hydrotherapy treatment.

WOUND CARE

Hydrotherapy has been shown to accelerate the healing of wounds of various etiologies, including diabetes mellitus, pressure, vascular insufficiency, or burns.[90-93] Hydrotherapy may also be used in the care of wounds from trauma, surgery, abscesses, dehisced incisions, necrotizing fasciitis, or cellulitis. Hydrotherapy is used for wound care because its cleansing properties facilitate the rehydration, softening, and **debridement** of necrotic tissue and the removal of exogenous wound debris, and the hydrostatic pressure of water immersion and the heat of warm water improve circulation (Fig. 9-12).[94] The use of hydrotherapy is also consistent with the current understanding that it is important to maintain a moist rather than a dry wound environment to optimize wound healing.[95]

The use of hydrotherapy for wound care is not new. As early as 1734, a German physician, Dr. Johann Hahn, recommended prolonged immersion in water for the treatment of leg sores.[95] Immersion hydrotherapy, using whirlpools, was still the most common method for applying wound hydrotherapy until recent years. Gradually, over the last 5 to 10 years, nonimmersion hydrotherapy techniques have largely replaced whirlpools for this type of treatment. This change in practice is a result of concerns about damaging regenerating tissue in wounds with the pressure exerted by water agitated by a whirlpool turbine and concerns that allowing wounds to soak in contaminated tank water for a prolonged period of time may promote infection.

It has been shown that excessive fluid pressure can cause wound trauma and drive bacteria into a wound.[96] Although the pressure of the water being applied to a wound in a whirlpool can be modified to some extent by moving the turbine output toward or away from the wound or by changing the degree of aeration, the absolute amount of pressure being exerted is not known and cannot be controlled and therefore too much or too little pressure may be applied with this type of device. It is recommended that whirlpool treatments be used only for cleansing wounds that contain extensive thick exudate, **slough** or necrotic tissue, gross **purulence**, or dry **eschar** when other, nonimmersion hydrotherapy devices may be ineffective or when nonimmersion hydrotherapy devices are not available. It is also recommended that all forms of hydrotherapy treatment be discontinued when a wound is clean.[21]

Concerns regarding the potential for wound **infection** with immersion hydrotherapy are the result of reports of outbreaks of wound infection, most commonly caused by *Pseudomonas aeruginosa* but also occasionally caused by *Staphylococcus aureus*, *Acinetobacter baumannii*, or *Candida albicans*, after whirlpool treatments.[97-101] Reports of contamination of hydrotherapy equipment with these microorganisms have been a cause for concern; however, a recent report found that only about 10% of whirlpools tested were contaminated.[98,100,102] Whirlpool tank water may become contaminated by microorganisms from the patient being treated at that time, or by microorganisms that become lodged in the crevices of the tank from prior treatments or between treatments. To reduce the risk of wound infection with hydrotherapy, a number of authors recommend the addition of antimicrobial additives to the water when treating wounds; however, this practice is controversial.[97,100-105] This controversy is based on the conflict between the potential benefits of improved infection control when antimicrobials are used and the potential for adverse effects because it has been found that many antimicrobial products are cytotoxic to regenerating tissue cells unless used at very dilute concentrations (Table 9-3).[106-113]

These conflicting findings on the benefits of using antimicrobial additives in hydrotherapy water lend support to the practice of either using an antimicrobial at the lowest effective concentration or using only clean water without additives when using a whirlpool to treat open wounds. The policy for the use of antimicrobials in whirlpools in most facilities is set by the infection control department of the facility, in accordance with regulatory guidelines, and should always be followed. Whether or not additives

TABLE 9-3	Toxicity Index for Wound and Skin Cleansers
Test Agent	**Toxicity Index***
Biolex	1 : 100
Saf Klenz	1 : 100
Ultra Klenz	1 : 100
Clinical Care	1 : 1000
Uniwash	1 : 1000
Ivory soap (0.5%)	1 : 1000
Constant Clens	1 : 10000
Dermal wound cleanser	1 : 10000
Puri-Clens	1 : 10000
Hibiclens	1 : 10000
Betadine surgical scrub	1 : 10000
Technicare scrub	1 : 100000
Bard Skin Cleanser	1 : 100000
Hollister	1 : 100000

*The dilution required to maintain white blood cell viability and phagocytic efficiency.
From Foresman PA, Payne DS, Becker D, et al: A relative toxicity index for wound cleaners, *Wounds* 5(5): 226-231, 1993.

are used during whirlpool treatment of open wounds, the tank and turbine should always be thoroughly cleaned and disinfected between uses. Recommendations for whirlpool cleaning procedures are provided in the section on safety issues regarding hydrotherapy. To avoid the infection risks associated with whirlpool use, most facilities use nonimmersion hydrotherapy techniques for wound care, thus avoiding soaking in potentially contaminated water inside a potentially contaminated tank.

A variety of devices can be used to apply hydrotherapy to wounds without immersion. Such devices must deliver fluid at a pressure between 4 and 15 pounds per square inch (psi) because below this level, bacteria and debris are not effectively removed, whereas at higher pressures, wound trauma may occur or bacteria may be driven into the tissue.[114-116]

> ⊚ **Clinical Pearl**
>
> Nonimmersion irrigation devices should deliver fluid at 4 to 15 psi to remove debris without causing tissue damage.

A number of devices deliver fluid within this pressure range (Table 9-4). These include a saline squeeze bottle with an irrigation cap or a 35-mL syringe with a 19-gauge needle. Electric **pulsed lavage** devices can also be set to deliver pressure within this range. The advantages of these devices are that they spray water onto the wound and then use suction or negative pressure to remove the contaminated water from the area, and they allow fine adjustable control of the water pressure.

A number of studies have compared infection and healing rates when different liquids are used to cleanse wounds by nonimmersion hydrotherapy. A randomized controlled trial found no difference in infection and healing rates between using drinkable tap water or sterile normal saline for wound cleansing.[117] A systematic review that included three studies also found no strong evidence for recommending a particular solution for wound cleansing for pressure ulcers.[118] However, one of the three studies included in this review did note that pressure ulcers healed faster when cleansed with a saline spray containing aloe vera, silver chloride, and decyl glucoside than when sprayed with isotonic saline alone.[119] A systematic review of studies on the use of different cleansing fluids for acute wounds found that wounds cleansed with clean potable tap water had infection and healing rates similar to wounds cleansed with sterile isotonic saline solution or wounds not cleansed at all.[120]

Generally, nonimmersion hydrotherapy is recommended for the treatment of wounds containing necrotic, nonviable tissue or debris. This type of treatment has been shown to facilitate the removal of necrotic tissue, promote healing, and increase patient comfort in hospital and home-bound patients.[121] It is recommended that nonimmersion hydrotherapy be continued until all necrotic, nonviable material has been removed and a full granulation bed is present.[122] A combination of immersion hydrotherapy, using a whirlpool to soften debris followed by nonimmersion hydrotherapy with a spray to remove this

TABLE 9-4	Irrigation Pressure Delivered by Various Devices	
Device	Irrigation Pressure (psi)	psi Level for Safe and Effective Wound Cleansing
Spray bottle—Ultra Klenz* (Carrington Laboratories Inc, Dallas, TX)	1.2	Too little
Bulb syringe* (Davol Inc, Cranston, RI)	2.0	Too little
Piston Irrigation Syringe, 60 mL, with catheter tip† (Premium Plastics Inc, Chicago, IL)	4.2	Appropriate
Saline Squeeze Bottle, 250 mL, with irrigation cap† (Baxter Healthcare Corp, Deerfield, IL)	4.5	Appropriate
Water Pik at lowest setting† (Teledyne Water Pik, Fort Collins, CO)	6.0	Appropriate
Irrijet DS Syringe with tip† (Ackrad Laboratories, Inc, Cranford, NJ)	7.6	Appropriate
35-mL syringe with 19-guage needle or angiocatheter†	8.0	Appropriate
Water Pik at middle setting† (Teledyne Water Pik, Fort Collins, CO)	42	Too much
Water Pik at highest setting† (Teledyne Water Pik, Fort Collins, CO)	50	Too much
Pressurized Cannister Dey Wash‡ (Dey Laboratories, Napa, CA)	50	Too much

From US Department of Health and Human Services: *Treatment of pressure ulcers: clinical practice guidelines*, Rockville, MD, 1994, USDHHS.
*Too little pressure for effective wound cleansing <4 psi.
†Appropriate pressure for safe and effective wound cleansing at 4 to 15 psi.
‡Too much pressure for safe wound cleansing >15 psi.

debris and bacteria, has been shown to be particularly effective for the removal of bacteria from wounds.[123]

When applying hydrotherapy to wounds, whether using immersion or nonimmersion techniques, it is important to balance the potential benefits to the wound with the potential for damaging regenerating **granulation tissue** in the wound bed by mechanical disruption, or for damaging the intact skin surrounding the wound by **maceration** as a result of excessive moisture. Therefore all forms of hydrotherapy should be discontinued when the wound base is fully covered with granulation tissue, and the intact skin surrounding a wound should always be thoroughly, though gently, dried immediately after completing any hydrotherapy treatment.

Clinical Pearl

Hydrotherapy should be discontinued when the wound base is fully covered with granulation tissue. The skin surrounding the wound should be dried immediately after hydrotherapy to avoid maceration.

Special Concerns Regarding the Use of Hydrotherapy in the Treatment of Burns

Hydrotherapy is considered an important component of the treatment of acute burn injuries in most burn centers in the United States.[99,124-126] The purposes and uses of hydrotherapy in burn care are generally the same as those for other types of wounds, except for a few noteworthy differences. As with other types of wounds, hydrotherapy is used as a component of early treatment to cleanse, soften, and loosen necrotic tissue before debridement and

to reduce bacterial load. However, in contrast to most other types of wounds, where such debridement is relatively painless, the debridement of burn wounds is frequently extremely painful because the wounds are less deep and many of the sensory nerves are still intact. Therefore high-dose analgesics are generally used during this procedure, necessitating closer monitoring of the patient during the treatment. Recently, virtual-reality distraction has also been used to reduce pain during this type of procedure.[127]

Because burn wounds are often extensive, covering a large area of the body, the larger **Hubbard tank** whirlpools have traditionally been used for this application, and, with the increasing concern for and awareness of the risks of **nosocomial infections** with the use of immersion hydrotherapy, special nonimmersion techniques for the treatment of burns have been developed.[99,125] These generally involve showering the patient while the patient is lying on a surface, such as a mesh net stretcher or trauma table, that allows the water to pour off into a suitable drain.[128] Although this may have less risk of infection, wound infections have also been associated with this type of hydrotherapy.[129] Nonimmersion hydrotherapy is also generally less painful and faster, and allows greater ease of patient handling. If immersion techniques are used for the hydrotherapy treatment of burns, it has been recommended that salt be added to the water to reduce sodium loss from the patient to the water and to reduce the risk of hyponatremia associated with the soaking of some patients with extensive burns in water.[130,131]

Hydrotherapy is used not only in the early treatment of burn wounds, when necrotic tissue is present, but also in the later stages of recovery after reepithelialization has occurred. In this circumstance, the risk of wound infection is eliminated and the water is used to provide a comfortable environment for exercise and for active ROM (AROM) and passive ROM (PROM), to help prevent contractures and to facilitate increased ROM in scarred areas.

Negative Pressure Wound Therapy (Vacuum-Assisted Wound Therapy)

Negative pressure wound therapy involves creating a vacuum over a wound bed that is filled with a foam dressing (Fig. 9-13). Although this is not a form of hydrotherapy, this modality is often used in conjunction with nonimmersion hydrotherapy in the treatment of wounds and was developed from electric pulsed lavage devices when it was realized that the suction these devices provide can promote wound healing. Negative pressure wound therapy is thought primarily to aid wound healing by removing fluid and mechanically deforming the wound.[132] A recent systematic review on the effects of negative pressure wound therapy included 6 studies with a total of 135 patients with pressure ulcers, full thickness wounds, nonhealing wounds, and diabetic foot wounds.[133] The studies included in the review compared negative pressure wound therapy to standard moist dressings changed once a day, with the exception of one study that compared negative pressure wound therapy to gel products. Negative pressure wound therapy was found to be superior to standard wound care in some studies but was no better in others. Outcomes included time to satisfactory healing, probability of complete healing, readiness for surgical closure, and changes in wound area and volume. The authors of this review concluded that the small size of the studies and their poor quality made it difficult to draw conclusions about the efficacy of negative pressure wound therapy. There are several better-designed, larger randomized trials of negative pressure wound therapy in progress at this time. Negative pressure wound therapy is currently recommended by the Association for the Advancement of Wound Care and the Wound, Ostomy and Continence Nurse Society for the treatment of venous ulcers and stage III and IV pressure ulcers that have failed to heal with standard wound care.[134,135]

CONTRAINDICATIONS AND PRECAUTIONS FOR HYDROTHERAPY

Although hydrotherapy is a relatively safe treatment modality, its use is contraindicated in some circumstances and it should be applied with caution in others.[136] When applying hot or cold water to a patient, all the contraindications and precautions that apply to the use of other superficial heating or cooling agents, described in detail in Chapter 6, apply to this mode of superficial heating or cooling. In addition, a number of contraindications and precautions apply specifically to the application of hydrotherapy, either by local immersion in a whirlpool or contrast bath, or by whole body immersion in a pool or Hubbard tank, or by nonimmersion methods. These are listed in the boxes and discussed in detail in the text that follows.

LOCAL IMMERSION FORMS OF HYDROTHERAPY

CONTRAINDICATIONS

for the Use of Local Immersion Forms of Hydrotherapy

- Maceration around a wound
- Bleeding

Maceration Around a Wound

Immersion hydrotherapy is contraindicated when there is maceration of intact skin around a wound because it is likely to increase the maceration and thus increase the size of the wound.

Assess

- Inspect the skin around the wound for signs of maceration, including pallor or other early indications of breakdown.

When there is maceration around a wound and when the cleansing benefits of hydrotherapy are desired, nonimmersion techniques should be used to avoid excessive or prolonged soaking of the macerated tissues.

Bleeding

Immersion hydrotherapy should not be applied if there is bleeding in or near an area being considered for treatment because immersion hydrotherapy may increase bleeding by increasing venous circulation as a result of the hydrostatic pressure and may increase arterial circulation as a result of vasodilation if warm or hot water is used.

Assess

- Check for bleeding in or near the area being considered for treatment.

If bleeding is mild and has been determined not to be dangerous to the patient, nonimmersion hydrotherapy may be used.

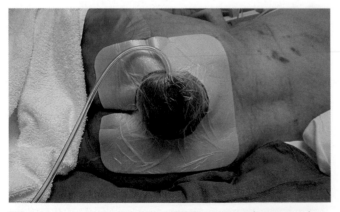

FIG 9-13 Vacuum-assisted closure (VAC) on a sacral pressure ulcer. *From Cameron MH, Monore LG: Physical Rehabilitation: Evidence-based Examination, Evaluation, and Intervention, St Louis, 2007, Saunders.*

PRECAUTIONS

for the Use of Local Immersion Forms of Hydrotherapy

- Impaired thermal sensation in the area to be immersed
- Infection in the area to be immersed
- Confusion or impaired cognition
- Recent skin grafts

Impaired Thermal Sensation in the Area to be Immersed

Areas with impaired thermal sensation are at increased risk for thermal burns. Therefore, to minimize this risk, the temperature of the water to be used for hydrotherapy should always be checked with a thermometer before the patient enters the water. It is also recommended that the clinician check the water temperature directly by placing a hand, wearing a clean rubber glove, in the water before the patient enters. Thermostatically controlled mixing valves should also be used to control the temperature of the incoming water.

Ask the Patient

- Can you feel heat and cold in this area?

Assess

- Thermal sensation can be tested by applying test tubes filled with cold or warm water to the area and asking the patient to report the sensation of the stimulus.

If the patient has impaired thermal sensation, only water at a temperature close to body temperature should be used for applying hydrotherapy.

Infection in the Area to be Immersed

Hydrotherapy is frequently applied to wounds when an infection is present in the area to be immersed. In such circumstances, additional infection control measures described in the sections on the use of hydrotherapy for the treatment of wounds and safety issues regarding the application of hydrotherapy should be used.

Assess

- Check the area to be treated for signs of infection. Signs of infection include induration, fever, erythema, and edema.

Since all open wounds are **colonized** with bacteria, when treating open wounds with immersion hydrotherapy, one should take the same precautions as when an infection is known to be present.[137]

Confusion or Impaired Cognition

Hydrotherapy is frequently applied when patients are confused or have impaired cognition. For example, many patients have open wounds, to some degree as a result of their impaired mental status, and many patients with burns are given high-dose analgesics to control pain during the debridement performed during or directly after hydrotherapy, which also results in impairment of mental status.

Assess

- The patient's level of cognition and alertness. Check if the patient can effectively communicate discomfort.

When a patient is confused or is unable to effectively report discomfort or other problems for any other reason, direct supervision should be provided throughout hydrotherapy treatment and only water at a temperature close to body temperature should be used.

Recent Skin Grafts

Extra care should be taken when treating recent skin grafts with hydrotherapy because a graft may not tolerate the mechanical agitation of a whirlpool or may not have a sufficient vascular response to compensate for extreme heat or cold. Therefore the whirlpool agitator should always be directed away from the area of a graft, and water with neutral warmth (33° to 35.5° C [92° to 96° F]) or mild warmth (35.5° to 37° C [96° to 98° F]) should be used when treating recent skin grafts.

FULL BODY IMMERSION HYDROTHERAPY

All the contraindications and precautions for partial body immersion hydrotherapy apply to full body immersion hydrotherapy.[138] In addition, a number of contraindications and precautions apply uniquely to full body immersion hydrotherapy because of the risks associated with deep water and the fact that most full body immersion occurs in a pool where the water is not changed between uses.

PRECAUTIONS

for the Use of Full Body Immersion in Hot or Very Warm Water

- Pregnancy
- Multiple sclerosis
- Poor thermal regulation

Pregnancy

Because maternal hyperthermia has been found to be teratogenic and is associated with a variety of central nervous system abnormalities in the child to minimize the possibility of maternal hyperthermia, full body immersion in a hot pool should be avoided during pregnancy, particularly during the first trimester, when the effects of heat are most hazardous to the fetus.[130,139] Full body immersion in normal temperature pool water is recommended during pregnancy because, as explained previously, this can be an ideal environment for exercise by the pregnant woman.

Ask the Patient

- Are you pregnant?
- Do you think you might be pregnant?

Multiple Sclerosis

Patients with multiple sclerosis should not be placed in a hot or warm pool because temperatures above 31° C (88° F) may increase fatigue and weakness in these patients.[130]

Poor Thermal Regulation

Thermal regulation in response to body heating is generally accomplished by a combination of conduction, convection, radiation, and evaporation. If a small area of the body is immersed in hot water, the patient with impaired thermal regulation may still be able to dissipate heat by conduction to areas in direct contact with the heated area and by direct radiation of heat from the skin; however, the dissipation of heat by convection by blood circulating through the area from other areas that have not been heated and the production of sweat may be impaired. Because all of these mechanisms are impaired when large areas of the body are heated, as occurs with full body immersion in hot or warm water, a patient with poor thermal regulation may be at risk for thermal shock if large areas of the body are immersed in hot water.[130]

Assess

- Check for any history of thermal shock or any other signs of poor thermal regulation.

Because thermal regulation is frequently impaired in the elderly and in infants, warm or hot water hydrotherapy should be limited to small areas in these individuals.

CONTRAINDICATIONS

for the Use of Full Body Immersion Hydrotherapy

- Cardiac instability
- Infectious conditions that may be spread by water
- Bowel incontinence
- Severe epilepsy
- Suicidal patients

Cardiac Instability

Full body immersion is contraindicated in cases of cardiac instability, such as uncontrolled hypertension or heart failure, because in such circumstances the heart may not be able to adapt sufficiently in response to the changes in circulation produced by the hydrotherapy to maintain cardiac homeostasis.

Assess

- Check with the patient's physician and review the patient's chart to determine if any cardiac instability is present.

Heart rate and blood pressure should also be monitored during and after immersion in all patients with a history of cardiac problems.

Infectious Conditions that May be Spread by Water

Patients with infectious conditions that may be spread by water should not use any type of hydrotherapy where the water is not changed between uses. Thus such patients should not use a pool but may use a Hubbard tank, where the water is changed between treatments, for full body immersion. Infectious conditions that may be spread by water include urinary tract infections, tinea pedis, plantar warts, and infections present in open wounds.

Ask the Patient

- Do you have a urinary tract infection, athlete's foot, plantar warts, or any open wounds? This question may be asked most readily in a written checkoff sheet given to all patients before any pool activities.

Bowel Incontinence

Patients with bowel incontinence may not be immersed in water that will be used by other patients. In patients with bowel incontinence and open wounds, care should also be taken to avoid contaminating the water used for hydrotherapy and thus the wound with bacteria from the patient's own feces.

Assess

- Check the patient's chart for any notation regarding bowel incontinence.

Nonimmersion forms of hydrotherapy are recommended for the treatment of open wounds in patients with bowel incontinence.

Severe Epilepsy

Full body immersion hydrotherapy should not be applied to patients with severe epilepsy because such patients have an increased risk of drowning.

Suicidal Patients

Full body immersion hydrotherapy should also not be applied to suicidal patients because they have an increased risk of drowning.

PRECAUTIONS

for the Use of Full Body Immersion Hydrotherapy

- Confusion or disorientation
- Alcohol ingestion by the patient
- Limited strength, endurance, balance, or ROM
- Medications
- Urinary incontinence
- Fear of water
- Respiratory problems

Confusion or Disorientation

Full body immersion is occasionally used for the treatment of confused or disoriented patients who have multiple or large open wounds or wounds that are difficult to access by other means. In such cases, extra care should be taken to monitor the water temperature and to be sure that the patient is well and safely secured, with the head above the water.

Alcohol Ingestion

Full body water immersion should be avoided after the ingestion of alcohol because the impairment of judgment and cognitive functions that occurs with intoxication and the hypotensive effects of alcohol ingestion can increase the risk of drowning.

Ask the Patient

- If you suspect that a patient has recently been drinking alcohol—for example, if you smell alcohol on the patient's breath, ask, "Have you had a drink of alcohol in the last few hours?"

Limited Strength, Endurance, Balance, or Range of Motion

Although hydrotherapy is frequently used for treating limitations of strength, endurance, balance, or ROM, extreme limitations in any of these areas can be a safety hazard for full body immersion hydrotherapy. Therefore, for full body immersion hydrotherapy treatment, a patient must have the ability to maintain the head above water or if unable to do so, must be well and safely secured so as to keep the head above water. Direct, hands-on assistance, with the therapist in the water, can also be provided for patients who have difficulty keeping their heads above water.

Assess

- Check strength, balance, and ROM before the patient enters the water.

If any of these are significantly limited, secure the patient so that the head cannot enter the water or accompany the patient into the water, at least for the first treatment, to assess the patient's safety in the water.

Medications

Some medications, particularly those used to treat cardiovascular disease, alter the cardiovascular response to exercise. It is therefore recommended that a physician be consulted to establish safe limits of cardiovascular response for each patient before initiating an aquatic exercise program with any patient taking medications.

Urinary Incontinence

A patient with urinary incontinence may be catheterized to allow full body immersion hydrotherapy; however, this is generally not recommended because immersion may increase the risk of urinary tract infection in a catheterized patient.

Fear of Water

Patients with a fear of water will generally refuse to participate in immersion hydrotherapy. For these patients, alternative treatments, such as immersing only the area requiring treatment, using nonimmersion hydrotherapy, or using an intervention such as dry land exercise that does not involve the use of water, should be considered.

Respiratory Problems

Although water-based exercise can provide respiratory and general conditioning for patients with exercise-induced asthma or other breathing problems, water immersion increases the work of breathing and patients with respiratory problems should be carefully monitored for signs of respiratory distress throughout the water immersion treatment. Some patients with asthma may also be sensitive to chlorine and other agents used to decontaminate exercise pools and whirlpools, and these patients should be closely monitored.

NONIMMERSION HYDROTHERAPY

PRECAUTIONS
for the Use of Nonimmersion Hydrotherapy

- Maceration
- May be ineffective

Maceration Around a Wound

Caution should be taken to minimize the wetting of intact skin surrounding a wound because of the risk of causing or aggravating maceration. The intact skin should also be gently and thoroughly dried after any type of hydrotherapy to minimize the risk of macerating this tissue.

Potential for Inefficaciousness

Because nonimmersion hydrotherapy does not provide buoyancy or hydrostatic pressure, it is effective for only a limited number of problems that can be addressed by immersion hydrotherapy. Thus it can be used for cleansing but should not be used when the cardiovascular, respiratory, musculoskeletal, or renal effects of immersion are desired. Nonimmersion hydrotherapy also produces little heat transfer because the water is in contact with the tissue for too brief a period. Therefore when considering the use of nonimmersion hydrotherapy, one must weigh these disadvantages against the advantages of reduced infection risk, increased ease of application, and reduced treatment times.

NEGATIVE PRESSURE WOUND THERAPY

CONTRAINDICATIONS
for the Use of Negative Pressure Wound Therapy

- Necrotic tissue
- Untreated osteomyelitis
- Malignancy
- Untreated malnutrition
- Exposed arteries, veins, nerves, or organs
- Nonenteric and unexplored fistulas

Necrotic Tissue

Negative pressure wound therapy should only be applied once a wound is cleaned and free of necrotic tissue and eschar so that it can then promote healing of potentially viable tissue.

Assess

- Examine the wound bed for necrotic tissue and debride as much as possible before applying negative pressure wound therapy.

Untreated Osteomyelitis

Negative pressure wound therapy should not be applied in an area of untreated osteomyelitis because this treatment may promote soft tissue growth over the infected bone.

Assess

• Examine all wounds for exposed bone.

If there is exposed bone, the physician should complete an evaluation for osteonecrosis before applying negative pressure wound therapy.

Malignancy

Because negative pressure wound therapy may promote growth of any tissue, including malignant tissue, it should not be applied in an area of malignancy.

Untreated Malnutrition

Wounds require adequate nutrition to provide the energy and substrates needed for healing. Therefore malnutrition should be treated before negative pressure wound therapy is initiated.

Assess

• Request evaluation by a nutritionist before initiating negative pressure wound therapy.

Exposed Arteries, Veins, Nerves, or Organs

Because of concerns that the force of negative pressure wound therapy may damage exposed arteries, veins, nerves, or organs, it is recommended that this intervention not be applied in such areas.

Nonenteric and Unexplored Fistulas

Application of negative pressure wound therapy over a fistula may cause excessive fluid loss and damage. Careful exploration of the fistula should be performed by a physician to determine if application of negative pressure wound therapy is appropriate. Occasionally, negative pressure wound therapy may be applied to enteric (bowel) fistulas.

Assess

• Examine the wound bed for exposed arteries, veins, or organs.

PRECAUTIONS

for the Use of Negative Pressure Wound Therapy

• Anticoagulant therapy
• Difficult hemostasis
• Confusion or disorientation

Anticoagulant Therapy

Negative pressure wound therapy should be applied with caution to patients taking anticoagulant therapy including warfarin (Coumadin) and heparin because these medications increase the risk of prolonged bleeding.

Ask the Patient

• Are you taking any anticoagulant or blood thinner? Which?

Assess

• If the patient is taking an anticoagulant check with his or her physician before initiating negative pressure wound therapy.

If negative pressure wound therapy is initiated, carefully check the area for signs of bleeding and discontinue treatment if bleeding occurs.

Difficult Hemostasis

If hemostasis is difficult to achieve, negative pressure wound therapy should be initiated with caution as the pressure of the treatment may cause some bleeding.

Confusion or Disorientation

Negative pressure wound therapy should be used with caution in patients who are confused or disoriented because such patients may inadvertently disrupt the operation of the dressing or the negative pressure suction device.

ADVERSE EFFECTS OF HYDROTHERAPY

DROWNING

The most severe potential adverse effect of hydrotherapy is death by drowning, and it is imperative that adequate precautions be taken to minimize this risk. The American Red Cross has identified the three most common causes of drowning to be failure to recognize hazardous conditions and practices, inability to get out of dangerous situations, and lack of knowledge of the safest ways to aid a drowning person.[140] Specific recommendations for safety precautions to be taken to minimize the risk of drowning are provided in the section on safety issues regarding hydrotherapy.

BURNS, FAINTING, AND BLEEDING

Treatment by immersion in a warm or hot whirlpool has the risks associated with other forms of superficial thermotherapy, including burning, fainting, and bleeding. To minimize the possibility of any of these adverse effects, the temperature of the water used for hydrotherapy should be kept within the appropriate range and should always be checked with a thermometer before the water touches the patient. Additionally, the therapist may check the water temperature by placing a gloved hand into the water. Because certain populations, including the elderly, the very young, and those with impaired sensation or other neurological deficits, are at an increased risk of suffering burns, the use of hot water should be avoided when treating these patients.[141]

The risk of fainting because of hypotension is greatest when large areas of the patient's body are immersed in warm or hot water. This risk may be further increased in patients taking antihypertensive medications. Therefore, to minimize the possibility of fainting, only the parts of the body requiring treatment in warm water should be immersed, and all patients taking antihypertensive medications should be closely monitored. Also, all patients should be well-supported during warm water immersion to prevent falling should the patient faint.

HYPONATREMIA

Immersion hydrotherapy has been associated with hyponatremia in patients with extensive burn wounds.[130]

Hyponatremia occurs because these patients can lose salt from the open wound areas into the whirlpool water when the salinity of the water is lower than that of the tissue fluids. Therefore, to minimize the possibility of this adverse consequence of hydrotherapy, salt should be added to the whirlpool water when treating patients with extensive burns or other extensive wounds.[131]

INFECTION

A number of reports have documented the association of hydrotherapy with infections in patients.[97-99] Such a risk can be minimized by using nonimmersion hydrotherapy techniques or, when using immersion techniques, strictly adhering to appropriate cleaning protocols and using antimicrobials in the water.

AGGRAVATION OF EDEMA

Immersion in hot or warm water has been shown to increase edema in the hands of patients with upper extremity disorders,[142] and this effect becomes more pronounced as the temperature of the water increases.[89] Therefore, to avoid aggravation of edema, only cool water should be used and dependency of the extremity in the water should be minimized when signs of acute inflammation are present.

ASTHMA EXACERBATION

While the humidity around exercise pools and whirlpools may help alleviate the symptoms of exercise-induced asthma, it has been found that exposure to chlorinated pools or whirlpools can cause a reduction in forced expiratory volume in patients with asthma even if they have no symptoms.[143] Additionally, one study suggests that children exposed to swimming pools with chlorinated water have an increased risk of developing asthma,[144] and there is a published report relating asthma in three swimming pool workers to the chlorine in the air around the pool.[145] Patients with asthma using chlorinated exercise pools or whirlpools should be closely monitored for asthma symptoms.

APPLICATION TECHNIQUES

This section provides guidelines for the sequence of procedures required for the safe and effective application of hydrotherapy. Application techniques for negative pressure wound therapy follow.

GENERAL HYDROTHERAPY

Hydrotherapy may be applied in several circumstances, but it must first be determined if this is the best modality for the patient. The following is a list of steps for the use of hydrotherapy in general.

APPLICATION TECHNIQUE 9-1	GENERAL HYDROTHERAPY

Procedure

1. Evaluate the patient and set the goals of treatment.
2. Determine if hydrotherapy is the most appropriate treatment.

   Hydrotherapy may be an appropriate treatment when progress toward the goals of treatment can be achieved by the use of superficial heat or cold, wound cleansing and débridement, exercise in a water environment, or where the goals of treatment include controlling pain or edema. Hydrotherapy is a particularly appropriate means of applying superficial heat or cold when the area to be treated is a distal extremity with varied contouring and when dependency of the limb will not aggravate the patient's symptoms. Hydrotherapy is the ideal intervention for wound cleansing and débridement when there is a moderate amount of debris or necrotic tissue in a wound. When a wound is clean, hydrotherapy is not indicated, although negative pressure wound therapy may be appropriate. When there is a large amount of necrotic tissue, more aggressive treatment, as can be provided by surgical débridement, may be required. Exercise in water is indicated for patients with load-sensitive conditions or where the benefits of resistance or hydrostatic pressure of water, as described above, can promote progress toward the goals of treatment.

3. Determine that hydrotherapy is not contraindicated for this patient or this condition.

   The treatment area should be inspected for the presence of any open wounds, rash, or other signs of infection, and sensation in the area should be assessed. The patient's chart should also be checked for any record of previous adverse responses to hydrotherapy, and the patient should be asked the appropriate questions regarding contraindications. It is also recommended that heart rate and blood pressure be measured and recorded if a large area of the body is going to be immersed.

4. Select the appropriate form of hydrotherapy according to the condition to be treated and the desired treatment effects. Select from the following list (see specific application recommendations for each hydrotherapy agent on the next pages):
   - Whirlpool
   - Hubbard tank
   - Contrast bath
   - Pool
   - Nonimmersion irrigation device

   The form of hydrotherapy selected should be one that produces the desired treatment effects, is appropriate for the size of the area to be treated, allows for adequate safety and control of infection, and is cost effective. The advantages and disadvantages of the different forms of hydrotherapy, based on treatment goals, are provided below, together with the directions for their application. Detailed information on safety and infection control is provided in the section on safety issues.

   Because most clinical settings have only a limited selection of forms of hydrotherapy, it is recommended that the available form be used if it is effective and safe. For example, if no nonimmersion devices are available for treating a small open wound on a patient's ankle, a whirlpool may be used as long as appropriate infection control measures are taken; however, treatment of this condition should not be provided in an exercise pool or Jacuzzi, where the same water will be used by other patients. In contrast, if hydrotherapy is being considered for cardiovascular conditioning but only nonimmersion hydrotherapy devices are available, hydrotherapy should not be performed because it will be ineffective. In this case, a land-based exercise program should be considered.

Continued

APPLICATION TECHNIQUE 9-1   GENERAL HYDROTHERAPY—*cont'd*

5. Explain to the patient the procedure, the reason for applying hydrotherapy, and the sensations the patient can expect to feel.

   During the application of hydrotherapy the patient may feel a sensation of warmth or cold, depending on the temperature of the water used. The patient will also feel gentle pressure if the water is being agitated. The patient should not feel excessively hot or cold, or excessive pressure, nor should the patient feel faint during the application of hydrotherapy. In general, hydrotherapy is not a painful procedure unless it is being used for the treatment of burns or other sensate wounds in conjunction with débridement. The pain associated with this procedure can usually be controlled to some extent by the administration of high-dose analgesics before the hydrotherapy treatment.

6. Apply the appropriate form of hydrotherapy.
7. When hydrotherapy is completed, assess the outcome(s) of the treatment. Remeasure and assess progress relative to the initial patient evaluation and the goals of treatment.
8. Document the treatment.

WHIRLPOOL

A whirlpool is composed of a tank that can hold water and a turbine that provides agitation and aeration to move the water in the tank. The tank is usually made of stainless steel, although fiberglass and plastic tanks are also available. Whirlpools are available in a number of different shapes and sizes to allow for treatment of different body parts. Extremity tanks are suitable for immersion of a distal extremity, such as a hand or a foot, whereas low-boy and high-boy tanks are intended for immersion of larger parts of the extremities and may be used for immersion up to the waist.

A whirlpool turbine is composed of a motor bracketed securely to the side of the whirlpool and pipes, for air and water circulation, suspended in the water (Fig. 9-14). The height and direction of the turbine can be adjusted to project the water pressure toward or away from the involved area. The turbine may be directed toward the involved area to apply maximum force, as may be desired to control pain or to remove tightly adhered wound debris. The turbine should be directed away from the involved area if the area is hypersensitive or if granulation tissue is present because the high direct pressure of water from the turbine can adversely affect such conditions. Most turbines also allow the clinician to open or close the aeration valve to further modify the pressure of the water flow.

Whirlpools are generally used for exercise or pain control in limited areas of the body, such as the leg and foot or arm and hand. They are also occasionally used for the treatment of open wounds, particularly in patients with extensive wounds, such as burns, or with wounds with much debris as occurs directly after a motor vehicle or bicycle crash (Fig. 9-15).

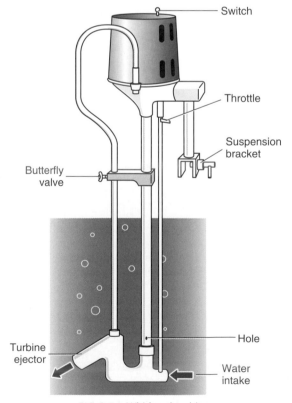

FIG 9-14 Whirlpool turbine.

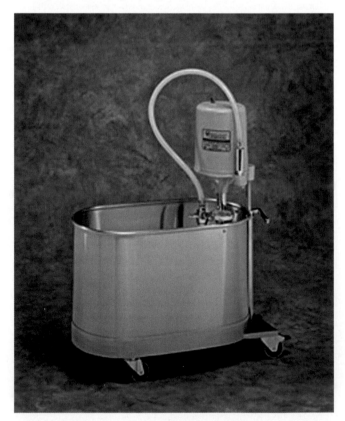

FIG 9-15 Whirlpool. *Courtesy Whitehall Manufacturing, City of Industry, CA.*

Whirlpool Water Temperature

A cold whirlpool, at 0° C to 26° C (32° F to 79° F), can be used in place of an ice pack or a cold pack, to treat acute inflammatory conditions of the distal extremities. The cold water provides better contact with the contoured distal extremity than a pack does. Low temperatures can be achieved by adding ice to the whirlpool water; however, very low temperatures should not be used on large areas due to the increased risk of tissue damage.

Tepid water, at 26° to 33° C (79° to 92° F), should be used in the whirlpool if the water is being used solely as a medium for exercise. Warmer temperatures are likely to produce fatigue and colder temperatures can inhibit muscle contraction. A tepid whirlpool may also be used when an inflammatory condition is present if lower temperatures are not tolerated.

A neutral warmth whirlpool, at 33° to 35.5° C (92° to 96° F), should be used for the treatment of open wounds and in patients with circulatory, sensory, or cardiac disorders. Neutral warmth may also be used to control tone in patients with neurologically based hypertonicity.

Mild warmth, at 35.5° to 37° C (96° to 98° F), may be used for the treatment of burns once epithelialization has begun. Such treatment promotes mobility and relaxation and minimizes energy loss by cooling or shivering.[131]

A hot whirlpool, at 37° to 40° C (99° to 104° F), or a very hot whirlpool, at 40° to 43° C (104° to 110° F), is recommended for the control of pain and/or to increase soft tissue extensibility because this temperature range of whirlpool water has been shown to increase the temperature of subcutaneous tissue to within the range required to produce these effects.[146] The higher end of this temperature range is recommended for the treatment of chronic conditions, such as osteoarthritis or rheumatoid arthritis in the nonacute phases, when small areas are being treated, while the lower end of this range is recommended when large areas of the body are to be immersed.

The whirlpool temperature should not exceed 43° C (110° F) at any time because higher temperatures may cause burns.

The tank should be filled with water immediately before it is used to prevent the water temperature from changing excessively between filling and patient immersion. If an antimicrobial is being used, it should be added to the water as the whirlpool is being filled.

APPLICATION TECHNIQUE 9-2	APPLICATION TECHNIQUE FOR WHIRLPOOL

Equipment Required

- Hot and cold water mixing valves
- Thermometer for checking the temperature of the water in the tank
- A turbine to agitate and aerate the water
- Seat or stretcher for the patient to sit either in or out of the water, depending on the area being treated and the configuration of the whirlpool
- Gravity drain
- Heated, well-ventilated space
- Towels and blankets

Procedure

1. Fill the tank with water. Select the appropriate temperature range according to the condition and treatment objectives as described previously and in Table 9-5.

2. Allow the patient to undress the area to be treated, and provide a gown or halter and pants as necessary for modesty. Do not allow any clothing to enter the water because it may be sucked into the turbine.

   When treating an open wound, the clinician must wear gloves, a waterproof gown, goggles, and a mask as universal precautions to protect the patient and the clinician from cross-infection by microorganisms that may be carried in the water or in airborne water droplets.

3. Remove wound dressings if any are present and if they are easy to remove without causing pain or damaging the tissue. Because adhered dressings may be easier to remove after brief soaking in the water, this may be done as long as the dressings are removed before the agitator turbine is turned on to avoid clogging the turbine. Inspect the skin and test it for thermal sensitivity. Vital signs should be checked and

---

TABLE 9-5	Clinical Applications and Sensations of Whirlpool Treatment at Different Temperature Ranges

Temperature Range (° C/° F)	Sensation	Clinical Applications
0 to 26/32 to 79	Cold	Acute inflammation
26 to 33/79 to 92	Tepid	Medium for exercise Acute inflammation if colder temperature not tolerated
33 to 35.5/92 to 96	Neutral warmth	Open wounds Medically compromised patients with circulatory, sensory, or cardiac disorders Decrease tone
35.5 to 37/96 to 98	Mild warmth	Increase mobility in burn patients
37 to 40/99 to 104	Hot	Control pain
40 to 43/104 to 110	Very hot	Increase soft tissue extensibility Chronic conditions Limited body area only
>43/>110	—	Should not be used

Continued

APPLICATION TECHNIQUE 9-2 | APPLICATION TECHNIQUE FOR WHIRLPOOL—*cont'd*

recorded before immersing any area of a patient with a current or recent cardiovascular abnormality in a whirlpool.

4. Position the patient comfortably, with the affected area immersed in the water. Try to avoid pressure of the limb on the edge of the whirlpool to avoid impairing circulation or nerve function or causing discomfort. Dry padding, such as a folded towel, may be placed on the rim of the tank to distribute pressure. Do not allow the patient's fingers or toes to be near the turbine ejector.

5. Adjust the direction and aeration of the turbine. The entire turbine can be moved from side to side and up and down to adjust its direction. The butterfly valve at the top of the shaft of the turbine adjusts the aeration of the water (see Fig. 9-14). The hole at the lower end of the pipe through which air is forced should always be immersed at least 2 inches below the surface of the water to avoid overheating the turbine.

6. Turn on the turbine.

7. Stay with the patient throughout the hydrotherapy treatment and monitor the patient's vital signs before, during, and after treatment as necessary. It is generally recommended that patients not be left alone during warm or hot hydrotherapy treatments because of the risk of fainting or other heat-related distress. Treatment should be discontinued if there are any abnormal or unsafe changes in vital signs.

8. The patient may exercise the affected part during the treatment. Movement is recommended when treatment is for joint stiffness or impaired ROM or when edema without acute inflammation is present.

9. Whirlpools are generally applied for 10 to 30 minutes; shorter periods may be sufficient for softening wound eschar,

whereas longer periods will increase the amount of heat transferred to the patient.

10. When the treatment is completed, remove the limb from the water, dry the intact skin thoroughly, and inspect the treated area. Keep the patient covered or wrapped after treatment to avoid chilling.

11. If the whirlpool is being used for the treatment of an open wound, a clean, pressurized rinse is recommended after the whirlpool to remove bacteria more effectively.

12. Reapply wound dressings if open wounds are present.

13. Drain, rinse, and clean the whirlpool according to the directions given in the section on safety issues regarding hydrotherapy.

Advantages

* Can be used for heat transfer, for cleansing and debriding open wounds, or for exercise.
* Patient can be positioned securely and comfortably.
* Weaker muscles can move more freely than on dry land.
* Allows movement while heat is being applied, unlike other conductive thermal agents such as hot packs.

Disadvantages

* Size of tank limits the amount of exercise and the size of the area that can be treated.
* Large quantity of water used.
* Risk of infection.
* Costs and time associated with cleaning the whirlpool.
* Costs associated with heating water.
* Time expended assisting the patient to dress and undress.

HUBBARD TANK

A Hubbard tank, named after the engineer who invented it, is a large whirlpool intended for full body immersion. These tanks vary somewhat in size but are generally about 8 feet long by 6 feet wide and 4 feet deep and hold approximately 425 gallons of water (Fig. 9-16). The tank is equipped with turbines, a stretcher, and a hoist to raise and lower the stretcher. This large tank is particularly suitable for debridement of burns covering large areas of the body and for the treatment of other painful conditions that affect large areas of the body. Hubbard tanks can also be used for ROM exercises for multiple areas or for ambulation if a walking trough is added; however, these procedures are more often performed in a pool, except in cases where pool use is specifically contraindicated because of the risk of infection.

The popularity of the Hubbard tank has waned in recent years because of the considerable expense associ-

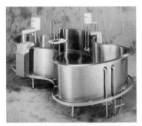

FIG 9-16 Hubbard tank. *Courtesy Whitehall Manufacturing, City of Industry, CA.*

ated with providing such a large volume of warm water and because of the time involved in cleaning this large pool. Hubbard tanks must be cleaned between each use in the same manner as whirlpools of other sizes, as described in the section on safety issues regarding hydrotherapy.

APPLICATION TECHNIQUE 9-3 — HUBBARD TANK

Equipment Required

- Hot and cold water mixing valves
- Thermometer for checking the temperature of the water in the tank
- A turbine to agitate and aerate the water
- Seat or stretcher for the patient to sit either in or out of the water, depending on the area being treated and the configuration of the whirlpool
- Gravity drain
- Heated, well-ventilated space
- Towels and blankets

Procedure

Treatment in a Hubbard tank is applied similarly to treatment in a whirlpool of any other size, as described above, except that the water temperature is generally kept in the slightly lower range of 36° to 39° C (97° to 100° F) because patients cannot dissipate the increase in tissue temperature as effectively when heat is applied to such a large area. Specific instructions for placing patients in a Hubbard tank and removing them from the tank are as follows:

1. Place the patient on the stretcher next to the tank, with the patient's weight evenly distributed.
2. Attach the hoist to the rings on the four corners of the stretcher.
3. Remove dressings if present and easy to remove without causing pain or damaging the tissue. If the dressings are adhered, they can be removed after brief soaking in the water before the turbines are turned on.
4. Raise the hoist to lift the patient. Gently swing the patient on the stretcher over the water and then slowly lower the patient to just above the water level.
5. Attach the head end of the stretcher to the support bracket.
6. Slowly lower the hoist until the foot end of the stretcher touches the bottom of the tank.
7. Remove the hoist.
8. Adjust the force and direction of the agitators.
9. Stay with the patient throughout the treatment to monitor the physiological responses to the treatment and to be sure that the patient does not slide down the stretcher into the water.
10. Patients generally stay in a Hubbard tank for about 20 minutes or until the procedure, such as débridement, is completed.
11. When the treatment is completed, reattach the hoist to the stretcher and remove the patient from the water.
12. Dry the patient quickly and thoroughly.
13. Wrap or cover the patient immediately to avoid chilling, leaving exposed any open wound areas requiring dressing.

Advantages

- Can treat large areas or multiple areas of the body.
- Can be used for heat transfer, for cleansing and débriding open wounds, or for water exercise.

Disadvantages

- Costly to provide treatment.
- Costly equipment and space requirements.
- Uses large amount of warm water.
- Time-consuming to fill, empty, and clean tank and to place patient in the tank.
- Requires extra caution with regard to possible systemic effects of overheating with a large body area exposed.

CONTRAST BATH

Contrast baths are applied by alternately immersing an area, generally a distal extremity, first in warm or hot water and then in cool or cold water (Fig. 9-17). Contrast baths have been shown to cause fluctuations in blood flow over a 20-minute treatment.[147] There are no other published research data on the effects of contrast baths. This form of hydrotherapy is frequently used clinically when a goal of treatment is to achieve the benefits of heat, including decreased pain and increased flexibility, while avoiding the risk of increased edema. The varying sensory stimulus is also thought to promote pain relief and desensitization. Thus treatment with a contrast bath may be considered when patients present with chronic edema; subacute trauma; inflammatory conditions such as sprains, strains, or tendonitis; or hyperalgesia or hypersensitivity caused by reflex sympathetic dystrophy or other conditions.

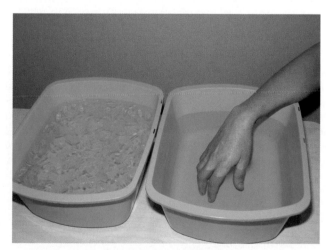

FIG 9-17 Contrast bath.

APPLICATION TECHNIQUE 9-4 | CONTRAST BATH

Equipment Required

- Two water containers
- Thermometer
- Towels

Procedure

1. Fill two adjacent containers with water. The containers may be whirlpools, buckets, or tubs. Fill one container with warm or hot water, at 38° to 44° C (100° to 111° F), and the other with cold or cool water, at 10° to 18° C (50° to 64° F). When using contrast baths for the control of pain or edema, it is recommended that the temperature difference between the warm and cold water be large; when using contrast baths for desensitization, it is recommended that the temperature difference between the two baths initially be small and then gradually increased for later treatments as the patient's sensitivity decreases.
2. First, immerse the area to be treated in the warm water for 3 to 4 minutes; then immerse the area in the cold water for 1 minute.

3. Repeat this sequence five or six times to provide a total treatment time of 25 to 30 minutes and end with immersion in the warm water.
4. When the treatment is completed, dry the area quickly and thoroughly.

Advantages

- May promote a more vigorous circulatory effect than heat or cold alone.
- Provides good contact with contoured distal extremities compared with other thermal agents.
- May help to provide pain control without aggravating edema.
- Allows movement in water for increased circulatory effects.

Disadvantages

- Limb is in a dependent position, which may aggravate edema.
- Some patients do not tolerate cold immersion.
- Lack of research evidence evaluating the effects of contrast baths.

EXERCISE POOL

To optimize the cardiovascular, respiratory, renal, or psychological benefits of hydrotherapy, the use of an exercise pool that allows full body immersion and exercise is recommended, unless immersion in water that will be used by other individuals is contraindicated. An exercise pool is also generally the optimal means for applying hydrotherapy to achieve the musculoskeletal benefits associated with water immersion, although a whirlpool may be used when only the extremities require immersion.

Swimming pools and purpose-designed hydrotherapy pools can be used for the application of hydrotherapy. Most swimming pools are at least 100 feet long and 25 feet wide and have a maximum depth of 8 feet, with a sloping bottom to produce a gradual descent. Most purpose-designed hydrotherapy pools are smaller and position the patient in the middle or at the edge of the pool to allow performance of specific types of exercises. Some hydrotherapy pools are equipped with an underwater treadmill,[148] an adjustable rate-of-water flow, and adjustable depths with movable floors to provide graded exercise activity (Fig. 9-18).[148] An exercise pool may be available for use in the clinical setting or the patient may be able to use a public or private swimming pool. Either type of pool may be used for individual or group treatment, depending on its size, with a therapist present, or for independent home exercise programs.

Pool Temperature

The temperature of the water in an exercise pool should be kept at 26° to 36° C (79° to 97° F). The amount of movement expected to be performed by the patient should be used to determine the optimal temperature within this range. The warmer end of the range, 34° to 36° C (93° to 97° F), should be used when low-intensity activities, such as light exercise by elderly deconditioned patients or by patients with arthritis, will be performed. This is because warmer temperatures are more comfortable and help patients who move less to conserve body heat while in the water. The cooler end of the range, 26° to 28° C (79° to 82° F), is recommended for recreational pools or where more intense exercise will be performed because the cooler temperature dissipates heat produced by the patients and therefore allows them to perform more exercise, or more vigorous exercise, with less fatigue. The water temperature should not be allowed to be below 18.5° C (65° F) because such low temperatures can impair the muscles' ability to contract.

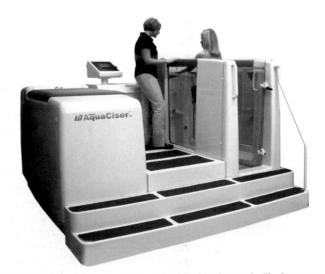

FIG 9-18 Purpose-designed exercise pool with treadmill. *Courtesy Ferno Performance Pools, Wilmington, OH.*

APPLICATION TECHNIQUE 9-5   POOL EXERCISE

Equipment Required

- Appropriate space for the pool—adequate size, support, ventilation, and heating
- Space to store auxiliary equipment, including chemicals and mechanical systems
- Space for patients to shower and change clothes
- Water supply
- Nonslip area around pool
- Safety equipment
- Infection control equipment, including pump and filter, chemicals, and testing kit
- Towels
- Thermometer

Procedure

1. The patient and the therapist should wear a bathing suit for pool exercise. The therapist may wear other light clothing over the bathing suit if not planning to enter the water except in the case of an emergency.
2. The therapist should assist the patient to enter the pool if necessary. Provide ramps, stairs, a ladder, or a lift to help patients get into and out of the pool.
3. The patient may perform activities to improve strength, cardiovascular fitness, endurance, or functional activities, as determined by the evaluation and plan of care. Activities may include upright exercise, walking in the pool, swimming, or other forms of exercise. The patient may use flotation devices, a tether, or other objects to alter the resistance or buoyancy effects of the water. Water-based exercise programs can be progressed by increasing the number of repetitions of an activity, increasing the speed of the activity, changing the length of the lever arm, decreasing the degree of stabilization

provided, or using larger floats to increase resistance. More detailed descriptions of water exercise programs are beyond the scope of this text and can be found in books devoted to aquatic therapy.
4. The therapist should stay with the patient throughout the treatment and monitor vital signs during exercise if the patient has risk factors or any history indicating that this may be necessary. For example, heart rate and blood pressure should be monitored in patients recovering from myocardial infarction, and heart rate should be monitored in pregnant patients.
5. After completion of the water activities, the therapist should help the patient to get out of the pool if necessary. The patient should dry the body and wrap up immediately to avoid chilling.

Advantages

- Patient can move freely, with less risk of falling during exercises.
- Decreases weight bearing on joints. With immersion in water 60 inches deep, weight bearing on the lower extremities is reduced by 88% to 95%.
- Buoyancy may assist weak muscles to allow increased performance of active exercise.

Disadvantages

- Risk of falling when the patient gets into and out of the water because water around the pool can make the floor slippery.
- Risk of infection from other individuals who have been in the water.
- Difficulty stabilizing or isolating body parts during exercise.
- Risk of drowning.
- Fear among some patients of water immersion.

NONIMMERSION IRRIGATION DEVICES

A variety of devices, including hand-held showers, syringes, and purpose-designed pulsatile irrigation units, can apply hydrotherapy without immersion of the area to be treated.[99,128,149] These devices apply water by spraying it on the treatment area. Nonimmersion irrigation devices are particularly well-suited for the application of hydrotherapy to open wounds because they involve less risk of infection than whirlpools and because some, although not all, of these devices can spray fluid onto an open wound within the appropriate, safe, and effective pressure limits of 4 to 15 psi (see Table 9-4). However, because water does not produce buoyancy or hydrostatic pressure without immersion and therefore does not reduce weight bearing or edema or increase circulation, the use of nonimmersion hydrotherapy is limited to situations where these are not required to achieve the goals of treatment.

Because electric pulsatile irrigation devices both deliver fluid at a controlled pressure and provide suction to remove contaminated fluid, they are ideally suited to the treatment of open wounds.[149] These devices pump an intermittent stream of fluid from an irrigation bag or bottle via tubing to a handpiece that directs the flow of fluid onto the wound (Fig. 9-19). The used and contaminated irrigation fluid is then removed from the treatment area by suction via the handpiece through other tubing

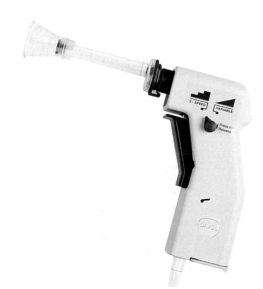

FIG 9-19 Pulsed lavage with suction handpiece with tip used to deliver water to the wound bed and suction contaminated wound. *Courtesy KCI, Inc, San Antonio, TX.*

APPLICATION TECHNIQUE 9-6 | NONIMMERSION IRRIGATION DEVICE

Equipment Required

- Nonimmersion irrigation device
- Tubing, handpiece, and tip for each treatment
- Irrigation fluid—usually bags of sterile saline
- Towels

Procedure

When applying nonimmersion irrigation, the following guidelines should be used. The clinician should always wear gloves, a waterproof gown, and eye, nose, and mouth protection during treatment because this type of treatment can spray contaminated fluid toward the clinician. To maximize comfort and optimize healing, clean, warm fluid should always be used for irrigation. Clean, warm water can be used for shower treatments, whereas sterile normal saline is recommended when irrigation is provided with other devices. It is recommended that treatment be applied once a day for 5 to 15 minutes or long enough to hydrate hard eschar or loosen debris. The appropriate frequency and duration of treatment will depend primarily on the size of the wound and the amount of necrotic tissue, exudate, or other debris present. In addition, when using an electric pulsatile irrigation device, the following treatment guidelines should be followed. Further specific directions for the use of different brands and models of these devices are provided by the manufacturers.

1. Although patients may be treated at the bedside with this type of device, to reduce the risk of transmitting infection, all irrigation treatments should be performed in an enclosed area separated from other patients. Pulsed lavage is also generally performed using sterile technique.
2. Sterile normal saline in 1000-mL bags is generally used as the irrigation fluid; in cases of wound infection, antimicrobials may be added to this fluid. It is recommended that the saline be warmed before it is used by placing it in a basin of hot tap water. Hang the bag(s) of fluid on the device.
3. Attach the tubing, suction canister, handpiece, and irrigation tip to the device.
4. Turn on the pump.
5. Select the treatment pressure. Most devices can spray fluid at pressures of between 0 and 60 psi and have a half-switch to limit the maximum pressure to 30 psi. Pressures of 4 to 8 psi are generally sufficient for cleansing or debriding most wounds; however, the pressure can be adjusted according to the nature of the wound, the tip used, and the sensitivity of the patient. It is recommended that the lowest pressure that effectively loosens and removes debris be used and that the pressure be decreased if the patient complains of pain, if

bleeding occurs, or if the tip is near a major or exposed vessel. The pressure may need to be increased in the presence of tough eschar or when there is a large amount of necrotic tissue.
6. Apply the treatment until adequate hydration or débridement is achieved.
7. This form of treatment may be followed by sharp débridement if necessary to remove adhered necrotic tissue.
8. Reapply the appropriate wound dressing.
9. Pulsed lavage is generally applied once a day but may be applied more frequently to wounds that have greater than 50% necrotic, nonviable tissue with purulent drainage or a foul odor and less frequently if the wound does not have purulent drainage or odor. Treatment with this type of device should result in a decrease in necrotic tissue and an increase in granulation within 1 week of initiating treatment. If this does not occur, the treatment approach should be reevaluated.

Advantages

- Control of fluid pressure to stay within a safe and effective range for application to open wounds.
- Reduced infection risk because the fluid and wound debris are removed from the wound by gravity and suction.
- Jet of fluid can be directed to stay within the wound bed.
- Less time-consuming to apply than a whirlpool.
- Saves the expense of filling, draining, and cleaning a whirlpool.
- Does not require the patient to be transferred to the whirlpool area.
- Uses less fluid than a whirlpool.
- Normal saline rather than water applied to the open wound reduces the risk of hyponatremia.
- Can be used where whirlpool treatment is not recommended, such as with an unresponsive or incontinent patient.
- Faster granulation of the wound bed reported in one study comparing pulsatile irrigation with whirlpool treatment of wounds.[150]

Disadvantages

- Treatment with a pulsatile irrigation device incurs the additional expense of using new tubing, handpiece, and tip for each application. These components cost between $100 and $140 per treatment.
- Does not provide the therapeutic benefits associated with the buoyancy and hydrostatic pressure of immersion hydrotherapy.

into a collection canister. The handpiece has a trigger to control the flow of fluid and can be fitted with a variety of tips to vary the fluid dispersion. With most of these devices, the tubing, handpiece, and tips are all intended to be discarded after each treatment in order to minimize the risk of cross-infection. Electric pulsatile irrigation devices are available in portable and clinical models. This type of treatment is known as pulsed lavage (Fig. 9-20).

NEGATIVE PRESSURE WOUND THERAPY

Negative pressure wound therapy is often used in conjunction with nonimmersion irrigation of wounds to promote wound healing. It may promote healing of chronic wounds of various etiologies, including pressure ulcers,

diabetic foot wounds, and large surgical wounds. Negative pressure wound therapy involves the application of continuous or intermittent negative (subatmospheric) pressure over a wound bed and foam dressing. Two companies manufacture this type of device. One company makes the V.A.C. (Vacuum Assisted Closure) devices (Kinetic Concepts, Inc, San Antonio, TX) and the other makes the Versatile 1 devices (BlueSky Medical Group, Carlsbad, CA) (Fig. 9-21). All devices include a 250 ml to 1000 ml canister to collect wound fluids and require electricity to operate, although some may have a rechargeable battery. Since the application technique for the two companies' devices are different they are described separately.

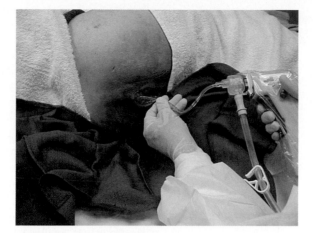

FIG 9-20 Using a nonimmersion hydrotherapy device to cleanse and debride a wound. *From Cameron MH, Monroe LG: Physical rehabilitation: evidence-based examination, evaluation, and intervention, St Louis, 2007, Saunders.*

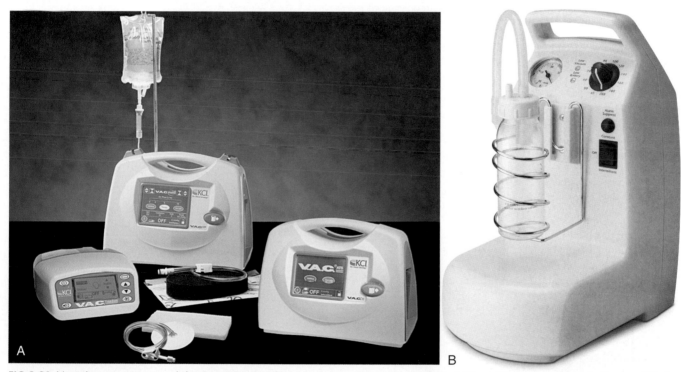

FIG 9-21 Negative pressure wound therapy units. **A,** KCI V.A.C. System; **B,** BlueSky Versatile 1 Wound Vacuum System. **A,** *Courtesy KCI, San Antonio, TX;* **B,** *Courtesy Smith & Nephew Wound Care, Largo, FL.*

APPLICATION TECHNIQUE 9-7A

NEGATIVE PRESSURE WOUND THERAPY (V.A.C. DEVICES)

Equipment Required

- V.A.C device, including drain (Therapeutic Regulated Accurate Care [T.R.A.C.] pad), drain tubing, canister
- Foam dressing (note that there are special foam and transparent film dressings intended only for use with the V.A.C device)
- Transparent film dressing (drape)
- Irrigation device and normal saline
- Gloves
- Nonadherent dressing (optional)

Procedure (Fig. 9-22)

1. Remove old wound dressings and clean the wound bed using an irrigation device and normal saline.
2. If the previous dressing adheres to wound, consider placing a nonadherent mesh dressing on the wound before placing the foam dressing for the VAC treatment. Cover superficial or retention sutures with a single layer of nonadherent dressing.
3. Make sure there is no bleeding in the wound. If there is bleeding do not use this type of treatment.
4. Protect vessels, organs, and nerves by covering with natural tissues or nonadherent mesh dressing.
5. Clean and dry the periwound area.
6. Assess wound size and shape, and cut the foam dressing to a size that will allow the dressing to be gently placed into the wound without overlapping onto intact skin. Be sure to cut the foam away from the wound site and remove loose fragments so that they do not fall into the wound.
7. Gently place the cut foam in the wound bed, ensuring contact with all wound surfaces. Do not force the foam dressing into any part of the wound. Do not place foam dressing into blind or unexplored tunnels where the distal aspect is not visible. Note and document the total number of pieces of foam used.
8. Trim and place the transparent film dressing (drape) to cover the foam dressing and an additional 3 to 5 cm of intact periwound skin. The dressing may be cut into multiple pieces if necessary.
9. Partially pull the backing off the transparent film to expose its adhesive.
10. Place the transparent film, adhesive side down, over the foam in the wound and over the periwound intact skin. Do

not pull or stretch the transparent film over the foam dressing. Minimize wrinkles to avoid pressure leaks.
11. Remove the remaining backing material and pat the transparent film to ensure a good seal.
12. Remove green-striped stabilization layer and blue handling tabs.
13. Choose T.R.A.C. pad application site, taking into consideration fluid flow and tubing position to allow for optimal drainage and avoid placement over bony prominences or within tissue creases.
14. Pinch the transparent film and cut a 2-cm hole through it. The hole should be large enough to allow for removal of fluid or exudate. It is not necessary to cut into the foam. Cut a hole rather than a slit because a slit may self-seal during therapy.
15. Apply the T.R.A.C. pad. Remove the pad's backing to expose adhesive. Place the T.R.A.C. pad directly over the hole in the transparent film. Apply gentle pressure on the T.R.A.C. pad and skirt to ensure complete adhesion. Remove the stabilization layer using the blue tab.
16. Remove canister from sterile packaging and insert into the V.A.C. unit until it locks in place. If the canister is not fully engaged, the unit will alarm.
17. Connect the T.R.A.C. pad tubing to the canister tubing and ensure the clamps on each tube are open.
18. Turn on the power to the V.A.C. unit and select the appropriate settings, depending on the type of wound and foam dressing.

The makers of the V.A.C. therapy system recommend continuous negative pressure for the first 48 hours followed by intermittent negative pressure (5 minutes on, 2 minutes off) for the rest of treatment for acute wounds, partial-thickness burns, pressure ulcers, diabetic foot ulcers, and chronic wounds. They recommend continuous negative pressure for the duration of treatment for surgical wound dehiscence, meshed grafts, dermal substitutes, flaps, and abdominal wounds.

Recommended pressures depend on the wound type and the kind of foam used in the wound. Target pressures range from 50 mm Hg to 175 mm Hg. See the manufacturer's recommendations for specific wound and foam types.

19. Assess dressing to ensure seal integrity. The dressing should be collapsed, and there should be no hissing sounds. Secure excess tubing to prevent interference with patient mobility. The dressing should be checked every 2 hours to make sure the seal is still intact and the device is running. Leaks may be patched with additional transparent film dressing. The dressing should be removed, the wound irrigated, and the dressing replaced if treatment is stopped for more than 2 hours. The unit may be disconnected for shorter periods of time without replacing the dressing.
20. Change the canister when it becomes full. The alarm will sound when the canister is full. If it does not fill sooner, the canister should be changed at least once a week to control odor. Large (1000 mL) canisters should not be used for patients at risk of bleeding or for patients, such as the elderly and children, who cannot tolerate a large loss of fluid volume.

It is recommended that V.A.C. therapy be on for 22 out of 24 hours for the best results. The dressing should be checked every 2 hours to ensure that the seal is still intact and that there is no bleeding. The dressing should be changed every 48 hours, or every 12 to 24 hours if the wound is infected. The wound should be reassessed at 2 weeks for signs of healing. The average length of treatment is 4 to 6 weeks.

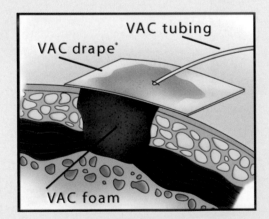

FIG 9-22 Diagram of V.A.C. negative pressure wound therapy application. *Courtesy KCI, Inc, San Antonio, TX.*

Adapted from *V.A.C. therapy clinical guidelines: A reference source for clinicians*, San Antonio, TX, 2007, KCI.

| APPLICATION TECHNIQUE 9-7B | NEGATIVE PRESSURE WOUND THERAPY (VERSATILE 1 DEVICES) |

Equipment Required

- Vacuum-assisted closure device, including drain, drain tubing, suction canister and fluid collection canister
- Transparent film dressing
- Non-adherent gauze
- Cotton gauze
- Normal saline solution, skin sealant, adhesive tape

Procedure (Fig. 9-23)

1. Irrigate the wound bed thoroughly.
2. Apply skin sealant to all skin that will be covered by the transparent dressing, a minimum of 1 inch beyond the wound margin. Allow the skin to dry.
3. Cut a single layer of non-adherent gauze to the size of the wound bed, and lay this gauze across the wound bed.
4. Place the drain in the wound bed. The drain should not come in direct contact with the wound bed, so if nonadherent gauze is not used, place gauze moistened with normal saline solution around the drain before placing it in the wound bed. Trim the drain so that it is confined to the wound bed.
5. Saturate cotton gauze with normal saline and place lightly in the wound to completely cover the drain and fill the wound to skin level. It is important that the gauze is moist, so that the wound stays moist.
6. Place the transparent dressing over the filled wound, ensuring contact with at least 1 inch of intact skin beyond the wound edges. Split one end of the transparent film dressing and bring each "arm" around the drain tubing. Crimp the edges of the transparent film dressing around the tubing.
7. At the tubing exit site apply a small amount of sealant paste where the dressing meets the tube to seal and ensure an airtight closure.
8. Reinforce this junction with adhesive tape.
9. Connect the drain tubing to the suction canister. Always use the smallest canister possible or fill the canister with water to reduce volume.
10. Adjust the pressure to between 40 and 80 mm Hg set at a continuous mode. Pressures should be as low as possible to still be effective, and the suction level should never cause patient discomfort.

   The dressing should contract noticeably. If the dressing fails to contract, the dressing has not been completely sealed. Reinforce the closure and/or adjust the drain and resume suction.
11. Check for dressing integrity every 6 to 8 hours by occluding the suction tubing. The surface of the dressing should appear wrinkled, indicating proper suction. If the dressing balloons but then contracts after releasing the tubing, check it for leaks. Reinforce the wound closure and/or adjust the drain and initiate suction again.
12. Change the fluid collecting canister when two-thirds full and dispose of according to the facility's guidelines for biohazardous materials.

Advantages

- Enhances wound healing.
- Provides continuous coverage to large wounds, reducing wound contamination and infection risk.
- Comfortable.
- Maintains optimally moist wound environment while keeping surrounding skin dry.
- Infrequent dressing changes reduces mechanical disruption and cooling of healing tissues.

Disadvantages

- More expensive in the short run than standard dressing changes.
- Patient is tethered to suction unit.
- Potential for skin irritation from the adhesive dressing.
- More time consuming to set up than standard dressing changes.
- Does not substitute for hydrotherapy.

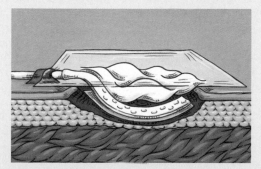

FIG 9-23 Diagram of Versatile 1 negative pressure wound therapy application. *Courtesy Smith & Nephew Wound Care, Largo, FL.*

Adapted from *BlueSky Medical Chariker-Jeter instructions for use,* BlueSky Medical Group, Inc, Carlsbad, CA, 2007.

SAFETY ISSUES REGARDING HYDROTHERAPY, INCLUDING INFECTION CONTROL AND POOL SAFETY

To optimize safety and infection control during hydrotherapy, the following general guidelines should be adhered to. A facility hydrotherapy safety and infection control program that addresses the specific needs of the facility should be developed in conjunction with an infection control specialist or in conjunction with the facility infection control committee. This program should take into account the specific safety hazards associated with this type of treatment and the types of microorganisms most commonly encountered at that time and place. The program must also be in compliance with the guidelines, rules, and regulations of the local public health department. Infection control experts should also be consulted if a problem with infection control, such as frequent patient infections after the use of hydrotherapy, arises.

SAFETY PRECAUTIONS AND INFECTION CONTROL FOR WHIRLPOOLS

These recommendations apply for whirlpools of all sizes and shapes, including Hubbard tanks.

Safety

1. The tank should be properly grounded, and the turbine must have a hospital-grade plug. The motor must be securely fastened to the outside of the tank. Whirlpools should also be inspected regularly for any breaks in wiring or insulation because of the high risk of severe electrical injury should any breach of electrical safety occur with this type of equipment.[151]
2. The turbine should not be run without water in the whirlpool because this can damage the turbine motor.
3. The treatment room should be comfortably warm and well-ventilated but not drafty. Ventilation is required to control the humidity of the room and to remove aerosolized additives or infectious agents from the air. A room temperature of 25° to 30° C (77° to 86° F) with a relative humidity of 50% is recommended.[152]

Infection Control

Hydrotherapy tanks, having numerous crevices and being in frequent contact with warm contaminated water under pressure, provide an ideal breeding ground for infectious organisms and are therefore particularly likely purveyors of infection. The primary goal of infection control is to reduce the number of microorganisms in the environment and thus to reduce the potential for infection.[152] For optimal infection control, there must be appropriate cleaning protocols and culturing of all relevant equipment, and protective garments should be worn by the individuals providing hydrotherapy care. Many facilities also add antimicrobials to the water being used for treatment in an attempt to reduce contamination with microorganisms. All of these precautions are intended to reduce the risk of patient or clinician contamination from waterborne bacteria, aerosolized mist, fomites, or blood-borne pathogens.

1. Generally, it is recommended that only clean water, without any antimicrobials, be used in a whirlpool when treating any type of open wound. As discussed previously, the use of antimicrobials in the water when treating open wounds is controversial because although these chemicals offer improved control of infection and cross-contamination, most have been found to be cytotoxic to healing tissue cells even when applied at low concentrations. When infection control is a priority, antimicrobials should be used only at the lowest concentration stated by the manufacturer to be effective for antimicrobial action. Soaps, detergents, or povidone-iodine should not be used for this application because their efficacy is reduced in the presence of blood or tissue debris.[153] Sodium hypochlorite, in the form of household bleach, can provide some control of infection during hydrotherapy; however, its application is limited because it corrodes stainless steel tanks and releases chlorine vapors, which are irritating to many individuals. The chloramine form of chlorine has been recommended for use as an antimicrobial in whirlpool water because it does not corrode stainless steel or release noxious vapors and is not inactivated in the presence of blood or tissue debris.

2. The whirlpool tank and turbines should be properly drained and cleaned after each use. Although there are slightly varying cleaning procedures at different facilities, all protocols are designed to optimize patient and clinician safety and minimize the risk of infection. In general, the cleaning procedure is as follows:

   a. The person cleaning the whirlpool should wear rubber gloves and goggles throughout the cleaning procedure.
   b. Drain the tank. Various drainage configurations or sumps are available to minimize the amount of water left at the bottom of the tank.
   c. Rinse the tank with clean water directly from a hose.
   d. Scrub the inside of the tank with a brush and detergent and then rinse the tank again.
   e. Disinfect the tank. A detergent must be used before the application of the disinfectant because most disinfectants are inactivated in the presence of blood or tissue debris.[153] At present there is no conclusive evidence to support the recommendation of one disinfectant over another; however, one should note that certain disinfectants are more effective against particular microorganisms and that some bromine-based disinfectants can cause allergic dermatitis.[154] It is also generally recommended that disinfecting agents be changed occasionally to reduce the risk of promoting the development of resistant strains. If the whirlpool was used only to treat areas with intact skin, then low-level disinfection of the whirlpool, using 70% to 90% ethyl or isopropyl alcohol, 100 parts per million (ppm) sodium hypochlorite (the active ingredient of household bleach), a phenolic germicidal detergent solution, or a quaternary ammonium germicidal solution, is sufficient. However, if areas where the skin was not intact have been treated, intermediate-level disinfection, using 70% to 90% ethyl or isopropyl alcohol, a phenolic germicidal detergent solution, or an iodophor germicidal detergent solution, has been recommended.[155] Chlorine-based products should not be used to clean stainless steel tanks because, with repeated use, these products corrode the tank surface. To apply the disinfectant, fill the tank with hot water, add the appropriate amount of disinfecting agent, and expose all the inside surfaces of the tank to the solution for 10 minutes.
   f. Clean and disinfect the turbine by running it for 5 minutes in a bucket with a detergent and then for 10 minutes in a bucket with disinfectant solution.

g. Drain the tank.

h. Rinse the tank with clean water.

i. Dry the tank thoroughly with clean towels.

j. Wipe all tank stretchers, hoist cables, and seats with disinfectant after each use.

3. Culture samples should be obtained periodically from the tank, the turbine, the tank drains, and the water supply in accordance with facility and governmental guidelines.[98]

SAFETY PRECAUTIONS AND INFECTION CONTROL FOR EXERCISE POOLS

Safety

Personnel Training. Individuals responsible for maintaining and cleaning an exercise pool must be trained in the use and hazards of the disinfecting and pesticide chemicals used. They should also be provided with the necessary protective clothing for handling these substances.

Staff working with individuals in the pool should have lifesaving and rescue training and knowledge of personal water safety techniques. At a minimum, they should be certified to perform cardiopulmonary resuscitation (CPR) and to provide advanced first aid. Ideally, a certified lifeguard should be present whenever anyone is in the pool. Staff should also be trained in emergency evacuation procedures and should know the emergency action plan.

Safety In and Around the Pool. To ensure safety around an exercise pool and to minimize the risk of a patient slipping and falling, the area surrounding the pool should have nonslip surfaces. Pool regulations, the water depth, emergency procedures, and phone numbers should all be clearly posted in the pool area. Means of entering the pool should be appropriate for patients' ambulatory ability and may include stairs, ramps, ladders, or lifts for nonambulatory or impaired patients. For safety in the pool, the depth of the water should be clearly marked at intervals around the pool edge, and there should be hand grip bars all the way around the edge of the pool.

The pool should be evacuated during power outages and floods, and outdoor pools should not be used during electrical storms. Emergency equipment should be kept near the pool at all times, and all such equipment should be inspected regularly. Emergency equipment should include a shepherd's crook, a life ring, a rescue tube, resuscitation equipment, a spine board, a blanket, and scissors. A first aid kit should also be available.

All chemicals for use in the pool should be kept in their original containers, off the floor, and in a locked cabinet. Material Safety Data Sheets for all chemicals must be maintained and filed to be in compliance with Occupational Safety and Health Administration (OSHA) and Environmental Protection Agency (EPA) regulations. Electrical shocks can be avoided by keeping electrical equipment, such as hair dryers, electrotherapy devices, and heaters, out of the wet environment of the pool and pool side.

Infection Control

Because water is not drained from an exercise pool between uses, the pool water must be filtered and treated with chemical additives at all times to prevent infection transmission. Coliform bacteria, *Giardia lamblia*, *Pseudomonas aeruginosa*, and various types of staphylococcal bacteria, which can cause intestinal, skin, or ear infections in exposed individuals, are commonly found in water, and the risk of excessive bacterial growth is elevated if the water is warm. Airborne endotoxins around a pool may also cause respiratory problems in susceptible individuals.

Adequate infection control of a pool can be achieved with continuous filtering and chemical disinfection of the pool water with chlorine or bromine. The pH and chlorine or bromine levels of the pool water should be tested at the beginning of each day and at least at two additional times during the day. The total alkalinity and calcium hardness of the water should also be checked twice a month. Chemical testing kits designed for this application indicate the safe levels for these tests. To minimize the risk of high bacterial levels in a pool, it is also essential that, as previously detailed in the section on contraindications, patients with conditions that may be a source of infection not be allowed to use an exercise pool that would be reused by themselves or by others.

DOCUMENTATION

Documentation of hydrotherapy should include the following:

- Type of hydrotherapy used
- Patient's position and/or activities
- Water temperature
- Duration of treatment
- Outcome of or response to treatment
- Fluid pressure, if applicable
- Water additives, if applicable

Documentation is typically written in the SOAP (Subjective, Objective, Assessment, Plan) note format. The following examples only summarize the modality component of treatment and are not intended to represent a comprehensive plan of care.

EXAMPLES

When applying a warm whirlpool (WP) to the right (R) ankle to promote increased motion, document the following:

S: Pt reports R ankle stiffness and difficulty with walking.

O: Intervention: Warm WP, 36° C, R ankle, 15 min. Pt performed AROM during immersion.

Posttreatment: PROM DF increased from −10 to −5 degrees, increased duration of heel strike during gait.

A: Pt tolerated WP without side effects

P: Continue WP as above, followed by gait training and therapeutic exercise.

When applying pulsatile irrigation to a sacral pressure ulcer, document the following:

S: Pt oriented to name but not date or place.

O: Intervention: Pulsed lavage, 1000 cc warm saline, pressure 25% of max to sacral pressure ulcer. Pt left side lying on gurney.

Posttreatment: Area of wound necrosis decreased from 50% to 20% since last week.

A: Pt appeared to tolerate irrigation well, with wound improvement.

P: Decrease treatment frequency of pulsed lavage from 2 × per day to 1 × per day.

When using pool exercise (ex) to increase the fitness of a patient with exercise-induced asthma and obesity, document the following:

S: Pt reports ambulation continues to be limited by asthma.

O: Intervention: Pool ex, pool at 30° C, forward and backward walking across pool, 20 min at slow pace with 1 min rest at each end of the pool.

Posttreatment: Functional ambulation tolerance increased from 30 min to 1 hr over the last month.

A: Pt tolerated ex without onset of asthma.

P: Continue pool ex program as above, increasing time from 20-25 min next session.

CLINICAL CASE STUDIES

The following case studies summarize the concepts of hydrotherapy discussed in this chapter. Based on the scenarios presented, an evaluation of the clinical findings and goals of treatment are proposed. These are followed by a discussion of the factors to be considered in the selection of hydrotherapy as an intervention and guidelines for the selection of the appropriate hydrotherapy device and application technique.

CASE STUDY 9-1

Bilateral Knee Pain
Examination
History

FR is a 45-year-old woman with osteoarthritis of both knees. She reports bilateral knee pain that is worse on the right (6/10) than on the left (4/10) and that worsens with standing or walking for more than 5 minutes. She uses a cane in her left hand to control her knee pain and to assist with balance during community and most household ambulation. She is able to walk approximately one-half block on a flat, level surface with her cane. She does not tolerate antiinflammatory medications because of gastric side effects. The pain in her right knee started about 5 years ago, without any known initiating event, and has gradually worsened since that time. The pain in her left knee started about 2 years ago, also without any known initiating event. She has had no prior treatment for her knee pain. As the patient's pain has worsened over the years, she has limited her activities, spending most of her time in her home or at work, where she is usually sitting. She cannot enjoy walks with friends and has not gone to church in 6 months because her knees hurt so much after walking from the parking lot to her seat. She used to attend church once or twice a week.

Tests and Measures

The patient is obese (265 lb), has bilateral genu valgum, bilateral foot pronation, and weakness and shortness of the quadriceps and hamstring muscles. Knee passive ROM is −5 degrees extension to 95 degrees flexion on the right and 0 degrees extension to 120 degrees flexion on the left. FR uses a step-to gait for ascending and descending stairs.

What kind of hydrotherapy is appropriate for this patient and why? What are some reasonable short- and long-term goals for her?

Evaluation, Diagnosis, Prognosis, and Goals
Evaluation and Goals

ICF Level	Current Status	Goals
Body structure and function	Bilateral knee pain Weak quadriceps and hamstrings Reduced knee PROM Obesity	Minimal knee pain (<2/10 bilaterally) Normal quadriceps and hamstring strength 0° extension to 120° flexion PROM of both knees 10 lb weight loss and actively involved in a home exercise program to lose further weight and improve fitness
Activity	Limited ability to stand (approx 5 minutes) and walk (approx ½ block)	Short-term (3 weeks): Increase standing tolerance to 20 minutes Increase walking tolerance to two blocks Discontinue use of a cane Long-term (3 months): Involved in a home exercise program to lose further weight and improve fitness
Participation	Not attending church because of knee pain	Able to attend church once a week without pain

CLINICAL CASE STUDIES—*cont'd*

Diagnosis

Preferred Practice Pattern 4D: Impaired joint mobility, motor function, muscle performance, and ROM associated with connective tissue dysfunction.

Prognosis/Plan of Care

Although many forms of exercise could be used to increase this patient's lower extremity strength and knee ROM, the best option is exercise with limited weight bearing. This will help avoid aggravation of the patient's symptoms, given her body weight and the reported degeneration of her knee joints. Non–weight-bearing exercises, such as straight leg raises, or reduced weight-bearing exercises, such as stationary cycling, could be used. However, water-based exercises are recommended because they have a number of advantages over non–weight-bearing, land-based exercises. These advantages include (1) allowing the patient to perform normal functional activities, such as walking without an assistive device, to train the muscles and develop the balance skills required for normal function; (2) providing some pain control during the exercise; (3) allowing fine grading of joint loading by varying the depth of the water; and (4) allowing fine grading of resistance by varying the speed of patient movement. Should the patient have lower extremity edema, as is common in inactive obese individuals, the hydrostatic pressure provided by immersion may also reduce edema.

From the examination described, it does not appear that hydrotherapy would be contraindicated for this patient. However, before initiating hydrotherapy, the clinician should ascertain that the patient is not afraid of being in water and that she does not have any infections that may be spread by water or any other medical conditions that would contraindicate the use of this form of treatment.

Intervention

Pool exercise is the only form of hydrotherapy that would address all of the proposed goals of intervention for this patient. Although soaking in a warm whirlpool may be comfortable and may temporarily decrease this patient's pain, and lower extremity active exercise in an extremity whirlpool may promote ROM to some degree, neither of these forms of hydrotherapy treatment is likely to provide sufficient resistance to motion to increase the patient's lower extremity strength and thus her functional standing and ambulation tolerance. For this patient's treatment the pool water should be kept slightly warmer than generally used for recreation, at 34° to 36° °C (93° to 95° F), to allow her to exercise comfortably at the slow pace to which she will probably be limited. A pool exercise program may include forward and backward walking, either holding or not holding on to the hand rail, as necessary for balance, partial squats, kicking, and a variety of other closed- and open-chain lower extremity activities. This water-based exercise program is likely to be most effective if provided in conjunction with land-based exer-

cises, active and passive stretching, joint mobilization, and a home exercise program.

Documentation

S: Pt reports ambulation and standing limited by knee pain.

O: Pretreatment: Standing and ambulation tolerance 5 minutes. Knee passive ROM –5 degrees extension to 95 degrees flexion on right and 0 degrees extension to 120 degrees flexion on left.

Intervention: Pool ex, pool at 30° C, forward and backward walking across pool, 15 minutes at slow pace with 1 minute rest at each end of the pool, 10 partial squats.

Posttreatment (after 2 weeks): Standing and ambulation tolerance 15 minutes. Knee ROM –5 degrees extension to 110 degrees flexion on right and –5 degrees extension to 130 degrees flexion on left.

A: Tolerated exercise without pain.

P: Continue pool ex program as above, increasing time to 20 minutes next session. Pt taught land-based exercises, active and passive stretching, and joint mobilization to incorporate into home routine. Next sessions to include home exercise plans.

CASE STUDY 9-2

Pressure Ulcers

Examination

History

ST is an 85-year-old woman with stage IV pressure ulcers near both femoral greater trochanters and a stage II pressure ulcer over her sacrum. The patient is bedridden, oriented to name and place, and not combative. She has a history of two strokes, one 3 years ago and the other 8 years ago, resulting first in right and then in left hemiplegia, with hypertonicity that is moderately severe and has not changed significantly in the last 2 years. She also has hypertension controlled by medication that generally keeps her blood pressure at or below 145/100. The pressure ulcers place her at risk for sepsis and limit safe positioning as sidelying on either side should be avoided in the presence of pressure ulcers over both greater trochanters.

Tests and Measures

The ulcer near the right greater trochanter is approximately 8 cm long and 8 cm wide and has no undermining. The ulcer near the left greater trochanter is approximately 9 cm long and 10 cm wide and has approximately 1 cm of undermining along the proximal border. Both of these wounds have yellow necrotic tissue and a heavy, thick exudate; no granulation tissue is visible. The ulcer over the sacrum is approximately 5 cm by 10 cm and has no necrotic tissue. No tunnels or sinus tracts are apparent in any of these wounds.

Hydrotherapy should be used for which of this patient's wounds? What type of hydrotherapy should be used and why? What precaution should be taken when using warm water for this patient?

Continued

Evaluation, Diagnosis, Prognosis, and Goals
Evaluation and Goals

ICF Level	Current Status	Goals
Body structure and function	Impaired soft tissue integrity Abnormal muscle tone Reduced functional mobility At risk for developing further pressure ulcers and systemic infection	Soften and remove necrotic tissue in trochanteric wounds Facilitate wound closure Reduce risk of infection and further tissue breakdown Improve circulation to wound areas
Activity	Unsafe to lie on either side	Safe lying in any position
Participation	Dependent	Dependent—no change expected

Diagnosis

Preferred Practice Pattern 7E: Impaired integumentary integrity associated with skin involvement extending into fascia, muscle, or bone and scar formation.

Prognosis/Plan of Care

Hydrotherapy is indicated for this patient because this intervention can soften and debride necrotic tissue, cleanse wound debris, and improve circulation by immersion in warm water. Removing necrotic tissue from a wound bed and improving the local circulation can accelerate wound healing and closure. For the best outcome, other interventions, such as pressure relief, electrical stimulation, exercise, appropriate wound dressings, and possibly other forms of debridement should be applied in conjunction with hydrotherapy.

The examination of this patient does not indicate that hydrotherapy would be contraindicated; however, the infection risk and safety concerns limit the types of hydrotherapy that are appropriate. Also, hydrotherapy is indicated only for the trochanteric wounds, where necrotic tissue is present, not for the sacral wound, where no necrotic tissue is apparent. Neither whirlpool immersion nor nonimmersion irrigation would be contraindicated, although care should be taken to ascertain that the patient can feel and report heat in the areas to be treated before warm or hot water is used. Since it is most likely that this patient has impaired sensation and circulation in the areas of the pressure ulcers, the water temperature should be no higher than 35.5° C (96° F).

Intervention

Either immersion or nonimmersion techniques could be used to apply hydrotherapy to this patient. Immersion techniques have the advantages of allowing all the wounds to receive hydrotherapy at the same time and providing potential circulatory benefits because of heat

transfer if warm water is used and hydrostatic pressure if the extremities are sufficiently immersed; however, because immersion techniques increase the risk of maceration of the intact tissue around the wounds, have a high infection risk, do not allow control of the water pressure at the wound bed, cannot restrict the hydrotherapy treatment to the trochanteric wounds, and require monitoring of vital signs during treatment, a nonimmersion technique would be more appropriate. A nonimmersion form of hydrotherapy would also be easier, quicker, and less costly to apply, although it would not have the circulatory benefits associated with immersion.

Although nonimmersion hydrotherapy can be provided with either a mechanical or electrical device, the use of an electric pulsatile irrigation device is recommended for the treatment of this patient because this will allow close control of fluid pressure and removal of contaminated fluid from the wound bed during treatment. Antimicrobials may be added to the fluid for either form of hydrotherapy. It is recommended that treatment with pulsed lavage be provided once each day until the wound bed is fully granulated. Hydrotherapy of these wounds should be discontinued if bleeding occurs, if the amount of necrotic tissue does not decrease, or if the amount of granulation does not increase within 1 week. If sharp debridement of necrotic tissue is indicated, it is recommended that this be performed after the hydrotherapy, when the necrotic tissue is likely to be softer and easier to remove.

Documentation

S: *Bedbound pt oriented to person and place.*

O: Pretreatment: *R greater trochanter ulcer 8 cm diameter, no undermining. L greater trochanter ulcer 9 cm × 10 cm with 1 cm of proximal border undermining. Both wounds have yellow necrotic tissue, thick exudate with no granulation tissue. Sacral ulcer 5 cm × 10 cm with no necrotic tissue.*

Intervention: *Pulsed lavage, 1000 cc warm saline, pressure 25% of max to R and L trochanteric pressure ulcers. Pt on gurney on L side for R ulcer treatment and on R side for L ulcer treatment.*

Posttreatment: *Both ulcers free of necrotic debris and exudate.*

A: *Pt tolerated irrigation without discomfort or bleeding.*

P: *Continue as above once daily until granulation tissue appears. Discuss optimization of pressure distribution and nutrition with team.*

CASE STUDY 9-3

Colles' Fracture
Examination
History

FS is a 65-year-old woman who sustained a closed Colles' fracture of her right arm 6 weeks ago. The fracture was initially treated with a closed reduction and cast fixa-

CLINICAL CASE STUDIES—*cont'd*

tion. This cast was removed 3 days ago, when radiographic reports indicated callus formation and good alignment of the fracture site. FS has been referred to therapy with an order to evaluate and treat. She has not received any prior rehabilitation treatment for this injury. FS reports severe pain, stiffness, and swelling of her right wrist and hand. She is wearing a wrist splint and is not using her right hand for any functional activities at this time because she is afraid that any activity may cause further damage. FS is retired and lives alone. She is unable to drive because of the dysfunctions of her right hand and wrist.

Tests and Measures

The examination is significant for decreased active and passive ROM of the right wrist. Active wrist flexion is 30 degrees on the right and 80 degrees on the left. Wrist extension is 25 degrees on the right and 70 degrees on the left. Wrist ulnar deviation is 10 degrees on the right and 30 degrees on the left, and wrist radial deviation is 0 degrees on the right and 25 degrees on the left. There is also moderate nonpitting edema of the right hand, and the skin of the right hand and wrist appears shiny. FS's functional grip on the right is limited by muscle weakness and restricted joint ROM. The patient is wearing a splint and is holding her hand across her abdomen. She reports severe pain when her hand is touched, even lightly. All other measures, including shoulder, elbow, and neck ROM, upper extremity sensation, and left upper extremity strength, are within normal limits for this patient's age and gender.

What type of hydrotherapy is best for this patient? What type of hydrotherapy would not be recommended?

Evaluation, Diagnosis, Prognosis, and Goals
Evaluation and Goals

ICF Level	Current Status	Goals
Body structure and function	R hand and wrist: Pain Weakness Hypersensitivity Restricted ROM Edema*	Control pt's pain, hypersensitivity, and fear Increase R wrist ROM by 20% to 50% in all planes in 2-4 weeks
Activity	Avoiding all use of R hand and wrist	Short-term: Hold hand in normal position with normal swing during gait Long-term: Regain use of R hand for functional activities
Participation	Unable to drive	Return to driving

*Although this patient's signs and symptoms are consistent with disuse after a fracture and immobilization, they also indicate that she has stage I reflex sympathetic dystrophy.

Diagnosis

Preferred Practice Pattern 4G: Impaired joint mobility, muscle performance, and ROM associated with fracture.

Prognosis/Plan of Care

Immersion hydrotherapy, using either a low level of water agitation in a neutral warmth whirlpool or a contrast bath with warm and cool water of similar temperatures, may reduce the hypersensitivity and hyperalgesia of this patient's hand while providing a suitable environment for active exercise to increase the ROM and functional use of her hand. The hydrostatic pressure provided by water immersion and the alternating vasoconstriction and vasodilation produced by a contrast bath may also help reduce edema in this extremity. Warm or hot water whirlpool use is not recommended because the resulting increase in tissue temperature, in conjunction with the dependent position of the extremity, is likely to aggravate the edema already present in this patient's hand. Although the evaluation of this patient does not indicate any contraindication for the use of hydrotherapy and because hot water may be used for the contrast bath during the later stages of desensitization, her ability to sense temperature should be assessed before initiating treatment with a contrast bath.

Intervention

Because immersion in water is required to provide the heat transfer, resistance, and hydrostatic pressure that will produce the therapeutic benefits of hydrotherapy for this patient, only immersion hydrotherapy techniques would be appropriate for her treatment. As noted, a contrast bath is likely to be most effective because it may assist with desensitization and edema reduction while providing a comfortable environment for active exercise. It is recommended that contrast bath treatments be provided both in the clinic and by the patient as part of her home program. It is also recommended that the water temperature of the two baths initially be similar and as the patient progresses, that the temperature difference gradually be increased.

Documentation

S: Pt reports R hand and wrist pain after a treated fracture.

O: Pretreatment: R wrist flexion 30 degrees, extension 25 degrees, ulnar deviation 10 degrees, radial deviation 0 degrees. L wrist flexion 80 degrees, extension 70 degrees, ulnar deviation 30 degrees, radial deviation 25 degrees. Restricted R grip. Nonpitting edema R hand.

Intervention: Contrast bath, 38° C (100° F) and 18° C (64° F). Warm × 3 min, then cold × 1 min. Sequence repeated 5 times.

Posttreatment: Decreased R hand edema, R wrist ROM improved with R wrist flexion 35 degrees, extension 30 degrees, ulnar deviation 20 degrees, radial deviation 5 degrees.

A: Pt tolerated contrast bath without pain or edema and gained increased ROM.

P: Continue contrast baths at home, gradually increasing the temperature difference. Pt given hand exercises to do at home.

CHAPTER REVIEW

1. Hydrotherapy is the application of water for therapeutic purposes. The unique physical properties of water, including its high specific heat and thermal conductivity, buoyancy, resistance, and hydrostatic pressure, all contribute to its therapeutic efficacy.

2. Water can be used therapeutically via immersion or nonimmersion techniques. Immersion in water can produce cardiovascular, respiratory, musculoskeletal, renal, and psychological changes. The clinical benefits of immersion hydrotherapy include controlling pain, modifying musculoskeletal demands, and reducing edema. Immersion hydrotherapy can be applied using a whirlpool, Hubbard tank, contrast bath, or exercise pool.

3. Nonimmersion hydrotherapy is used for cleansing wounds to reduce bacterial load and remove debris during wound care. Nonimmersion hydrotherapy can be applied with a shower or a specialized irrigation device. Because immersion can be associated with increased risks of infection or drowning and can be time-consuming to apply, nonimmersion hydrotherapy techniques are generally recommended when only the cleansing effects of hydrotherapy are desired.

4. Negative pressure wound therapy is often used in conjunction with nonimmersion hydrotherapy in the treatment of wounds. This therapy involves the application of vacuum suction to the wound and can further promote wound healing.

5. Contraindications and precautions for immersion hydrotherapy include wound maceration, bleeding, impaired cognition or thermal sensation, infection, cardiac instability, and pregnancy. Contraindications and precautions for nonimmersion hydrotherapy and negative pressure wound therapy contraindications include wound maceration, exposed vessels, malignancy in the wound bed, and bleeding.

6. To optimize the outcome of hydrotherapy treatments, the treatment plan and equipment selection should take into account the risks and benefits associated with the various means of applying hydrotherapy, and all appropriate precautions should be taken to provide a safe environment for such treatment.

7. The reader is referred to the Evolve web site for further exercises and links to resources and references.

ADDITIONAL RESOURCES evolve

Web Sites

AquaJogger: In addition to selling products for water exercise, this web site has information on how to exercise in a pool, as well as links to several other water exercise resources. www.aquajogger.com

Aquatic Physical Therapy Section of the American Physical Therapy Association (APTA): This section of the APTA web site answers common questions about aquatic physical therapy and has some links to articles and guidelines. www.aquaticpt.org

BlueSky Medical Group: This web site includes information on the company's negative pressure wound therapy device, including instructions for use. www.blueskymedical.com

Davol: Davol sells a pulsed lavage system among other products. The web site has limited information and a few case studies. www.davol.com

DeRoyal: DeRoyal has a pulsed lavage system. The web site includes their pulsed lavage product insert, with instructions for the use of their product. www.deroyal.com

Kinetic Concepts Inc: Web site includes information on the company's negative pressure wound therapy device and an excellent list of abstracts from research on negative pressure wound therapy. There are also detailed instructions for the use of their V.A.C. system, including parameters based on wound type and type of foam used. www.kci1.com

Zimmer: Zimmer sells orthopedic products and a pulsed lavage system. The web site is unwieldy, but medical professionals can register and obtain access to product brochures. www.zimmer.com

GLOSSARY evolve

General Terms

Buoyancy: An upward force on an object immersed in a fluid that is equal to the weight of the fluid it displaces, enabling it to float or to appear lighter.

Closed-chain exercises: Exercises where the distal extremity is stationary on a stable support. When closed-chain exercises are performed in a pool, the distal extremity is supported on the bottom or side of the pool.

Contrast baths: Alternating immersion in hot and cold water.

Edema: Swelling that results from accumulation of fluid in the interstitial space.

Hubbard tank: A large, stainless steel whirlpool designed for immersion of the entire body that is used primarily for the treatment of patients with extensive burn wounds.

Hydrostatic pressure: The pressure exerted by a fluid on a body immersed in the fluid. Hydrostatic pressure increases with increased depth of immersion.

Hydrotherapy: The therapeutic use of water.

Open-chain exercises: Exercises where the distal extremity is free to move. Open-chain exercises can be performed in a pool if the distal extremity is not touching the side or bottom of the pool.

Pressure: Force per unit area, generally measured in pounds per square inch (psi).

Resistance: A force counter to the direction of movement. The resistance to a body's movement in water is proportional to the relative speed of the body and water's motion and to the frontal areas of the body part(s) in contact with the water.

Specific gravity: The ratio of the density of a material to the density of water.

Specific heat: The amount of energy required to raise the temperature of a given weight of a material by a given number of degrees, usually expressed in $J/g/°C$.

Thermal conductivity: The rate at which a material transfers heat by conduction, usually expressed in $(cal/sec)/(cm^2 \times °C/cm)$.

Viscosity: The thickness or resistance to flow of a liquid, caused by friction between the molecules of the liquid. A more viscous liquid is thick and pours slowly. Water, a liquid with a relatively low viscosity, pours quickly and easily.

Wound-Related Terms

Colonization: The establishment and growth of microorganisms in a wound.

Debridement: Removal of foreign material or dead, damaged, or infected tissue from a wound to expose healthy tissue.

Eschar: Dead tissue or a scab that forms on a wound.

Exudate: Wound fluid composed of serum, fibrin, and white blood cells.

Granulation tissue: Tissue composed of new blood vessels, connective tissue, fibroblasts, and inflammatory cells that fills an open wound when it starts to heal; typically appears deep pink or red with an irregular, berrylike surface.

Infection: Establishment and growth of microorganisms causing disease. With infection, there are more microorganisms or more pathological microorganisms than with colonization.

Maceration: Softening of tissues from excessive soaking in liquid.

Necrotic tissue: Dead tissue.

Negative pressure wound therapy: The application of continuous or intermittent subatmospheric-pressure vacuum suction to an open wound to promote wound healing; also known as vacuum-assisted wound closure.

Nosocomial infection: Infection acquired in a hospital.

Pulsed lavage: Nonimmersion pulsatile irrigation, often used to clean and debride wounds and thereby promote wound healing.

Purulence: Pus; opaque wound fluid that is thicker than exudate and contains white blood cells, tissue debris, and microorganisms.

Slough: Necrotic tissue in the process of separating from viable, living tissue.

REFERENCES *evolve*

1. Bettmann OL: City life: beware of contagion. In Bettmann OL, Hench PC, eds: *A pictorial history of medicine*, Springfield, IL, 1956, Charles C Thomas.
2. Shepard CH: Insanity and the Turkish bath, *JAMA* 34:604-606, 1900.
3. Kenney E, Ostenso M: *And they shall walk*, New York, 1943, Dodd Mead and Co.
4. Roberts P: Hydrotherapy: its history, theory and practice, *Occup Health Safe* 33(5):235-244, 1982.
5. Becker BE: The biological aspects of hydrotherapy, *J Back Musculoskel Rehabil* 4(4):255-264, 1994.
6. Robson MC, Heggers JP: Bacterial quantification of open wounds, *Mil Med* 134:19-24, 1969.
7. Winter GD: Formation of scab and the rate of epithelialization in superficial wounds of the domestic pig, *Nature* 193:293-294, 1962.
8. Trengove NJ, Stacey MC, McGechie DF, et al: Qualitative bacteriology and leg ulcer healing, *J Wound Care* 5(6):277-280, 1996 Jun.
9. Wade J: Sports splash, *Rehab Mgmt* 10(4):64-70, 1997.
10. Gwinup G: Weight loss without dietary restriction: efficacy of different forms of aerobic exercise, *Am J Sport Med* 15:275-279, 1987.
11. Kieres J, Plowman S: Effect of swimming and land exercises on body composition of college students, *J Sport Med Phys Fitness* 31:192-193, 1991.
12. Ruoti RG, Troup JT, Berger RA: The effects of nonswimming water exercises on older adults, *J Orthop Sports Phys Ther* 19(3):140-145, 1994.
13. Gehlsen GM, Grigsby S, Winant D: The effects of an aquatic fitness program on the muscular strength and endurance of patients with multiple sclerosis, *Phys Ther* 64(5):653-657, 1984.
14. Henker L, Provast-Craig M, Sestili P, et al: Water running and the maintenance of maximum oxygen consumption and leg strength in runners, *Med Sci Sport Exerc* 24:3-5, 1991.
15. Gusi N, Tomas-Carus P, Hakkinen A, et al: Exercise in waist-high warm water decreases pain and improves health-related quality of life and strength in the lower extremities in women with fibromyalgia, *Arthritis Rheum* 55(1):66-73, 2006.
16. Balldin UI, Lundgren CEG, Lundvall J, et al: Changes in the elimination of 133 Xenon from the anterior tibial muscle in man induced by immersion in water and by shifts in body position, *Aerospace Med* 42(5):489-493, 1971.
17. Arborelius M, Balldin UI, Lilja B, et al: Hemodynamic changes in man during immersion with the head above water, *Aerospace Med* 43(3):593-599, 1972.
18. Risch WD, Koubenec HJ, Beckmann U, et al: The effect of graded immersion on heart volume, central venous pressure, pulmonary blood distribution and heart rate in man, *Pfleugers Arch* 374:115-118, 1978.
19. Haffor AA, Mohler JG, Harrison AAC: Effects of water immersion on cardiac output of lean and fat male subjects at rest and during exercise, *Aviation Space Environ Med* 62:123-127, 1991.
20. McMurray RG, Katz VL, Berry MJ, et al: Cardiovascular responses of pregnant women during aerobic exercise in water: a longitudinal study, *Int J Sports Med* 9(6): 443-447, 1988.
21. Katz VL, McMurray R, Goodwin WE, et al: Nonweight-bearing exercise during pregnancy on land and during immersion; a comparative study, *Am J Perinatol* 7(3):281-284, 1990.
22. Svendenhag J, Serger J: Running on land and in water: comparative exercise physiology, *Med Sci Sports Exerc* 24:1155-1160, 1992.
23. Butts NK, Tucker M, Smith R: Maximal responses to treadmill and deep water running in high school female cross country runners, *Res Q Exer Sports* 62:236-239, 1991.
24. Butts NK, Tucker M, Greening C: Physiologic responses to maximal treadmill and deep water running in men and women, *Am J Sports Med* 19:612-614, 1991.
25. Michaud T, Brennan D, Wilder R, et al: Aquarun training and changes in treadmill running maximal oxygen consumption, *Med Sci Sports Exerc* 24:5-7, 1991.
26. Hamer TW, Morton AR: Water-running: training effects and specificity of aerobic, anaerobic and muscular parameters following an eight week interval training programme, *Aust J Sci Med Sport* 22(1):13-22, 1990.
27. Cider A, Svealv BG, Tang MS, et al: Immersion in warm water induces improvement in cardiac function in patients with chronic heart failure, *Eur J Heart Fail* 8(3):308-313, 2006.
28. Cider A, Sunnerhagen KS, Schaufelberger M, et al: Cardiorespiratory effects of warm water immersion in elderly patients with chronic heart failure, *Clin Physiol Funct Imaging* 25(6):313-7, 2005.
29. Cider A, Schaufelberger M, Sunnerhagen KS, et al: Hydrotherapy—a new approach to improve function in the older patient with chronic heart failure, *Eur J Heart Fail* 5(4):527-535, 2003.
30. Michalsen A, Ludtke R, Buhring M, et al: Thermal hydrotherapy improves quality of life and hemodynamic function in patients with chronic heart failure, *Am Heart J* 146(4):728-733, 2003.
31. Abramson D, Brunnet C, Bell Y, et al: Changes in blood flow, oxygen uptake, and tissue temperatures produced by a topical application of wet heat, *Arch Phys Med Rehabil* 42:305-318, 1961.

32. Gleim GW, Nicholas JA: Metabolic costs and heart rate responses to treadmill walking in water at different depths and temperatures, *Am J Sports Med* 17(2):248-252, 1989.

33. Evans BW, Cureton KJ, Purvis JW: Metabolic and circulatory responses to walking and jogging in water, *Res Q* 49(4):442-449, 1978.

34. Hong SK, Cerretelli P, Cruz JC, et al: Mechanics of respiration during submersion in water, *J Appl Physiol* 27(4):535-536, 1969.

35. Perk J, Perk L, Boden C: Adaptation of COPD patients to physical training on land and in water, *Eur Respir J* 9(2):248-252, 1996.

36. Agostoni E, Gurtner G, Torri G, et al: Respiratory mechanics during submersion and negative pressure breathing, *J Appl Physiol* 21(1):251-258, 1966.

37. Bar-Yishay E, Gur I, Inbar O, et al: Differences between swimming and running as stimuli for exercise-induced asthma, *Eur J Appl Physiol* 48:387-397, 1982.

38. Fitch KD, Morton AR: Specificity of exercise in exercise-induced asthma, *Br Med J* 4:577-581, 1971.

39. Bar-Or O, Inbar I: Swimming and asthma benefits and deleterious effects, *Sports Med* 14:397-405, 1992.

40. Epstein M: Cardiovascular and renal effects of head out water immersion in man, *Circ Res* 39(5):620-628, 1976.

41. Katz VL, McMurray R, Berry MJ, et al: Renal responses to immersion and exercise in pregnancy, *Am J Perinatol* 7(2):118-121, 1990.

42. Epstein M, Pins DS, Silvers W, et al: Failure of water immersion to influence parathyroid hormone secretion and renal phosphate handling in normal man, *J Lab Clin Med* 87(2):218-226, 1976.

43. Pechter U, Ots M, Mesikepp S, et al: Beneficial effects of water-based exercise in patients with chronic kidney disease, *Int J Rehabil Res* 26(2):153-156, 2003 Jun.

44. Braslow JT: Punishment or therapy: patients, doctors, and somatic remedies in the early twentieth century, *Psych Clin North Am* 17(3):493-513, 1994.

45. Benfield RD, Herman J, Katz VL, et al: Hydrotherapy in labor, *Res Nurs Health* 24(1):57-67, 2001.

46. Holmes G: Hydrotherapy as a means of rehabilitation, *Br J Phys Med* 5:93-95, 1942.

47. Bates A, Hanson N: *Aquatic therapy: a comprehensive approach to use of aquatic exercise in treatment of orthopaedic injuries*, Westbank, BC, Canada, 1992, Swystun & Swystun.

48. Hoyrup G, Kjorvel L: Comparison of whirlpool and wax treatments for hand therapy, *Physiother Can* 38:79-82, 1986.

49. Templeton MS, Booth DL, O'Kelly WD: Effects of aquatic therapy on joint flexibility and functional ability in subjects with rheumatic disease, *J Orthop Sport Phys Ther* 23(6):376-381, 1996.

50. Genuario SE, Vegso JJ: The use of a swimming pool in rehabilitation and reconditioning of athletic injuries, *Contemp Orthop* 4:381-387, 1990.

51. Cole AJ, Eagleston RE, Moschetti M, et al: Spine rehabilitation aquatic rehabilitation strategies, *J Back Musculoskel Rehabil* 4(4):273-286, 1994.

52. Triggs M: Orthopedic aquatic therapy, *Clin Mgmt* 11:30-31, 1991.

53. Konlian C: Aquatic therapy: making a wave in the treatment of low back injuries, *Orthop Nurs* 18(1):11-18, 1999.

54. Foley A, Halbert J, Hewitt T, et al: Does hydrotherapy improve strength and physical function in patients with osteoarthritis—a randomised controlled trial comparing a gym based and a hydrotherapy based strengthening programme, *Ann Rheum Dis* 62(12):1162-1167, 2003.

55. Wyatt FB, Milam S, Manske RC, et al: The effects of aquatic and traditional exercise programs on persons with knee osteoarthritis, *J Strength Cond Res* 15:337-340, 2001.

56. Suomi R, Collier D: Effects of arthritis exercise programs on functional fitness and perceived activities of daily living measures in older adults with arthritis, *Arch Phys Med Rehabil* 84(11):1589-1594, 2003.

57. Hinman RS, Heywood SE, Day AR: Aquatic physical therapy for hip and knee osteoarthritis: results of a single-blind randomized controlled trial, *Phys Ther* 87(1):32-43, 2007.

58. Stener-Victorin E, Kruse-Smidje C, Jung K: Comparison between electro-acupuncture and hydrotherapy, both in combination with patient education and patient education alone, on the symptomatic treatment of osteoarthritis of the hip, *Clin J Pain* 20(3):179-185, 2004.

59. Tsukahara N, Toda A, Goto J, et al: Cross-sectional and longitudinal studies on the effect of water exercise in controlling bone loss in Japanese postmenopausal women, *J Nutr Sci Vitaminol Tokyo* 40(1):37-47, 1994.

60. Ay A, Yurtkuran M: Influence of aquatic and weight-bearing exercises on quantitative ultrasound variables in postmenopausal women, *Am J Phys Med Rehabil* 84(1):52-61, 2005.

61. Bravo G, Gauthier P, Roy PM, et al: A weight-bearing, water-based exercise program for osteopenic women: its impact on bone, functional fitness, and well-being, *Arch Phys Med Rehabil* 78(12):1375-1380, 1997.

62. Mannerkorpi K, Nyberg B, Ahlmen M, et al: Pool exercise combined with an education program for patients with fibromyalgia syndrome. A prospective, randomized study, *J Rheumatol* 27:2473-2481, 2000.

63. Assis MR, Silva LE, Alves AM, et al: A randomized controlled trial of deep water running: clinical effectiveness of aquatic exercise to treat fibromyalgia, *Arthritis Rheum* 55(1):57-65, 2006.

64. Vitorino DF, Carvalho LB, Prado GF: Hydrotherapy and conventional physiotherapy improve total sleep time and quality of life of fibromyalgia patients: randomized clinical trial, *Sleep Med* 7(3):293-6, 2006.

65. Mannerkorpi K, Ahlmen M, Ekdahl C: Six- and 24-month follow-up of pool exercise therapy and education for patients with fibromyalgia, *Scand J of Rheumatol* 31(5):306-310, 2002.

66. Hurley R, Turner C: Neurology and aquatic therapy, *Clin Mgmt* 11:26-29, 1991.

67. Johnson CR: Aquatic therapy for an ALS patient, *Am J Occup Ther* 42(2):115-120, 1988.

68. Simmons V, Hansen PD: Effectiveness of water exercise on postural mobility in the well elderly: an experimental study on balance enhancement, *J Gerontol A Biol Sci Med Sci* 51(5):M233-M238, 1996.

69. Kesiktas N, Paker N, Erdogan N, et al: The use of hydrotherapy for the management of spasticity, *Neurorehabil Neur Repair* 18(4):268-273, 2004.

70. Driver S, O'Connor J, Lox C, et al: Evaluation of an aquatics programme on fitness parameters of individuals with a brain injury, *Brain Inj* 18(9):847-859, 2004.

71. Harris SR: Neurodevelopmental treatment approach for teaching swimming to cerebral palsied children, *Phys Ther* 58(8):979-983, 1978.

72. Boyle AM: The Bad Ragaz ring method, *Physiotherapy* 67:265-268, 1981.

73. Eyestone ED, Fellingham G, George J, et al: Effect of water running and cycling on the maximum oxygen consumption and 2 mile run performance, *Am J Sports Med* 21:41-44, 1993.

74. Wadell K, Sundelin G, Henriksson-Larsen K, et al: High intensity physical group training in water—an effective training modality for patients with COPD, *Respir Med* 98(5):428-438, 2004.

75. McMurray RG, Fieselman CC, Avery KE, et al: Exercise hemodynamics in water and on land in patients with coronary artery disease, *Cardiopulm Rehabil* 8:69-75, 1986.

76. Tei C, Tanaka N: Thermal vasodilation as a treatment of congestive heart failure: a novel approach, *J Cardiol* 21(1):29-30, 1996.

77. Kurabayashi H, Machida I, Yoshida Y: Clinical analysis of breathing exercise during immersion in 38 degrees C water for obstructive and constrictive pulmonary diseases, *J Med* 30(1-2):61-66, 1999.

78. Kurabayashi H, Machida I, Kubota K: Improvement in ejection fraction by hydrotherapy as rehabilitation in patients with chronic pulmonary emphysema, *Physiother Res Int* 3(4):284-291, 1998.

79. Watson WJ, Katz VL, Hackney AC, et al: Fetal response to maximal swimming and cycling exercise during pregnancy, *Obstet Gynecol* 77(3):382-386, 1991.

80. Smith SA, Michel Y: A pilot study on the effects of aquatic exercises on discomforts of pregnancy, *J Obstet Gynecol Neonatal Nurs* 35(3):315-323, 2006.

81. American College of Obstetricians and Gynecologists: *Exercise during pregnancy and postnatal period: ACOG Home Exercise Programs*, Washington, DC, 1985, ACOG.

82. Ward EJ, McIntyre A, van Kessel G, et al: Immediate blood pressure changes and aquatic physiotherapy, *Hyperten Pregnancy* 24(2):93-102, 2005.

83. Huang SW, Veiga R, Sila U, et al: The effect of swimming in asthmatic children participants in a swimming program in the city of Baltimore, *J Asthma* 26:117-121, 1989.

84. Svenonius E, Kautto R, Arborelius M Jr: Improvement after training of children with exercise-induced asthma, *Acta Paediatr Scand* 72:23-30, 1983.

85. Tsourlou T, Benik A, Dipla K, et al: The effects of a twenty-four-week aquatic training program on muscular strength performance in healthy elderly women, *J Strength Cond Res* 20(4):811-818, 2006 Nov.

86. Devereux K, Robertson D, Briffa NK: Effects of a water-based program on women 65 years and over: a randomised controlled trial, *Austral J Physiother* 51(2):102-108, 2005.

87. Takeshima N, Rogers ME, Watanabe E, et al: Water-based exercise improves health-related aspects of fitness in older women, *Med Sci Sports Exerc* 34(3):544-551, 2002.

88. Tovin BJ, Wolf SL, Greenfield BH, et al: Comparison of the effects of exercise in water and on land on the rehabilitation of patients with intraarticular anterior cruciate ligament reconstructions, *Phys Ther* 74(8):710-719, 1994.

89. Magnes J, Garret T, Erickson D: Swelling of the upper extremity during whirlpool baths, *Arch Phys Med Rehabil* 51:297-299, 1970.

90. Feedar JA, Kloth LC: Conservative management of chronic wounds. In Kloth LC, McCulloch JM, Feedar JA, eds: *Wound healing: alternatives in management*, Philadelphia, 1990, FA Davis.

91. Neiderhuber S, Stribley R, Koepke G: Reduction in skin bacterial load with the use of therapeutic whirlpool, *Phys Ther* 55(5):482-486, 1975.

92. Walter PH: Burn wound management, *AACN Clin Issues Crit Care Nurs* 4(2):378-387, 1993.

93. Burke DT, Ho CH, Saucier MA, et al: Effects of hydrotherapy on pressure ulcer healing, *Am J Phys Med Rehabil* 77(5):394-398, 1998.

94. McCulloch J: Physical modalities in wound management: ultrasound, vasopneumatic devices and hydrotherapy, *Ostomy Wound Mgmt* 41(5):30-32, 35-37, 1995.

95. Hahn JS: *Lecture on the power and effect of fresh water on the human body*, 1734, Germany.

96. Wheeler CB, Rodeheaver GT, Thacker JG, et al: Side effects of high-pressure irrigation, *Surg Gynecol Obstet* 143(5):775-778, 1976.

97. McGuckin M, Thorpe R, Abrutyn E: Hydrotherapy: an outbreak of *Pseudomonas aeruginosa* wound infections related to Hubbard tank treatments, *Arch Phys Med Rehabil* 62:283-285, 1981.

98. Tredget EE, Shankowsky HA, Joffe AAM, et al: Epidemiology of infections with *Pseudomonas aeruginosa* in burn patients: the role of hydrotherapy, *Clin Infect Dis* 15(6):641-649, 1992.

99. Shankowsky HA, Callioux LS, Tredget EE: North American survey of hydrotherapy in modern burn care, *J Burn Care Rehabil* 15(2):143-146, 1994.

100. Richard P, LeFoch R, Chamoux C, et al: *Pseudomonas aeruginosa* outbreak in a burn unit: role of antimicrobials in the emergence of multiply resistant strains, *J Infect Dis* 170(2):377-383, 1994.

101. Wisplinghoff H, Perbix W, Seifert H: Risk factors for nosocomial bloodstream infections due to *Acinetobacter baumannii*: a case-control study of adult burn patients, *Clin Infect Dis* 28(1):59-66, 1999.

102. Stanwood W, Pinzur MS: Risk of contamination of the wound in a hydrotherapeutic tank, *Foot Ankle Int* 19(3):173-176, 1998.

103. Myers RS: *Saunders manual of physical therapy practice*, Philadelphia, 1995, WB Saunders.

104. Walsh MT: Hydrotherapy: the use of water as a therapeutic agent. In Michlovitz SL, ed: *Thermal agents in rehabilitation*, ed 3, Philadelphia, 1996, FA Davis.

105. Steve L, Goodhart P, Alexander J: Hydrotherapy burn treatment: use of chloramine-T against resistant microorganisms, *Arch Phys Med Rehabil* 60(7):301-303, 1979.

106. Custer J, Edlich RF, Prusak M, et al: Studies in the management of the contaminated wound: V. An assessment of the effectiveness of pHisoHex and Betadine surgical scrub solutions, *Am J Surg* 121:572-575, 1971.

107. Johnson AR, White AC, McAnalley B: Comparison of common topical agents for wound treatment: cytotoxicity for human fibroblasts in culture, *Wounds* 1(3):186-192, 1989.

108. Rodeheaver GT, Kurtz L, Kircher BJ, et al: Pluronic F-68: a promising new wound cleanser, *Ann Emerg Med* 9(11):572-576, 1980.

109. Rydberg B, Zederfeldt B: Influence of cationic detergents on tensile strength of healing skin wounds in the rat, *Acta Chir Scand* 134(5):317-320, 1968.

110. Burkey JL, Weinberg C, Branden RA: Differential methodologies for the evaluation of skin and wound cleansers, *Wounds* 5(6):284-291, 1993.

111. Foresman PA, Payne DS, Becker D, et al: A relative toxicity index for wound cleansers, *Wounds* 5(5):226-231, 1993.

112. Henderson JD, Leming JT, Melon-Niksa DB: Chloramine-T solutions: effect on wound healing in guinea pigs, *Arch Phys Med Rehabil* 70(8):628-631, 1989.

113. Rabenberg VS, Ingersoll CD, Sandrey MA, et al: The bactericidal and cytotoxic effects of antimicrobial wound cleansers. *J Athl Train* 37(1):51-54, 2002.

114. Winter GD: Formation of a scab and the rate of epithelialization of superficial wounds in the skin of the young domestic pig, *Nature* 193:293-294, 1962.

115. Bhaskar SN, Cutright DE, Gross A: Effect of water lavage on infected wounds in the rat, *J Periodontol* 40(11):671-672, 1969.

116. Brown LL, Shelton HT, Bornside GH, et al: Evaluation of wound irrigation by pulsatile jet and conventional methods, *Ann Surg* 187(2):170-173, 1978.

117. Griffiths RD, Fernandez RS, Ussia CA: Is tap water a safe alternative to normal saline for wound irrigation in the community setting? *J Wound Care* 10(10):407-411, 2001.

118. Moore ZE, Cowman S: Wound cleansing for pressure ulcers, *Cochrane Database System Rev* 4:CD004983, 2005.

119. Bellingeri R, Attolini C, Fioretti O, et al: Evaluation of the efficacy of a preparation for the cleansing of cutaneous injuries, *Minerva Medica* 95:1-9, 2004.

120. Fernandez R, Griffiths R, Ussia C: Water for wound cleansing, *Cochrane Database System Rev* 4:CD003861, 2002.

121. Morgan D, Hoelscher J: Pulsed lavage: promoting comfort and healing in home care, *Ostomy Wound Manage* 46(4):44-49, 2000.

122. University Medical Center Physical Therapy Department: *Wound care protocol using the Pulsavac wound debridement system*, Lubbock, TX, 1994, University Medical Center.

123. Bohannon RW: Whirlpool versus whirlpool rinse for removal of bacteria from a venous stasis ulcer, *Phys Ther* 62(3):304-308, 1982.

124. Bingham HG, Hudson D, Popp J: A retrospective review of the burn intensive care unit admissions for a year, *J Burn Care Rehabil* 16(1):56-58, 1995.

125. Thomson PD, Bowden ML, McDonald K, et al: A survey of burn hydrotherapy in the United States, *J Burn Care Rehabil* 11(2):151-155, 1990.

126. Staley M, Richard R: Management of the acute burn wound: an overview, *Adv Wound Care* 10(2):39-44, 1997.

127. Hoffman HG, Patterson DR, Magula J, et al: Water-friendly virtual reality pain control during wound care, *J Clin Psychol* 60(2):189-195, 2004.

128. Neville C, Dimick AR: The trauma table as an alternative to the Hubbard tank in burn care, *J Burn Care Rehabil* 8(6):574-575, 1987.

129. Embil JM, McLoed JA, Al-Barak AM, et al: An outbreak of methicillin resistant *Staphylococcus aureus* on a burn unit: potential role of contaminated hydrotherapy equipment, *Burns* 27(7):681-688, 2001.

130. Said RA, Hussein MM: Severe hyponatremia in burn patients secondary to hydrotherapy, *Burns Incl Thermal Inj* 13(4):327-329, 1987.

131. Headley BJ, Robson MC, Krizek TJ: Methods of reducing environmental stress for the acute burn patient, *Phys Ther* 55(1):5-9, 1975.

132. Morykwas MJ, Simpson J, Punger K, et al: Vacuum-assisted closure: state of basic research and physiologic foundation, *Plast Reconstr Surg* 117(7 suppl):121S-126S, 2006.

133. Samson D, Lefevre F, Aronson N: *Wound healing technologies: low-level laser and vacuum-assisted closure. Summary. Evidence Report/Technology Assessment No. 111*, AHRQ Publication No. 05-E005-1, Rockville, MD, 2004AHRQ. http://www.ahrq.gov/downloads/pub/evidence/pdf/woundtech/woundtech.pdf.

134. Association for the Advancement of Wound Care (AAWC): Summary algorithm for venous ulcer care with annotations of available evidence, Malvern, PA,2005,AAWC.http://www.guideline.gov/summary/summary.aspx?doc_id=7109&nbr=004280&string=vacuum+AND+assisted+AND+wound+AND+closure.

135. Wound, Ostomy, and Continence Nurses Society (WOCN): *Guideline for prevention and management of pressure ulcers*, Glenview IL, 2003, WOCN. http://www.guideline.gov/summary/summary.aspx?doc_id=3860&nbr=003071&string=vacuum+AND+assisted+AND+wound+AND+closure.

136. Gleck J: Precautions for hydrotherapeutic devices, *Clin Mgmt* 3:44, 1983.

137. US Department of Health and Human Services: *Treatment of pressure ulcers: clinical practice guidelines*, Rockville, MD, 1994, US Department of Health and Human Services.

138. Moschetti M: Aquatics risk management strategies for the therapy pool, *J Back Musculoskel Rehabil* 4(4):265-272, 1994.

139. McMurray RG, Katz VL: Thermoregulation in pregnancy: implications for exercise, *Sports Med* 10(3):146-158, 1990.

140. American National Red Cross: *Lifesaving rescue and water safety*, Washington, DC, 1989, Water Safety Program.

141. Hwang JCF, Himel HN, Edlich RF: Bilateral amputations following hydrotherapy tank burns in a paraplegic patient, *Burns* 21(1):70-71, 1995.

142. Byl N, Cameron M, Kloth L, et al: Treatment and prevention goals and objectives. In Myers RS, ed: *Saunders manual of physical therapy practice*, Philadelphia, 1995, WB Saunders.

143. Stav D, Stav M: Asthma and whirlpool baths, *N Engl J Med* 353(15):1635-1636, 2005.

144. Bernard A, Carbonnelle S, Michel O, et al: Lung hyperpermeability and asthma prevalence in schoolchildren: unexpected associations with the attendance at indoor chlorinated swimming pools, *Occup Environ Med* 60:385-394, 2003.

145. Thickett KM, McCoach JS, Gerber JM, et al: Occupational asthma caused by chloramines in indoor swimming pool air, *Eur Respir J* 19:827-832, 2002.

146. Borell PM, Parker R, Henley EJ, et al: Comparison of in vivo temperatures produced by hydrotherapy paraffin wax treatment and fluidotherapy, *Phys Ther* 60:1273-1276, 1980.

147. Fiscus KA, Kaminski TW, Powers ME: Changes in lower-leg blood flow during warm-, cold-, and contrast-water therapy, *Arch Phys Med Rehabil* 86(7):1404-1410, 2005.

148. Hall J, MacDonald IA, Maddison PJ, et al: Cardiorespiratory responses to underwater treadmill walking in healthy females, *Eur J Apply Physiol* 77(3):278-284, 1998.

149. Loehne HB: Enhanced wound care using the Pulsavac system: case studies, *Acute Care Perspect* 3(2), 1995.

150. Luedtke-Hoffman KA, Schafer DS: Pulsed lavage in wound cleansing, *Phys Ther* 80(3):292-300, 2000.

151. Arledge RL: Prevention of electrical shock hazards in physical therapy, *Phys Ther* 58(10):1215-1217, 1978.

152. Atkinson G, Harrison A: Implications of the Health and Safety At Work Act in relation to hydrotherapy departments, *Physiotherapy* 67:263-265, 1981.

153. Bloomfield SF, Miller EA: A comparison of hypochlorite and phenolic disinfectants for disinfection of clean and soiled surfaces and blood spillages, *J Hosp Infect* 13:231-239, 1989.

154. Loughney E, Harrison J: Irritant contact dermatitis due to 1-bromo-3-chloro-5,5-dimethylhydantoin in a hydrotherapy pool. Risk assessments: the need for continuous evidence-based assessments, *Occup Med* (Lond) 48(7):461-463, 1998.

155. American Physical Therapy Association: *Hydrotherapy/therapeutic pool infection control guidelines*, Alexandria, VA, 1994, APTA.

Traction

Traction is a mechanical force applied to the body in a way that separates the joint surfaces and elongates the surrounding soft tissues. **Traction** can be applied manually by the clinician or mechanically by a machine. Traction can also be applied by the patient using body weight and gravity to apply a force. Traction can be applied to the spinal or peripheral joints. This chapter focuses on the application of **mechanical traction** to the cervical and lumbar spine and briefly discusses the application of traction to the spine by other means. Information on the application of traction to the peripheral joints is not pro-vided in this book because such traction is generally pro-vided manually by the therapist and is therefore considered to be manual therapy rather than a physical agent. For further information on the application of traction to the peripheral joints, the reader should consult a manual therapy text.

Spinal traction gained popularity in the 1950s and 1960s in response to James Cyriax's recommendations regarding the efficacy of this technique for the treatment of back and leg pain caused by disc protrusions.[1] A range of studies suggest that spinal traction is more effective for reducing back pain and returning patients to activity than infrared radiation, corset and bed rest, hot packs and rest, hot packs, massage and mobilization, and bed rest.[2-5] A number of studies, however, have failed to demonstrate that traction is more effective than other treatments, such as isometric exercises, or that high-force traction is any more effective than low-force traction.[6,7] A systematic review of 24 randomized controlled trials with 2,177 patients looked at traction for mixed groups of patients with low back pain with and without sciatica.[8] They found (1) strong evidence that there is no significant difference in short- or long-term outcomes between traction (con-tinuous or intermittent) as a single treatment and placebo, sham, or no treatment; (2) moderate evidence that trac-tion as a single treatment is no more effective than other treatments; and (3) limited evidence that adding traction to a standard physiotherapy program does not result in significantly different outcomes. There was moderate evi-dence that autotraction was more effective than mechani-cal traction for global improvement. However, many of the trials on traction are of poor quality, so the effective-ness of traction is still not known, and traction continues to be used and recommended for patients with symptoms attributable to spinal disorders with reports of good success. This chapter presents what is known about the efficacy of traction and makes recommendations for inter-ventions that are most likely to be effective.

EFFECTS OF SPINAL TRACTION

Spinal traction can distract joint surfaces, reduce protru-sions of nuclear discal material, stretch soft tissue, relax muscles, and mobilize joints.[1,9] Low-force traction, of 10 to 20 lb, applied for a long duration, ranging from hours to a few days, can also be used to temporarily immo-bilize a patient. All of these effects may reduce the pain

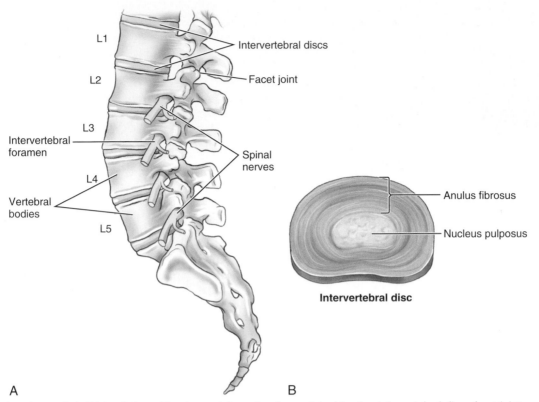

FIG 10-1 Spinal anatomy. **A,** Left lateral view of lumbar vertebrae showing vertebral bodies, intervertebral discs, facet joints, and intervertebral foramen, and spinal nerves. **B,** Cross-section of an intervertebral disc (showing anulus fibrosus and nucleus pulposus).

associated with spinal dysfunction. The stimulation of sensory mechanoreceptors by traction may also gate the transmission of pain along afferent neural pain pathways.

A basic understanding of spinal anatomy is helpful when thinking about how traction works and its effects on the joints of the spine. The spine consists of 24 vertebrae stacked on top of each other and connected by ligaments. Between the bodies of each vertebra is a disc that connects one vertebra to another and that serves as a shock absorber (Fig. 10-1, *A*). The disc has a soft center called the **nucleus pulposus** surrounded by the tough, fibrous **anulus fibrosus** (Fig. 10-1, *B*). The spinal cord is posterior to the discs and the spinal bodies and runs through the spinal canal. The primary joints of the spine are the facet joints, also known as spinal apophyseal or zygapophyseal joints, which connect the posterior elements of the vertebrae. There are foramina, or holes, between the posterior elements of each of the vertebrae that serve as exit points for spinal nerve roots coming off the spinal cord. Spinal traction pulls longitudinally on the spine, potentially reducing pressure on the discs and facet joints, enlarging the intervertebral foramina, and stretching the ligaments, tendons, and muscles running along the spine.

JOINT DISTRACTION

Joint distraction is defined as "the separation of two articular surfaces perpendicular to the plane of the articulation."[10] Distraction of the spinal apophyseal joints help

the patient who has signs and symptoms related to loading of these joints or compression of the spinal nerve roots as they pass through the intervertebral foramina. Joint distraction reduces compression on the joint surfaces and widens the intervertebral foramina, potentially reducing pressure on articular surfaces, intraarticular structures, or the spinal nerve roots.[11] Thus joint distraction may reduce pain originating from joint injury or inflammation or from nerve root compression.

It has been proposed that the application of a traction force to the spine can cause distraction of the spinal apophyseal joints.[1] One study showed approximately 3 mm joint distraction of the L2 to S1 intervertebral joints with gravitational traction in both healthy subjects and patients with low back pain.[12] For distraction to occur, the force applied must be great enough to cause sufficient elongation of the soft tissues surrounding the joint to allow the joint surfaces to separate. Smaller amounts of force will increase the tension on, or elongate, the soft tissues of the spine without separating the joint surfaces. For example, a force equal to 25% of the patient's body weight has been shown to be sufficient to increase the length of the lumbar spine; however, a force equal to 50% of the patient's body weight has been found to be necessary to distract the lumbar apophyseal joints.[13,14] The amount of force required to distract the spinal joints also varies with the location and health of the joints. In general, the larger lumbar joints, which have more and tougher surrounding soft tissues, require more force to achieve

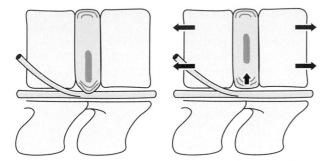

FIG 10-2 Suction caused by traction causing realignment of nuclear discal material.

joint distraction than do the smaller cervical joints. As mentioned, distraction of the lumbar apophyseal joints has been demonstrated with a force equal to 50% of total body weight; in contrast, a force equal to approximately 7% of total body weight has been reported to be sufficient to distract the cervical vertebrae.[15] It has also been shown that the same magnitude of force produces greater vertebral separation in healthy spines than in spines with signs of disc degeneration.[16]

REDUCTION OF DISC PROTRUSION

According to Cyriax, "traction is the treatment of choice for small nuclear protrusions."[1] The proposed mechanisms for disc realignment include clicking back of a disc fragment, suction caused by decreased intradiscal pressure pulling displaced parts of the disc back toward the center, or tensing of the posterior longitudinal ligament at the posterior aspect of the disc, thereby pushing any posteriorly displaced discal material anteriorly toward its original position[1,17] (Fig. 10-2).

A number of studies have shown that spinal traction can reduce spinal discal protrusions, and a number of authors have proposed that the relief of back pain and related symptoms that occurs with the application of traction is the result of a reduction in protrusions of nuclear discal material.[18,19] Studies using a variety of diagnostic imaging techniques, including discography, epidurography, and computed tomography (CT), have demonstrated that lumbar traction, using a force of 27 to 55 kg (60 to 120 lb), can reduce a disc prolapse, cause retraction of herniated discal material, reduce the size of a disc herniation, increase space within the spinal canal, widen the neural foramina, and result in clinical improvement in those patients in whom the discal defects are reduced.[17,20-23] One small study also showed an increase in straight leg raise (SLR) immediately after traction using 30% and 60% of body weight and little effect on SLR after traction using 10% of body weight.[24] It has been reported that symptoms generally do not improve when traction is applied to patients with large discal herniations that fill the spinal canal or when it is applied to those with calcification of the disc protrusion.[17]

Although studies support the belief that high-force traction can reduce nuclear discal protrusions, some reports indicate that lower forces may not produce this effect.[19] Andersson et al reported that intradiscal pressure was not reduced when **self-traction** was applied by the patient pulling on an overhead bar while lying down, wearing a pelvic harness attached to a spring force scale, or when **manual traction** was applied by one therapist pulling on the subject's pelvis while another pulled under the arms.[25] Also, Lundgren and Eldevik found that autotraction, in which the traction force is limited by the patient's ability to pull with the arms, caused no change in the appearance of herniated lumbar discs on CT scan.[26]

Although the evidence for the effects of traction on discal protrusions is not conclusive, it appears that with sufficient traction force, of at least 27 kg (60 lb) to the lumbar spine, some disc protrusions are reduced by spinal traction and that traction can reduce symptoms in patients with local back or neck pain or radicular spinal symptoms caused by a disc protrusion, if the protrusion is reduced. These symptomatic improvements may be the result of reducing the discal protrusion or may be caused by concurrent changes in other associated structures such as increased size of the neural foramina, changes in the tension on soft tissues or nerves, or modification of the tone of the low back muscles.

SOFT TISSUE STRETCHING

Traction has been reported to elongate the spine and increase the distance between the vertebral bodies and the facet joint surfaces.[27-29] It is proposed that these effects are a result of increased length of the soft tissues in the area, including the muscles, tendons, ligaments, and discs. Soft tissue stretching using a moderate-load, prolonged force, such as that provided by spinal traction, has also been shown to increase the length of tendons and to increase joint mobility.[30-32] Increasing the length of the soft tissues of the spine may provide clinical benefits by contributing to spinal joint distraction or reduction of disc protrusion, as described previously, or by increasing spinal range of motion (ROM) and decreasing the pressure on the facet joint surfaces, discs, and intervertebral nerve roots even when complete joint surface separation is not achieved.

MUSCLE RELAXATION

Spinal traction has been reported to facilitate relaxation of the paraspinal muscles.[18,33] It has been proposed that this effect may be the result of pain reduction caused by reduced pressure on pain-sensitive structures or gating of pain transmission by stimulation of mechanoreceptors by the oscillatory movements produced by **intermittent traction**.[34] As explained in detail in Chapter 3, reduction of pain by any means can facilitate muscle relaxation and a reduction of muscle spasms by interrupting the pain-spasm-pain cycle. It has also been proposed that **static traction** may cause muscle relaxation as a result of the depression in monosynaptic response caused by stretching the muscles for several seconds and that intermittent traction may cause small changes in muscle tension to produce muscle relaxation by stimulating the Golgi tendon organs (GTOs) to inhibit alpha motor neuron firing.[35]

JOINT MOBILIZATION

Traction has been recommended as a means to mobilize joints in order to increase joint mobility or decrease joint-related pain.[36,37] Joint mobility is thought to be increased by high-force traction because of stretching of the surrounding soft tissue structures. When lower levels of force are applied, the repetitive oscillatory motion of intermittent spinal traction may also move the joints sufficiently to stimulate the mechanoreceptors and thus decrease joint-related pain by gating the afferent transmission of pain stimuli. In this manner, the effects of spinal traction may be similar to those produced by manual joint mobilization techniques, except that with most traction techniques a number of joints are mobilized at one time, whereas with manual techniques the mobilizing force can be more localized.

CLINICAL INDICATIONS FOR THE USE OF SPINAL TRACTION

The clinical indications for the use of spinal traction include back or neck pain, with or without radiating symptoms when caused by a disc bulge or herniation, nerve root impingement, joint hypomobility, subacute joint inflammation, or paraspinal muscle spasm. Although substantial evidence demonstrates the mechanical effects of spinal traction, limitations in the data from clinical studies concerning its use for the treatment of back and neck pain have caused its use for these problems to be controversial.[8,38]

Because treatment with traction has frequently been associated with a reduction or elimination of spinal pain, with or without radiating symptoms, and because spinal traction has been shown to reduce mechanical dysfunctions associated with such symptoms, the use of spinal traction is recommended for consideration as an intervention for such problems. The indications and recommendations for the selection of traction as a treatment modality, which are provided in the following section, and the guidelines for selection of treatment parameters, are based on the available data and an understanding of the spinal pathologies that can cause signs and symptoms in patients. If a patient's signs and symptoms are known to be caused by a disc bulge or herniation, nerve root impingement, subacute joint inflammation, or paraspinal muscle spasm and if these are aggravated by joint loading and eased by distraction or reduction of joint loading, then traction may be effective in reducing or controlling the symptoms. Traction is less likely to be effective when there is a large disc herniation that protrudes into the spinal canal or when herniated or protruding discal material has become calcified.

Clinical Pearl

Traction is less effective for large or calcified disc herniations.

DISC BULGE OR HERNIATION

In a number of clinical studies, spinal traction has been shown to relieve symptoms associated with a disc bulge or **herniated nucleus pulposus**.[2,17,39] A prospective randomized trial found that lumbar traction can improve symptoms and clinical findings in patients with lumbar disc herniation and decrease the size of the **herniated disc** material as measured by CT.[40] The primary proposed mechanism of symptom relief is reduction of the disc bulge or protrusion and thus reduction of compression on the spinal nerve roots. Traction is most likely to improve the patient's outcome if it is applied soon after a discal injury when there is protrusion of soft nuclear discal material.

Clinical Pearl

Traction is most effective when applied soon after discal injury.

This improvement occurs because traction can reduce not only the protrusion that has occurred but can also reduce the risk of further protrusion.[19]

In contrast, a number of studies have failed to demonstrate a significant clinical benefit in response to the application of traction to patients with discal injuries.[4,6,8,41] This lack of positive effect may be related to the severity of the disc protrusions in the subjects studied, the use of insufficient traction force, or the use of sample sizes that were too small to detect a treatment effect. Despite these equivocal findings, spinal traction remains a common intervention for treating patients with discal protrusions and back or neck pain with or without radicular symptoms.

Because it is likely that any correction of a discal protrusion produced by spinal traction may be quickly lost if the patient returns to his or her prior activities, it is recommended that all patients be instructed in other techniques for reducing stresses on the spine after treatment with traction to avoid a rapid recurrence of symptoms.

Clinical Pearl

To maintain the effects of spinal traction, patients should also use other techniques to reduce stress on the spine.

Such techniques may include correction of posture and body mechanics, lumbar stabilization through exercise or use of a corset, self-traction, and a cautious, gradual return to prior activities. Other exercises and mobilization techniques may also assist in maintaining the symptom relief and correction of discal positioning achieved with spinal traction.

NERVE ROOT IMPINGEMENT

Traction has been reported to help alleviate signs and symptoms associated with spinal nerve root impingement, particularly if it is applied shortly after the onset of such symptoms.[2] Traction is generally recommended as the treatment of choice for patients with neurological deficits from spinal nerve root impingement.[42] Such impingement may be caused by bulging or herniation of discal material, as described previously, or by ligament encroachment, narrowing of the intervertebral foramen, osteophyte encroachment, spinal nerve root swelling, or **spondylo-**

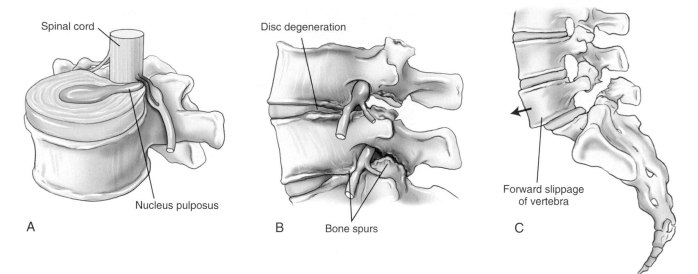

FIG 10-3 Causes of spinal nerve root compression. **A,** Disc herniation. **B,** Osteophyte encroachment and disc degeneration causing narrowing of the intervertebral foramen. **C,** Spondylolisthesis.

listhesis (Fig. 10-3). In the latter cases, if sufficient traction force is applied, the size of the neural foramen may temporarily be increased, reducing pressure on the spinal nerve root.[14,16,43] For example, when cervical lateral flexion and rotation to the same side, which both narrow the intervertebral foramina, are markedly limited by arm pain on the same side, indicating impingement of cervical nerve roots, the application of traction may effectively reduce the arm pain by increasing the size of the neural foramina and decreasing pressure on the involved nerve(s).

Some studies have reported good results when using traction for the treatment of pain and other related neurological symptoms associated with nerve root impingement, whereas others have failed to demonstrate greater benefits with traction than with sham traction.[41,44-46] Although the available data do not readily indicate which patients will benefit from spinal traction, clinically, in general, those patients who report aggravation of symptoms with increased spinal loading and casing of symptoms with decreased spinal loading are more likely to respond well to treatment with traction.

Clinical Pearl

Patients who have worsening symptoms with spinal loading and improved symptoms with decreased spinal loading are good candidates for traction.

It has also been recommended that traction be considered for patients with symptoms of radiating pain or paresthesia that do not improve with trunk movements.[47]

JOINT HYPOMOBILITY

Because longitudinal spinal traction can glide and distract the spinal facet joints and stretch the soft tissues sur-rounding these joints, spinal traction may prove beneficial in the treatment of symptoms caused by joint hypomobility. However, spinal traction is not generally the optimal treatment if only individual segments are hypomobile because it applies a mobilizing force to multiple rather than single spinal levels. Such nonspecific mobilization could prove deleterious to the patient with hypomobility of one segment and hypermobility of adjoining segments. In such patients, the mobilizing force applied by traction would most probably cause the greatest increase in motion in the most extensible areas, the hypermobile segments, resulting in joint laxity, while having no effect on the mobility of the less mobile segments causing the patient's symptoms. Adjusting the degree of spinal flexion during the application of traction localizes the mobilizing effect of the force to some degree and thus may help to alleviate this problem.[48] For example, positioning the lumbar spine in more flexion localizes the force to the upper lumbar and lower thoracic spine, whereas positioning it in neutral or extension localizes the force to the lower lumbar area. Similarly, for the cervical spine, the flexed position focuses the forces on the lower cervical area, and the neutral or slightly extended position focuses the forces on the upper cervical area.[48] More detailed recommendations for patient positioning are provided in the section on application techniques.

SUBACUTE JOINT INFLAMMATION

Traction has been recommended for reducing the pain and limitations of function associated with subacute joint inflammation.[37] The force of traction can be used to reduce the pressure on inflamed joint surfaces, whereas the small movements of intermittent traction may control pain by gating transmission at the spinal cord level. These movements may also help to maintain normal fluid exchange in the joints to relieve edema in or around the joints caused by chronic inflammation.[49] Spinal traction can be used safely in the subacute or chronic stages of joint inflammation; however, intermittent traction should be avoided immediately after an injury, during the acute inflammatory phase, when the repetitive motion may cause further injury or amplify the inflammatory response.

Clinical Pearl

Intermittent traction should be avoided immediately after an injury, during the acute inflammatory phase, and when repetitive motion may worsen an injury or increase inflammation. Static traction may be used at this time.

PARASPINAL MUSCLE SPASM

The maintained stretch of static traction or the repetitive motion of low-load, intermittent traction may help to reduce paraspinal muscle spasm.[18,33] As noted previously, this effect may be a result of a reduction in pain and the consequent interruption of the pain-spasm-pain cycle or may be caused by inhibition of alpha motor neuron firing from depression of the monosynaptic response or stimulation of the GTOs.[34] Higher load spinal traction may also alleviate protective paraspinal muscle spasms by reducing the underlying cause of pain, such as a disc protrusion or herniation or a nerve root impingement, thus interrupting the pain-spasm-pain cycle.

CONTRAINDICATIONS AND PRECAUTIONS FOR USE OF SPINAL TRACTION

The application of spinal traction is contraindicated in some circumstances, and it should be applied with extra caution in other circumstances.[50] To minimize the probability of adverse consequences in all cases, traction should first be applied using a small amount of force, and the patient's response to treatment should be closely monitored.

Clinical Pearl

Traction should always be applied with a low force at first, and the patient should be monitored for adverse responses.

If the patient's condition worsens in response to traction, with symptoms becoming more severe, peripheralizing, increasing in distribution, or progressing to other domains (e.g., from pain to numbness or weakness), the treatment approach should be reevaluated and changed. If the patient's signs or symptoms do not improve within two or three treatments, the treatment approach should be reevaluated and changed or the patient should be referred to a physician for further evaluation.

PATIENT RECOMMENDATIONS AND INSTRUCTIONS

The patient should be instructed to try to avoid sneezing or coughing while on full traction because these activities increase intraabdominal pressure and can thus increase intradiscal pressure. It is also recommended that the patient empty the bladder and not have a heavy meal before lumbar traction because the constriction of the pelvic belts may cause discomfort on a full bladder or stomach.

CONTRAINDICATIONS FOR THE USE OF TRACTION

CONTRAINDICATIONS
for the Use of Traction

- Where motion is contraindicated
- Acute injury or inflammation
- Joint hypermobility or instability
- Peripheralization of symptoms with traction
- Uncontrolled hypertension

Where Motion is Contraindicated

Traction should not be used if motion is contraindicated in the area to be affected. Examples include an unstable fracture, cord compression, or immediately after spinal surgery.

Ask the Patient
- Have you been instructed not to move your neck or back? If so, by whom?
- If wearing a brace or corset: Have you been instructed not to remove your brace at any time?
- How recent was your injury or surgery?

Any form of traction should not be used if motion in the area is contraindicated. Direct treatment with other physical agents, such as heat or cold, should be considered or other involved areas where motion is allowed can be treated.

Acute Injury or Inflammation

Acute inflammation may occur immediately after trauma or surgery or as the result of an inflammatory disease such as rheumatoid arthritis or osteoarthritis. Because intermittent or static traction may aggravate acute inflammation or interfere with the healing of an acute injury, traction should not be applied under these conditions.

Ask the Patient
- When did your injury occur?
- When did your pain start?

If the injury or onset of pain was within the last 72 hours, the injury is likely to still be in the acute inflammatory phase and traction should not be used. As inflammation resolves, static traction may be used initially, with progression to intermittent traction as the area tolerates more motion.

Assess
• Palpate and inspect the area to detect signs of inflammation, including heat, redness, and swelling.

If signs of acute inflammation are present, it is recommended that the application of traction be delayed until they resolve.

Hypermobile or Unstable Joint

High-force traction should not be used in areas of joint hypermobility or instability because it may further increase the mobility of the area. Therefore the mobility of joints in the area to which one is considering applying traction should be assessed before the traction is applied. Joint hypermobility may be the result of a recent fracture, joint dislocation, or surgery, or it can be caused by an old injury, high relaxin levels during pregnancy and lactation, poor posture, or congenital ligament laxity. Joint hypermobility and instability, particularly of the C1-C2 articulations, is also common in patients with rheumatoid arthritis, Down syndrome, and Marfan syndrome as a result of degeneration of the transverse atlantar ligament. Therefore cervical traction should not be applied to patients with these diagnoses until the integrity of the transverse atlantar ligament and the stability of the C1-C2 articulations have been ascertained.

Ask the Patient
• Have you dislocated a joint in this area?
• Do you have rheumatoid arthritis or Marfan's syndrome?
• Are you pregnant?

Assess
• Assess joint mobility in the area that will be affected by the traction. All levels of the cervical or lumbar spine, depending on which is being treated, should be assessed, not just the symptomatic ones, since traction can affect the mobility of multiple levels.
• Check the patient's chart for any diagnosis of rheumatoid arthritis, Marfan syndrome, or Down syndrome and request radiographic studies to rule out C1-C2 instability before applying traction.

Traction should not be applied in areas where joint hypermobility is detected on manual or radiographic examination or to areas that have been previously dislocated. When some segments are hypomobile and adjacent segments are hypermobile, it is recommended that the hypomobile segments be treated with manual techniques rather than mechanical traction because manual techniques can mobilize individual spinal segments more specifically.

Peripheralization of Symptoms

Traction should be discontinued or modified immediately if it causes peripheralization of symptoms because, in general, progression of spinal symptoms from a central area to a more peripheral area indicates worsening nerve function and increasing compression. Continuing treatment when symptom peripheralization occurs could result in aggravation of the initial injury and prolonged worsening of signs and symptoms.

Tell the Patient
• Let me know immediately if you get more pain or other symptoms further down your arms or legs. Stop the traction if this occurs.

Assess
• Recheck sensation, motor function, and reflexes in the appropriate extremity or extremities, if the patient complains of peripheralization of symptoms.

Traction should be discontinued or modified if signs or symptoms peripheralize. Traction may be modified by decreasing the load or changing the patient's position. Modified traction may be continued if peripheralization of symptoms no longer occurs. Mild aggravation of central symptoms alone in a patient with prior central and peripheral symptoms should not be a cause for discontinuation of treatment.

Uncontrolled Hypertension

Inversion traction should be avoided in patients with uncontrolled hypertension since inversion has been found to significantly increase blood pressure.[51] In addition, one study found that in 40 patients with no history of hypertension, 10 minutes of cervical traction at 10% body weight caused increases in blood pressure (9 mm Hg increase in systolic and 5 mm Hg increase in diastolic pressure) and heart rate (7 beats per minute [bpm] increase).[52] Although this mild increase in blood pressure may not be problematic in healthy individuals, it is recommended that clinicians assess a patient's cardiovascular status before applying cervical traction to avoid exacerbating poorly controlled hypertension in some patients.

Ask the Patient
• Do you have high blood pressure? If so, is it well-controlled with medications?

Assess
• Take the patient's blood pressure.

In a patient with a resting blood pressure of more than 140/90, blood pressure and heart rate should be checked after application of cervical traction and treatment discontinued if systolic or diastolic BP increases by more than 10 mm Hg or heart rate increases by more than 10 bpm.

PRECAUTIONS FOR THE USE OF TRACTION

PRECAUTIONS

for the Use of Traction

- Structural diseases or conditions affecting the spine (e.g., tumor, infection, rheumatoid arthritis, osteoporosis, or prolonged systemic steroid use)
- When pressure of the belts may be hazardous (e.g., with pregnancy, hiatal hernia, vascular compromise, osteoporosis)
- Displaced anular fragment
- Medial disc protrusion
- When severe pain fully resolves with traction
- Claustrophobia or other psychological aversion to traction
- Inability to tolerate the prone or supine position
- Disorientation

In cases where traction should be applied with caution, the referring physician should be consulted before initiating traction. First, a low level of force should be applied, then progress slowly and monitor the patient's response to the treatment closely at all times.

Structural Diseases or Conditions Affecting the Bones of the Spine

Traction should be applied with caution when the structural integrity of the spine may be compromised. Such structural compromise can occur with a tumor, infection, rheumatoid arthritis, osteoporosis, or prolonged systemic steroid use. In these circumstances, the spine may not be strong enough to sustain the forces of traction, and injury may result from the application of strong traction forces. Radiographic reports and other studies that may indicate the nature and severity of the structural compromise should be checked before deciding to apply traction to patients with these conditions.

Ask the Patient

- Do you have any disease affecting your bones or joints?
- Do you have cancer, an infection in your bones, rheumatoid arthritis, or osteoporosis?
- Do you take steroid medications? If so, how long have you taken them?

Only low-force traction should be applied to patients with structural compromise of the spine. For these patients, manual traction, which allows more direct monitoring of patient response, may be more appropriate.

When the Pressure of the Belts May Be Hazardous

The pelvic belts used for the application of mechanical lumbar traction may apply excessive abdominal pressure to pregnant patients or to those with hiatal hernia and may place excessive pressure on the inguinal region on those with femoral artery compromise. Compression of the femoral arteries in the inguinal region can be avoided

by ensuring that the pelvic belt is positioned with its lower edge superior to the femoral triangle and by tightly securing the belt and keeping it in direct contact with the skin to prevent it from slipping down during treatment. There is also concern that pelvic or thoracic belts may apply excessive pressure to the pelvis or ribs of patients with osteoporosis. Because the thoracic belts used for fixation of the patient during the application of lumbar traction may constrict respiration, it is also recommended that lumbar traction be applied with caution to patients with cardiac or pulmonary disorders.[53]

Cervical traction should be applied with caution to patients with cerebrovascular compromise, as indicated by a positive vertebral artery test, because poor placement of the halter may further compromise circulation to the brain. The halter should be positioned away from the carotid arteries in patients with compromise of these arteries. This is most easily achieved by using a halter that distracts via the occiput rather than one that applies force to both the occiput and the mandible.

Ask the Patient

- Are you pregnant?
- Do you have a hiatal hernia?
- Have you had any trouble with blocked arteries?
- Do you get pain in your calves when walking a short distance? This is a sign of intermittent claudication, indicating possible arterial insufficiency to the lower extremities.
- Do you have osteoporosis?
- Do you have problems with your breathing?
- Have you had a stroke?
- Do you get dizzy when you put your head back?

If compression by the belts used for mechanical traction is hazardous to the patient, one should consider using other forms of traction, such as self-traction or manual traction, that do not require the use of these belts. Fastening the belts less tightly is generally not recommended because they can slip during treatment, rendering the treatment ineffective or increasing pressure in the inguinal region. If the patient's responses indicate possible compromise of the cervical or lower extremity vessels, it is essential that the halter or belts used for traction be positioned so that they do not compress these vessels.

Displaced Anular Fragment

Once a fragment of anulus has become displaced and is no longer connected to the body of the disc, traction is not likely to change the position of the disc fragment and therefore treatment with traction is not likely to improve the patient's symptoms.

Ask the Patient

- Has a magnetic resonance imaging (MRI) or CT scan of your spine been performed? Please bring me the report(s) from that (those) test(s).

Traction should not be used to treat symptoms resulting from a displaced disc fragment that is no longer attached to the body of the disc.

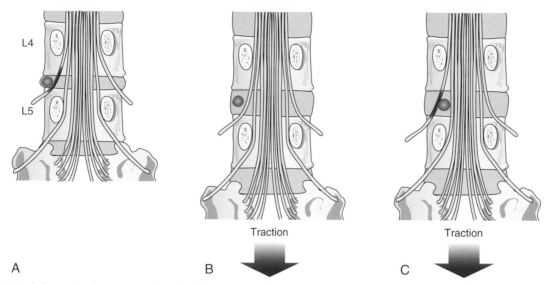

FIG 10-4 A, Lateral disc protrusion compressing the L4 nerve root. **B,** L4 nerve root compression by lateral disc protrusion relieved by traction caused by elongation of the lumbar spine and a consequent medial movement of the nerve root. **C,** L4 nerve root compression by medial disc protrusion aggravated by traction caused by medial movement of the nerve root.

Medial Disc Protrusion

It has been proposed that traction may aggravate symptoms caused by a medial disc protrusion because, in such circumstances, the medial movement of the nerve root caused by a traction force may increase the impingement of the disc on the nerve root (Fig. 10-4).[54]

Ask the Patient

• Has an MRI or CT scan of your spine been performed? Please bring me the report(s) from that (those) test(s).

When Severe Pain Resolves Fully with Traction

If severe pain resolves fully with traction, this may indicate that the traction has increased rather than decreased compression on a nerve root, causing a complete nerve block.

Ask the Patient

• After a few minutes of traction: Have your symptoms changed?

If the patient had severe pain and reports that the pain has decreased: Has the pain completely gone away or is it just less severe?

Assess

Test sensation, reflexes, and strength before treatment. Also, if the patient reports complete resolution of severe pain during treatment, check these again and assess for any changes.

If severe pain is fully relieved by traction, it is recommended that the clinician immediately recheck other indicators of nerve conduction, including sensation, reflexes, and strength, to rule out increasing nerve compression. If these are worse, traction should be stopped immediately. If these are not worse, the force of traction may be reduced by 50%, or the direction of the traction force modified, and traction may be continued. If traction is maintained at a level that causes a

nerve block, the patient may sustain a severe nerve injury as the result of the treatment.

Claustrophobia or Other Psychological Aversion to Traction

A number of patients are psychologically averse to the use of traction because this procedure generally involves considerable restriction of movement and loss of control. In particular, patients with claustrophobia may not tolerate the restriction of movement required for the application of mechanical lumbar traction. In such cases, other forms of traction that do not require immobilization with belts, such as manual or **positional traction**, may be better tolerated.

Inability to Tolerate the Prone or Supine Position

Some patients cannot tolerate the prone or supine position for the period of time necessary for the application of traction. Such limitations may be the result of their spinal condition or other medical problems such as reflux esophagitis. In such cases, the use of supports, such as a lumbar roll, may allow the patient to tolerate the position; cervical traction may be applied in the sitting position; or for lumbar traction, some of the self-traction techniques may be effective.

Ask the Patient

• Does lying on your back with your knees bent for 15 to 20 minutes cause any problems for you?
• Does lying on your stomach for 15 to 20 minutes cause any problems for you?

Disorientation

It is recommended that mechanical traction not be applied to disoriented patients because they may move in the halter or belts, becoming entangled or altering the amount of force they receive. It is recommended that only manual traction techniques be used to treat disoriented patients.

PRECAUTIONS FOR THE USE OF CERVICAL TRACTION

PRECAUTIONS

for the Use of Cervical Traction

- Temporomandibular joint (TMJ) problems
- Dentures

Temporomandibular Joint Problems

In patients with TMJ problems, or a history of such problems, it is recommended that a halter that only applies pressure through the occiput be used rather than one that applies pressure through both the mandible and the occiput because the latter may place pressure on the TMJs and thus aggravate preexisting joint pathology. Many clinicians use an occipital halter with all patients to avoid the possibility of causing TMJ problems in patients who did not have such problems previously.

Ask the Patient

- Do you have problems with your jaw?

Dentures

The patient who wears dentures should be instructed to keep the dentures in place during treatment with cervical traction because their removal can alter the alignment of the TMJs and may cause problems if pressure is applied to these joints through the mandible. An occipital halter should be used to protect dentures and the teeth, as well as the TMJ.

Ask the Patient

- Do you wear dentures?
- Do you have them in now?

ADVERSE EFFECTS OF SPINAL TRACTION

Although no systematic research has been performed on the adverse effects of spinal traction, some case reports suggest that prior symptoms may be increased by the application of lumbar traction exceeding 50% of the patient's total body weight or by the application of cervical traction exceeding 50% of the weight of the patient's head.[37,55] These reports stand in contrast to the finding that the force of traction must be at least 50% of the patient's body weight to achieve separation of the lumbar vertebrae.[14] Because a rebound increase in pain after the initial application of high-force traction can occur, it is generally recommended that traction force be kept low for the initial treatment and then be gradually increased until maximum benefit is obtained.

◎ Clinical Pearl

Traction force should be kept low for the initial treatment and then gradually increased, within the recommended range, to the point of maximum benefit.

Specific recommendations for the amount of traction force to be used for different regions of the spine and different spinal conditions are given in the section on application techniques.

It has been reported that some patients experience lumbar radicular discomfort after receiving treatment with intermittent cervical traction for cervical radicular symptoms.[56,57] Thirty-three percent of the patients who were reported to experience this adverse effect had transitional lumbar vertebrae evident on radiographs, and 83% had evidence of spinal osteoarthritis. The onset of lumbar radiculopathy after cervical traction suggests that axial tension induced in the spinal cord's dural covering was transmitted from the cervical spine to the lumbar nerve roots and that limitations in nerve root excursion caused by structural abnormalities and degenerative changes in these patients probably resulted in excessive tension being placed on the nerve roots, provoking lumbar radicular symptoms.

Other adverse effects of spinal traction have been described in detail in the section describing contraindications and precautions.

APPLICATION TECHNIQUES

Traction can be applied in many ways. At this time, traction is applied using electrical and weighted mechanical devices, self-traction, positional traction, and manual traction. In the past, traction was also applied using inversion techniques and purpose-built autotraction tables and for prolonged periods with very low loads.

Inversion traction, which is applied by placing the patient in a device that requires a head-down position, uses the weight of the patient's upper body to apply traction to the lumbar spine. This form of traction was fairly popular in the past 10 to 20 years; however, most inversion traction devices have been removed from the United States market by their manufacturers because of concerns regarding potential adverse effects in patients with hypertension. Significant increases in systolic and diastolic blood pressure and ophthalmic artery pressure have been documented in subjects without cardiovascular disease or a history of hypertension in response to the application of inversion traction; therefore it is thought that the application of this type of traction could increase the risk of a stroke or myocardial infarction in the patient with uncontrolled hypertension.[51,58,59] Because of these possible risks, the use of inversion traction is not recommended, and therefore instructions for its application are not provided in this book.

Autotraction, a form of self-traction that requires the use of a purpose-built table with sections that can be moved apart by the patient during treatment, was also popular for a number of years; however, this type of table is no longer being manufactured, thus directions for its application are also not provided in this book.

Patient immobilization using very low-load, prolonged static traction applied for hours to days was used to relieve symptoms aggravated by spinal motion.[14] The benefits of this treatment were thought to come from the limited mobility and bedrest forced on the patient rather than from the traction force.[60] Although the application of traction in the hospital for this purpose was popular only a decade or two ago, it has fallen out of favor because of the growing awareness that most patients with back pain do not benefit from prolonged bed rest and inactivity.[61] The significant cost of providing this treatment also limits its application.

When selecting the type of spinal traction, patient position, traction force, and duration and frequency of treatment to be used, the effects of these different parameters of treatment, the nature of the patient's problem, and the patient's response to prior treatments should be considered. Guidelines for the standard application technique for each of these types of traction and the advantages and disadvantages of each are provided in the next sections. However, if the clinician understands the principles underlying the application of this type of treatment, many of these techniques can be modified or adapted to suit individual clinical situations such as when a patient does not tolerate the standard position(s) used for treatment or when preferred equipment is not available.

For all forms of traction, the clinician should first determine if the presenting symptoms and problems are likely to respond to treatment with traction. The clinician should also determine that traction is not contraindicated for this patient or condition. Traction can be applied to the lumbar or cervical spine; however, some forms of traction are appropriate for only one area or the other, whereas others can be applied to either with appropriate modifications.

MECHANICAL TRACTION

Mechanical traction can be applied to the lumbar or cervical spine. A variety of belts and halters, as well as different patient treatment positions, can be used to apply traction to particular areas of the spine and to focus the effect on different segments or structures. Types of mechanical traction devices include electrical traction units, over-the door cervical traction devices, and other home traction devices. Traction can be applied continuously (static traction) or intermittently. Electrical mechanical traction units can apply static or intermittent traction of varying force. With static traction, the same amount of force is applied throughout the treatment session. With intermittent traction, the traction force alternates between two set points every few seconds throughout the treatment session. The force is held at a maximum for a number of seconds, the hold period, and is then reduced, usually by about 50%, for the following relaxation period. The newest electrical mechanical traction devices also allow the user to control the rate of force application and allow for finer control of the force to more closely mimic forces applied during manually applied traction or other manual joint mobilization techniques. Although the manufacturers of these newer devices claim that these features improve outcomes, as yet no studies have been published evaluating the effects of these devices.

Weighted mechanical traction units apply static traction only, with the amount of force being determined by the amount of weight used.

Advantages of Mechanical Traction

- Force and time well-controlled, readily graded, and replicable.
- Once applied, does not require the clinician to be with the patient throughout the treatment.
- Electrical mechanical traction units allow the application of static or intermittent traction.
- Static weighted devices, such as over-the-door cervical traction, are inexpensive and convenient for independent use by the patient at home.

Disadvantages of Mechanical Traction
- Expensive electrical mechanical devices.
- Time-consuming to set up.
- Lack of patient control or participation.
- Restriction by belts or halter poorly tolerated by some patients.
- Mobilizes broad regions of the spine rather than individual spinal segments, potentially inducing hypermobility in normal or hypermobile joints.

Electrical Mechanical Traction Units
Most clinics have one or more electrical mechanical traction units available. These units use a motor to apply traction forces to the lumbar or cervical spine, statically or intermittently, and can be used to apply forces of up to 70 kg (150 lb). These units have the advantage of being able to apply static or intermittent traction to the lumbar or cervical spine, and they allow fine, accurate control of the forces being applied.

> **◎ Clinical Pearl**
>
> Electrical mechanical traction units can apply static or intermittent traction to the lumbar or cervical spine with precise control and allow the patient to be in a variety of positions.

These units also allow considerable variation in patient position. The newer computerized models can finely control the speed of traction application, store a number of clinician- or patient- specific protocols, and track each patient's pain severity and location over time. The most significant limitations of electrical mechanical traction devices are their cost and size (Fig. 10-5).

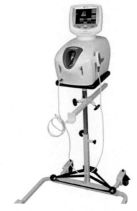

FIG 10-5 Mechanical traction unit. *Courtesy Chattanooga Group, Hixson, TN.*

Over-the-Door Cervical Traction Devices

Over-the-door cervical traction units can be used for the application of static cervical traction only. The limited treatment flexibility of these devices makes them appropriate primarily for home use. In this setting, they have the additional advantages of being inexpensive, easy to set up, and compact (Fig. 10-6). Before using this device at home, the patient should be educated on positioning and the amount and duration of force to use.

Other Home Traction Devices

A number of other spinal traction devices are also available for home application of static or intermittent lumbar or cervical traction (Fig. 10-7). These devices offer more treatment options but are more expensive than over-the-door devices, are more complex to use, and take up more space in the home.

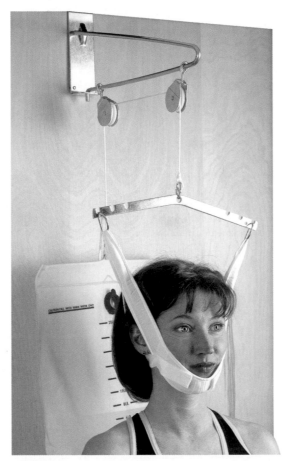

FIG 10-6 Over-the-door traction device. *Courtesy Chattanooga Group, Hixson, TN.*

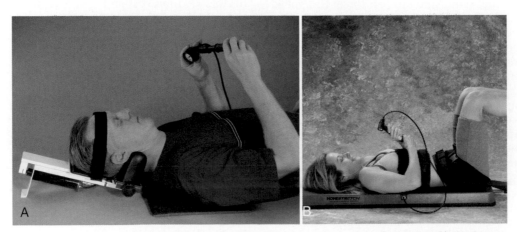

FIG 10-7 Examples of home traction devices. **A,** *Courtesy The Saunders Group, Chaska, MN.* **B,** *Courtesy Glacier Cross, Inc, Kalispell, MT.*

APPLICATION TECHNIQUE 10-1   MECHANICAL LUMBAR TRACTION

Equipment Required for Electrical Mechanical Traction

- Traction unit
- Thoracic and pelvic belts
- Spreader bar
- Extension rope
- Split traction table (optional)

Equipment Required for Weighted Mechanical Traction

- Traction device (ropes, pulley, weights)
- Thoracic and pelvic belts
- Spreader bar
- Weight bag for water, weights, or sand

Procedure for Mechanical Lumbar Traction

1. Select the appropriate mechanical traction device.

Various devices are available for applying mechanical traction to the lumbar spine in the clinic or home setting. The choice depends on the amount of force to be applied, whether static or intermittent traction is desired, and the setting in which the treatment will be applied.

2. Determine optimal patient position.

When positioning the patient, try to achieve a comfortable position that allows muscle relaxation while maximizing the separation between the involved structures. The relative degree of flexion or extension of the spine during traction determines which surfaces are most effectively separated.[37] The flexed position results in greater separation of the posterior structures, including the facet joints and intervertebral foramina, whereas the neutral or extended position results in greater separation of the anterior structures, including the disc spaces (Fig. 10-8). In most cases, a symmetrical central force is used, in which the direction of force is in line with the central sagittal axis of the patient (Fig. 10-9); however, if the patient presents with unilateral symptoms, a unilateral traction force that applies more force to one side of the spine than to the other may prove to be more effective.[62] A unilateral force can be applied by offsetting the axis of the traction in the direction that most reduces the patient's symptoms. For example, if the patient presents with right low back and lower extremity pain that is aggravated by right sidebending and is relieved by left sidebending, the traction should be offset to apply a left sidebending force.

For the application of traction to the lumbar spine, the patient may be positioned prone or supine (Fig. 10-10). Supine positioning is more commonly used; however, prone positioning may be advantageous if the patient does not tolerate flexion or being supine, or if the symptoms are reduced by extension or by being in the prone position. Greater lumbar paraspinal muscle relaxation and less EMG activity have also been reported during traction in the prone rather than the supine position.[63] Clinically, symptoms of discal origin are also usually most reduced in the prone position, when the lumbar spine is in neutral or extension and the disc space is most separated (see Fig. 10-8), whereas symptoms caused by facet joint dysfunction are most reduced when the patient is positioned supine with the hips flexed, the lumbar spine is flexed, and the facet joints are most separated.[37] Prone neutral positioning of the lumbar spine also localizes the force of the traction to the lower lumbar segments, whereas supine flexed positioning localizes the traction force to the upper lumbar and lower thoracic segments.

The patient should lie on a split traction table, with the area of the spine to be distracted positioned over the split, and if supine, with the lower extremities supported on a stool that does not

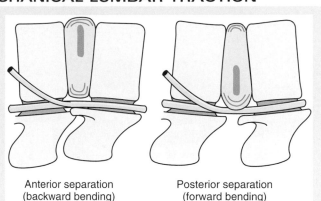

Anterior separation   Posterior separation
(backward bending)   (forward bending)

FIG 10-8 Effects of anterior and posterior separation on the spinal disc.

interfere with the motion of the traction rope. A split traction table separates into two sections, with one section sliding away from the other when the sections are unlocked and traction is applied (Fig. 10-11). This type of table reduces the amount of traction force lost to friction between the patient and the table because the lower half of the patient's body moves with the lower section of the table. Thus less traction force is needed when a split table is used than when a nonsplit table is used to provide the same amount of distractive force to the lumbar spine.[64] Initially the patient should be positioned with the sections of the table locked together so that the table does not move as the patient moves into the treatment position. The sections should then be slowly unlocked, after the traction force has been applied, to control the speed at which the initial traction force is applied.

3. Apply the appropriate belts or halter.

Heavy-duty nonslip thoracic and pelvic belts should be used to secure the patient during the application of mechanical lumbar traction (Fig. 10-12, *A*). These belts must be placed with the nonslip surface directly in contact with the patient's skin and not over the clothing, and both belts must be securely tightened to prevent slipping when the traction force is applied.

Clinical Pearl

The nonslip belt surface should be placed directly in contact with the patient's skin and not over clothing.

The belts can either be placed on the table at the appropriate level and then adjusted when the patient lies down on them, or they can be secured around the patient first and then secured to the table after the patient lies down. The thoracic belt is used to stabilize the upper body above the level at which traction force is desired to prevent the patient from being pulled down the table by the force on the pelvic belt and isolate the traction force to the appropriate spinal segments. The thoracic belt should be placed so that its lower edge aligns with the superior limit at which the traction force is desired, and with its upper edge aligned approximately with the xiphoid immediately below the greatest diameter of the thorax. The pelvic belt should be placed so that its superior edge aligns with the inferior limit at which traction force is desired, generally just superior to the iliac crests (or superior to the superior edge of the sacrum if the patient is prone) (see Fig. 10-9).

Newer belts, shaped to be more comfortable than the older models, and with Velcro attachments are also available (Fig. 10-12,

Continued

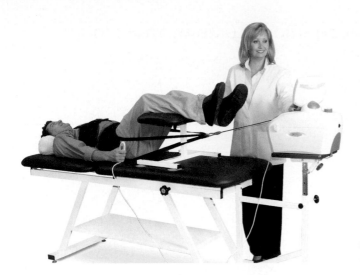

FIG 10-9 Central axis lumbar traction. *Courtesy Chattanooga Group, Hixson, TN.*

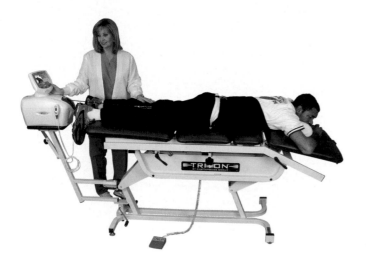

FIG 10-10 Prone lumbar traction with spine in neutral or slight extension. *Courtesy Chattanooga Group, Hixson, TN.*

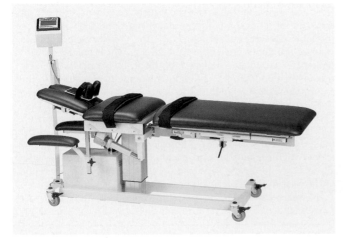

FIG 10-11 Split traction table. *Courtesy The Saunders Group, Chaska, MN.*

APPLICATION TECHNIQUE 10-1   MECHANICAL LUMBAR TRACTION—*cont'd*

B). Their placement is slightly different than for the standard belt, and it is best to follow the manufacturer's instructions when applying these belts. Instructions for applying the type of belt shown in Figure 10-12, *B*, are included on the Evolve web site.

When the patient is supine with the lumbar spine in slight flexion, as recommended to maximize distraction of the posterior spinal structures, the pelvic belt should be placed with the fastening anteriorly and the rope posteriorly so that the pull is primarily from the posterior aspect of the pelvis (see Fig. 10-9). When the patient is prone, with the lumbar spine in neutral or slight extension, as recommended to maximize distraction of the anterior spinal structures, the pelvic belt may be placed with the fastening posteriorly and the rope anteriorly so that the pull is primarily from the anterior aspect of the pelvis.[65]

4. Connect the belts or halter to the traction device. Fasten the thoracic belt to the table above the patient's head and connect the pelvic belt to the traction unit using a rope and a spreader bar.
5. Set the appropriate traction parameters (Table 10-1). See also the discussion of parameters in the next section. Select static or intermittent traction and then for static traction, set the maximum traction force and the total traction duration, or for intermittent traction, set the maximum and minimum traction force, hold and relax times, and the total traction duration.
6. Start the traction.

When applying traction to the lumbar spine, if a split table is being used, first allow the traction to pull for one hold cycle to take up the slack in the belt and rope and then during the following relaxation of the traction, release the sections of the table slowly. If static traction is being used, the sections of the table may be released after the traction force is applied. The therapist should manually control the rate of separation of the sections to prevent sudden motion of the patient and the lower section of the table. If a split table is not available, the traction device will take up the slack in the belt and rope during the first hold cycle. When using a split table, once the sections are released, the force of the traction pulls the patient and the lower section of the table simultaneously and so does not have to overcome friction between the patient and the surface of the table. For this to occur, it is essential that the lower section of the table actually move back and forth during the hold and relax cycles, rather than being stationary at its position of maximal excursion, where it will act as a static surface. The clinician should observe the traction being applied and the movement of the table for a few cycles and then make any necessary adjustments to ensure that the traction is producing the desired effect.

7. Assess the patient's response.

It is recommended that the clinician assess the patient's initial response to the application of traction within the first 5 minutes of treatment so that any adjustments can be made at that time if needed.

8. Give the patient a means to call you and to stop the traction.

Most electrical mechanical traction units are equipped with a patient safety cutoff switch that turns off the unit and rings a bell when activated. Instruct the patient to use this switch if he or she experiences any increase in or peripheralization of pain or other symptoms.

9. Release traction and assess the patient's response.

When the traction time is completed, lock the split sections of the table, release the tension on the traction ropes, and allow the patient to rest briefly before getting up and recompressing the joints. Then reexamine the patient.

TABLE 10-1   Recommended Parameters for the Application of Lumbar Spinal Traction

Area of Spine and Goals of Treatment	Force	Hold/Relax Times (seconds)	Total Traction Time (minutes)
Initial/acute phase	13-20 kg (29-44 lbs)	Static	5 to 10
Joint distraction	22.5 kg (50 lbs); 50% of body weight	15/15	20 to 30
Decrease muscle spasm	25% of body weight	5/5	20 to 30
Disc problems or stretch soft tissue	25% of body weight	60/20	20 to 30

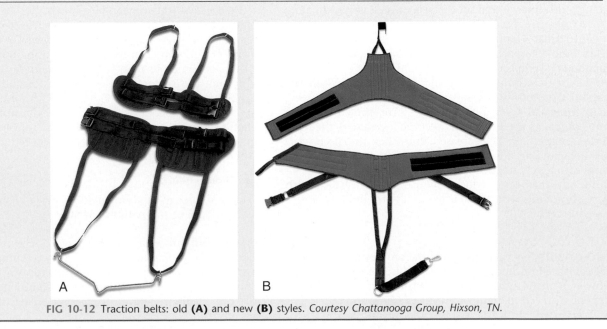

A   B

FIG 10-12 Traction belts: old **(A)** and new **(B)** styles. *Courtesy Chattanooga Group, Hixson, TN.*

MECHANICAL LUMBAR TRACTION

Parameters for Mechanical Lumbar Traction

Static Versus Intermittent Traction. Mechanical traction may be administered statically, with the same force throughout the treatment, or intermittently, with the force varying every few seconds throughout the treatment. Some authors recommend that only static traction be applied to avoid a stretch reflex of the muscles[11]; however, others report that static and intermittent traction are equally effective but that higher forces can be used with intermittent traction.[66] No differences in lumbar sacrospinalis electromyographic (EMG) activity or vertebral separation have been found when static and intermittent traction of the same force have been compared.[67,68] It is generally recommended that static traction be used if the area being treated is inflamed, if the patient's symptoms are easily aggravated by motion, or if the patient's symptoms are related to a disc protrusion.[11] Intermittent traction with long hold times may also be effective for treatment of symptoms related to disc protrusion, whereas shorter hold and relax times are recommended for symptoms related to joint dysfunctions.

> ### ◎ Clinical Pearl
>
> Static traction is useful for inflammation, symptoms aggravated by motion, and symptoms caused by a disc protrusion. Intermittent traction is useful for symptoms caused by a disc protrusion or joint dysfunction.

Hold and Relax Times. If intermittent traction is selected, the maximum traction force is applied during the hold time and a lower traction force is applied during the relax time. The recommended ratio and duration of the hold and relax times depend on the patient's condition and tolerance. In general, if intermittent traction is used for treatment of a disc problem, longer hold times, approximately 60 seconds, and shorter relax times, approximately 20 seconds, are recommended, whereas if traction is being used to treat a spinal joint problem, shorter hold and relax times of approximately 15 seconds each are recommended.[13] Symptom severity should also be used as a guide for determining hold and relax times. When the patient's symptoms are severe, both long hold and long relax times are recommended to limit the amount of movement. As the symptoms become less severe, the relax time can gradually be decreased, and when the discomfort has decreased to a local ache rather than a pain, the hold time can also be reduced so that when the symptoms are mild, the traction produces an oscillatory motion with very short hold and relax times of approximately 3 to 5 seconds each.

Force. Authors vary in their recommendations with regard to the amount of force to be used for traction; however, most agree that the optimal amount of force depends on the patient's clinical presentation, the goals of treatment, and the patient's position during treat-

ment.[11,19,20] For all applications, the force should be kept low during the initial traction session to reduce the risk of reactive muscle guarding and spasms and to determine if traction is likely to aggravate the patient's symptoms. The traction force can be increased gradually in subsequent sessions as the patient becomes used to the procedure. It is recommended that, for all applications, the traction force to the lumbar spine start at between 13 and 20 kg (30 and 45 lb).

> ### ◎ Clinical Pearl
>
> The traction force to the lumbar spine should start at between 13 and 20 kg (30 and 45 lb).

When the goal is to decrease compression on a spinal nerve root or facet joint, sufficient force to separate the facet joints in the area being treated must be used. In the lumbar spine, it has been shown that this requires a force of between 22.5 kg (50 lb) and approximately 60% of the patient's body weight.[13,67,69]

When the goal is to decrease muscle spasm, stretch soft tissue, or exert a centripetal force on the disc by spinal elongation without joint surface separation, lower forces of 25% of total body weight for the lumbar spine are generally effective. When this is the goal, the application of a hot pack in conjunction with the traction may result in greater spinal elongation and thus more effective relief of symptoms.

Higher traction forces are needed when patient positioning, or the harness or table, requires the traction force to overcome gravity or friction between the patient and the table. For example, when lumbar traction is applied without a split table and the traction has to overcome the friction between the patient's body and the surface of the table, higher traction forces may be necessary, whereas when gravity and friction are reduced, as occurs with lumbar traction when a split table is used, lower traction forces may be sufficient.

The force of traction can be adjusted during or between treatments. The force should be decreased during the treatment if there is any peripheralization of signs or symptoms or, as mentioned in the section on precautions, if there is complete relief of severe pain. If the patient's symptoms are moderately decreased by traction, the force can be increased by 2 to 5 kg (5 to 15 lb) for lumbar traction at each subsequent treatment session until maximal relief of symptoms is achieved. Traction force to the lumbar spine should generally not exceed 50% of the patient's body weight.

> ### ◎ Clinical Pearl
>
> Traction force to the lumbar spine should generally not exceed 50% of the patient's weight.

When intermittent traction is used, the relaxed force should be approximately 50% of the maximum force or less; however, total release of the force during the relaxed phase of intermittent traction is not recommended because this can result in rebound aggravation of the patient's symptoms.

Total Treatment Duration. There are no published studies comparing the effects of different traction treatment durations; however, most authors recommend that the duration of a patient's first treatment with traction be brief (i.e., about 5 minutes if the initial symptoms are severe and 10 minutes if the initial symptoms are moderate) to assess the patient's response.[13,70] If severe symptoms are significantly relieved by brief low-force traction, the duration of treatment should be kept short; otherwise, symptom exacerbation after the treatment is likely. If the patient's symptoms are partially relieved after 10 minutes of traction, it is recommended that the duration of the initial treatment not be extended; however, if symptoms are unchanged after 10 minutes, the hold force may be increased slightly or the angle of pull modified, and treatment may be continued for a further 10 minutes. Recommendations for the duration of subsequent treatments vary from as short as 8 to 10 minutes for treatment of a disc protrusion[13] to as long as 20 to 40 minutes for this and other indications.[41] Treatment for longer than 40 minutes is generally thought to provide no additional benefit.

Treatment Frequency. Some authors state that spinal traction must be administered daily to be effective; however, there are no published studies evaluating the outcome of different treatment frequencies.[13,41]

APPLICATION TECHNIQUE 10-2 | MECHANICAL CERVICAL TRACTION

Equipment Required for Electrical Mechanical Traction

- Traction unit
- Cervical traction halter
- Spreader bar
- Extension rope

Equipment Required for Weighted Mechanical Traction

- Traction device (ropes, pulley, weights)
- Cervical traction halter
- Weight bag for water, weights, or sand

Procedure for Mechanical Cervical Traction[71]

1. Select the appropriate mechanical traction device.

    Various devices are available for applying mechanical traction to the cervical spine in the clinic or home setting. The choice depends on the region of the body to be treated, the amount of force to be applied, whether static or intermittent traction is desired, and the setting in which the treatment will be applied.

2. Determine optimal patient position.

    When positioning the patient, try to achieve a comfortable position that allows muscle relaxation while maximizing the separation between the involved structures. The relative degree of flexion or extension of the spine during traction determines which surfaces are most effectively separated.[37] The flexed position results in greater separation of the posterior structures, including the facet joints and intervertebral foramina, whereas the neutral or extended position results in greater separation of the anterior structures, including the disc spaces (see Fig. 10-8). In most cases, a symmetrical central force is used, in which the direction of force is in line with the central sagittal axis of the patient; however, if the patient presents with unilateral symptoms, a unilateral traction force that applies more force to one side of the spine than to the other may prove to be more effective.[62] A unilateral force can be applied by offsetting the axis of the traction in the direction that most reduces the patient's symptoms. For example, if the patient presents with right neck or arm pain that is aggravated by right side bending and is relieved by left side bending, the traction should be offset so as to apply a left side bending force.

    For the application of traction to the cervical spine, the patient may be in the supine or the sitting position (Fig. 10-13 and see Fig. 10-6). Certain cervical traction devices can only be used in one of these positions, whereas others can be used in either position. For example, over-the-door cervical traction units must be applied with the patient sitting, whereas the Saunders occipital cervical traction halter can only be used with the patient supine. In the supine position, the cervical spine is supported and non–weight-bearing, resulting in increased patient comfort and muscle relaxation and greater separation between the cervical segments than when the same amount of traction force is applied with the patient in the sitting position.[15] When the patient is supine, cervical flexion, rotation, and sidebending can be adjusted for patient comfort and to focus the traction force on the involved area. When cervical traction is applied in the sitting position, cervical flexion and extension can be controlled to a limited degree by placing the patient facing toward (more flexion) or away from (neutral or more extension) the traction force; however, cervical sidebending and rotation are difficult to adjust in the sitting position. Placing the cervical spine in a neutral or slightly extended position focuses the traction forces on the upper cervical spine, whereas placing the cervical spine in a flexed position focuses the traction forces on the lower cervical spine.[48,72] Maximum posterior elongation of the cervical spine is achieved when the neck and angle of pull are approximately 25 to 35 degrees of flexion, as shown in Figure 10-13.[48,73]

3. Apply the appropriate halter.

    Different cervical halters have been developed to maximize patient comfort and avoid excessive pressure on the TMJs during

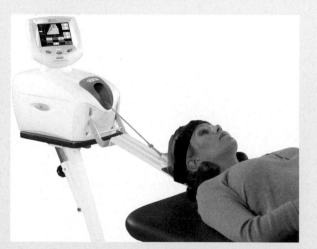

FIG 10-13 Supine cervical traction with soft occipital halter with approximately 20- to 30-degree angle of pull to maximize separation of the intervertebral foramina and disc spaces. *Courtesy Chattanooga Group, Hixson, TN.*

Continued

the application of cervical traction (see Figs. 10-7 and 10-13). There are soft fabric halters that apply pressure through both the mandibles and the occiput, and soft fabric halters that apply pressure only through the occiput. The Saunders frictionless traction halter, which is solid and padded, is also designed to apply pressure only through the occiput. The adjustability of the halter, the patient position, and the status of the TMJs should all be considered in selecting the most appropriate cervical halter for a particular patient. The halter should be adjustable to accommodate variations in the shape and size of patients' heads and necks and to allow for different angles of traction pull. A halter that applies force through the mandibles and the occiput should allow adjustment of the distance between the occiput and spreader bar, the chin and spreader bar, and the mandibles and occiput. The tension on the straps should be adjusted so that the pull is comfortably and evenly applied to both the occiput and the mandibles. A halter that only applies pressure through the occiput should allow size adjustment and should be adjusted to fit snugly enough to stay on during the application of traction. The soft halters can be used in the sitting or supine position, whereas the Saunders halter can only be used in the supine position; however, the soft halters that apply pressure through the occiput tend to slip off the patient's head when traction is applied, even when appropriately adjusted for size, whereas the Saunders halter, which also avoids pressure on the TMJs, generally remains securely in place when traction is applied. The Saunders halter is also designed with a low-friction sliding component for the patient's head so that the traction force does not have to overcome friction between the patient's head and the table. Therefore slightly less force should be applied when using this type of halter than when using a soft fabric halter.

4. Connect the belts or halter to the traction device.

For cervical traction, all types of soft fabric halters are connected to the traction device by a rope and spreader bar, and the Saunders halter is connected directly to the traction device by a rope.

5. Set the appropriate traction parameters (Table 10-2; see parameter discussion in the next section).

Select static or intermittent traction and then for static traction, set the maximum traction force and the total traction duration, or for intermittent traction, set the maximum and minimum traction force, hold and relax times, and the total traction duration.

6. Start the traction.

The patient should be observed for the first few cycles of cervical traction to ensure that the halter is staying in place and exerting force through the appropriate areas and to ensure that the patient is comfortable and not experiencing any adverse effects from the treatment.

7. Assess the patient's response.

It is recommended that the clinician assess the patient's initial response to the application of traction within the first 5 minutes of treatment so that any adjustments can be made at that time if needed.

8. Give the patient a means to call you and to stop the traction.

Most electrical mechanical traction units are equipped with a patient safety cutoff switch that turns off the unit and rings a bell when activated. Instruct the patient to use this switch if he or she experiences any increase in or peripheralization of pain or other symptoms.

9. Release traction and assess the patient's response.

When the traction time is completed, lock the split sections of the table, release the tension on the traction ropes, and allow the patient to rest briefly before getting up and recompressing the joints. Then reexamine the patient.

TABLE 10-2	Recommended Parameters for the Application of Cervical Spine Traction			
Area of the Spine and Goals of Treatment	**Total Traction Force**	**Hold/Relax Times (seconds)**	**Total Traction (minutes)**
Initial/acute phase	3 to 4 kg (7 to 9 lbs)	Static	5 to 10
Joint distraction	9 to 13 kg (20 to 29 lbs); 7% of body weight	15/15	20 to 30
Decrease muscle spasm	5 to 7 kg (11 to 15 lbs)	5/5	20 to 30
Disc problems or stretch soft tissue	5 to 7 kg (11 to 15 lbs)	60/20	20 to 30

MECHANICAL CERVICAL TRACTION

Parameters for Mechanical Cervical Traction

The principles for selecting parameters for mechanical cervical traction are similar to those used for lumbar traction, with a few exceptions mentioned in the next section. For a detailed discussion of the principles for selecting treatment parameters for mechanical cervical traction, see the previous section on mechanical lumbar traction. It should be noted that cervical traction uses far less force than lumbar traction.

Intermittent traction may be most effective for reducing pain and increasing cervical ROM in a variety of cervical conditions[74] and may be particularly helpful for reducing symptoms associated with mechanical neck disorders.[75]

Force. The greatest difference between parameters used for lumbar and cervical traction is the amount of force. For all cervical traction applications, the traction force should start at 3 to 4 kg (8 to 10 lb).

When the goal is to decrease compression on a spinal nerve root or facet joint, sufficient force to separate the facet joints in the area being treated must be used. In the cervical spine, 9 to 13 kg (20 to 30 lb), or approximately 7% of the patient's body weight, is generally sufficient to achieve this outcome.[13,67,69] When the goal is to decrease muscle spasm, stretch soft tissue, or exert a centripetal force on the disc by spinal elongation without joint surface separation, 5 to 7 kg (12 to 15 lb) of force will generally be effective. Applying a hot pack in conjunction with the traction may result in greater spinal elongation and thus more effective relief of symptoms.

Higher traction forces are needed when patient positioning, or the harness or table, requires the traction force to overcome gravity or friction. For cervical traction, higher forces are needed when the patient is sitting and the traction has to overcome the force of gravity on the patient's head. In contrast, when the patient is supine, gravity is not opposing the force of the traction and if the Saunders frictionless halter is used, there is little friction, so lower traction forces may be sufficient.

The force of traction can be adjusted during or between treatments. The force should be decreased during the treatment if there is any peripheralization of signs or symptoms or, as mentioned in the section on precautions, if there is complete relief of severe pain. If the patient's symptoms are moderately decreased by mechanical cervical traction, the traction force can be increased by 1.5 to 2 kg (3 to 5 lb) at each subsequent treatment session until maximal relief of symptoms is achieved. Traction force to the cervical spine should generally not exceed 13.5 kg (30 lb).

SELF-TRACTION

Self-traction is a form of traction that uses gravity and the weight of the patient's body, or force exerted by the patient, to exert a distractive force on the spine. Self-traction can be used for the lumbar but not the cervical spine.

Self-traction of the lumbar spine is appropriate for home use by the patient whose symptoms are relieved by low loads of mechanical traction or that are associated with mild to moderate compression of spinal structures. Because the amount and duration of force that can be applied by self-traction is limited by the upper body strength of the patient and the weight of the lower body, self-traction is not generally effective when high forces are required to relieve symptoms with mechanical traction or when distraction of the spinal joints is necessary. Self-traction can be applied in a several ways, a few of which are described in Application Technique 10-3. All methods of self-traction attempt to fix the patient's upper body and use either the body weight or the force of the arms to pull on the lumbar spine. Positions and ways to apply self-traction other than those described can be developed by the clinician or the patient who is familiar with the principles of self-traction.

APPLICATION TECHNIQUE 10-3 — SELF-TRACTION

Procedure for Self-Traction: Sitting

The patient should do the following:
1. Sit in a sturdy chair with arms.
2. Hold on to the arms of the chair and push down with the arms, lifting the trunk to reduce the weight on the spine (Fig. 10-14). The patient may grade the force of the traction by varying the force of the downward pressure on the arms of the chair and thus the degree of unweighting of the spine; however, the patient should keep the feet on the floor at all times in order to control lumbopelvic position.

Procedure for Self-Traction: Between Corner Counters

The patient should do the following:
1. Stand in a corner with solid counter surfaces behind the patient.
2. Place the forearms on the counter and push down with the arms in order to decrease the weight on the spine by unweighting the feet (Fig. 10-15). The patient should leave the feet on the ground in order to control lumbopelvic position.

Procedure for Self-Traction: Overhead Bar

The patient should do the following:
1. Stand in a partial squat under a horizontal bar.
2. Hold onto the bar and pull to reduce the weight on the spine (Fig. 10-16). The patient should leave the feet on the ground in order to control lumbopelvic position.

Advantages

- Minimal or no equipment needed.
- Easy for patient to perform.
- Easy for patient to control.
- Can be performed in many environments and thus many times during the day.

Disadvantages

- Low maximum force, therefore may not be effective.
- Requires strong, injury-free upper extremities.
- Cannot be used for the cervical spine.
- No research data to support the efficacy of this form of traction.
- Patient must have adequate postural awareness and control to position the body appropriately for maximum benefit.

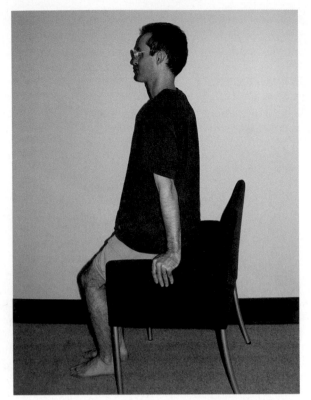

FIG 10-14 Sitting self-traction for the lumbar spine.

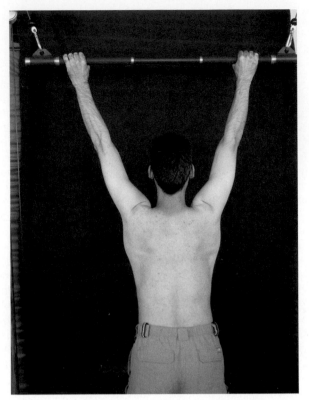

FIG 10-16 Self-traction with overhead bar.

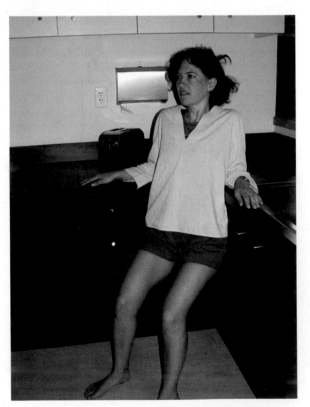

FIG 10-15 Self-traction between corner counters.

POSITIONAL TRACTION

Positional traction involves prolonged placement of the patient in a position that places tension on one side of the lumbar spine only (Fig. 10-17). This type of traction gently stretches the lumbar spine by applying a prolonged low-load longitudinal force to one side of the spine. Although the low force associated with this form of traction is unlikely to cause joint distraction, it may effectively decrease muscle spasm, stretch soft tissue, or exert a centripetal force on the disc by spinal elongation without joint surface separation. Positional traction may be used to treat unilateral symptoms originating from the lumbar spine and can be a valuable component of a patient's home program during the early stages of recovery when symptoms are severe and irritable.

MANUAL TRACTION

Manual traction is the application of force by the therapist in the direction of distracting the joints. It can be used for the cervical and lumbar spine, as well as for the peripheral joints. There are many techniques for applying manual traction; however, because manual traction is generally classified as manual therapy rather than as a physical agent, only a few basic techniques for applying manual traction to the spine are described here. For more detailed descriptions of these and other techniques for applying manual traction to the spine or to the peripheral joints, please consult a manual therapy text.[11,76]

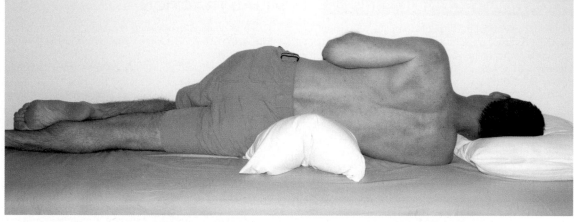

FIG 10-17 Positional traction to stretch and distract the left lumbar area.

APPLICATION TECHNIQUE 10-4 — POSITIONAL LUMBAR TRACTION

Equipment Required

- Pillow(s)

Procedure

The patient should do the following:
1. Lie on the side, with the involved side up and a pillow under the waist at approximately the level of the dysfunction. The pillow acts to sidebend the lumbar spine away from the involved side, opening the joints and disc spaces on the involved side.
2. Rotate toward the involved side by moving the lower shoulder forward and the upper shoulder back.
3. Rotate further toward the involved side by straightening the inferior lower extremity, bending the superior lower extremity, and hooking the superior foot behind the inferior leg. Rotation toward the involved side further stretches and opens the involved area.

4. Adjust flexion/extension to the position of greatest comfort and symptom relief.
5. Maintain the position for 10 to 20 minutes.

Advantages

- Requires no equipment or assistance.
- Inexpensive.
- Can be applied by the patient at home.
- Low force, thus not likely to aggravate an irritable condition.
- Position readily adjustable.

Disadvantages

- Low force, thus not likely to be effective where joint distraction is required.
- Requires agility and skill by the patient to perform correctly.
- No research data to support the efficacy of this form of traction.

APPLICATION TECHNIQUE 10-5 — MANUAL TRACTION

Procedure for Manual Lumbar Traction

1. Position the patient in the position of least pain. This is usually supine, with the hips and knees flexed.
2. Position yourself. Kneel at the patient's feet, facing the patient.
3. Place your hands in the appropriate position, behind the patient's proximal legs, over the muscle belly of the triceps surae (Fig. 10-18).
4. Apply traction force to the patient's spine by leaning your body back and away from the patient, keeping your spine in a neutral position.
5. Maintain this force for at least 15 seconds. Apply the force for 5 minutes or longer, for static traction, if the patient's symptoms are relieved by traction and aggravated by motion. Apply the force for 15 to 30 seconds, then release for 15 to 30 seconds, for intermittent traction, for patients whose symptoms are relieved by traction and motion.
   Adjust the force of the traction according to the desired outcome and the patient's report.

Procedure for Manual Cervical Traction: Patient Supine

1. Position the patient supine.
2. Position yourself. Stand at the head of the patient, facing the patient.
3. Place your hands in the appropriate position. Supinate your forearms so your hands are facing up; place the lateral border of your second finger in contact with the patient's occiput and your thumbs behind the patient's ears.
4. Apply traction. Apply force through the occiput by leaning back, keeping your spine in a neutral position (Fig. 10-19).

Procedure for Manual Cervical Traction: Patient Sitting

1. Position the patient in the sitting position.
2. Stand behind the patient.
3. Place your hands in the appropriate position. With your arms in a neutral position, place your thumbs under the patient's occiput and the rest of your hands along the side of the patient's face.

Continued

| APPLICATION TECHNIQUE 10-5 | MANUAL TRACTION—*cont'd* |

4. Apply traction. Apply traction through the patient's occiput by lifting up (Fig. 10-20).

Adjust the force of the traction according to the desired outcome and the patient's report. Manual traction to the cervical spine may also be static or intermittent.

Advantages

- No equipment required.
- Short setup time.
- Force can be finely graded.
- Clinician is present throughout treatment to monitor and assess the patient's response.

- Can be applied briefly, before setting up mechanical traction, to help determine if longer application of traction will be beneficial.
- Can be used with patients who do not tolerate being placed in halters or belts.

Disadvantages

- Limited maximum traction force, probably not sufficient to distract the lumbar facet joints.
- Amount of traction force cannot be easily replicated or specifically recorded.
- Cannot be applied for a prolonged period of time.
- Requires a skilled clinician to apply.

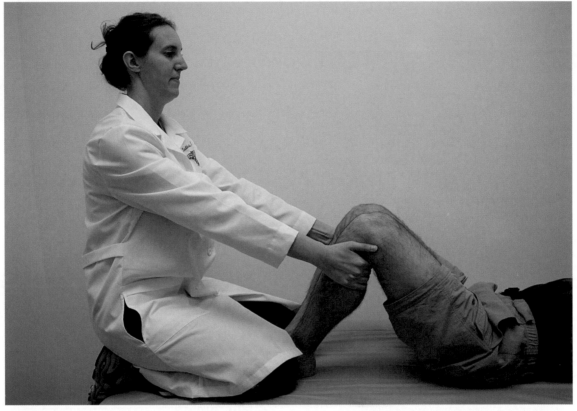

FIG 10-18 Manual lumbar traction.

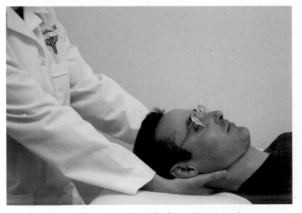

FIG 10-19 Manual cervical traction—supine.

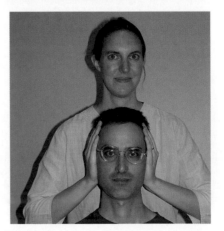

FIG 10-20 Manual cervical traction—sitting.

DOCUMENTATION

When applying traction, document the following:
- Type of traction
- Area of the body where traction is applied
- Patient's position
- Type of halter if one is used
- Maximum force
- Total treatment time
- Response to treatment

With intermittent traction, also document the following:
- Hold time
- Relax time
- Force during the relax time

Documentation is typically written in the SOAP (Subjective, Objective, Assessment, Plan) note format. The following examples only summarize the modality component of treatment and are not intended to represent a comprehensive plan of care.

EXAMPLES

When applying intermittent (int) mechanical (mech) cervical (cerv) traction (txn) to an upper extremity (UE), document the following:

S: Pt reports R UE pain from shoulder to wrist aggravated by turning his neck to the right or bending his neck backward.

O: Pretreatment: R UE pain 6/10 from shoulder to wrist. Cervical ROM 20% backward bend, 20% R sidebend, aggravating R UE pain.

Intervention: Int mech cerv txn, pt supine, soft occipital halter. 10 kg/5 kg, 60 sec/20 sec, 15 min.

Posttreatment: R UE pain 4/10 from shoulder to elbow. Cervical ROM 40% backward bend, 50% R sidebend.

A: Pt tolerated cerv txn well, with decreased pain and increased cervical ROM.

P: Continue int mech cerv txn, pt supine, soft occipital halter. Increase force to 12 kg/7 kg next treatment.

When instructing a patient in the application of self-traction to a lower extremity (LE), document the following:

S: Pt reports low back and L LE pain that increases with sitting.

O: Pretreatment: Pt unable to sit >30 min without low back and L LE pain increasing to 8/10.

Intervention: Pt instructed in self-traction in chair with arms. Pt unweighted approx 50% of body weight, 30 sec hold/relax × 3.

Posttreatment: Low back and L LE pain decreased 50% for 2-3 hr after self-traction, pt able to continue working in sitting position for 2 hr without getting out of his chair.

A: Pt able to perform self-traction appropriately and had improved symptoms.

P: Pt advised to perform self-traction as above every 20 min at work.

When applying lumbar positional traction, document the following:

S: Pt reports low back pain that awakens her 3-5 × per night.

O: Pretreatment: Low back pain 5/10 when lying in bed at night.

Intervention: Lumbar positional traction, R sidelying with pillow at waist, R sidebend, L rotation × 20 minutes.

Posttreatment: Pain decreased to 2/10.

A: Pt had successful trial of positional traction with decreased pain.

P: Pt to perform traction as above at home 2-3 × per day, including immediately before sleeping.

CLINICAL CASE STUDIES

The following case studies summarize the concepts of spinal traction discussed in this chapter. Based on the scenario presented, an evaluation of the clinical findings and goals of treatment are proposed. These are followed by a discussion of the factors to be considered in the selection of spinal traction as the indicated intervention and in selection of the ideal patient position, traction technique, and traction parameters to promote progress toward the goals.

CASE STUDY 10-1

Radiating Lower Back Pain
Examination
History

TR is a 45-year-old man who has been referred to physical therapy with a diagnosis of a right L5, S1 radiculopathy. He reports constant mild to moderately severe (4-7/10) right low back pain that radiates to his right buttock and lateral thigh after sitting for more than 20 minutes and that is relieved to some degree by walking or lying down. He reports no numbness, tingling, or weakness of the lower extremities. The pain started about 6 weeks ago, the morning after TR spent a day stacking firewood, at which time he woke up with severe low back pain and right lower extremity pain down to his lateral calf; he also had difficulty standing up straight. He had similar problems in the past; however, they always resolved fully after a couple of days of bed rest and a few aspirins. TR first saw his doctor regarding his present problem 5 weeks ago and at that time was prescribed a nonsteroidal antiinflammatory drug (NSAID) and a muscle relaxant and was told to take it easy. His symptoms improved to their current level over the next 2 weeks but have not changed since that time. He has also been unable to return to his job as a telephone installer since the onset of symptoms 6 weeks ago. An MRI scan last week showed a mild posterolateral disc bulge at L5-S1 on the right. The patient has had no previous physical therapy for his back problem.

Tests and Measures

The patient's weight is 91 kg (200 lb). The objective examination is significant for a 50% restriction of lumbar ROM in forward bending and right sidebending, both of

Continued

which cause increased right low back and lower extremity pain. Left sidebending decreases the patient's pain. Passive straight leg raising is 35 degrees on the right, limited by right lower extremity pain, and 60 degrees on the left, limited by hamstring tightness. Palpation reveals stiffness and tenderness to right unilateral posterior-anterior pressure at L5-S1 and no notable areas of hypermobility. All other tests including lower extremity sensation, strength, and reflexes are within normal limits.

What is the likely cause of this patient's problem? What symptoms point to this as the cause? What type of traction would be most suitable? Why did you select this type of traction?

Evaluation, Diagnosis, Prognosis, and Goals
Evaluation and Goals

ICF Level	Current Status	Goals
Body function and structure	Right low back pain with radiation to right buttock and lateral thigh Restricted lumbar ROM Restricted lumbar nerve root mobility on the right (limited right straight leg raise) Bulging L5-S1 disc	Decrease pain to 1/10-3/10 in 1 week Eliminate pain completely in 3 weeks Return lumbar ROM and SLR to normal
Activity	Decreased sitting tolerance Unable to stand straight or lift	Increase sitting tolerance to 1 hour in 1 week Stand straight in 1 week Lift 20 lbs in 2 weeks
Participation	Unable to work	Return to limited work duties within 2 weeks Return to full work duties within 1 month

Diagnosis
Preferred Practice Pattern 4F: Impaired joint mobility, motor function, muscle performance, ROM, and reflex integrity associated with spinal disorders.

Prognosis/Plan of Care
The distribution of this patient's pain and its response to changes in loading indicate that his symptoms are probably related to the mild posterolateral disc bulge at L5-S1 on the right noted on his MRI scan. Traction is an indicated intervention for reducing symptoms associated with a disc bulge or lumbar nerve root compression and therefore should be considered for this patient. Studies have shown that lumbar traction can reduce disc protrusions and effectively relieve related symptoms. Traction is most likely to be effective for this patient if it is applied in conjunction with other treatment techniques, including strengthening, stabilization and stretching exercises, joint mobilization, and body mechanics training. Treatment in the clinic should be integrated with a complete home program. The use of spinal traction is not contraindicated in this patient because there is no displaced fragment of anulus or areas of hypermobility and there are no indications of a hiatal hernia or a cardiac or pulmonary condition that may be aggravated by use of the belts for mechanical traction.

Intervention
Electric mechanical traction is the best option for this patient because this type of traction allows the greatest control of lumbar traction force and the application of sufficient force to distract the lumbar vertebrae. Prone positioning, if tolerated, will place the spine in a neutral or slightly extended position and thus provide greater separation of the disc spaces anteriorly and to localize the force to the lower lumbar segments.

A traction force of 25% of the patient's body weight may be sufficient to help this patient reach the set goals of treatment because this amount of traction force can produce a centripetal force on the lumbar disc and reduce a disc displacement. However, traction force as much as 50% of the patient's body weight may be needed if joint distraction is required to alleviate this patient's symptoms. Initial treatment should use a low force of approximately 25% of the patient's body weight, or 13 to 20 kg (25 to 50 lb), to allow assessment of the patient's response to the intervention and minimize the risk of protective muscle spasms. The traction force may then be increased for subsequent treatments, if necessary, until a level is reached at which the patient responds with approximately a 50% reduction in symptom severity after treatment. The application of a hot pack in conjunction with traction may improve the patient's response to the intervention by increasing superficial tissue extensibility and decreasing pain.[31,32]

Intermittent traction with a long hold time, approximately 60 seconds, and a short relax time, approximately 20 seconds, is likely to have most effect on the discs. Static traction may also be effective. The initial treatment should be limited to 10 minutes if the patient reports some reduction of symptoms in this time. If this does not reduce the patient's symptoms, the treatment time may be extended to up to 20 to 40 minutes for subsequent treatments.

If the application of mechanical traction in the manner described relieves this patient's symptoms and particularly if lower forces and lower durations of treatment are effective, the use of self-traction or positional traction at home, with the patient lying on the left side with the left side bent and right rotation, may also help this patient progress toward his treatment goals.

CLINICAL CASE STUDIES—*cont'd*

Documentation

S: Pt reports constant 4-7/10 R low back pain radiating to the R buttock and lateral thigh after sitting for more than 20 minutes, relieved somewhat by walking or lying down.

O: Pretreatment: 50% restricted lumbar ROM with forward bend and R sidebend, limited by R low back and R LE pain 7/10. L sidebend decreases pain. Passive SLR 35 degrees on R, limited by R LE pain, and 60 degrees on L, limited by hamstring tightness. Tenderness to palpation R posterior-anterior pressure at L5-S1.

Intervention: Intermittent mech lumbar txn, pt prone. 22 kg/11 kg (48 lb/24 lb), 60 sec/20 sec, 10 minutes.

Posttreatment: 30% restricted lumbar ROM with R forward and sidebend. Pain 4/10 with R sidebend.

A: Pt tolerated txn well, and symptoms improved.

P: Continue intermittent mech txn at these parameters once daily. Teach patient positional lumbar txn.

CASE STUDY 10-2

Osteoarthritis with Facet Joint Degeneration

Examination

History

AW is a 75-year-old woman who has been referred to physical therapy with a diagnosis of osteoarthritis with moderately severe facet joint degeneration at C4 through C6 observed on x-ray. She complains of bilateral neck pain that is worse on the right than on the left. She also reports that her neck is stiff first thing in the morning, loosening up throughout the day but becoming stiff and sore late in the afternoon and for the rest of the evening. She has no complaints of upper extremity pain or stiffness; however, the neck stiffness makes her feel unsafe while driving, and when the pain is severe, she is unable to participate in her sewing class at the local senior center. She has had similar but gradually worsening symptoms intermittently for the past 20 years, and her symptoms are always more severe during the winter. In the past, AW has been referred to physical therapy for treatment of these symptoms, and her treatment has included traction, heat, massage, and a few exercises. Within four to six visits this combination of interventions helps relieve her symptoms for about a year until the following winter.

Tests and Measures

The objective examination reveals a kyphotic thoracic posture with a forward head position. Cervical ROM is restricted by approximately 50% in all planes, and there is moderate hypertonicity of the cervical paraspinal muscles and stiffness of all the cervical facet joints on passive intervertebral motion testing, with the lower cervical joints being stiffer than the upper cervical joints. Shoulder flexion and abduction are limited to 140 degrees bilaterally, and all other objective tests, including upper extremity sensation, strength, and reflexes, are within normal limits for this patient's age.

What are the indications for spinal traction in this patient? What other physical agent would be useful for this patient in conjunction with traction? How would you improve her long-term benefits? What should you examine (including elements of the history, as well as tests and measures) before applying traction to this patient?

Evaluation, Diagnosis, Prognosis, and Goals
Evaluation and Goals

ICF Level	Current Status	Goals
Body function and structure	Neck pain and stiffness	Decrease pain by 50%
	Kyphotic thoracic posture	Improve posture
	Loss of neck movement in all planes	Prevent symptom recurrence
	Hypertonic paraspinal cervical muscles	Increase active and passive cervical ROM to 75% of normal
	Limited bilateral shoulder flexion and abduction	Improve soft tissue mobility
		Improve shoulder ROM
Activity	Unable to turn head to see far to the side or behind	Improve ability to turn head so patient can see all the way to the side
	Unable to look down to write or sew for >10 minutes	Increase tolerance for looking down to 30 minutes
Participation	Able to drive but feels unsafe	Improve ability to drive safely within 2 weeks
	Unable to participate in sewing class	Return to full participation in sewing class within 2 weeks

Diagnosis

Preferred Practice Pattern 4B: Impaired posture.

Prognosis/Plan of Care

Cervical spinal traction is indicated for the treatment of joint hypomobility, particularly when multiple spinal segments are involved, and for the relief of symptoms caused by subacute joint inflammation. Spinal traction may also help alleviate this patient's spinal pain by gating its transmission at the spinal cord or by reducing joint compression and inflammation. Intermittent traction may help to reduce symptoms resulting from inflammation by facilitating normal fluid exchange in the joints to relieve edema caused by chronic inflammation. This change, combined with stretching of the periarticular soft tissue structures, may increase spinal joint and soft tissue mobility and cervical active ROM. Applying a deep or superficial heating agent to this patient's neck, before or during the application of traction, may optimize the benefits of the treatment by increasing soft tissue extensibility to facilitate greater increases in soft

Continued

CLINICAL CASE STUDIES—*cont'd*

tissue length. As in previous years, traction and other passive modalities alone are likely to result in only temporary control of this patient's symptoms; however, more long-lasting benefits may be achieved by additionally addressing her posture and thoracic mobility and by modifying her home activities.

At the age of 75, this patient should be cleared for impairment of vertebral or carotid artery circulation and for osteoporosis before the application of cervical traction. If she normally wears dentures, she should wear them during the treatment. It is important to not assume that because this patient has tolerated traction well in the past, she will tolerate it equally well at this time, particularly if she has experienced any medical events, such as a cerebrovascular accident, since she was last treated with traction.

Intervention

Once this patient is cleared for the application of traction, a trial of manual traction is recommended to assess her response to traction and to help determine the ideal position before considering the use of other forms of traction. If manual traction affords her some relief of symptoms, then electrical mechanical traction should be used in the clinic to provide optimal efficiency and consistency of treatment. An occipital halter should be used to avoid compression on the temporomandibular joints (TMJs), and the patient should be positioned supine, with her cervical spine in about 24 degrees of flexion, to achieve maximum separation of the lower cervical joints and elongation of the posterior spinal structures.

As with all traction treatments, the force of traction should initially be low, at approximately 4 kg (10 lb), for the first session. The amount of force may then be increased by 1.5 to 2 kg (3 to 5 lb) at each subsequent session until optimal symptom control is achieved. A low amount of force, of 5 to 7 kg (12 to 15 lb), which can elongate the cervical spine without distracting the joints, will probably be sufficient to alleviate this patient's symptoms, and the use of more force will probably not provide greater benefit. The traction force should not exceed 13 kg (30 lb) at any time. Intermittent traction should employ short hold and relax times of approximately 15 seconds each because this ratio is generally effective at reducing symptoms associated with the joints. The total duration of the traction treatment should be between 10 and 40 minutes, depending on the patient's response.

Because this patient presents with recurrent symptoms that are probably a result of progressive and chronic osteoarthritis, it is also recommended that she obtain and be instructed in the use of a simple mechanical traction device, such as an over-the-door cervical traction unit, for use at home. She may then use this device to treat aggravations of similar symptoms that she may experience in the future.

Documentation

S: Pt reports neck stiffness and pain that is worse in the morning and evening.

O: Pretreatment: Pain 7/10. Kyphotic thoracic posture. Cervical ROM restricted by 50% in all planes. Moderate hypertonic cervical paraspinal muscles. Stiff cervical facet joints on passive intervertebral motion testing. Bilateral shoulder flexion and abduction active ROM 140 degrees.

Intervention: Hot pack to neck before txn. After trial of manual txn, intermittent mech cervical txn applied, pt supine, soft occipital halter, cervical spine approx 24 degrees flexion. 4 kg/2 kg (10 lb/5 lb), 15 sec/15 sec, 10 min.

Posttreatment: Pain 3/10. Cervical ROM restricted by 40% in all planes. Cervical paraspinal muscles mildly hypertonic. Shoulder flexion and abduction unchanged.

A: Pt tolerated txn well, with some improvement in symptoms.

P: Continue intermittent mech txn 3x week for the next week, gradually increasing weight or length of time txn is applied. Give pt exercises to improve posture, suggest use of home txn device.

CASE STUDY 10-3

Neck Pain in a Patient with Rheumatoid Arthritis

Examination

History

MS is a 30-year-old female high school teacher. She was diagnosed with rheumatoid arthritis at the age of 22 and has been referred to physical therapy for treatment of neck pain. She complains of constant and severe pain in her neck that is aggravated by all neck movement, and she reports intermittent dizziness that is brought on by moving from sitting to standing or by looking up. The neck pain started about 3 or 4 years ago and has gradually become more severe, while the dizziness started only a few weeks ago. MS reports that at this time the pain keeps her awake at night and the dizziness interferes with her ability to write on the chalkboard when she is at work. MS has no numbness or tingling of her extremities and reports that no x-ray films have been taken of her neck in the last 3 years.

Tests and Measures

Her objective exam reveals postural abnormalities, including standing with approximately 20 degrees of hip and knee flexion bilaterally, bilateral genu valgum, a moderately increased lumbar lordosis, a flat thoracic spine, and a forward head position. The flat thoracic spine and forward head position are maintained in sitting. Cervical ROM testing was deferred at the initial evaluation due to the severity of the patient's reports of pain with motion. Her upper extremity strength was 4+/5 throughout within the available ROM, and her upper extremity sensation and reflexes were within normal limits.

CLINICAL CASE STUDIES—*cont'd*

What part of this patient's history needs further evaluation before the use of traction? Would you expect complete relief of symptoms in this patient?

Evaluation, Diagnosis, Prognosis, and Goals
Evaluation and Goals

ICF Level	Current Status	Goals
Body function and structure	Neck pain and stiffness Dizziness Abnormal posture Limited cervical ROM	Ascertain the ligamentous stability and bony integrity of her upper cervical spine Relieve pain and dizziness Improve cervical ROM
Activity	Unable to sleep Unable to write on chalkboard	Improve sleep until pt able to sleep through night Improve chalkboard writing to 100% of normal in 1 month
Participation	Decreased ability to teach	Return to teaching full time without restrictions in 1 month

Diagnosis
Preferred Practice Pattern 4D: Impaired joint mobility, motor function, muscle performance, and ROM associated with connective tissue dysfunction.

Plan of Care
Although treatment goals could include resolving any of the above impairments or functional limitations, this patient's reports of dizziness associated with neck pain and the diagnosis of rheumatoid arthritis should alert the clinician to the possibility that this patient may have an unstable C1-C2 articulation as a result of ligamentous instability or, she may have osteoporosis as a result of prolonged systemic steroid use. Because instability at C1-C2 poses a significant risk to the patient, and because the presence of osteoporosis requires special caution with the application of traction, the initial goal, before applying traction or any other treatment, should be to ascertain the ligamentous stability and bony integrity of her upper cervical spine. Because these both require radiographic studies that must generally be ordered by a physician, the patient should be referred back to her physician for further evaluation.

If all radiographic reports indicate that her upper cervical spine is stable and that she does not have osteoporosis, she may return to physical therapy for treatment of her complaints, with goals as listed in the previous table. Because this patient has a systemic disease that affects the joints and that appears to have caused permanent changes in other joints, including her hips and knees, complete relief of symptoms or return of ROM will probably not occur.

Prognosis
If all tests indicate that spinal traction is not contraindicated, then traction may improve this patient's cervical mobility and decrease her neck pain. Distraction or mobilization of the cervical joints or relaxation of the cervical paraspinal muscles can achieve these effects. Cervical traction may also help alleviate this patient's dizziness because she associates this symptom with neck motion; however, her dizziness may be a result of an inner ear or vestibular dysfunction, which would also be affected by head position, in which case this symptom would probably not respond to treatment with traction. Although traction may reduce this patient's symptoms sufficiently to allow her to write on a chalkboard, it is recommended that job site adaptations, such as the use of an overhead projector, also be instituted to reduce the stress on her cervical spine.

Intervention
To constantly monitor this patient's severe symptoms and to allow adjustment of the traction force and direction during the treatment, manual traction should be used initially. If the patient reports moderate relief of her pain with manual traction, then optimal cervical positioning for traction should be determined, and static mechanical traction may be substituted if it is thought that a longer duration of treatment would be beneficial. Static cervical traction may be provided by an electrical or weighted device, but in either case, it is recommended that the patient be treated supine rather than sitting, to achieve maximum muscle relaxation, and it is recommended that low forces be used initially because of the severity of the patient's symptoms.

As treatment progresses, the force of traction may be increased up to a maximum of 13 kg (30 lb) to achieve joint distraction if necessary, and intermittent traction may be used if this is more comfortable as the patient tolerates more motion. Treatment with spinal traction should occur in conjunction with postural education and recommendations for home or work site modifications to minimize the risk of symptom reaggravation or progression.

Documentation
S: Pt reports neck pain worsening over the last 4 years and dizziness that began 3 weeks ago, which is worse when looking up and moving from sitting to standing.

O: Pretreatment: Neck pain 8/10. 20 degree hip and knee flexion bilaterally, bilateral genu valgum, lumbar lordosis, flat thoracic spine, and forward head position when standing. Flat thoracic spine and forward head position when sitting. Cervical ROM testing deferred. UE strength 4+/5 throughout.

Continued

CLINICAL CASE STUDIES—*cont'd*

Intervention: Manual txn applied initially. Static cervical mech txn, pt supine, soft occipital halter. 4 kg (10 lb), 10 min.

Posttreatment: Neck pain 6/10. Continued exacerbation of neck pain with neck movement.

A: Pt tolerated txn well, with mildly reduced neck pain.

P: Continue static cervical mech txn and increase weight gradually, as tolerated for further symptom reduction. Postural education. Discuss home and work site modifications with pt.

CHAPTER REVIEW

1. Traction is a mechanical force applied to the body to distract joints, stretch soft tissue, relax muscles, or mobilize joints. Types of spinal traction used today include electrical mechanical traction, weighted mechanical traction, over-the-door cervical traction, various home traction devices, self-traction, positional traction, and manual traction.

2. Traction may be static (continuous force) or intermittent (varying force). Static traction is recommended when the area being treated is inflamed, if the patient's symptoms are aggravated by motion, or if the patient's symptoms are related to a disc protrusion. All the types of spinal traction listed can be used to apply static traction. Intermittent traction is used for symptoms related to disc protrusion and joint dysfunction. Electrical mechanical traction units and manual techniques can be used to apply intermittent traction.

3. Spinal traction can be used to relieve signs, symptoms, and functional limitations associated with disc bulge or herniation, nerve root impingement, joint hypomobility, subacute joint inflammation, and paraspinal muscle spasm. The effects and clinical benefits of spinal traction depend on the amount of force used, the direction of the force, and the status of the area to which the traction is applied.

4. Selection of a spinal traction technique depends on the nature of the problem being treated, specific contraindications, and whether the treatment is to be applied in the clinic or at home.

5. Spinal traction is contraindicated where motion is contraindicated, with an acute injury or inflammation, with joint hypermobility or instability, with peripheralization of symptoms with traction, and with uncontrolled hypertension. Precautions for the application of spinal traction include structural diseases or conditions affecting the spine, when the pressure of the belts may be hazardous, displacement of an anular fragment, medial disc protrusion, severe pain fully relieved by traction, claustrophobia, intolerance of the prone or supine position, disorientation, TMJ problems, and dentures.

6. The reader is referred to the Evolve web site for further exercises and links to resources and references.

ADDITIONAL RESOURCES *evolve*

Web Sites

Chattanooga Group: Chattanooga supplies a variety of physical agents, including traction devices. The web site has product photos and information, including instructions for the use of some products. It is possible to search for products by body part or by modality. www.chattgroup.com

The Saunders Group: Saunders supplies rehabilitation products for musculoskeletal pain. They specialize in patented traction devices, back supports and exercise equipment for neck and back disorders. www.thesaundersgroup.com

GLOSSARY *evolve*

Anulus fibrosus: A ring of fibrocartilage that forms the outer layer of the intervertebral disc.

Herniated disc: Bulging of the intervertebral disc into the spinal canal.

Herniated nucleus pulposus: Bulging of the nucleus pulposus of the intervertebral disc into the spinal canal.

Intermittent traction: Traction in which the force varies every few seconds.

Intervertebral disc: Structure located between the vertebrae that acts as a shock absorber for the spine.

Joint distraction: The separation of two articular surfaces perpendicular to the plane of articulation; the widening of a joint space.

Manual traction: Application of force by the therapist in the direction of distracting the joints.

Mechanical traction (electrical mechanical traction): Application of static or intermittent force by an electrical motor, through belts or a halter, in the direction of distracting the joints of the spine.

Nucleus pulposus: Elastic, pulpy substance found at the center of an intervertebral disc.

Over-the-door cervical traction: Application of static force to the neck, through a halter, using a device hung on a door that can be adjusted to provide differing amounts of distractive force.

Positional traction: Prolonged specific positioning to place tension on one side of the lumbar spine.

Self-traction: A form of traction that uses gravity and the weight of the patient's body, or force exerted by the patient, to exert a distractive force on the spine.

Spondylolisthesis: Forward displacement of one vertebra on another that can cause nerve root compression and pain.

Static traction: Traction in which the same force is applied throughout treatment.

Traction: A mechanical force applied to the body in a way that separates, or attempts to separate, joint surfaces and elongate soft tissues surrounding a joint.

REFERENCES *evolve*

1. Cyriax J: *Textbook of orthopedic medicine*, volume Diagnosis of soft tissue lesions, London, 1982, Bailliere Tindall.
2. Mathews JA, Mills SB, Jenkins YM, et al: Back pain and sciatica: controlled trials of manipulation, traction, sclerosant and epidural injections, *Br J Rheumatol* 26:416-423, 1987.
3. Larsson U, Choler U, Lindstrom A, et al: Auto-traction for treatment of lumbago-sciatica, *Acta Orthoped Scand* 51:791-798, 1980.
4. Lidstrom A, Zachrisson M: Physical therapy on low back pain and sciatica, *Scand J Rehabil Med* 2:37-42, 1970.
5. Moret NC, van der Stap M, Hagmeijer R, et al: Design and feasibility of a randomized clinical trial of vertical traction in patients with a lumbar radicular syndrome, *Man Ther* 3:203-211, 1998.
6. Weber H, Ljunggren E, Walker L: Traction therapy in patients with herniated lumbar intervertebral discs, *J Oslo City Hosp* 34:61-70, 1984.
7. Beurskens AJ, de Vet HC, Koke AJ, et al: Efficacy of traction for nonspecific low back pain: 12-week and 60-month results of a randomized clinical trial, *Spine* 22:2756-2762, 1977.
8. Clarke J, van Tulder M, Blomberg S, et al: Traction for low back pain with or without sciatica: an updated systematic review within the framework of the Cochrane collaboration, *Spine* 31(14):1591-1599, 2006.
9. Goldish GD: Lumbar traction. In Tolison CD, Kriegel ML, eds: *Interdisciplinary rehabilitation of low back pain*, Baltimore, 1989, Williams & Wilkins.
10. Paris SV, Loubert PV: *Foundations of clinical orthopedics*, St Augustine FL, 1990, Institute Press.
11. Maitland GD: *Vertebral manipulation*, ed 5, London, 1986, Butterworth.
12. Tekeoglu I, Adak B, Bozkurt M, et al: Distraction of lumbar vertebrae in gravitational traction, *Spine* 23(9):1061-1063, 1998.
13. Judovich B, Nobel GR: Traction therapy: a study of resistance forces, *Am J Surg* 93:108-114, 1957.
14. Judovich B: Lumbar traction therapy, *JAMA* 159:549, 1955.
15. Deets D, Hands KL, Hopp SS: Cervical traction: a comparison of sitting and supine positions, *Phys Ther* 57:255-261, 1977.
16. Twomey LT: Sustained lumbar traction: an experimental study of long segments, *Spine* 10:146-149, 1985.
17. Onel D, Tuzlaci M, Sari H, et al: Computed tomographic investigation of the effect of traction on lumbar disc herniations, *Spine* 14:82-90, 1989.
18. Grieve GP: *Mobilization of the spine*, ed 4, New York, 1984, Churchill Livingstone.
19. Cyriax J: *Textbook of orthopaedic medicine*, vol II, ed 11, Eastbourne, UK, 1984, Balliere Tindall.
20. Krause M, Refshauge KM, Dessen M, et al: Lumbar spine traction: evaluation of effects and recommended application for treatment, *Man Ther* 5(2):72-81, 2000.
21. Mathews J: Dynamic discography: a study of lumbar traction, *Ann Phys Med* 9:275-279, 1968.
22. Gupta R, Ramarao S: Epidurography in reduction of lumbar disc prolapse by traction, *Arch Phys Med Rehabil* 59:322-327, 1978.
23. Sari H, Akarimak U, Karacan I, et al: Computed tomographic evaluation of lumbar spinal structures during traction, *Physiother Theory Pract* 21(1):3-11, 2005.
24. Meszaros TF, Olson R, Kulig K, et al: Effect of 10%, 30%, and 60% body weight traction on the straight leg raise test of symptomatic patients with low back pain, *J Orthop Sports Phy Ther* 30(10):595-601, 2000.
25. Andersson GBJ, Schultz AB, Nachemson AL: Intervertebral disc pressures during traction, *Scand J Rehabil Med* 9:88-91, 1983.
26. Lundgren AE, Eldevik OP: Auto-traction in lumbar disc herniation with CT examination before and after treatment, showing no change in appearance of the herniated tissue, *J Oslo City Hosp* 36:87-91, 1986.
27. Basmajian JV: *Manipulation, traction and massage*, ed 3, Baltimore, 1985, Williams & Wilkins.
28. Coalchis SC, Strohm BR: Cervical traction relationship of time to varied tractive force with constant angle of pull, *Arch Phys Med Rehabil* 46:815-819, 1965.
29. Worden RE, Humphrey TL: Effect of spinal traction on the length of the body, Arch *Phys Med Rehabil* 45:318-320, 1964.
30. LaBan MM: Collagen tissue: Implications of its response to stress in vitro, *Arch Phys Med Rehabil* 43:461-466, 1962.
31. Lehmann J, Masock A, Warren C, et al: Effect of therapeutic temperatures on tendon extensibility, *Arch Phys Med Rehabil* 51:481-487, 1970.
32. Lentall G, Hetherington T, Eagan J, et al: The use of thermal agents to influence the effectiveness of a low-load prolonged stretch, *J Orthop Sport Phys Ther* 16(5):200-207, 1992.
33. Mathews JA: The effects of spinal traction, *Physiotherapy* 58:64-66, 1972.
34. Wall PD: The mechanisms of pain associated with cervical vertebral disease. In Hirsch C, Zollerman Y, eds: *Cervical pain: proceedings of the International Symposium in Wenner-Gren Center*, Oxford, 1972, Pergamon.
35. Seliger V, Dolejs L, Karas V: A dynamometric comparison of maximum eccentric, concentric and isometric contractions using EMG and energy expenditure measurements, *Eur J Appl Physiol* 45:235-244, 1980.
36. Swezey RL: The modern thrust of manipulation and traction therapy, *Semin Arthritis Rheum* 12:322-331, 1983.
37. Saunders HD: Use of spinal traction in the treatment of neck and back conditions, *Clin Orthop* 179:31-38, 1983.
38. Van der Heijden GJMG, Beurskens AJHM, Assendelft WJJ, et al: The efficacy of traction for back and neck pain: a systematic, blinded review of randomized clinical trial methods, *Phys Ther* 75(2):93-104, 1995.
39. Hood LB, Chrisman D: Intermittent pelvic traction in the treatment of the ruptured intervertebral disc, *Phys Ther* 48:21-30, 1968.
40. Ozturk B, Gunduz OH, Ozoran K, et al: Effect of continuous lumbar traction on the size of herniated disc material in lumbar disc herniation, *Rheumatol Int* 26(7):622-6, 2006 May.
41. Weber H: Traction therapy in sciatica due to disc prolapse, *J Oslo City Hosp* 23:167-176, 1973.
42. Grieve G: *Common vertebral joint problems*, Edinburgh, 1981, Churchill Livingstone.
43. Saunders HD, Saunders R: *Evaluation, treatment and prevention of musculoskeletal disorders*, Bloomington, MN, 1993, Educational Opportunities.
44. Mathews JA, Hickling J: Lumbar traction: a double-blind controlled study of sciatica, *Rheum Rehabil* 14:222-225, 1975.
45. Buerskens AJ, de Vet HC, Koke AJ, et al: Efficacy of traction for non-specific low back pain: a randomized clinical trial, *Lancet* 346(8990):1596-1600, 1995.
46. Buerskens AJ, van der Heijden GJ, de Vet HC, et al: The efficacy of traction for lumbar back pain: design of a randomized clinical trial, *J Manip Physiol Ther* 18(3):141-147, 1995.
47. Pellecchia GL: Lumbar traction: A review of the literature, *J Orthop Sports Phys Ther* 20(5):262-267, 1994.
48. Coalchis SC, Strohm BR: A study of tractive forces and angle of pull on vertebral interspaces in the cervical spine, *Arch Phys Med Rehabil* 46:820-824, 1965.
49. McDonough A: Effect of immobilization and exercise on articular cartilage: a review of the literature, *J Orthop Sport Phys Ther* 3:2-9, 1981.
50. Yates DAH: Indications and contraindications for spinal traction, *Physiotherapy* 54:55-57, 1972.
51. Haskvitz EM, Hanten WP: Blood pressure response to inversion traction, *Phys Ther* 66:1361-1364, 1986.
52. Utti VA, Ege S, Lukman O: Blood pressure and pulse rate changes associated with cervical traction, *Niger J Med* 15(2):141-143, 2006.
53. Quain MB, Tecklin JS: Lumbar traction: its effect on respiration, *Phys Ther* 65:1343-1346, 1985.

54. Frymoyer JW, Moskowitz RW: Spinal degeneration: pathogenesis and medical management. In Frymoyer JW, ed: *The adult spine: principles and practice*, New York, 1991, Raven Press.

55. Eie N, Kristiansen K: Complications and hazards of traction in the treatment of ruptured lumbar intervertebral disks, *J Oslo City Hosp* 12:5-12, 1962.

56. LaBan MM, Macy JA, Meerschaert JR: Intermittent cervical traction: a progenitor of lumbar radicular pain, *Arch Phys Med Rehabil* 73:295-296, 1992.

57. Laban MM, Mahal BS: Intraspinal dural distraction inciting spinal radiculopathy: cranial to caudal and caudal to cranial, *Am J Phys Med Rehabil* 84(2):141-4, 2005.

58. Giankopoulos G, Waylonis GW, Grant PA, et al: Inversion devices: their role in producing lumbar distraction, *Arch Phys Med Rehabil* 66(2):100-102, 1985.

59. Zito M: Effect of two gravity inversion methods on heart rate, systolic brachial pressure, and ophthalmic artery pressure, *Phys Ther* 68:20-25, 1988.

60. Cheatle MD, Esterhai JL: Pelvic traction as treatment for acute back pain, *Spine* 16:1379-1381, 1991.

61. Pal B, Mangion P, Hossain MA, et al: A controlled trial of continuous lumbar traction in the treatment of back pain and sciatica, *Br J Rheumatol* 25:181-183, 1986.

62. Saunders HD: Unilateral lumbar traction, *Phys Ther* 61:221-225, 1981.

63. Weatherell VF: Comparison of electromyographic activity in normal lumbar sacrospinalis musculature during static pelvic traction in two different positions, *J Orthop Sport Phys Ther* 8:382-390, 1987.

64. Goldish GD: A study of mechanical efficiency of split table traction, *Spine* 15:218-219, 1989.

65. Saunders HD: Lumbar traction, *J Orthop Sport Phys Ther* 1:36-41, 1979.

66. Rogoff JB: Motorized intermittent traction. In Basmajian JV, ed: *Manipulation, traction, and massage*, Baltimore, 1985, Williams & Wilkins.

67. Coalchis SC, Strohm BR: Effects of intermittent traction on separation of lumbar vertebrae, *Arch Phys Med Rehabil* 50:251-253, 1969.

68. Hood CJ, Hart DL, Smith HG, et al: Comparison of electromyographic activity in normal lumbar sacrospinalis musculature during continuous and intermittent pelvic traction, *J Orthop Sports Phys Ther* 2:137-141, 1981.

69. Meszaros TF, Olson R, Kulig K, et al: Effect of 10%, 30%, and 60% body weight traction on the straight leg raise test of symptomatic patients with low back pain, *J Orthop Sports Phys Ther* 30(10):595-601, 2000.

70. Hickling J: Spinal traction technique, *Physiother* 58:58-63, 1972.

71. Harris PR: Cervical traction: review of literature and treatment guidelines, *Phys Ther* Aug;57(8):910-914, 1977.

72. Daugherty RJ, Erhard RE: Segmentalized cervical traction. In Kent BE, ed: *International Federation of Orthopaedic Manipulative Therapists Proceedings*, Vail, CO. 1977.

73. Hseuh TC, Ju MS, Chou YL: Evaluation of the effects of pulling angle and force on intermittent cervical traction with the Saunders Halter, *J Formos Med Assoc* 90(12):1234-1239, 1991.

74. Zylbergold RS, Piper MC: Cervical spine disorders: a comparison of three types of traction, *Spine* 10(10):867-871, 1985.

75. Graham N, Gross AR, Goldsmith C, the Cervical Overview Group: Mechanical traction for mechanical neck disorders: a systematic review, *J Rehabil Med* 38(3):145-152, 2006.

76. Maitland GD: *Peripheral manipulation*, ed 3, London, 1991, Butterworth.

Compression

Compression is a mechanical force that increases external pressure on the body or a body part. It is generally used to improve fluid balance and circulation or to modify scar tissue formation. Fluid balance is improved by increasing **hydrostatic pressure** in the intersitial space so that the pressure becomes greater in the interstitial space than in the vessels. This can limit or reverse outflow of fluid from blood vessels and lymphatics. Keeping fluid in, or returning it to, the vessels allows it to circulate rather than accumulate in the periphery. **Compression** can be static, exerting a constant force, or intermittent, with the force varying over time. With **intermittent compression** the pressure may be applied to the entire limb all at one time, or it may be applied sequentially, starting distally and progressing proximally.

The primary clinical application for compression is the control of peripheral **edema** caused by vascular or lymphatic dysfunction; however, this physical agent can also be applied to help prevent the formation of deep venous thromboses, for residual limb shaping after amputation, or to facilitate the healing of venous ulcers.[1-3]

EFFECTS OF EXTERNAL COMPRESSION

IMPROVES VENOUS AND LYMPHATIC CIRCULATION

The controlled application of external compression has a variety of effects on the body that vary with the pressure applied and the nature of the device used.[4] Both static and intermittent compression devices can increase circulation by increasing the hydrostatic pressure in the interstitial space outside the blood and lymphatic vessels. Increasing extravascular pressure can limit the outflow of fluid from the vessels into the interstitial space, where it tends to pool, keeping it in the circulatory system, where it can circulate. Intermittent compression may improve circulation more effectively than **static compression** because the varying amount of pressure is thought to milk fluids from the distal to the proximal vessels.[5,6] When the venous and lymphatic vessels are compressed, the fluid in them is pushed proximally. When compression is then reduced, the vessels open and refill with new fluid from the interstitial space, ready to be pushed proximally at the next compression cycle. Sequential compression is thought to provide more effective milking than single-chamber, intermittent compression because it can cause a wave of vessel constriction moving in a proximal direction to ensure that fluid is pushed along the vessels toward the heart rather than in a distal direction.[5-7] Improving circulation can benefit patients with edema, may help prevent the formation of deep venous thromboses in high-risk patients, and may facilitate the healing of ulcers caused by venous stasis.

LIMITS THE SHAPE AND SIZE OF TISSUE

Static compression garments or bandaging can provide a form to limit the shape and size of new tissue formation.

This type of compression device acts as a second skin, which, having an elastic compression element or being less extensible than skin, limits the shape and size of the tissue. This effect of compression is exploited when compression bandaging or garments are used over residual limbs after amputation, when compression garments are applied over burn-damaged skin, and when compression bandaging or garments are applied to edematous limbs.

INCREASES TISSUE TEMPERATURE

Most compression devices, except those with built-in cooling mechanisms, increase superficial tissue temperature because the device insulates the area to which it is applied. A heavy compression stocking or an air-filled sleeve will act as an insulator, preventing loss of body heat, thereby increasing local superficial tissue temperature. Although the increase in temperature produced by compression garments is not a direct effect of the compressive forces, it has been proposed that the warmth produced by these garments increases the activity of temperature-sensitive enzymes which break down collagen, such as collagenase.[8] It is possible that this is how compression garments control scar formation.

CLINICAL INDICATIONS FOR THE USE OF EXTERNAL COMPRESSION

EDEMA
Causes of Edema

Edema is caused by increased fluid in the interstitial spaces of the body. Normal fluid equilibrium in the tissues is maintained by the balance between the hydrostatic and **osmotic pressure** inside and outside the blood vessels. Hydrostatic pressure is determined by blood pressure and the effects of gravity, whereas osmotic pressure is determined by the concentration of proteins inside and outside the vessels. The higher hydrostatic pressure inside the vessels acts to push fluid out of the vessels, whereas the higher protein concentration and osmotic pressure inside the vessels acts to keep fluid inside the vessels (Fig. 11-1).

> ### ◎ Clinical Pearl
>
> In a healthy body, hydrostatic pressure pushing fluid out of the blood vessels and osmotic pressure keeping fluid in the blood vessels are almost balanced.

Under normal circumstances, the hydrostatic pressure pushing fluid out of the veins is slightly higher than the osmotic pressure keeping fluid in, resulting in a slight loss of fluid into the interstitial space. The fluid that is pushed out of the veins into the interstitial space is then taken up by the lymphatic capillaries to be returned to the venous circulation at the subclavian veins. This fluid, known as **lymphatic fluid** or lymph, is rich in protein, water, and macrophages.

A healthy diet, vascular system, and muscular contraction act together to ensure that the appropriate amount of fluid exits the veins and flows back toward the heart.

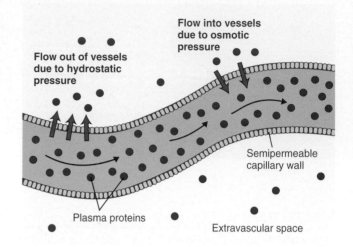

FIG 11-1 Effects of hydrostatic and osmotic pressure on tissue fluid balance.

Dysfunction in any of these mechanisms can result in increased movement of fluid from the vessels into the extravascular space, or reduced flow of venous blood or lymph back toward the heart, and thus the formation of edema.

Major causes of edema include venous or lymphatic obstruction or insufficiency, increased capillary permeability, and increased plasma volume due to sodium and water retention.[9] Edema caused by venous or lymphatic insufficiency or dysfunction can be helped by compression, thus these forms of edema are discussed in detail in the following sections.

Edema may also occur after exercise, trauma, surgery, or burns, or with infection, because of the increase in blood flow and vascular capillary permeability that occurs with the acute inflammation associated with these events. Increased vascular capillary permeability increases the fluid flow out of the capillaries, causing an accumulation of fluid at the site of trauma or infection. Edema caused by acute inflammation is described in detail in Chapter 2.

Airline travel can also cause edema, probably as a result of the prolonged sitting and the reduced external air pressure. A systematic review of 10 randomized trials with a total of 2,856 subjects showed that wearing compression stockings for flights of at least 7 hours significantly reduced the incidence of edema associated with flying.[10] Pregnancy is also associated with edema formation. There are multiple contributors to edema formation during pregnancy including increased blood volume, altered venous smooth muscle tone, and increased pressure within the veins caused by the gravid uterus reducing venous return from the lower body leading to **venous insufficiency** and leg edema. Intermittent pneumatic compression may be helpful for reducing ankle edema in pregnancy, although edema during pregnancy may also signal preeclampsia, which needs careful monitoring by a physician.[11]

A variety of diseases and other medical conditions, including congestive heart failure (CHF), cirrhosis, acute

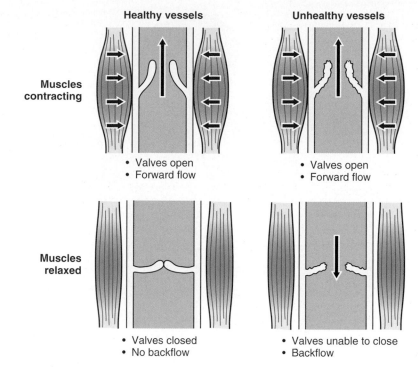

Healthy vessels   **Unhealthy vessels**

Muscles contracting

- Valves open
- Forward flow

- Valves open
- Forward flow

Muscles relaxed

- Valves closed
- No backflow

- Valves unable to close
- Backflow

FIG 11-2 Normal and abnormal valves in venous and lymphatic vessels and their relation to backflow.

renal disease, diabetic glomerulonephritis, malnutrition, and radiation injury, may cause peripheral and central edema by altering circulation or osmotic pressure balance. Edema from these causes should not be treated with compression as compression is not likely to reduce the edema and may in fact worsen the overall health of the patient.

Edema Caused by Venous Insufficiency

The peripheral veins' function is to carry deoxygenated blood from the periphery back to the heart. In a healthy vascular system, the resting hydrostatic venous pressure at the entrance to the right atrium of the heart averages 4.6 mm Hg, and this pressure increases by 0.77 mm Hg for each centimeter below the right atrium to reach an average of 90 mm Hg at the ankle.[12] When the calf muscles contract, they exert a pressure of about 200 mm Hg on the outside of the veins, which pushes the blood proximally through the veins. After the contraction, the pressure on the veins falls to about 10 to 30 mm Hg, allowing the veins to refill. A healthy amount of skeletal muscle activity, such as occurs with walking or running or with rhythmic isometric muscle contraction, provides a milking action to propel the blood in the veins from the periphery back toward the heart. Muscle contraction is the primary factor propelling both lymphatic and venous flow, and valves within the vessels prevent backflow of the fluid, ensuring that it moves proximally toward the heart rather than being pushed toward the distal extremities (Fig. 11-2).

Lack of physical activity, dysfunction of the venous valves caused by degeneration, or mechanical obstruction of the veins by a tumor or inflammation can result in venous insufficiency and accumulation of fluid in the periphery.

> **Clinical Pearl**
>
> Lack of physical activity, valve dysfunction, and venous obstruction can result in peripheral edema.

The most common cause of venous insufficiency is inflammation of the veins, known as **phlebitis**, which causes thickening of the vessel walls and damage to the valves. Thickening and loss of elasticity of the vessel walls elevates the hydrostatic pressure in the venous system, and damage to the valves allows blood to flow in both proximal and distal directions, rather than just proximally through the veins, when the muscles contract (see Fig. 11-2). The retrograde flow reduces circulation of deoxygenated blood out of the veins and thus increases pressure in the venous system if fluid inflow from the arterial system is unchanged. The elevated venous pressure pushes fluid into the extravascular space causing edema. If the limbs are in a dependent position, the edema will worsen further because of increased hydrostatic pressure caused by gravity.

Lymphedema

As explained previously, the hydrostatic pressure that pushes fluid out of the veins normally exceeds the osmotic pressure keeping fluid inside them. This results in a net flow of fluids and proteins into the interstitial space, producing lymph. To prevent the lymph from accumulating

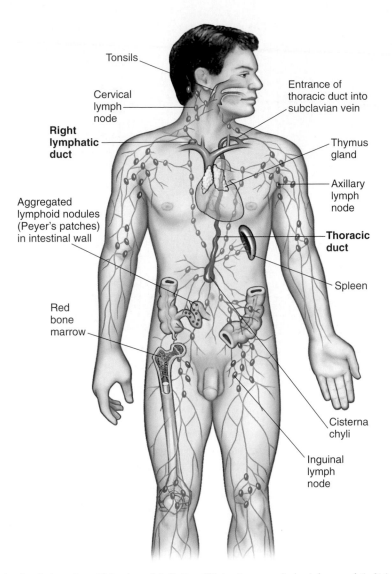

Tonsils

Cervical
lymph
node

**Right
lymphatic
duct**

Aggregated
lymphoid nodules
(Peyer's patches)
in intestinal wall

Red
bone
marrow

Entrance of
thoracic duct into
subclavian vein

Thymus
gland

Axillary
lymph
node

**Thoracic
duct**

Spleen

Cisterna
chyli

Inguinal
lymph
node

FIG 11-3 Lymphatic circulation. *From Thibodeau GA, Patton KT:* Anatomy and physiology, *ed 6, St Louis, 2006, Mosby.*

in the interstitial space, the **lymphatic system**, acting as an accessory channel, returns this fluid to the blood circulation. The lymphatic system consists of a large network of vessels and nodes through which the lymphatic fluid flows. Lymphatic vessels are found in almost every area where there are blood vessels, and lymph flows along these vessels, passing through numerous lymph nodes, to empty into the subclavian veins (Fig. 11-3). The lymph nodes are concentrated in the axillary, throat, groin, and paraaortic areas and filter the lymph, removing bacteria and other foreign particles. The lymphatic vessels of the right arm terminate in the right lymphatic duct and empty into the right subclavian vein, and the lymphatic vessels from all other areas terminate in the thoracic duct and empty into the left subclavian vein. Once the lymphatic fluid reenters the circulatory system, it is processed through the kidneys, along with other fluids, waste products, and electrolytes, and is eliminated.

Fluid flows into the lymphatic system because the concentration of proteins inside the lymphatic vessels is gen-

erally higher than in the interstitial space. As with the veins, flow along the lymphatic vessels in a proximal direction depends on muscle activity, such as walking or running, which compresses the vessels and their valves and prevents backflow. Decreased levels of plasma proteins, particularly albumin, mechanical obstruction of the lymphatics, abnormal distribution of lymphatic vessels or lymph nodes, or reduced activity can result in reduced lymphatic flow and the formation of **lymphedema**.

Clinical Pearl

Low albumin, lymphatic obstruction, abnormal vessel distribution, and reduced activity can cause lymphedema.

Decreased levels of plasma proteins cause fluid to accumulate in the extravascular space because the osmotic pressure that normally keeps fluid in the lymphatic vessels and the veins is reduced. If the plasma protein level drops

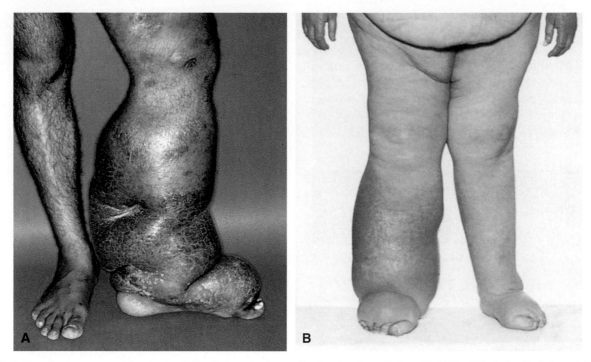

FIG 11-4 **A,** Lymphedema caused by elephantiasis. **B,** Lymphedema affecting function. **A,** *From Goldstein B (ed): Practical dermatology, ed 2, St Louis, 1997, Mosby.* **B,** *From Browse N, Burnand K, Mortimer P: Diseases of the lymphatics, London, 2003, Arnold.*

below the normal range of 6 to 8 gm/dL or the plasma albumin levels fall below 3.3 gm/dL, lymphedema is likely to result. A healthy diet and adequate protein absorption are required to keep plasma protein at an appropriate level. When lymphedema is caused by hypoproteinemia, this underlying problem should be addressed first to prevent further edema formation and other adverse consequences.

Lymphedema can be primary or secondary, although in most cases, it is secondary. Primary lymphedema is caused by a congenital disorder of the lymphatic vessels, whereas secondary lymphedema is caused by some other disease or dysfunction. An example of primary lymphedema is Milroy's disease, in which the individual has hypoplastic, aplastic, or varicose and incompetent lymphatic vessels. Patients with primary lymphedema often have backflow in the lymphatic vessels, and the rate of protein reabsorption across the vessel walls is also usually slowed. In secondary lymphedema, lymphatic flow is impaired by blockage or insufficiency of the lymphatics. Infection, neoplasm, radiation therapy, trauma, surgery, arthritis, chronic venous insufficiency, and lipedema are common causes of secondary lymphatic obstruction in the developed world.[13] However, the most common cause of secondary lymphedema worldwide is filariasis, a disease characterized by infestation of the lymphatics and obstruction of the lymph vessels and nodes by microscopic filarial worms. Although this disease is common in Asia, it is rarely seen in the United States (US), Australia, or Europe. In the US, secondary lymphedema is usually the result of cancer treatment with lymph node removal or radiation,

both of which can cause fibrosis. Other common causes of lymphedema in the US include mechanical obstruction of the vessels by a tumor or inflammation, dysfunction of the valves caused by degeneration, or accidental damage to the lymphatics during non–cancer-related surgery.

Adverse Consequences of Edema

Edema of any origin can result in impaired range of motion (ROM), limitations of function, or pain. Reducing edema has been shown to increase joint ROM and to decrease pain and joint stiffness.[14,15] Persistent chronic edema, particularly lymphedema, can cause collagen to be laid down in the area, leading to subcutaneous tissue fibrosis and hard induration of the skin. This edema may eventually cause disfiguring and disabling contractures and deformities (Fig. 11-4). Chronic edema also increases the risk of infection because tissue oxygenation is reduced; this risk is further elevated with lymphedema because of the presence of a protein-rich environment for bacterial growth.[13,16] Advanced chronic lymphatic or venous obstruction may result in cellulitis, ulceration, and if unmanaged, partial limb amputation.[16] These more serious sequelae are more likely to occur if the pressure of the excess fluid accumulated in the interstitial extravascular spaces causes arterial obstruction. Chronic venous insufficiency often causes itching due to stasis dermatitis, and brown pigmentation of the skin due to hemosiderin deposition. These signs are commonly seen on the medial lower leg (Fig. 11-5). Early control of edema can help prevent the progression and development of the signs and symptoms of chronic edema and its associated complications.

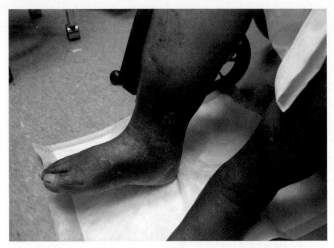

FIG 11-5 Venous stasis ulcer. Note the areas of darkened skin around the ulcer caused by hemosiderin deposits. *From Cameron MH, Monroe LG: Physical rehabilitation: evidence-based examination, evaluation, and intervention, St Louis, 2007, Saunders.*

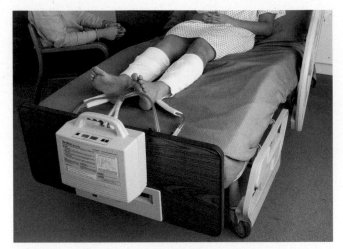

FIG 11-6 Use of intermittent pneumatic compression to prevent DVT formation in a bedridden patient. *Courtesy DJO, Vista, CA.*

Clinical Pearl

Edema can lead to restricted ROM, functional impairment, pain, disfiguration, infection, ulceration, amputation, itching, and brown skin pigmentation.

How Compression Reduces Edema

Compression controls edema by increasing extravascular hydrostatic pressure and by promoting circulation. If the patient has underlying causes of edema, such as infection, malnutrition, inadequate physical activity, or organ dysfunction, these must also be addressed to achieve an optimal outcome and prevent recurrence of the edema.

Compression of a limb with a static or intermittent device increases the pressure surrounding the extremity to counterbalance any increased osmotic or hydrostatic pressure, causing fluid to flow out of the vessels into the extravascular space. If sufficient pressure is applied, the hydrostatic pressure in the interstitial spaces becomes greater than that in the veins and lymphatic vessels, reducing outflow from the vessels and causing fluid in the interstitial spaces to return to the vessels.[17] Once fluid is in the vessels it can be circulated out of the periphery, preventing or reversing edema formation. If an intermittent compression device is used this may help to move the fluid proximally through the vessels.

PREVENTION OF DEEP VENOUS THROMBOSIS

Deep venous thrombosis (DVT) is a blood clot (thrombus) in the deep veins. The risk for DVT formation increases when local circulation is reduced because blood flowing slowly can coagulate and form a thrombus. Any intervention that increases the circulatory rate may therefore reduce the risk of thrombus formation. Risk factors for DVT include older age, surgery, trauma, hospital or nursing home confinement, cancer, central vein catheterization, transvenous pacemaker, prior superficial vein thrombosis, varicose veins, paralysis, use of oral contraceptives, pregnancy, and hormone therapy.[18] DVT formation is most common in immobilized patients, and greater than 50% of all DVTs occur in hospitalized or nursing home patients. Other known risk factors account for 25% of DVTs, and 25% are of unknown cause.[19]

DVTs can cause a postthrombotic syndrome, characterized by pain, swelling, and skin changes in the area of the thrombus, but a more significant health risk can occur if the thrombus becomes dislodged and moves to block the blood supply of the lungs, causing a pulmonary embolus. Such blockage may cause shortness of breath, respiratory failure, or death. Therefore preventing the formation of DVTs in at-risk patients is imperative.

A number of approaches, including external compression, as well as calf muscle electrical stimulation and various anticoagulant medications, have been found to reduce the risk of DVT formation. A recent systematic review and metaanalysis found that 81 (13%) of 624 patients who used graded compression stockings developed DVTs, compared to 154 (27%) in the control group of 581 patients.[20] This is approximately a 60% reduction in risk of DVT formation. External compression devices applied to the foot and calf (Fig. 11-6) have specifically been shown to reduce the incidence of DVTs in patients hospitalized for surgery and after trauma.[21-25] However, the studies on the effects of external compression on DVT formation after acute stroke have been few and inconclusive. A systematic review, based on two randomized controlled trials, did not find that physical methods significantly reduced the frequency of DVT immediately after stroke.[21]

A number of studies have compared the effectiveness of compression with that of anticoagulant medication (generally heparin) for DVT prophylaxis. Randomized clinical trials have found that intermittent pneumatic compression is at least as effective as low molecular weight heparin in preventing DVTs in patients immobilized after trauma.[24,25] Metaanalyses have found that compression is as effective, if not more effective, than heparin in reducing the risk of DVTs and pulmonary emboli,[26,27] and there is some evidence that combining these two approaches may be even more effective.[28] A recent systematic review found that external compression devices, such as graduated compression stockings, intermittent pneumatic compression, and footpumps, all resulted in an approximately two-thirds reduction in DVT risk when used alone and reduced the risk by an additional 50% when added to pharmacological DVT prophylaxis.[23]

External compression stockings reduce not only the incidence of DVT formation but have also been found to reduce the incidence of postthrombotic syndrome after a DVT has formed.[29]

Recently, there has been interest in the idea that long air flights increase the risk of DVT formation. Current evidence indicates that the risk of DVT formation during flights is only increased in people with additional risk factors who are on flights lasting 8 hours or longer.[29] However, a recent systematic review found that wearing compression stockings during flights of at least 7 hours duration substantially reduces the number of asymptomatic DVTs that form in all persons.[10]

Compression is thought primarily to reduce DVT formation by improving venous flow and thus reducing venous stasis and the opportunity for thrombus formation.[30,31] Intermittent compression may also inhibit tissue factor pathways that initiate blood coagulation or may degrade thrombi by enhancing fibrinolytic activity.[32-35]

Although early studies suggested that application of intermittent pneumatic compression (IPCs) devices to the arms reduced the incidence of DVTs in the legs, more recent studies have found this approach to be less effective than application to the legs.[24] Therefore, when possible, compression should be applied to both legs to optimize outcome.

VENOUS STASIS ULCERS

Venous stasis ulcers are areas of tissue breakdown and necrosis that occur in areas of impaired venous circulation (see Fig. 11-5). The exact mechanism by which poor venous circulation causes ulcers is still not known. The current understanding is that the elevation in venous pressure caused by impaired venous circulation leads to endovascular and inflammatory changes, which provide a setting for ulcer formation.[36] Skin changes associated with inflammation can then cause fibrosis, impaired wound healing, and ulceration.[37-39] Deep venous reflux may also contribute to the formation of venous stasis ulcers.[39-41] It used to be thought that venous stasis ulcers were caused by poor tissue oxygenation in areas of poor venous circulation, but this is unlikely because studies show that tissue oxygen levels are generally in the normal range in the area of venous ulcers.[36] Because compression can improve venous circulation and because improving circulation may reduce adverse effects of poor venous flow, diminish the risk of vascular ulcer formation, and facilitate healing of previously formed ulcers, compression is the treatment of choice for venous stasis ulcers.

Compression has been shown to increase the rate of healing of venous stasis ulcers when compared with no compression.[42] Multilayered compression is more effective than single-layer compression, and high pressure compression is more effective than low pressure compression.[43] Compression stockings may also reduce the rate of venous stasis ulcer recurrence, although the evidence for this benefit is weak, with no studies specifically comparing ulcer recurrence rates with and without compression.[44,45] Studies evaluating patient compliance with compression stockings have found that venous ulcer recurrence rates are lower in patients who wear compression stockings more often.[46-48] IPC has been recommended for treatment of venous stasis ulcers that do not heal using other methods, and patient compliance is higher with IPC than with other methods of compression, such as bandaging.[40] Compression therapy is considered to be the most important aspect of the treatment of venous stasis ulcers.[49]

> ◎ **Clinical Pearl**
>
> Compression therapy is the cornerstone of treatment of venous stasis ulcers.

Standard treatment involves bandaging to promote ulcer healing and compression stockings to prevent recurrence. For patients with venous insufficiency and a history of ulcers, compression should be continued even after an ulcer has healed in order to control edema and increase patient comfort, in addition to preventing ulcer recurrence.[50]

Position affects how well compression works, especially in the legs, because gravity increases the hydrostatic pressure in the veins when standing. For the leg veins to be compressed effectively, the external pressure has to exceed the hydrostatic pressure in the vein. When a person stands, the veins' hydrostatic pressure is much higher than when lying down. Therefore higher compression is needed in the standing position than when lying down, and compression is most effective in the supine position. One small study found that external pressure delivered by elastic compression stockings was not sufficient to effectively compress leg veins in the upright position. This study found that the pressure needed to occlude the leg veins when subjects were supine was 20 to 25 mm Hg, whereas the pressure needed to occlude leg veins when subjects were standing was approximately 70 mm Hg.[51] Another study found that in the standing position graduated compression stockings that provided 20 to 30 mm Hg did not compress the deep or superficial veins of the calf.[52]

The proposed mechanisms by which compression facilitates the healing of venous stasis ulcers include improved venous circulation, reduced venous pooling and reflux, improved tissue oxygenation, altered white cell adhesion, and reduced edema.[53-56]

Although compression is generally contraindicated in the presence of arterial insufficiency because compression of the arterial vessels may further impair arterial flow, aggravating the condition, compression has been found to facilitate the healing of arterial insufficiency ulcers.

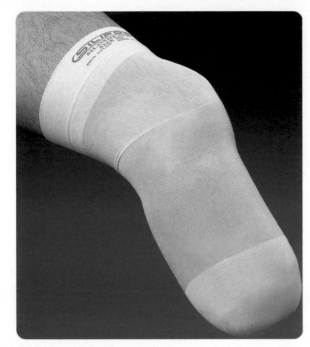

FIG 11-7 Compression for residual limb shaping. *Courtesy Silipos, New York, NY.*

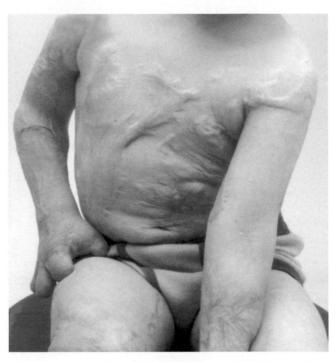

FIG 11-8 Hypertrophic scarring. *From Cameron MH, Monroe LG: Physical rehabilitation: evidence-based examination, evaluation, and intervention, St Louis, 2007, Saunders.*

A metaanlysis found that some studies demonstrated improved wound healing with intermittent pneumatic compression in patients with severe peripheral arterial disease who were not candidates for surgery.[57] It is possible that compression helped these patients by reducing chronic edema that places pressure on the arterial vessels. However, because of the risk of further impairing arterial flow with compression, in most cases compression should not be used on patients with peripheral arterial disease.

RESIDUAL LIMB SHAPING AFTER AMPUTATION

Compression can be used for residual limb reduction and shaping after amputation to help prepare the limb for prosthetic fitting (Fig. 11-7). Both static and intermittent compression are used for limb shaping, although intermittent compression has been shown to reduce the residual limb in approximately half of the time required by other techniques.[58] When intermittent compression is used for limb shaping it is applied in conjunction with an elastic bandage. Compression reduces residual limb size because it controls postsurgical edema and prevents stretching of the soft tissues by excessive fluid accumulation. Residual limb reduction and shaping is required to prepare for functional weight bearing on a prosthetic device. The residual limb must be shaped so that the prosthesis maintains its position and alignment and promotes weight bearing on the appropriate structures. Excessive pressure on unprotected bony prominences should be avoided to promote comfort and function and to limit the risk of tissue breakdown.

CONTROL OF HYPERTROPHIC SCARRING

Hypertrophic scarring is a common complication of deep burns and other extensive skin and soft-tissue injuries.[59,60] Normal skin is pliable and aesthetically pleasing and has clearly identifiable layers, whereas hypertrophic scars are not pliable, have a raised and ridged appearance, and have loss of identity of the skin layers (Fig. 11-8).[61] Hypertrophic scars result in poor cosmesis and the development of contractures that may restrict ROM and function. The risk of hypertrophic scarring is increased with delayed healing, a deep wound, repeated trauma, infection, or a foreign body present and in individuals with a genetic predisposition. Hypertrophic scarring is most common in the areas of the sternum, upper back, and shoulders.[62]

Although many approaches, including surgery, pharmaceuticals, passive stretch with positioning, massage, and silicone gel, are used to control hypertrophic scar formation, compression is the most common.[62-65] Larson and colleagues first published a report in the US of this application of compression in 1971. They demonstrated that compression garments decreased the height and vascularity of scar tissue and increased its pliability.[66]

Many mechanisms for the effect of compression on hypertrophic scarring have been proposed. Compression may directly shape the scar tissue by acting as a mold for the new tissue, decreasing local edema formation, and facilitating improved collagen orientation. One study found that compression of hypertrophic scars makes the extracellular matrix organization more similar to that seen in normal scar tissue.[67] It has also been proposed that compression reduces scar formation by increasing collagenase activity, either as a result of increased skin temperature or as a result of increased prostaglandin E_2 release, both of which have been shown to be induced by compression.[8,63,68] Alternatively, compression may control scar formation by inducing local tissue hypoxia.[64] Compression has been shown to induce apoptosis (cell death) and regulate cytokine release in hypertrophic scars, thus reducing the hyperproliferation underlying excessive scarring.[69]

When applying compression to control hypertrophic scar formation, treatment is generally initiated once the new epithelium has formed and is then continued for 8 to 12 months or longer, until the scar is no longer growing and has reached maturity. Compression can be applied with elastic bandages, self-adherent wraps, tubular elastic cotton supports, or elastic custom-fit garments. With any of these approaches, the compression pressure is maintained at approximately 20 to 30 mm Hg. It is recommended that the compression device be worn 24 hours a day, except when bathing, to achieve maximum benefit. Common complications of this treatment include skin irritation, constriction of circulation, and restriction of joint motion.[62]

CONTRAINDICATIONS AND PRECAUTIONS FOR THE USE OF EXTERNAL COMPRESSION

There are few contraindications that apply to all compression devices; however, when compression is used to treat edema or impaired circulation, the underlying cause of these problems should be ascertained and addressed before compression therapy is initiated. Compression therapy will be ineffective and contraindicated in cases where edema is caused by a blockage of the circulation or when there is active infection or malignancy in the affected extremity. When peripheral edema is caused by cardiovascular disease, such as CHF or cardiomyopathy, one must make sure that the increased fluid load that could be placed on the heart by the shifting of fluid from the periphery in response to treatment with compression will not be detrimental to the patient. In such cases, the patient's physician should always be consulted before the initiation of compression therapy.

All forms of compression are contraindicated in patients with symptomatic heart failure (because of the risk of system overload) and those with a thrombus (because of the risk of dislodgment) and may not be appropriate if an arterial revascularization has been performed on the involved limb. In addition, the clinician must evaluate for the presence and severity of arterial insufficiency before compressing a limb. This is most often determined by calculating the ankle brachial index (ABI). If the ABI is less than 0.6, all forms of static compression are contraindicated. If the ABI is greater than 0.8, standard or full compression (30 to 40 mm Hg) may be used. When the ABI is between 0.5 and 0.8, the compression pressure should be reduced to between 23 and 27 mmHg. If the patient also has neuropathy, careful monitoring is necessary because

he or she may fail to recognize symptoms of ischemia, such as pain, numbness, or tingling.

Particular care should be taken when donning and doffing compression bandages and garments to avoid trauma to healing tissue or fragile skin. Details of contraindications and precautions for the use of compression pumps are provided next.

CONTRAINDICATIONS FOR THE USE OF INTERMITTENT OR SEQUENTIAL COMPRESSION PUMPS

> **CONTRAINDICATIONS**
>
> **for the Use of Intermittent or Sequential Compression Pumps**
>
> - Heart failure or pulmonary edema
> - Recent or acute DVT, thrombophlebitis, or pulmonary embolism
> - Obstructed lymphatic or venous return
> - Severe peripheral arterial disease or ulcers resulting from arterial insufficiency
> - Acute local skin infection
> - Significant hypoproteinemia (protein levels less than 2 gm/dL)
> - Acute trauma or fracture
> - Arterial revascularization

Heart Failure or Pulmonary Edema

Although edema of the dependent parts of the body is a common consequence of CHF, compression pumps should not be used to treat edema of this etiology because the shift of fluid from the peripheral to the central circulation may increase stress on the failing organ system. CHF results from a decrease in the ability or efficiency of cardiac muscle contraction and subsequent decreased cardiac output. This stimulates an increase in venous pressure and increased sodium and water retention, which cause edema. Treatment of CHF requires decreasing the load on the heart, whereas compression increases the cardiac load by increasing the amount of fluid in the veins. Thus compression tends to aggravate the underlying condition, resulting in worsening edema and potentially causing other more serious side effects, such as pulmonary edema, as CHF progresses. Peripheral edema caused by CHF is usually bilateral and symmetrical.

Pulmonary edema occurs with prolonged or severe CHF. It is the result of elevated lung capillary pressure causing fluid to leave the circulation and accumulate in the alveolar air spaces in the lungs. Compression is contraindicated when pulmonary edema is present because compression increases the fluid load of the vascular system and the pressure in the lung capillaries, potentially aggravating this serious medical condition.

Ask the Patient

- Do you have any heart or lung problems?
- Do you have difficulty breathing?

- Are you taking any medications for your heart or blood pressure?
- Do you have swelling in both legs?

Assess
- Check for the presence of bilateral edema.

Compression should not be used to treat edema until the clinician has ascertained that the edema is not a result of CHF or pulmonary edema.

Recent or Acute Deep Vein Thrombosis, Thrombophlebitis, or Pulmonary Embolism

Compression, particularly intermittent compression, should not be used when the patient is known to have a DVT, thrombophlebitis, or a pulmonary embolus because the thrombus may become dislodged or the embolus may travel. This can occur because of direct mechanical agitation of the clot by the compression or because of increased circulation produced by compression. If a thrombus or embolus becomes dislodged, it may travel in the bloodstream to a distant site and lodge in a location where it impairs blood flow to an organ sufficiently to cause organ damage, severe morbidity, or even death. For example, an embolus in the pulmonary arteries produces approximately a 30% mortality rate, whereas an embolus that lodges in the arteries supplying the brain may cause a stroke or death.[59] Compression can help prevent the formation of DVTs, but it should not be used when it is thought that a thrombus may already be present.

Ask the Patient
- Do you have pain in your calves?
- How long have you not been walking?

Assess
- Check for Homan's sign (discomfort in the calf on forced dorsiflexion of the foot), a sign of thrombosis in the leg.

Further evaluation by a physician should be requested if the clinician suspects that there may be a thrombus in the deep veins of the leg. The use of compression should be delayed until the patient has been cleared for the presence of thromboses or thrombophlebitis in the area to be treated.

Obstructed Lymphatic or Venous Return

Compression is contraindicated when lymphatic or venous return is totally obstructed because, in such cases, increasing the fluid load of the vessels cannot reduce the edema until the obstruction has been removed. Lymphatic or venous return may be obstructed by a thrombus, radiation damage to the lymph nodes, an inguinal or abdominal tumor, or other masses. With partial obstruction of the vessels or complete occlusion of only a few of the vessels, treatment with compression may enhance the functioning of the intact collateral vessels.

Ask the Patient
- Do you know why you have swelling in your legs/arms?
- Is something obstructing your circulation?

If there is complete lymphatic or venous obstruction, compression should not be used. Such obstruction may need to be treated surgically. When there is partial obstruction, compression may be used in conjunction with careful monitoring of the patient's response to the treatment to ensure that the treatment is helping to resolve the edema rather than just shifting the fluid to a more proximal area of the affected limb.

Severe Peripheral Arterial Disease or Ulcers Resulting from Arterial Insufficiency

Compression should not be used in patients with severe peripheral arterial disease or where there are ulcers resulting from arterial insufficiency because it can aggravate these conditions by closing down the diseased arteries and further impairing circulation in the area.

Ask the Patient
- Do you get pain in your calves when walking?
- If an ulcer is present: Have you had problems with your arteries; for example, heart bypass surgery or bypass surgery in your legs?

Pain in the calves while walking can be the result of intermittent claudication, a sign of peripheral arterial disease. A history of bypass surgeries suggests the presence of arterial disease in other areas.

Assess
- If an ulcer is present, try to determine if it is the result of arterial insufficiency. Ulcers caused by arterial insufficiency are usually small and round, with definite borders, and painful. They occur most often on the interdigital spaces between the toes or on the lateral malleolus.
- Request that an ABI be obtained. This is generally performed by vascular services and is a measure of the ratio of the systolic blood pressure in the lower extremity to the systolic blood pressure in the upper extremity. Compression should not be applied if the ABI is less than 0.8, indicating that the blood pressure at the ankle is less than 80% of that in the upper extremity.

> ### ◎ Clinical Pearl
> Compression should not be applied if the ABI is less than 0.8.

Acute Local Skin Infection

A local skin infection is likely to be aggravated by the application of compression because the sleeves and skin coverings used increase the moisture and temperature of the area, encouraging the growth of microorganisms. If a chronic skin infection is present, single-use sleeves that avoid cross-contamination from one patient to another or reinfection of the same patient may be used for the application of intermittent compression.

Ask the Patient
- Do you have any skin infections in the area to be treated?

Assess

- Inspect the skin for rashes, redness, or skin breakdown indicating the possible presence of infection.

Significant Hypoproteinemia

Although peripheral edema is a common symptom of severe hypoproteinemia, when the serum protein level is less than 2 gm/dl, the resulting edema should not be treated with compression because returning fluid to the vessels will further lower the serum protein concentration, potentially resulting in severe adverse consequences, including cardiac and immunological dysfunction. Severe hypoproteinemia can occur because of inadequate food intake, increased nutrient losses, or increased nutrient requirements resulting from an underlying disease.

Ask the Patient

- Have you recently lost weight?
- Have you changed your diet?
- Do you have any other disease?

Assess

- Check the laboratory values section of the patient's chart for the serum protein level.

The use of compression should be delayed until the patient's serum protein level is above 2 gm/dL.

Acute Trauma or Fracture

Intermittent compression is contraindicated immediately after an acute trauma because compression may cause excessive motion at the site of trauma, increasing bleeding, aggravating the acute inflammation, or destabilizing an acute fracture. Such effects can cause further damage at the site of injury and impair healing. Intermittent compression should be used for treating posttraumatic edema only after the initial acute inflammatory phase has passed, bleeding has stopped, and the area is mechanically stable. Static compression, as provided by stockings or wraps, may be used immediately after an acute trauma to prevent edema and reduce bleeding. Directly after an injury, static compression is frequently applied in conjunction with rest, ice, and elevation to optimize the control of pain, edema, and inflammation.

⊚ Clinical Pearl

Static compression can be applied immediately after trauma, but intermittent compression is contraindicated immediately after trauma.

Ask the Patient

- When did your injury happen?
- Do you know if a bone was broken?

Arterial Revascularization

Intermittent compression is contraindicated after arterial revascularization surgery because there is a risk of occluding the arterial vessels and preventing blood from reaching the extremities, leading to ischemia. If the patient has had recent arterial revascularization, elevation of the extremity and exercise may be used to decrease edema.

Ask the Patient

- Have you had surgery on your arteries?

Assess

- Look for scars that would indicate vascular surgery, especially on the legs.

PRECAUTIONS FOR THE USE OF INTERMITTENT OR SEQUENTIAL COMPRESSION PUMPS

PRECAUTIONS

for the Use of Intermittent or Sequential Compression Pumps

- Impaired sensation or mentation
- Uncontrolled hypertension
- Cancer
- Stroke or significant cerebrovascular insufficiency
- Superficial peripheral nerves

Impaired Sensation or Mentation

Compression should be applied with caution to patients with impaired sensation or mentation because such patients may be unable to recognize or communicate when pressure is excessive or painful.

Ask the Patient

- Do you have normal feeling in this area?

Assess

- Sensation in the area.
- Alertness and orientation.

Compression garments or low levels of intermittent compression may be used if the patient has impaired sensation or mentation; however, such patients must be carefully monitored for adverse effects, such as skin irritation or any aggravation of edema caused by constriction of the garments in tight areas.

Uncontrolled Hypertension

Compression should be applied with caution to patients with uncontrolled hypertension because compression can further elevate blood pressure by increasing the vascular fluid load. Blood pressure should be monitored frequently during treatment of these patients, and treatment should be stopped if their blood pressure increases above the safe level determined by their physician.

Ask the Patient

- Do you have high blood pressure? If so, is it well controlled with medication?

Assess

- Resting blood pressure.

The clinician should check with the patient's physician for guidelines on blood pressure limits.

Cancer

Compression can increase circulation, which may disturb or dislodge metastatic tissue promoting metastasis, or may improve tissue nutrition promoting tumor growth. Although there have been no reports of metastasis or accelerated tumor growth caused by the use of compression, it is generally recommended that compression not be applied where a tumor is present or when it is thought that an increase in circulation may cause a tumor to move or grow more rapidly. However, compression is frequently used to control lymphedema that results from the treatment of breast cancer with mastectomy or radiation. Experts in this field vary in their opinions regarding the safety of this treatment and the precautions to be applied.[70-72] Although some experts do not consider the presence or history of malignancy to be a contraindication for the use of compression, others recommend avoiding the use of compression in areas close to the malignancy and still others recommend not applying this type of intervention until the patient has been cancer-free for 5 years. In general, most agree that the use of compression need not be restricted during the time that patients are receiving chemotherapy, hormone therapy, or biological response modifiers for treatment of their cancer.

Ask the Patient

• If edema results from the treatment of breast cancer, ask the patient if he or she is receiving chemotherapy, hormone therapy, or biological response modifiers for treatment of the cancer.

Assess

• Determine how recent the cancer diagnosis was made.

If the cause of edema is unknown and the patient has signs of cancer, such as recent unexplained changes in body weight or constant pain that does not change, treatment with compression should be deferred until a follow-up evaluation to rule out malignancy has been performed by a physician.

Stroke or Significant Cerebrovascular Insufficiency

Compression should be applied with caution to patients who have had a stroke or have signs of significant cerebrovascular insufficiency, such as a history of transient ischemic attacks. Caution is required because the hemodynamic changes caused by the compression may alter circulation to the brain.

Ask the Patient

• Have you had a stroke?
• Do you have lapses in consciousness?

Superficial Peripheral Nerve

Peroneal nerve palsy has been documented after the application of intermittent sequential compression.[73-75] Signifi-

cant weight loss, resulting in loss of fat and muscle mass around the peroneal nerves, may predispose these nerves to injury from compression devices. When compression is applied over an area where there is a superficial nerve, particularly in a patient with significant weight loss, the clinician should monitor closely for symptoms of nerve compression, including distal changes in or loss of sensation or strength.

ADVERSE EFFECTS OF EXTERNAL COMPRESSION

The potentially adverse effects of compression generally relate to aggravating a condition that is causing edema or impairing circulation if excessive pressure is used. When edema is the result of heart, kidney, or liver failure or circulatory obstruction compression may aggravate the underlying condition. Also, if too much pressure is used, the compression device may act as a tourniquet, impairing arterial circulation and causing ischemia and edema. If ischemia is prolonged, impaired healing or tissue death can occur. When compression is effective in reducing edema in an extremity, it is recommended that if this fluid accumulates at the proximal end of the extremity or where the extremity attaches to the trunk, it should be mobilized using massage.[16,76] To minimize the probability of adverse circulatory effects from treatment with compression, it is also recommended that the patient always be monitored closely for undesired changes in blood pressure or edema, particularly with the first application of the treatment or with changes in treatment parameters.

APPLICATION TECHNIQUES

Compression can be applied in several ways, depending on the patient's clinical presentation and the goals of treatment. Static compression can be applied with bandages or garments, and intermittent compression can be applied with electric pneumatic pumps. Static compression can be used to help control edema caused by venous or lymphatic dysfunction or inflammation, to form the shape of amputated residual limbs in preparation for the use of a prosthetic device, or to control scar formation after burn injury. Both static and intermittent compression, used either alone or together, can be applied to help prevent the development of DVT in bedridden patients (see Fig. 11-6). Intermittent compression is used primarily to prevent or reduce edema formation in limbs with poor venous or lymphatic drainage, with static compression being applied after this treatment to maintain edema control.

COMPRESSION BANDAGING

Compression bandages work by applying resting or working pressure, or a combination of the two. **Resting pressure** is exerted by elastic when it is put on stretch. An elastic bandage exerts this pressure whether the patient is moving or immobile. **Working pressure** is produced by active muscles pushing against an inelastic bandage (Fig. 11-9) and is only produced when the patient is moving and contracting the muscles. Compression bandages come in varying degrees of extensibility and may be applied as a single layer or in multiple layers. Types of

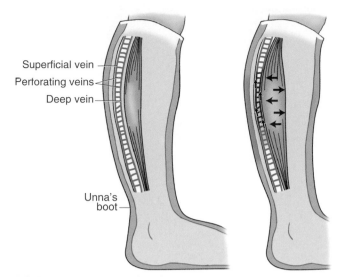

FIG 11-9 Development of working pressure. **A,** Muscle relaxed. **B,** Calf muscle contracting and pressing against the Unna's boot to compress the veins.

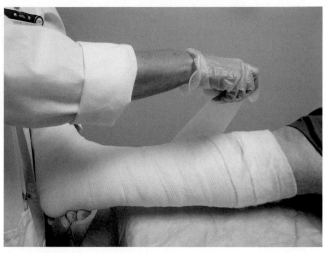

A

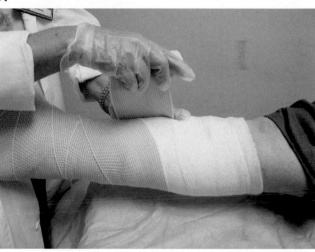

B

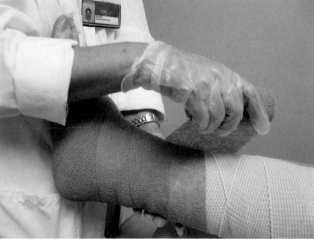

C

FIG 11-10 Application of a four-layer compression bandage. *From Cameron MH, Monroe LG: Physical rehabilitation: evidence-based examination, evaluation, and intervention, St Louis, 2007, Saunders.*

compression bandages include long-stretch, short-stretch, multilayered, and semirigid bandages.

Long-stretch(also known as high-stretch) bandages can extend by 100% to 200%. These bandages provide the greatest resting pressure because they exert the greatest restoring force. When stretched, a **long-stretch bandage** typically applies approximately 60 to 70 mm Hg pressure. These highly elastic bandages provide little to no working pressure because they stretch rather than resist when the muscles expand. Long-stretch bandages are most effective for applying compression for immobile patients or limbs. Examples of long-stretch bandages include Ace wraps and Tubigrip (ConvaTec). In general, it is recommended that if high-stretch bandages, such as a new Ace wrap, are used to control edema, they should be applied with only moderate tension to avoid excessive resting pressure because, without activity, the high resting pressure provided by this type of bandage may impair circulation.

Short-stretch (also known as low-stretch) bandages have low elasticity, with 30% to 90% extension. These bandages produce a low resting pressure but cause resistance and high working pressure during muscle activity. Since low-stretch bandages provide a degree of both resting and working pressure, they can be somewhat effective during activity or at rest. For an inelastic bandage to produce working pressure, the patient must have a functional calf muscle and a functional gait pattern. **Short-stretch bandages** are most useful during exercise when the activity of the muscles results in high working pressure, and generally they do not control edema effectively or improve circulation in a flaccid or inactive limb. An example of a short-stretch bandage is Comprilan (Smith & Nephew/Beiersdorf).

Multilayered bandage systems use a combination of inelastic and elastic layers to apply moderate to high resting pressure through the use of two, three, or four layers of different bandages (Fig. 11-10). For example, one type of multilayered bandage system (Profore, Smith & Nephew) provides approximately 40 mm Hg of resting

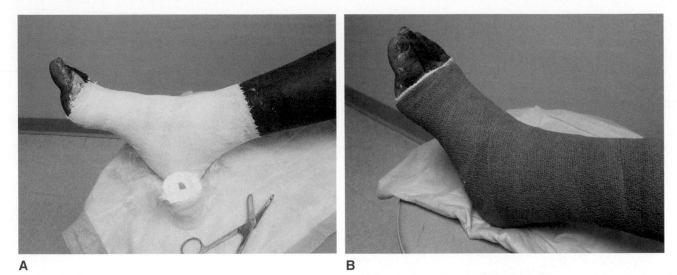

A   **B**

FIG 11-11 Unna's boot. *From Cameron MH, Monroe LG:* Physical rehabilitation: evidence-based examination, evaluation, and intervention, *St Louis, 2007, Saunders.*

pressure at the ankle, graduating to 17 mm Hg at the knee.[77] The layers of bandages provide protection and absorption, as well as compression. This type of bandage system is most commonly used for the treatment and prevention of venous leg ulcers and can maintain high compression for up to 1 week after application. One randomized controlled trial with 89 patients with venous stasis ulcers found that ulcers treated with multilayered bandages healed faster than those treated with short-stretch bandages. Additionally, treatment costs were lower with the multilayered bandage.[43] A systematic review of 22 trials found that multilayered compression is more effective than single-layered compression in the treatment of venous leg ulcers.[42] Examples of multilayered bandages include Profore and Dyna-Flex (Johnson & Johnson, New Brunswick, NJ).

A semirigid bandage formed of zinc oxide–impregnated gauze is commonly used to exert working pressure. When this type of bandage is applied to the lower extremity, it is known as an **Unna's boot** (Fig. 11-11). This bandage is typically used for the treatment of venous stasis ulcers.[78] Zinc oxide–impregnated gauze bandages become soft when wet, to allow molding around the involved limb, and then harden as they dry to form a semirigid boot. The boot is left on the patient for 1 to 2 weeks and is then removed and replaced. An Unna's boot is reported to provide a sustained compression force of 35 to 40 mm Hg.[75]

Compression bandages are generally applied by wrapping them around the limb in a figure-8 manner, starting distally and progressing proximally. Circular, circumferential, and spiral wrapping are generally not recommended because these configurations can result in uneven pressure, thus uneven control of edema. The bandage should be applied tightly enough to apply moderate, comfortable compression without impairing circulation. To avoid the compression bandage slipping on the skin, cohesive gauze or foam bandages are often applied under the compression bandages directly against the patient's skin. Soft cotton

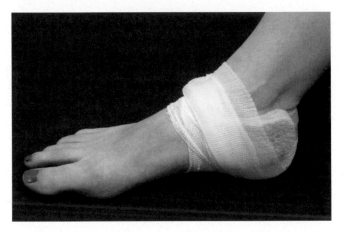

FIG 11-12 Foam padding around anatomical indentations.

may also be used as an underwrapping to absorb sweat and to help distribute pressure more evenly.

> ◎ **Clinical Pearl**
>
> Cohesive gauze, foam bandages, or soft cotton should be applied against the patient's skin under a compression bandage to prevent slippage.

For all types of bandages, it is recommended that tension and thus compression should be greatest distally and gradually decrease proximally to achieve an appropriate pressure gradient. To maintain consistency of pressure around anatomical indentations, such as the ankles, pieces of foam or cotton cut to size should be placed in these indentations before the bandage is applied (Fig. 11-12).

> ◎ **Clinical Pearl**
>
> Compression should be greatest distally and gradually decrease proximally.

APPLICATION TECHNIQUE 11-1   COMPRESSION BANDAGE

Equipment Required

- Cohesive gauze, foam, or cotton under-bandage
- Bandages of appropriate elasticity
- Cotton or foam for padding

Procedure

1. Remove clothing and jewelry from the area to be treated.
2. Inspect the skin in the area.
3. Apply foam or cotton padding around anatomical indentations.
4. Dress and cover any wound according to the treatment regimen being used for that wound.
5. Apply a cohesive gauze, foam, or cotton under bandage to protect the skin from the compression bandage and minimize slipping of the compression bandage. Start distally and progress proximally.
6. Apply the compression bandage, starting distally and progressing proximally. When applying a bandage to the lower extremity, first apply it around the ankle to fix the bandage in place, then wrap the foot, and then bandage the leg and thigh. Wrapping around the foot should be from medial to lateral when on the dorsum of the foot, in the direction of pronation.[79] When applying a bandage to the upper extremity, first apply it to the wrist to fix it in place, then wrap the hand and bandage the forearm and arm. For all areas, slightly more tension should be applied distally than proximally, and the bandage should be applied in a figure-8 manner (Fig. 11-13).

Advantages

- Inexpensive.
- Quick to apply once skill is mastered.
- Readily available.
- Extremity can be used during treatment.
- Safe for acute conditions.

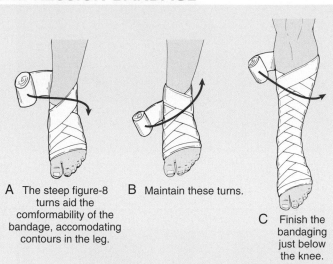

A The steep figure-8 turns aid the comformability of the bandage, accomodating contours in the leg.

B Maintain these turns.

C Finish the bandaging just below the knee.

FIG 11-13 Elastic compression wrap of the foot, ankle, and leg. Note the figure-8 wrap at the ankle. *Redrawn from Morrison M, Moffat C: A Colour Guide to the Assessment and Management of Leg Ulcers, ed 2, London, 1994, Mosby.*

Disadvantages

- When used alone, does not reverse edema.
- Effective only for controlling edema formation.
- Requires moderate skill, flexibility, and level of cognition to apply.
- Compression not readily quantifiable or replicable.
- Bulky and unattractive.
- Inelastic bandages do not control edema in a flaccid limb.

COMPRESSION GARMENTS

Compression garments provide various degrees of compression and are available in custom-fit sizes for all areas of the body and in standard off-the-shelf sizes for the limbs. They are generally made of washable Lycra spandex and nylon and have moderate elasticity to provide a combination of moderate resting and working pressure. Inelastic or low-stretch garments, which provide more working pressure, are not made because these are too difficult to put on and take off; however, low-stretch Velcro-closure static compression devices that are easier to use are available.

Off-the-shelf stockings, known as **antiembolism stockings**, provide a low compression force of about 16 to 18 mm Hg and are used to prevent DVTs in bedridden patients (Fig. 11-14).[80] These stockings are not intended to provide sufficient compression to prevent DVT formation or alter circulation when the lower extremities are in a dependent position. These stockings should fit snugly but comfortably around the lower extremities, and they should be worn by the patient 24 hours per day, except when bathing. Knee-high and thigh-high stockings have been found to be similarly efficient at reducing venous stasis,

and knee-high stockings are more comfortable to wear and wrinkle less than thigh-high stockings.[81]

Custom-fit and off-the-shelf compression garments that provide sufficient compression to control edema and counteract the effects of gravity on circulation in active patients or to modify scar formation after burns are also available (Fig. 11-15). These garments are available in dif-

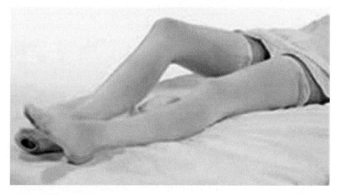

FIG 11-14 Antiembolism stockings. *Courtesy Carolon, Rural Hall, NC.*

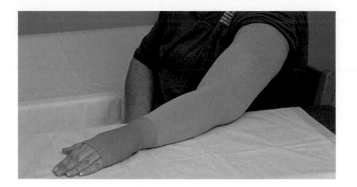

FIG 11-15 Upper extremity compression garment. *From Pierson FM, Fairchild SL:* Principles and Techniques of Patient Care, ed 4, *St Louis, 2008, Saunders.*

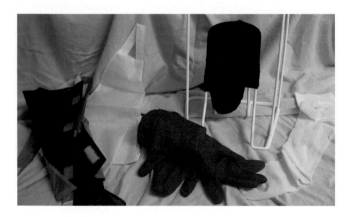

FIG 11-16 Stocking butler and rubber gloves to assist with donning compression stockings. *From Cameron MH, Monroe LG:* Physical rehabilitation: evidence-based examination, evaluation, and intervention, *St Louis, 2007, Saunders.*

ferent thicknesses and with different degrees of pretensioning to provide pressure ranging from 10 to 50 mm Hg.[80] A pressure of 20 to 30 mm Hg is generally appropriate for the control of scar tissue formation, whereas 30 to 40 mm Hg pressure will control edema in most ambulatory patients.

Clinical Pearl

In general, compression of 20 to 30 mm Hg is used for scar tissue control and 30 to 40 mm Hg for edema control.

Lower pressure may be sufficient in mild cases of edema, and higher pressure may be necessary in more severe cases. Some garments provide a pressure gradient so that the compression is greatest distally and decreases proximally. Although off-the-shelf stockings can improve venous circulation and control edema in most patients, custom-fit garments may be necessary in severe conditions or when an individual's limb contours do not match off-the-shelf sizing. Custom-fit garments may include options such as zippers and reinforced padded areas to improve ease of use and fit, and are effective in normalizing venous flow in many cases in which off-the-shelf garments are ineffective.[82] For sizing to be appropriate, both custom-fit and off-the-shelf compression garments should be fitted when

edema is minimal. This is generally first thing in the morning or after treatment with an intermittent compression pump. Garments are available for both the upper and lower extremities, as well as for the trunk and head (see Fig. 11-15). They are also available in a number of colors.

Compression garments are sometimes difficult for patients to put on and take off, especially for patients with poor vision, manual dexterity, coordination, or balance, or for those who are weak or cannot reach their feet. Assistive devices, such as the stocking butler and rubber gloves, can assist with donning compression stockings, but many people still have difficulty wearing compression devices as recommended (Fig. 11-16). In a study that reviewed adherence to compression stocking regimens, Jull and colleagues found that 52% of 129 participants reported wearing stockings every day for the first 6 months after the healing of an ulcer, 16% reported they wore stockings "most days," 5% reported they "occasionally" wore stockings, 22% reported they did not wear compression stockings at all once the ulcer had healed, and 4% did not report data.[82] The authors of this study concluded that the patient's belief that wearing stockings was worthwhile and the belief that the stockings were comfortable to wear were the greatest determinants of adherence 75% of the time.

APPLICATION TECHNIQUE 11-2 | COMPRESSION GARMENT

Compression garments should be applied by gathering them up, placing them on the distal area first, and then gradually unfolding them proximally. Because higher compression garments have more pretensioning, some patients have difficulty putting them on. A number of devices have been developed to assist with donning these garments, or the patient may wear two sets of lower-compression garments to provide a total compression equal to the sum of both of them. For example, the patient could wear two pairs of 20 mm Hg compression stockings instead of one pair of 40 mm Hg stockings to achieve the same effect.

Compression garments need to be worn every day throughout the day, except for bathing, to control edema, improve circulation, or control scar formation most effectively. In general, with proper care, these garments last about 6 months, after which time they lose their elasticity and no longer exert the appropriate amount of pressure.

Advantages

- Compression quantifiable (unlike bandaging).
- Extremity can be used during treatment (unlike a pump).

- Less expensive than intermittent compression devices for short-term use.
- Thin and attractive, available in various colors.
- Safe for acute condition.
- Can be used 24 hours per day.
- Preferred by patients to compression bandages.[54]

Disadvantages

- When used alone, may not reverse edema that is already present.
- More expensive than most bandages.
- Need to be fitted appropriately.
- Require strength, flexibility, and dexterity to put on.
- Hot, particularly in warm weather.
- Expensive for long-term use because they need to be replaced at least every 6 months, and the patient requires at least two identical garments so that one is available when the other is being laundered.

© **Clinical Pearl**

Compression garments must be worn all day, every day, and they last approximately 6 months.

Garments also need to be replaced if there is a significant change in limb size, which may occur with changes in edema or in body weight. For the compression device to be effective and to avoid the expense of purchasing many sets of garments, it is recommended that a patient use bandages to treat edema initially, while limb size is still diminishing, and that compression garments be ordered when the limb size appears to have stabilized.

VELCRO-CLOSURE DEVICES

Readily removable and adjustable compression devices that fasten with Velcro straps are also available (Fig. 11-17). Although this can improve patient acceptance, the ease of removal can also decrease adherence. A review of studies comparing these devices with Unna's boots, below-the-knee stockings, and 4-layer and short-stretch bandages found them to be a viable, low-cost option for compression therapy.[83] It should be noted that these devices provide inelastic compression similar to an Unna's boot, but that the amount of pressure can be adjusted by the patient to change compression during daily activities. With optimal use, companies claim that these devices provide 30 to 40 mm Hg gradient compression.[84] Because the Velcro bands are nonstretch, the amount of compression does not decrease with the age of the device.

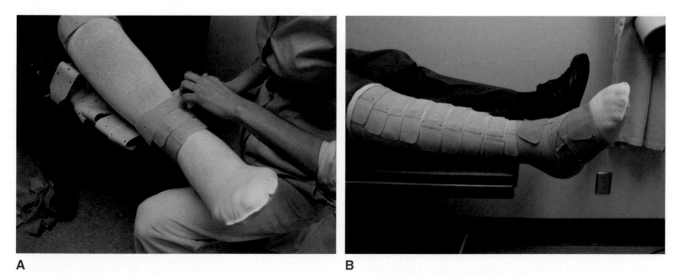

A   **B**

FIG 11-17 Velcro-closure compression device. *From Cameron MH, Monroe LG: Physical rehabilitation: evidence-based examination, evaluation, and intervention, St Louis, 2007, Saunders.*

APPLICATION TECHNIQUE 11-3 | **VELCRO-CLOSURE COMPRESSION DEVICES**

Equipment Required

- Stockinette
- Velcro-closure device

Procedure

1. Remove clothing and jewelry from the area to be treated.
2. Inspect skin for infection and wounds.
3. Dress and cover any wound according to the treatment regimen being used for that wound.
4. Apply stockinette.
5. Apply Velcro-closure device and close it, starting at the foot and working upward toward the knee.

Advantages

- Easier for patient to apply than compression garments providing comparable compression.
- Does not lose effectiveness with use or washing.
- Can adjust the tightness of the device depending on activity.

Disadvantages

- Easy to remove, with decreased effectiveness if patient removes device.
- Loosening the Velcro straps reduces compression to levels that may be insufficient for controlling edema.

INTERMITTENT PNEUMATIC COMPRESSION PUMP

IPC pumps are used to provide the force for intermittent compression. The pump is attached, via a hose, to a chambered sleeve placed around the involved limb (Fig. 11-18). The methods of application differ slightly among pumps, and specific instructions for the application of intermittent compression are provided with all pumps. General instructions for the application of most pumps are given in Application Technique 11-4. Although intermittent compression is suitable for home use, the patient should always begin the course of therapy under medical supervision.

Once satisfactory reduction of edema has been achieved with the pump, the clinician should determine if control will be maintained with continued use of the pump or if better results would be obtained with a compression garment or bandaging. In general, because a compression pump is used for only a number of hours each day, the patient should use a static compression device between treatments with the pump to maintain the reversal of edema produced by the pump.[58] In patients with chronic venous insufficiency and resulting edema and leg ulcers, intermittent compression is recommended if compression stockings have been used unsuccessfully for 6 months.[85] Intermittent compression is not generally used for the control of scar tissue formation because, for this effect, compression is required at all times.

There is some controversy in the current literature regarding the use of compression pumps for the treatment of lymphedema. One recent systematic review found that only one study compared IPC with no treatment, and the results were inconclusive. Other smaller, less well-designed studies had mixed results, some finding that edema was reduced more with intermittent pneumatic compression than with elastic compression and others finding no difference.[86] Further study is needed on the treatment of lymphedema with pneumatic compression, but at this time it may be best to combine treatments such as complete decongestive therapy (massage, compression bandaging, exercise, or skin and nail care) with IPC.[87]

PARAMETERS FOR INTERMITTENT PNEUMATIC COMPRESSION PUMPING

Inflation and Deflation Times. The inflation time is the period during which the compression sleeve is being inflated or is at the maximal inflation pressure, and the deflation time is the period during which the compression sleeve is being deflated or is fully deflated. For the treatment of edema or venous stasis ulcers or for DVT prevention, the inflation time is generally between 80 and 100 seconds, and the deflation time is generally between 25 and 50 seconds to allow for venous refilling after compression. For residual limb reduction, these periods are generally shorter, with inflation time being between 40 and 60 seconds and deflation time being between 10 and 15 seconds. Usually, the pressure is applied in approximately a 3 : 1 ratio of inflation to deflation time and then adjusted if necessary according to the patient's tolerance and response.

Inflation Pressure. Inflation pressure is the maximum pressure during the inflation time and is measured in millimeters of mercury (mm Hg). Most units can deliver between 30 and 120 mm Hg of inflation pressure. When

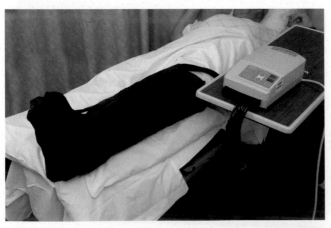

FIG 11-18 Intermittent pneumatic compression being applied for treatment of lymphedema. *From Pierson FM, Fairchild SL:* Principles and Techniques of Patient Care, *ed 4, St Louis, 2008, Saunders.*

TABLE 11-1	Recommended Parameters for the Application of Intermittent Compression		
Problem	Inflation/Deflation Time in Seconds (ratio)	Inflation Pressure (mm Hg)	Treatment Time (hours)
Edema, DVT prevention, venous stasis ulcer	80-100/25-35 (3:1)	30-60 UE 40-80 UE	2-3
Residual limb reduction	40-60/10-15 (4:1)	30-60 UE 40-80 UE	2-3

DVT, Deep venous thrombosis; *UE*, upper extremity.

a single-chamber sleeve is used to provide intermittent compression, the chamber inflates to the maximum pressure and then deflates. When a multichamber sleeve is used to provide sequential compression, the distal segment inflates first to the maximum pressure and then, as it deflates, the more proximal segments inflate sequentially, generally to slightly lower levels of pressure. Some recommend that inflation pressure not exceed diastolic blood pressure in the belief that higher pressures may impair arterial circulation; however, because the tissues of the body protect the arterial vessels from collapse, higher pressures may be used if this is necessary to achieve the desired clinical outcome and does not cause pain, although close patient supervision is recommended when higher pressures are used. For all indications, inflation pressure is generally between 30 and 80 mm Hg and frequently just below the patient's diastolic blood pressure. Because venous pressure is usually lower in the upper extremities than in the lower extremities, the lower end of the pressure range, 30 to 60 mm Hg, is generally used for the upper extremities, while the higher end of the

range, 40 to 80 mm Hg, is generally used for the lower extremities. Lower pressures are generally recommended for residual limb reduction and shaping and for the treatment of posttraumatic edema rather than for the treatment of problems caused by venous insufficiency. Although high pressures have been recommended for the treatment of lymphedema, current guidelines indicate that lower pressures are safer and may still be effective for this condition.[88] Treatment with inflation pressures below 30 mm Hg is not likely to affect circulation or tissue form and is therefore not recommended for any condition.

Total Treatment Time. Total treatment time recommendations vary from 1 to 4 hours per treatment, with treatment frequency ranging from 3 times per week to 4 times per day. For most applications, treatments of 2 to 3 hours once or twice a day are recommended. The frequency and duration of treatment should be the minimum necessary to maintain good edema control or satisfactory progress toward the goals of treatment (Table 11-1).

APPLICATION TECHNIQUE 11-4 — INTERMITTENT PNEUMATIC COMPRESSION PUMP

Equipment Required

- Intermittent pneumatic compression unit
- Inflatable sleeves for upper and lower extremities
- Stockinette
- Blood pressure cuff
- Stethoscope
- Tape measure

Procedure

1. Determine that compression is not contraindicated for the patient or the condition. Be certain to check for signs of DVT, including calf pain or tenderness associated with swelling. Take the patient's history or check the chart for CHF, pulmonary edema, or other contraindications that may be the cause of the edema.
2. Remove jewelry and clothing from the treatment area and inspect the skin. Cover any open areas with gauze or an appropriate dressing.
3. Place the patient in a comfortable position, with the affected limb elevated. Limb elevation reduces both the pain and the edema caused by venous insufficiency, if applied soon after the development of these symptoms, because elevation allows gravity to accelerate the flow of blood in the veins toward the heart. With chronic venous insufficiency or lymphatic dysfunction, elevation of the limbs is generally less effective in reducing edema because the fluid is trapped

within fibrotic tissue and cannot return as readily to the venous or lymphatic capillaries, from where it can flow back to the central circulation.

4. Measure and record the patient's blood pressure.
5. Measure and record the limb circumference at a number of places with reference to bony landmarks[89] or take volumetric measurements by displacement of water from a graduated cylinder.
6. Place a stocking or stockinette over the area to be treated and smooth out all the wrinkles (Fig. 11-19).
7. Apply the sleeve from the unit (Fig. 11-20). Reusable sleeves made of washable Neoprene and nylon are generally used, although vinyl sleeves intended for single use are also available for application when there is concern about cross-contamination. The Neoprene and nylon sleeves can be machine washed in warm water and air dried or dried at low heat in a drier. The sleeves provide intermittent or sequential compression, depending on their design. Single-chamber sleeves provide intermittent compression only, while sleeves composed of a series of overlapping chambers can inflate sequentially, starting distally and progressing proximally, to produce a milking effect on the extremity. As noted, sequential compression has been shown to result in more complete emptying of the deep veins and a greater increase in fibrinolytic activity than single-chamber, intermittent compression and is therefore preferred for most applications,[31,54] although it has not been shown to result in

Continued

APPLICATION TECHNIQUE 11-4 | INTERMITTENT PNEUMATIC COMPRESSION PUMP—*cont'd*

greater acceleration of venous blood flow than single-chamber compression.[31]

Both single-chamber and multichamber sleeves are available in a variety of lengths and widths for treatment of upper or lower extremities of various sizes. When using a compression pump for the treatment of edema, it is recommended that the sleeve be long enough to cover the entire involved limb so that fluid does not accumulate in areas of the limb proximal to the end of the sleeve. When using a compression pump for the prevention of DVT formation, either calf-high or thigh-high sleeves can be used because both have been found to be effective for this application.[30,90]

8. Attach the hose from the pneumatic compression pump to the sleeve. The pumps vary in size and complexity from small home units intended for the treatment of one extremity to larger clinical units that can be used to treat four extremities at different settings all at one time (Fig. 11-21).

9. Set the appropriate compression parameters, including inflation and deflation times, inflation pressure, and total treatment time. At this time, there are little research data to guide precise selection of any of these parameters. Thus the parameters used clinically are derived from an understanding of the pathology being treated, measures of the patient's blood pressure, comfort, and observed efficacy in the individual patient. Most protocols use an inflation pressure slightly below the patient's diastolic blood pressure, although higher pressures can be used, and all units come with guidelines for treatment parameters based on their design and manufacture. The parameter ranges provided and listed in Table 11-1 cover the ranges suggested by most manufacturers for most pumps.

10. Provide the patient with a means to call you during the treatment. Measure and record the patient's blood pressure during the treatment, and discontinue treatment if either the systolic or diastolic pressure exceeds the limits set for the patient by the physician.

11. When the treatment is complete, turn off the unit, disconnect the tubing, and remove the sleeve and the stockinette.

12. Remeasure and record limb volume in the same manner as in step 5.

13. Reinspect the patient's skin.

14. Remeasure and document the patient's blood pressure.

15. Apply a compression garment or bandage to maintain the reduction in edema between treatments and after discontinuing the use of a compression pump. Maximum reduction of edema is usually achieved with use of the pump for 3 to 4 weeks.

Advantages

- Actively moves fluids and therefore may be more effective than static devices, particularly for a flaccid limb.
- Compression quantifiable.
- Can provide sequential compression.
- Requires less finger and hand dexterity to apply than compression bandages or garments.
- Can be used to reverse as well as control edema.
- Use can be supervised in a patient who is noncompliant with static compression.

Disadvantages

- Used only for limited times during the day and therefore not appropriate for modification of scar formation.
- Generally requires a static compression device to be used between treatments.
- Expensive to purchase unit or to pay for regular treatments in a clinic.
- Requires moderate comfort using machinery to apply.
- Requires electricity.
- Extremity cannot be used during treatment.
- Patient cannot move about during treatment.
- Pumping motion of device may aggravate an acute condition.

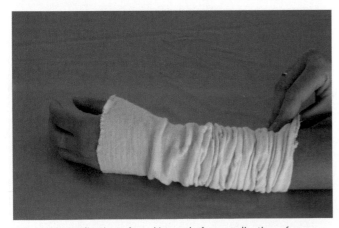

FIG 11-19 Application of stockinette before application of compression sleeve.

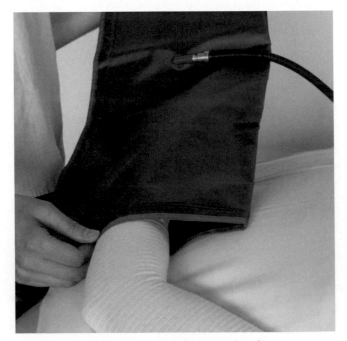

FIG 11-20 Application of compression sleeve.

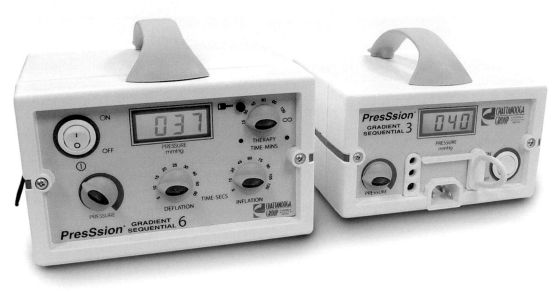

FIG 11-21 Intermittent compression units. *Courtesy Chattanooga Group, Hixson, TN.*

DOCUMENTATION

When applying external compression, document the following:

- Type of compression device
- Area of the body being treated
- Inflation and deflation times
- Compression or inflation pressure
- Total treatment time
- Patient's response to the treatment

Documentation is typically written in the SOAP (Subjective, Objective, Assessment, Plan) note format. The following examples only summarize the modality component of treatment and are not intended to represent a comprehensive plan of care.

EXAMPLES

When applying a compression bandage to the left (L) ankle after an acute sprain, document the following:

S: Pt reports L ankle swelling that increases in the PM.

O: Ankle girth R 9", L 10½", 3 days ago, before placement of elastic bandage.
Today, L ankle girth 10".

Treatment: Replaced elastic bandage to L ankle and leg, figure 8, and instructed pt in bandage application.

A: Pt responding to treatment, with reduced edema 3 days after injury.

P: Continue high stretch elastic bandage to L ankle and leg, figure 8. Pt to keep LE elevated.

When applying IPC to the right (R) arm to treat lymphedema, document the following:

S: Pt reports decreasing R UE edema in the past 2 wks and is now able to use a key with her R hand.

O: Pretreatment arm volume to elbow: R 530 cc, L 410 cc.

BP pretreatment: 135/80, during and immediately after treatment: 140/85. No overall change in pretreatment blood pressure during 2-wk course of treatment.

Treatment: IPC R UE, 80 sec/30 sec, 50 mm Hg, 2 hr BID twice daily. After 1 treatment: R 500 cc; after 2 wks of treatment R: 450 cc.

A: Pt tolerating treatent well, with decreased edema, increased R hand function, and no change in BP over 2 wks.

P: Continue IPC R UE, 80 sec/30 sec, 50 mm Hg, 2 hr BID daily. When R UE volume stabilizes consider fitting for compression garment.

When applying compression hose to prevent DVT formation, document the following:

S: Pt not oriented; bedridden.

O: Negative Homan's sign. No other signs of DVT formation.

Treatment: Compression hose both LEs, approx 20 mm Hg compression.

A: Bedridden pt at risk for DVT.

P: Pt to wear compression hose 24 hr/day while in bed. Instruct other caregivers in compression hose program.

CLINICAL CASE STUDIES

The following case studies summarize the concepts of compression discussed in this chapter. Based on the scenarios presented, an evaluation of the clinical findings and goals of treatment are proposed. These are followed by a discussion of the factors to be considered in selection of compression as the indicated intervention and in selection of the ideal compression device and treatment parameters to promote progress toward the goals of treatment.

CASE STUDY 11-1

Chronic Lymphedema
Examination
History

FR is a 40-year-old carpenter. She has chronic lymphedema of her right upper extremity and complains of pain and swelling in this extremity that worsens with use and that is moderately alleviated by elevation and avoiding use of the extremity. She rates her pain severity 4-8/10. She first noticed the swelling 2 or 3 years ago, but at that time it occurred only after extensive use of her upper extremity at work; the swelling was mild and resolved with a night's rest. Over the last year, the swelling has worsened. Now, it never resolves fully and is easily aggravated by even light activity at work or by yard work, and she has reduced her work hours by 50%.

FR reports that 8 years ago she had a right mastectomy and 16 lymph nodes removed as part of her treatment for breast cancer. She was also treated with chemotherapy and radiation therapy at that time and has had no recurrence of the malignancy. FR has been advised by her physician to reduce the use of her right arm and elevate it when possible to control the swelling. At her request, she has been referred to therapy for further management of her lymphedema.

Tests and Measures

The objective examination reveals moderate pitting edema of the right arm and forearm, with circumferential measurements of 7 inches at the right wrist compared with 6 inches at the left wrist, 11 inches at the right elbow compared with $9\frac{1}{2}$ inches at the left elbow, and 14 inches at the right midbiceps compared with 11 inches at the same level on the left. The swelling also causes moderate restriction of elbow, wrist, hand, and finger ROM. Passive elbow ROM was measured as 130 degrees flexion and −10 degrees extension on the right compared with 145 degrees flexion and full extension on the left. The skin of the patient's right upper extremity appears thin, flaky, and red, and her blood pressure is 120/80. All other tests, including shoulder ROM and upper extremity sensation, are within normal limits.

Based on the patient's history, is the lymphatic system in her right upper extremity blocked? What parts of the history lead you to this conclusion? Is malignancy a concern when considering compression as an intervention for this patient?

Evaluation, Diagnosis, and Prognosis
Evaluation

ICF Level	Current Status	Goals
Body structure and function	Increased girth and loss of motion of the R UE	Control and reduce edema until measurement of R arm girth equals L arm girth Restore ROM so that R UE ROM becomes equal her L UE ROM within 3 months
Activity	Reduced tolerance for using and lifting with her right arm	Able to use R UE for all daily activities and to lift 40 lb
Participation	Reduced work hours by 50%	Improve work hours to 100% of normal over next 3 months

Diagnosis

Preferred Practice Pattern 6H: Impaired circulation and anthropometric dimensions associated with lymphatic systems disorders.

Prognosis/Plan of Care

Although experts in the field of lymphedema vary in their recommendations for treatment of this condition, most agree that some form of compression is indicated. Compression can provide working or resting pressure to control fluid flow out of the venous circulation and into the lymphatic circulation and can also promote the movement of fluid through the lymphatic vessels. Some experts recommend the use of special massage techniques in conjunction with compression to promote lymphatic flow, particularly in proximal areas such as the axilla and the trunk, to aid or divert flow in areas where lymphatic function is compromised and where most compression devices are not effective. Without such additional treatment, compression alone may result in the accumulation of fluid proximal to the compression device, particularly if proximal lymphatic function is impaired.

Although the use of compression is generally not recommended in the presence of malignancy, because this patient has had no recurrence of her disease after more than 5 years, most experts agree that compression may be used. Although the lymphatic circulation in this patient is clearly impaired, the fact that the severity of her edema varies, resolving to some extent with rest and elevation, indicates that the lymphatic circulation in the right upper extremity is not completely blocked and therefore compression is not contraindicated for this reason.

CLINICAL CASE STUDIES—*cont'd*

Intervention

Initially, an intermittent sequential pneumatic pump was to apply compression. This form of compression is likely to produce the fastest and most effective reversal of edema because it provides both compression and the milking action of sequential distal to proximal compression. To control the formation of edema between treatments with the pneumatic device, an inelastic bandage was applied during the day to provide a high working pressure. When the reduction of edema plateaus, which usually takes 2 to 3 weeks, pumping can be gradually discontinued. The patient should continue to use the bandages when working or exercising her upper extremity. If the patient is not compliant with long-term use of bandages, a compression garment may be used. However, since this type of garment is made of a moderately elastic material, which develops limited working pressure, it may not be as effective as an inelastic bandage in maintaining edema control during exercise or other heavy upper extremity activity. The patient should not be measured for fitting of a compression garment at the initiation of treatment because a garment fitted at that time will soon be too big if any edema reversal is achieved with pumping or bandaging. Measurement for fitting of the garment should be performed when limb volume stabilizes.

Optimal treatment parameters at the initiation of treatment, when the sequential intermittent pneumatic compression pump is being used, are 80 to 100 seconds of inflation and 25 to 35 seconds of deflation, with a maximum inflation pressure of 30 to 60 mm Hg. The lowest inflation pressure that achieves reduction of edema should be used to minimize the risk of collapsing the superficial lymphatic or venous vessels. For most patients, treatment with the pump for 2 to 3 hours once or twice per day is sufficient. All parameters may be adjusted within these ranges to achieve optimal edema control without pain and with the least disruption of the patient's regular activities. Compression bandages or garments should be worn at all times, except for bathing, when the pump is not being used.

Appropriate use of massage, exercise, and activity modification should also be considered, in addition to treatment with compression, to achieve the optimal outcome for this patient. The patient's blood pressure should be monitored before, during, and after the use of the compression pump. If it becomes excessively elevated, the pressure, and if necessary the duration, of pumping should be reduced. During pumping, the patient's upper extremity should also be elevated above the level of her heart. This is most readily achieved if the patient lies supine and places her arm on a pillow.

Documentation

S: Pt reports swelling and pain, severity 4-8/10, in R UE that worsens with use and at the end of the day.

O: Pretreatment: Moderate pitting edema R arm and forearm. R wrist circumference 7 in, R midbiceps 14″ L wrist circumference 6″, L midbiceps 11″. Passive ROM R elbow 130 degrees flexion, −10 degrees extension.

Treatment: IPC to R UE 80 sec inflation, 25 sec deflation for total treatment time 2 hours.

Posttreatment: Minimal edema R arm and forearm. R wrist circumference 6 ½″, R midbiceps 12″. Passive ROM R elbow 140 degrees flexion, −5 degrees extension.

A: Good response to compression with IPC, with reduced edema, increased functional ROM, decreased pain.

P: Instruct pt on home use of IPC device 2 hr once daily. Instruct pt on application of bandages or compression garment to R UE after IPC. Follow-up 1 week for reassessment.

CASE STUDY 11-2

Venous Stasis Ulcer
Examination
History

JU is a 65-year-old man with a full-thickness venous stasis ulcer on his distal medial left leg. He reports that the ulcer is minimally painful at 1/10 on the pain scale but requires frequent dressing changes because a large amount of fluid leaks from it. The ulcer has been present for 4 to 6 months and is gradually getting larger. The only treatment being provided for the ulcer is gauze dressing application, which the patient changes two or three times a day when he notices seepage.

This wound has significantly impacted JU's acitivities. He stopped attending biweekly bingo games and weekly church services 4 months ago because he found that the prolonged sitting made his left leg swell and hurt and because he was embarrassed by his weeping ulcer. He has also decreased his physical activity at home, spending most of the day sitting indoors in his recliner with his legs up rather than gardening for 2 hours when the weather permitted. He reports that his ankle is often uncomfortable to move and that swelling worsens when he is upright for more than an hour.

He had coronary artery bypass surgery 2 years ago, at which time the left saphenous vein was removed to be used for the graft. He is currently taking medication to control hypertension.

Tests and Measures

JU has a shallow, flat ulcer with a red base fully covered with granulation tissue, approximately 5 cm × 10 cm in area on the distal medial left leg, with darkening of the intact skin around the ulcer. There is also edema of the left foot, ankle, and leg. Ankle girth, measured at the medial malleolus, is 9 inches on the right and 10½ inches on the left. There are no signs of edema in the right lower extremity. Ankle ROM is +10 degrees of dorsiflexion to 60 degrees on the right and 0 degrees of dorsiflexion to 50 degrees of plantar flexion on the left. The patient's blood pressure is 140/100.

Continued

Why does this patient have a venous stasis ulcer? What other aspect of the patient's examination is concerning? What would you tell this patient about the lifetime use of compression? What measurement needs to be made before compression is applied to this patient?

Evaluation, Diagnosis, Prognosis, and Goals

Evaluation and Goals

ICF Level	Current Status	Goals
Body function and structure	Enlarging L LE venous stasis ulcer Increased girth L lower distal extremity Restricted L ankle ROM	Heal the ulcer Reduce edema so that L ankle girth matches R ankle girth and prevent ulcer recurrence Increase left ankle ROM to match right ankle ROM
Activity	Sitting with LE dependent and walking limited to 60 minutes	Sitting with LE dependent and walking tolerated for up to 2 hours
Participation	Decreased gardening, bingo, church attendance	Return to prior level of gardening, bingo, and church attendance within 2 months

Diagnosis

Preferred Practice Pattern 7D: Impaired integumentary integrity associated with full-thickness skin involvement and scar formation.

Prognosis/Plan of Care

JU presents with loss of skin and subcutaneous tissue integrity requiring him to change wound dressings frequently and placing him at risk for local infection and possible sepsis. His ulcer and edema of the distal lower extremity are probably a result of poor venous circulation. Compression is an indicated intervention because it can improve venous circulation to facilitate wound healing and edema control. Specialized dressings that are more absorbent and less adherent than gauze should be used to reduce the frequency of dressing changes and thus reduce the potential for wound trauma and inconvenience to the patient. Contraindications for the use of compression, including arterial insufficiency, heart failure, and DVT, should be ruled out before the initiation of treatment with compression. The patient's history of cardiac bypass surgery suggests the possibility of arterial insufficiency in the lower extremities, although the presence of edema and the conformation of the leg ulcer indicate that it is probably a result of venous rather than arterial insufficiency. To rule out arterial insufficiency, an ABI should be obtained and compression should be applied only if this is above 0.8. The presence of unilateral rather than bilateral edema indicates that this patient's edema is probably not from cardiac failure.

Assessment for Homan's sign should be performed to rule out a DVT before treatment with compression is initiated.

Intervention

Initally, JU was treated with intermittent compression applied with an intermittent sequential pneumatic pump twice per week, with static compression with an Unna's boot applied between pumping sessions. This combination of compression interventions promotes healing of venous stasis ulcers and has been found to double the speed of wound healing as compared with static compression with an Unna's boot alone.[91] It is proposed that this combination of types of compression produces such rapid, complete wound healing and resolution of edema because the edema is reduced by the milking action associated with sequential distal to proximal intermittent compression and then edema control is maintained by the continuous compression of the rigid Unna's boot. Recommended treatment parameters for the sequential IPC pump to promote circulation and control edema are 80 to 100 seconds of inflation and 25 to 35 seconds of deflation, with a maximum inflation pressure of 30 to 60 mm Hg and a treatment duration of 2 to 3 hours. Adjustments within these ranges should be made to achieve optimal edema control without pain and with the least disruption of the patient's regular activities. The Unna's boot should be worn at all times between intermittent compression treatments. If an Unna's boot is not available, then compression stockings providing 30 to 40 mm Hg of pressure may be worn between pumping treatments. Because these stockings are easier to remove and reapply than the Unna's boot, the frequency of pumping may be increased to once or twice per day. A Velcro-closure compression device would also be a good option between intermittent compression treatments. The patient's blood pressure should be monitored before, during, and after use of the compression pump. If his blood pressure increases the force, and if necessary the duration, of pumping should be reduced. An appropriate dressing should be placed on the ulcer site before the compression sleeve, boot, or stocking are applied. A single-use sleeve should be used for pumping, or an occlusive barrier should be placed over the ulcer during pumping to avoid cross-contamination.

It is essential that the patient continue to wear a compression stocking after the ulcer has healed because his circulatory compromise puts him at high risk for recurrence of edema and tissue breakdown in this extremity.

Documentation

S: Pt reports a nonhealing ulcer present for 4-6 months on his left medial lower extremity and increased edema of his L LE.

O: **Pretreatment:** 5 cm × 10 cm shallow ulcer on the distal medial L leg, with darkening of the intact skin around the ulcer. L ankle girth measured at the medial malleolus is 10½" and R ankle girth is 9". L ankle ROM 0-50 degrees, R ankle ROM +10-60 degrees.

Treatment: IPC to L leg at 80 sec inflation and 35 sec deflation, and maximum inflation pressure of 50 mm Hg × 2 hr.

Posttreatment: Ulcer unchanged in size after one treatment. L ankle girth 10".

A: Good response to treatment. No adverse effects.

P: Continue twice weekly treatments with intermittent sequential pneumatic compression at 80 sec inflation and 35 sec deflation, and maximum inflation pressure of 50 mm Hg for 2 hr. Pt should wear Unna's boot between intermittent compression treatments and may switch to compression stockings when ulcer begins to heal. Reassess each time patient comes for intermittent compression treatment and Unna's boot application.

CASE STUDY 11-3

Acute Ankle Sprain

Examination

History

ND is a 20-year-old man who sustained an inversion sprain of his right ankle within the last hour while playing football. He complains of ankle pain, stiffness, and swelling. The pain is primarily at the lateral ankle and increases when he bears weight on his right lower extremity when walking. He rates the pain as 7/10. He is unable to run because of the pain and walks with a limp.

Tests and Measures

There is mildly increased temperature, swelling, and restricted passive ROM of the right ankle. Ankle girth at the level of the medial malleolus is 12 inches on the right and 11 inches on the left. Passive ankle ROM was as follows:

Direction of Motion	Right	Left
Inversion	30 degrees, limited by pain	50 degrees
Eversion	20 degrees	25 degrees
Plantarflexion	0 degrees	15 degrees
Dorsiflexion	40 degrees	50 degrees

During ambulation, ND protected his right ankle by decreasing the duration of stance phase on the right, decreasing dorsiflexion of the right ankle during midstance, and decreasing plantar flexion of the right ankle during terminal stance.

Other than compression, what interventions could help prevent further swelling and injury? What type of compression would be most useful in the short term? In the long term?

Evaluation, Diagnosis, Prognosis, and Goals
Evaluation and Goals

ICF Level	Current Status	Goals
Body function and structure	R ankle pain Increased girth and temperature Decreased ROM	Short-term: Normalize temperature and swelling, prevent further injury Long-term: Regain normal girth and ROM of right ankle
Activity	Gait deviations Reduced ambulation tolerance and unable to run	Short-term: Painfree ambulation with appropriate use of assistive devices Long-term: Return to normal ambulation and running
Participation	Unable to play football	Return to playing football without limitations or pain

Diagnosis

Preferred Practice Pattern 4D: Impaired joint mobility, motor function, muscle performance, and ROM associated with connective tissue dysfunction.

Prognosis/Plan of Care

Compression should be a component of this patient's intervention because this treatment can help to control the formation of edema; however, it will not be optimally effective in promoting the achievement of this or other goals of treatment if used alone. When edema is caused by acute inflammation, compression is likely to be most effective if it is applied in conjunction with rest, ice, and elevation. Local rest can be achieved by the appropriate use of crutches; ice may be applied as described in Chapter 6, and. for optimal benefit, the patient's ankle should be elevated above the level of his heart. The use of crutches will also reduce the risk of further injury to other areas as a result of stresses of an abnormal gait pattern. Although the use of compression is not contraindicated in this patient, the use of intermittent compression is not recommended because, with such an acute trauma, the motion produced by intermittent compression may aggravate bleeding or displace a fracture if one is present.

Intervention

Because the movement associated with intermittent compression may exacerbate inflammation after an acute injury, static compression should be used to control edema in this patient. Static compression can be provided most readily with an elastic compression bandage. This type of bandage provides high resting pressure, is readily available, can easily be used by the patient at

Continued

CLINICAL CASE STUDIES—*cont'd*

home, and is inexpensive. The bandage should be wrapped in a figure-8 manner to provide consistent and comfortable compression in all areas. It should be snug but not so tight that it limits circulation. For optimal control of edema, slightly more compression should be applied distally than proximally. To apply cryotherapy in conjunction with the compression, the bandage may be applied over or under an ice pack or cold pack. Because compression should be maintained at all times until the edema resolves, whereas cryotherapy should generally be applied for 15 minutes every 1 to 2 hours, placing the pack over the compression bandage may be more time efficient. The patient should also elevate his lower extremity above the level of his heart when possible to achieve the most rapid resolution of the edema. Compression should be applied at all times until the edema resolves. As the patient recovers and the edema is reduced, an elastic compression brace may be used in place of the compression bandage.

Documentation

S: Pt reports R ankle pain at 7/10, stiffness, and swelling after a football injury in the past hour.

O: Pretreatment: R ankle has increased temperature, swelling. R ankle girth 12″ at the medial malleolus, L ankle 11″. R ankle passive ROM 30 degrees of inversion limited by pain and 20 degrees of eversion. L ankle 50 degree inversion and 25 degrees eversion. R ankle dorsiflexion 0 degrees, L ankle 15 degrees. R ankle plantar flexion 40 degrees, L ankle 50 degrees.

Treatment: Ace bandage applied to R foot and ankle, R leg elevated, ice applied × 15 minutes.

Post-treatment: Pain decreased to 3/10. R ankle girth 11½″. R ankle passive ROM mildly improved.

A: Pt responded well to treatment.

P: Continue compression with Ace bandage until edema is reduced, then replace with elastic compression brace. Cryotherapy 15 min each hr until edema is reduced. Elevate R LE above heart for next 2 hrs.

CHAPTER REVIEW

1. Compression applies an inwardly directed force to the tissues, increasing extravascular pressure and venous and lymphatic circulation.
2. External compression can be used to control edema, prevent the formation of DVTs, facilitate venous stasis ulcer healing, and shape residual limbs after amputation.
3. Compression devices include compression bandages, compression garments, Velcro-closure devices, and pneumatic pumps. Bandages and garments provide static compression and can be worn throughout the day, whereas pneumatic pumps provide intermittent compression for limited periods of time.
4. The choice of compression device depends on the problem being treated and the ability of the patient to comply with the treatment.
5. The use of compression is contraindicated in heart failure, pulmonary edema, DVT, thrombophlebitis, pulmonary embolism, obstructed lymphatic or venous return, peripheral arterial disease, skin infection, hypoproteinemia, and trauma. Caution should be used in patients with impaired sensation or mentation, uncontrolled hypertension, cancer, or stroke and in the application of compression over superficial peripheral nerves.
6. The reader is referred to the Evolve web site for further exercises and links to resources and references.

ADDITIONAL RESOURCES *evolve*

Web Sites

Healthy Legs: Retailer selling support hose and compression stockings. The web site has links to companies that make these products, information on keeping legs healthy, and videos on topics such as measuring for compression stockings and understanding venous disease: www.healthylegs.com

Heller Socks: Manufacturer of compression socks for residual limbs after amputation: www.hellersocks.com

Lymph Notes: Online resource for patients with lymphedema that provides information, support groups, lists of clinics and product manufacturers: www.lymphnotes.com

National Lymphedema Network: A nonprofit organization established in 1988 to provide education and guidance to patients with lymphedema, health care professionals, and the general public by disseminating information on the prevention and management of primary and secondary lymphedema. This web site includes general information, position papers, resources, and research: www.lymphnet.org

Teufel International: Manufacturer of orthotics, prosthetics and residual limb compression products: www.teufel-international.com

Textbooks

Sparks-DeFriese B: Vascular ulcers. In Cameron MH, Monroe LM: *Physical rehabilitation: evidence-based examination, evaluation, and intervention,* St Louis, 2007, Elsevier

Sussman C, Bates-Jensen BM, eds: *Wound care: a collaborative practice manual for health professionals,* ed 3, Philadelphia, 2007, Lippincott, Williams & Wilkins.

GLOSSARY *evolve*

Antiembolism stockings: Knee-high or thigh-high stockings that provide low compression force to prevent DVT formation.

Compression: The application of a mechanical force that increases external pressure on a body part to reduce swelling, improve circulation, or modify scar tissue formation.

Deep venous thrombosis (DVT): Blood clot in a deep vein.

Edema: Swelling caused by increased fluid in the interstitial spaces of the body.

Hydrostatic pressure: Pressure exerted by a fluid, for example, in the blood vessels, it is determined by the force of the heart and gravity and contributes to movement of fluid into or out of blood vessels and lymphatics.

Hypertrophic scarring: Excessive scarring with a raised and ridged appearance that does not extend beyond the boundaries of the original site of skin injury. This type of scar has poor flexibility and can result in contractures and poor cosmesis

Intermittent compression: Pressure that is alternately applied and released and usually applied by a pneumatic compression pump.

Keloid: Excessive scarring that extends beyond the boundaries of the original site of skin injury.

Long-stretch bandage: An elastic bandage that can extend by 100% to 200% and provides high resting pressure; also called a high-stretch bandage.

Lymphatic fluid: Fluid rich in protein, water, and macrophages that is removed from the interstitial space by the lymphatic system and returned to the venous system; also called lymph.

Lymphatic system: A system of vessels and nodes designed to carry excess fluid from the interstitial space to the venous system and to filter the fluid, removing bacteria and other foreign particles.

Lymphedema: Swelling caused by excess lymphatic fluid in the interstitial space.

Osmotic pressure: Pressure determined by the concentration of proteins inside and outside blood vessels that contributes to movement of fluid into or out of blood vessels and lymphatics; also known as oncotic pressure when the term is applied to blood.

Phlebitis: Inflammation of the veins; the most common cause of venous insufficiency.

Resting pressure: Pressure exerted by elastic when put on stretch.

Short-stretch bandage: A bandage with low elasticity and 30% to 90% extension that provides a low resting pressure but a high working pressure during muscle activity; also called a low-stretch bandage.

Static compression: Steady application of pressure.

Unna's boot: A semirigid bandage made of zinc oxide–impregnated gauze that is applied to the lower extremity to exert pressure.

Venous insufficiency: Decreased ability of the veins to return blood to the heart.

Venous stasis ulcer: An area of tissue breakdown and necrosis that occurs as a result of impaired venous return.

Working pressure: Pressure produced by active muscles pushing against an inelastic bandage.

REFERENCES *evolve*

1. Ramos R, Salem BI, DePawlikowski MP, et al: The efficacy of pneumatic compression stockings in the prevention of pulmonary embolism after cardiac surgery, *Chest* 109(1):82-85, 1996.
2. Samson RH: Compression stockings and non-continuous use of polyurethane foam dressings for the treatment of venous ulceration: a pilot study, *J Dermatol Surg Oncol* 19(1):68-72, 1993.
3. Chen AH, Frangos SG, Kilaru S, et al: Intermittent pneumatic compression devices—physiological mechanisms of action, *Eur J Vasc Endovasc Surg* 21(5):383-392, 2001.
4. Whitelaw GP, Oladipo OJ, Shah BP, et al: Evaluation of intermittent pneumatic compression devices, *Orthopedics* 24(3):257-261, 2001.
5. Kamm RD: Bioengineering studies of periodic external compression as prophylaxis against deep venous thrombosis. I. Numerical studies, *J Biomech Eng* 104:87-95, 1982.
6. Olson DA, Kamm RD, Shapiro AH: Bioengineering studies of periodic external compression as prophylaxis against deep venous thrombosis. II. Experimental studies on a simulated leg, *J Biomech Eng* 104:96-104, 1982.
7. Wakim KG, Martin GM, Krusen FH: Influence of centripetal rhythmic compression on localized edema of an extremity, *Arch Phys Med Rehabil* 36:98-103, 1955.
8. Lee RC, Capelli-Schellpfeffer M, Astumian RD: A review of thermoregulation of tissue repair and remodeling, 1995, Abstract Soc Phys Rev Biol Med 15th Ann Mtg, Washington, DC.
9. O'Brien JG, Chennubhotla SA: Treatment of edema, *Am Fam Phys* 71(11):2111-2117, 2005.
10. Clarke M, Hopewell S, Juszczak E, et al: Compression stockings for preventing deep vein thrombosis in airline passengers, *Cochrane Database Syst Rev* 2:CD004002, 2006.
11. Young GL. Jewell D: Interventions for varicosities and leg oedema in pregnancy, *Cochrane Database Syst Rev* 2:CD001066, 2000.
12. Ganong WF: *Review of medical physiology*, Norwalk, CT, 1987, Appleton & Lange.
13. Szuba A, Rockson SG: Lymphedema: classification, diagnosis, and therapy, *Vasc Med* 3:145-156, 1998.
14. Airaksinen O: Changes in posttraumatic ankle joint mobility, pain, and edema following intermittent pneumatic compression therapy, *Arch Phys Med Rehabil* 70(4):341-344, 1989.
15. Chleboun GS, Howell JN, Baker HL, et al: Intermittent pneumatic compression effect on eccentric exercise-induced swelling, stiffness and strength loss, *Arch Phys Med Rehabil* 76(8):744-749, 1995.
16. Boris M, Weindorf S, Lasinski B, et al: Lymphedema reduction by noninvasive complex lymphedema therapy, *Oncology* 8(9):95-106, 1994.
17. Gilbart MK, Ogilvie-Harris DJ, Broadhurst C, et al: Anterior tibial compartment pressures during intermittent sequential pneumatic compression therapy, *Am J Sports Med* 23(6):769-772, 1995.
18. Heit JA, The epidemiology of venous thromboembolism in the community: implications for prevention and management, *J Thrombos Thrombol* 21(1):23-29, 2006.
19. Heit JA, O'Fallon WM, Petterson TM, et al: Relative impact of risk factors for deep vein thrombosis and pulmonary embolism: a population-based study, *Arch Int Med* 162(11):1245-1248, 2002.
20. Amarigiri SV, Lees TA: Elastic compression stockings for prevention of deep vein thrombosis, *Cochrane Database Syst Rev* 3:CD001484, 2000.
21. Mazzone C, Chiodo Grandi F, Sandercock P, et al: Physical methods for preventing deep vein thrombosis in stroke, *Cochrane Database Syst Rev* 4:CD001922, 2004.
22. Handoll HH, Farrar MJ, McBirnie J, et al: Heparin, low molecular weight heparin and physical methods for preventing deep vein thrombosis and pulmonary embolism following surgery for hip fractures, *Cochrane Database Syst Rev* 4:CD000305, 2002.
23. Roderick P, Ferris G, Wilson K, et al: Towards evidence-based guidelines for the prevention of venous thromboembolism: systematic reviews of mechanical methods, oral anticoagulation, dextran and regional anaesthesia as thromboprophylaxis, *Health Technol Assess* 9(49):1-94, 2005.
24. Ginzburg E, Cohn SM, Lopez J, et al: Randomized clinical trial of intermittent pneumatic compression and low molecular weight heparin in trauma, *Br J Surg* 90:1338-1344, 2003.
25. Kurtoglu M, Yanar H, Bilsel Y, et al: Venous thromboembolism prophylaxis after head and spinal trauma: intermittent pneumatic compression devices versus low molecular weight heparin, *World J Surg* 28:807-811, 2004.
26. Freedman KB, Brookenthal KR, Fitzgerald RH Jr, et al: A meta-analysis of thromboembolic prophylaxis following elective total hip arthroplasty, *J Bone Joint Surg* 82A(7):929-938, 2000.

27. Westrich GH, Haas SB, Mosca P, et al: Meta-analysis of thromboembolic prophylaxis after total knee arthroplasty, *J Bone Joint Surg* 82B(6):795-800, 2000.

28. Wille-Jorgensen P, Rasmussen MS, Andersen BR, et al: Heparins and mechanical methods for thromboprophylaxis in colorectal surgery, *Cochrane Database Syst Rev* 4:CD001217, 2003.

29. Kolbach DN, Sandbrink MW, Hamulyak K: Non-pharmaceutical measures for prevention of post-thrombotic syndrome, *Cochrane Database Syst Rev* 1:CD004174, 2004.

30. Adi Y, Bayliss S, Rouse A, Taylor RS. The association between air travel and deep vein thrombosis: systematic review and meta-analysis, *BMC Cardiovasc Dis* 4(7):1-8, 2004.

31. Pidala MJ, Donovan DL, Kepley RF: A prospective study on intermittent pneumatic compression in the prevention of deep vein thrombosis in patients undergoing total hip or total knee replacement, *Surgery* 175:47-51, 1992.

32. Flam E, Berry S, Coyle A, et al: Blood-flow augmentation of intermittent pneumatic compression systems used for the prevention of deep vein thrombosis before surgery, *Am J Surg* 171:312-315, 1996.

33. Tarnay TJ, Rohr PR, Davidson AG, et al: Pneumatic calf compression, fibrinolysis, and the prevention of deep venous thrombosis, *Surgery* 88:489-495, 1980.

34. Knight MTN, Dawson R: Effect of intermittent compression of the arms on deep venous thrombosis in the legs, *Lancet* 2(7998):1265-1268, 1976.

35. Salzman EW, McManama GP, Shapiro AH, et al: Effect of optimization of hemodynamics on fibrinolytic activity and antithrombotic efficacy of external calf compression, *Ann Surg* 206:636-641, 1987.

36. Chouhan VD, Comerota AJ, Sun L, et al: Inhibition of tissue factor pathway during intermittent pneumatic compression: a possible mechanism for antithrombotic effect, *Arterioscler Thromb Vasc Biol* 19(11):2812-2817, 1999.

37. Abbade LP, Lastória S: Venous ulcer: epidemiology, physiopathology, diagnosis and treatment, *Int J Dermatol* 44 (6): 449-456, 2005.

38. Smith PD: Update on chronic-venous-insufficiency-induced inflammatory processes, *Angiology* 52 (suppl 1):S35-42, 2001.

39. Stvrtinova V, Jahnova E, Weissova S, et al: Inflammatory mechanisms involving neutrophils in chronic venous insufficiency of lower limbs, *Bratislavske Lekarske Listy* 102(5):235-239, 2001.

40. White JV, Ryjewski C: Chronic venous insufficiency, *Perspect Vasc Surg Endovasc Ther* 17(4):319-327, 2005.

41. Danielsson G, Eklof B, Grandinetti A, et al: Deep axial reflux, an important contributor to skin changes or ulcer in chronic venous disease, *J Vasc Surg* 38(6):1336-1341, 2003.

42. Stanley AC, Fernandez NN, Lounsbury KM, et al: Pressure-induced cellular senescence: a mechanism linking venous hypertension to venous ulcers, *J Surg Res* 124(1):112-117, 2005.

43. Cullum N, Nelson EA, Fletcher AW, et al: Compression for venous leg ulcers, *Cochrane Database Syst Rev* 2:CD000265, 2001.

44. Ukat A, Konig M, Vanscheidt W, et al: Short-stretch versus multilayer compression for venous leg ulcers: a comparison of healing rates, *J Wound Care* 12(4):139-143, 2003.

45. Nelson EA, Bell-Syer SE, Cullum NA: Compression for preventing recurrence of venous ulcers, *Cochrane Database Syst Rev* 4: CD002303, 2000.

46. Poore S, Cameron J, Cherry G: Venous leg ulcer recurrence: prevention and healing, *J Wound Care* 11(5):197-199, 2002.

47. Mayberry JC, Moneta GL, Taylor LM Jr, et al: Fifteen-year results of ambulatory compression therapy for chronic venous ulcers, *Surgery* 109(5):575-581, 1991.

48. Erickson CA, Lanza DJ. Karp DL, et al: Healing of venous ulcers in an ambulatory care program: the roles of chronic venous insufficiency and patient compliance, *J Vasc Surgery* 22(5):629-636, 1995.

49. Samson RH, Showalter DP: Stockings and the prevention of recurrent venous ulcers, *Dermatol Surg* 22(4):373-376, 1996.

50. Berliner E, Ozbilgin B, Zarin DA: A systematic review of pneumatic compression for treatment of chronic venous insufficiency and venous ulcers, *J Vasc Surg* 37(3):539-544, 2003.

51. Kunimoto B, Cooling M, Gullinver W, et al: Best practices for the prevention and treatment of venous leg ulcers, *Ostomy Wound Manage* 47(2):34-46, 48-50, 2001.

52. Registered Nurses Association of Ontario Professional Association: Assessment and management of venous leg ulcers, 2004. http://www.guideline.gov/summary/summary.aspx?ss=15&doc_id=5309&nbr=003632&string=ulcer. Accessed August 9, 2006.

53. Partsch B, Partsch H: Calf compression pressure required to achieve venous closure from supine to standing positions, *J Vasc Surg* 42(4):734-738, 2005.

54. Lord RS, Hamilton D: Graduated compression stockings 20-30 mmHg. do not compress leg veins in the standing position, *ANZ J Surg* 74: 581-585,2004.

55. Pekanmaki K, Kolari PJ, Kirstala U: Intermittent pneumatic compression treatment for post-thrombotic leg ulcers, *Clin Exp Dermatol* 12:350-353, 1987.

56. Coleridge Smith PD, Thomas PRS, Scurr JH, et al: The aetiology of venous ulceration:a new hypothesis, *Br Med J* 296:1726-1728, 1988.

57. Agu O, Baker D, Seifalian AM: Effect of graduated compression stockings on limb oxygenation and venous function during exercise in patients with venous insufficiency, *Vascular* 12(1):69-76, 2004.

58. Ibegbuna V, Delis KT, Nicolaides AN, et al: Effect of elastic compression stockings on venous hemodynamics during walking, *J Vasc Surg* 37(2):420-5, 2003.

59. Labropoulos N, Wierks C, Suffoletto B: Intermittent pneumatic compression for the treatment of lower extremity arterial disease: a systematic review, *Vasc Med* 7(2):141-148, 2002.

60. The Jobst Extremity Pump: *Clinical applications with an overview of the pathophysiology of edema,* Charlotte, NC, 1996, Beiersdorf-Jobst.

61. Deitch EA, Wheelahan TM, Rose MP, et al: Hypertrophic burn scars: analysis of variables, *J Trauma* 23:895-898, 1983.

62. Hunt TK: Disorders of wound healing, *World J Surg* 4:271-277, 1980.

63. Sullivan T, Smith J, Kermode J, et al: Rating the burn scar, *J Burn Care Rehabil* 11:256-260, 1990.

64. Ward RS: Pressure therapy for the control of hypertrophic scar formation after burn injury: a history and review, *J Burn Care Rehabil* 12:257-262, 1991.

65. Reno F, Grazianetti P, Cannas M: Effects of mechanical compression on hypertrophic scars: prostaglandin E2 release, *Burns* 27(3):215-218, 2001.

66. Berman B, Flores F: The treatment of hypertrophic scars and keloids, *Eur J Dermatol* 8(8):591-595, 1998.

67. Staley MJ, Richard RL. Use of pressure to treat hypertrophic burn scars, *Adv Wound Care* 10(3):44-46, 1997.

68. Larson DL, Abston S, Evans EB, et al: Techniques for decreasing scar formation and contractures in the burned patient, *J Trauma* 11:807-823, 1971.

69. Costa AM, Peyrol S, Porto LC, et al: Mechanical forces induce scar remodeling. Study in non-pressure-treated versus pressure-treated hypertrophic scars, *Am J Pathol* 155(5):1671-1679, 1999.

70. Kircher CW, Shetlar MR, Shetlar CL: Alteration of hypertrophic scars induced by mechanical pressure, *Arch Dermatol* 111:60-64, 1975.

71. Reno F, et al: In vitro mechanical compression induces apoptosis and regulates cytokines release in hypertrophic scars, *Wound Repair Regen* 11(5):331-336, 2003.

72. Swedborg I: Effects of treatment with an elastic sleeve and intermittent pneumatic compression in post-mastectomy patients with lymphoedema of the arm, *Scand J Rehabil Med* 26:35-41, 1984.

73. Brennan MJ, DePompolo RW, Garden FH: Focused review: postmastectomy lymphedema, *Arch Phys Med Rehabil* 77:S74-S80, 1996.

74. Reynolds JP: Lymphedema: an "orphan" disease, *PT Magazine* June, 1996, pp 54-63.

75. McGrory BJ, Burke DW: Peroneal nerve palsy following intermittent sequential pneumatic compression, *Orthopedics* 23(10):1103-1105, 2000.

76. Pittman GR: Peroneal nerve palsy following sequential pneumatic compression, *JAMA* 261:2201-2202, 1989.

77. Lachmann EA, Rook JL, Tunkel R, et al: Complications associated with intermittent pneumatic compression, *Arch Phys Med Rehabil* 73(5):482-485, 1992.

78. Harris R: An introduction to manual lymphatic drainage: the Vodder method, *Massage Ther J* 5:55-66, 1992.

79. Profore product description, Smith & Nephew, http://wound.smith-nephew.com/no/Product.asp?NodeId=857. Accessed August 16, 2006.

80. Hiatt WR: Contemporary treatment of venous lower limb ulcers, *Angiology* 43(10):852-855, 1992.

81. Staudinger P: *Compression step by step*, Nuremberg, 1991, Beiersdorf Medical Bibliothek.

82. *The at-a-glance guide to vascular stockings*, Charlotte, NC, 1991, Jobst.

83. Benko T, Cooke EA, McNally MA, et al: Graduated compression stockings: knee length or thigh length, *Clin Orthop* 383:197-203, 2001.

84. Samson RH: Compression stocking therapy for patients with chronic venous insufficiency, *J Cardiovasc Surg* 26:10, 1985.

85. Jull AB, Mitchell N, Arroll J, et al: Factors influencing concordance with compression stockings after venous leg ulcer healing, *J Wound Care* 13(3): 90-92; 2004.

86. Bergan JJ, Sparks SR: Non-elastic compression: an alternative in management of chronic venous insufficiency, *J Wound Ostomy Cont Nurs* 27(2):83-89, 2000.

87. CompreFit: http://www.compressiondesign.com/products2/productscomprefit.html. Accessed September 20, 2006.

88. Swedborg I: Voluminometric estimation of the degree of lymphedema and its therapy by pneumatic compression, *Scand J Rehabil Med* 9:131-135, 1977.

89. Harris SR, Hugi MR, Olivotto IA, et al: Clinical practice guidelines for the care and treatment of breast cancer: lymphedema, *Can Med Assoc J* 164(2):191-199, 2001.

90. Holcomb SS: Identification and treatment of different types of lymphedema, *Adv Skin Wound Care* 19(2):103-108, 2006.

91. Caprini JA, Scurr JH, Hasty JH: The role of compression modalities in a prophylactic program for deep vein thrombosis, *Semin Thromb Hemostat* 14:77-87, 1988.

92. Jacobs L: Lymphedema: the debate continues, *PT Magazine* November, 1996, p 11.

93. Foldi M: Treatment of lymphedema, *NLN Newsletter* 7(3):1,2,6,8, 1995.

Chapter 12

Electromagnetic Radiation: Lasers and Light

TERMINOLOGY

It is recommended that the first time reader and student carefully review the glossary of useful terms and concepts before reading the text because much of the terminology used to describe **laser** and light therapy is unique to this area.

INTRODUCTION TO ELECTROMAGNETIC RADIATION

Electromagnetic radiation is composed of electric and magnetic fields that vary over time and are oriented perpendicular to each other (Fig. 12-1). Physical agents that deliver **energy** in the form of **electromagnetic radiation** include various forms of visible and invisible light and radiation in the shortwave and microwave ranges. All living organisms are continuously exposed to electromagnetic radiation from natural sources, such as the magnetic field of the earth and **ultraviolet (UV) radiation** from the sun. We are also exposed to electromagnetic radiation from manufactured sources, such as light bulbs, domestic electrical appliances, computers, and power lines.

This chapter serves as an introduction to the application of electromagnetic radiation in rehabilitation and provides specific information on the therapeutic application of lasers and other light therapy. The therapeutic use of electromagnetic radiation in the UV, radiowave, and microwave ranges are covered in Chapters 13 and 14. Because infrared (IR) radiation produces superficial heating, the clinical application of IR lamps and other superficial heating agents is described in Chapter 6.

PHYSICAL PROPERTIES OF ELECTROMAGNETIC RADIATION

Electromagnetic radiation is categorized according to its **frequency** and **wavelength**, which are inversely proportional to each other (Fig. 12-2). Lower-frequency electromagnetic radiation, including extremely low-frequency (ELF) waves, shortwaves, microwaves, IR radiation, visible light, and UV, is nonionizing, cannot break molecular bonds or produce ions, and can therefore be used for therapeutic medical applications. Higher-frequency electromagnetic radiation, such as x-rays and gamma rays, is ionizing and can break molecular bonds to form ions.[1,2] **Ionizing radiation** can also inhibit cell division and is therefore either not used clinically or is used in very small doses for imaging, or in larger doses to destroy tissue. Approximate frequency ranges for the different types of electromagnetic radiation are shown in Fig. 12-3 and are provided in the sections concerning each type of radiation. Approximate ranges are given because the reported values differ slightly among texts.[3]

The intensity of any type of electromagnetic radiation that reaches the patient from a radiation source is proportional to the energy output from the source, the inverse square of the distance of the source from the patient, and the cosine of the angle of incidence of the beam with the tissue. The intensity of energy reaching the body is greatest when the energy output is high the radiation source is close to the patient and the beam is perpendicular to the surface of the skin.

> ### ◎ Clinical Pearl
>
> The intensity of any type of electromagnetic radiation reaching the body is greatest when the energy output is high, the radiation source is close to the patient, and the beam is perpendicular to the surface of the skin.

As the distance from the skin, or the angle with the surface, increase, the intensity of the radiation reaching the skin falls.

Electromagnetic radiation can be applied to a patient to achieve a wide variety of clinical effects. The nature of these effects is determined primarily by the frequency and wavelength range of the radiation[4] and to some degree by the intensity of the radiation.

> ### ◎ Clinical Pearl
>
> The clinical effects of electromagnetic radiation are determined primarily by the radiation's frequency and wavelength range.

The frequencies of electromagnetic radiation used clinically can be in the IR, visible light, UV, shortwave, or microwave range. Far IR radiation, which is close to the microwave range, produces superficial heating and can be used for the same purposes as other superficial heating agents. It has the advantage over other superficial heating agents of not requiring direct contact with the body. UV radiation produces erythema and tanning of the skin and epidermal hyperplasia and is essential for vitamin D synthesis. It is used primarily for the treatment of psoriasis and other skin disorders. Shortwave and microwave energy can be used to heat deep tissues and, when applied at a low-average intensity using a pulsed signal, may decrease pain and edema and facilitate tissue healing by nonthermal mechanisms. Low-intensity lasers and other light sources in the visible and near IR frequency ranges are generally used to promote tissue healing and control pain and inflammation by nonthermal mechanisms.

With the exception of lasers and light, electromagnetic agents are currently not in widespread use by therapists in the United States (US). However, most are commonly used in other countries and some are effective for the treatment of disorders not related to the musculoskeletal system and are therefore more commonly used by other health professionals. For example, **diathermy** is commonly used in other countries as a thermal agent to heat larger deeper areas but is unpopular in the US because of the risks associated with its misuse and the size of most devices. UV radiation has proven beneficial in the treatment of many skin disorders and is therefore most frequently used by dermatologists.

HISTORY OF ELECTROMAGNETIC RADIATION

Electromagnetic agents have been used for therapy to varying degrees at different times. Until recently, most electromagnetic agents were used in a limited manner by therapists. However, since 2002, when the Food and Drug Administration (FDA) cleared the use of a laser device for the treatment of carpal tunnel syndrome, the use of lasers

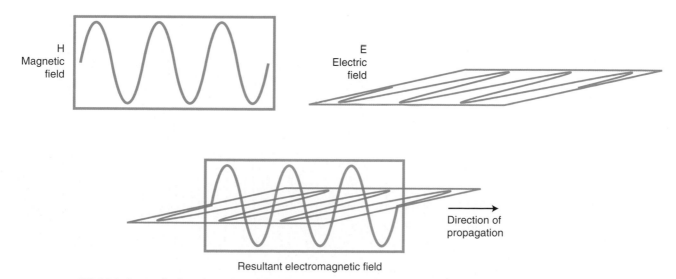

FIG 12-1 Perpendicular orientation of the electric and magnetic components of an electromagnetic field.

and other forms of light for therapy has gained much popularity.

Sunlight was the earliest form of electromagnetic energy therapy. As noted previously, sunlight includes electromagnetic radiation in the UV, visible and IR range of the spectrum. Prehistoric man believed that sunlight could drive out the evil spirits that caused disease. The ancient Greeks praised Helios, their god of light, sun, and healing. It is from the word Helios that the term for treatment with sunlight, *heliotherapy*, is derived. Although the exact purpose and effectiveness of heliotherapy, as recommended by the ancient Greeks and Romans, are hard to judge, their prominent physicians, Celsus and Galen, recommended sunbathing for a many conditions including seizures, arthritis, and asthma, as well for preventing a wide range of problems and disorders.

Sunlight exposure, with a particular emphasis on exposure to UV light, regained therapeutic popularity in the 19th century when its value for preventing rickets (a bone disorder caused by vitamin D deficiency) in people exposed to a small amount of light because of dark living and working conditions, and its effectiveness in the treatment of tuberculosis, were recognized.[5] Today, although rickets and tuberculosis are rare, UV therapy remains popular for the treatment of psoriasis and other skin disorders, and lasers and similar forms of light, generally in the red and IR range, are used clinically, particularly for the treatment of pain and to promote tissue healing.

Other forms of treatment with electromagnetic radiation gained popularity in the 20th century when electrically driven devices that could deliver controlled wavelengths and intensities of electromagnetic energy were produced. These included diathermy devices that output energy in the shortwave or microwave wavelength range to produce heat in patients and fluorescent and incandescent lights that output energy in the UV, visible,

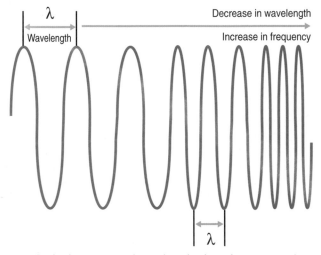

FIG 12-2 The frequency and wavelength of an electromagnetic wave are inversely related. As the frequency increases, the wavelength decreases.

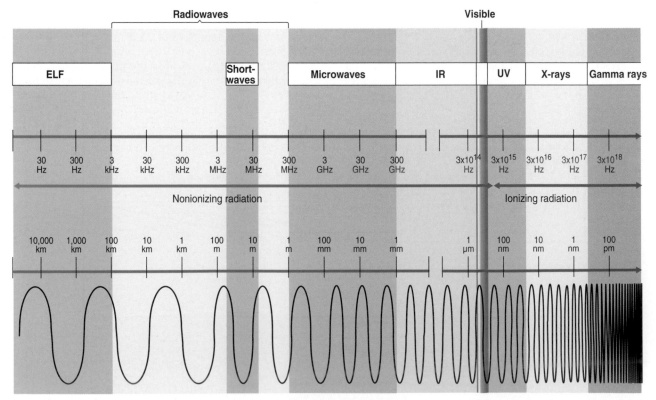

FIG 12-3 The electromagnetic spectrum ranges from low frequencies in the hertz range to over 1023 Hz, with wavelengths varying from over 10,000 km to less than 1 pm.

and IR parts of the spectrum. Diathermy was a popular heating device worldwide but has fallen out of favor in the US since the advent of ultrasound, which is a deep heating device that is safer, smaller, and easier to use. UV light continues to be used for the treatment of certain skin disorders, but this area of practice is now generally the domain of dermatologists rather than therapists. IR lamps were popular in the mid-20th century as heating devices. Although they have the advantage of not requiring contact with the body, their safety is limited by the fact that the amount of heat delivered to an area varies with the distance of the body from the lamp, so that closer placement may produce too much heating and burns and further placement may be ineffective. This is a particular challenge when trying to treat contoured body areas. Therefore conductive heating devices, such as hot packs, have become a much more popular thermal agent.

Today, laser and other light devices are probably the most common form of electromagnetic therapy. The section on the history of light and laser therapy later in this chapter includes additional details about the development of this physical agent.

PHYSIOLOGICAL EFFECTS OF ELECTROMAGNETIC RADIATION

When electromagnetic radiation is absorbed by tissues it can affect them via thermal or nonthermal mechanisms. Because IR radiation and continuous shortwave and microwave diathermy delivered at sufficient intensity can increase tissue temperature, these agents are thought to affect tissues primarily by thermal mechanisms. IR lamps can be used to heat superficial tissues, whereas continuous shortwave and microwave diathermy heat deep and superficial tissues. The physiological and clinical effects of these thermal agents are generally the same as those of the superficial heating agents (see Chapter 6), except that the tissues affected are different.

UV radiation and low levels of pulsed diathermy or light do not increase tissue temperature and are therefore thought to affect tissues by nonthermal mechanisms. It has been proposed that these types of electromagnetic energy cause changes at the cellular level by altering cell membrane function and permeability and intracellular organelle function.[6] Nonthermal electromagnetic agents may also promote binding of chemicals to the cell membrane to trigger complex sequences of cellular reactions. Because these agents are thought to promote the initial steps in cellular function, this mechanism of action could explain the wide variety of stimulatory cellular effects that have been observed in response to the application of nonthermal levels of electromagnetic energy. Electromagnetic energy may also affect tissues by causing proteins to undergo conformational changes to promote active transport across cell membranes and to accelerate adenosine triphosphate (ATP) synthesis and use.[7]

Many researchers have invoked the Arndt-Schulz law to explain the effects of low, nonthermal levels of electromagnetic radiation. According to this law, a certain minimum stimulus is needed to initiate a biological process. In addition, although a slightly stronger stimulus may produce greater effects, beyond a certain level, stronger stimuli will have a progressively less positive effect and higher levels will become inhibitory. For example, a low level of mechanical stress during childhood promotes normal bone growth, whereas too little or too much stress can result in abnormal growth or fractures. Similarly, with some forms of electromagnetic radiation, such as diathermy or laser light, although too low a dose may not produce any effect, the optimal dose to achieve a desired physiological effect may be lower than that which produces heat. If excessive doses are used, they may cause tissue damage.

INTRODUCTION TO LASERS AND LIGHT

Light is electromagnetic energy in or close to the visible range of the electromagnetic spectrum. Most light is polychromatic, or made up of light of various wavelengths within a wide or narrow range. Laser (an acronym for *l*ight *a*mplification by *s*timulated *e*mission of *r*adiation) light is also electromagnetic energy in or close to the visible range of the electromagnetic spectrum. Laser light differs from other forms of light in that it is **monochromatic** (made up of light that is only a single wavelength [Fig. 12-4]),

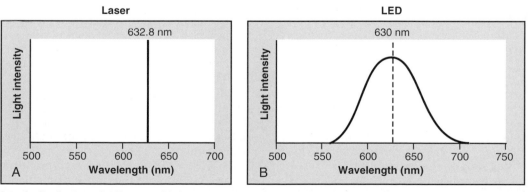

FIG 12-4 Wavelength distribution of different red light sources. **A,** Light from a He-Ne laser with a wavelength of 632.8 nm. This monochromatic light has a single wavelength. **B,** Light from a red LED. This light concentrates around a wavelength of 630 nm but has a range of wavelengths.

Coherent versus noncoherent light

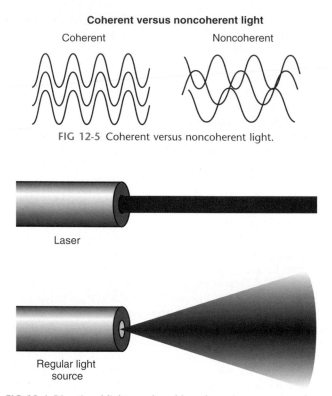

FIG 12-5 Coherent versus noncoherent light.

Laser

Regular light source

FIG 12-6 Directional light produced by a laser, in contrast to the divergent light produced by other sources.

coherent (i.e., in phase [Fig. 12-5]), and **directional** (Fig. 12-6).

BRIEF HISTORY OF LASERS AND LIGHT

The earliest records of using light for clinical purposes involved the use of sunlight as described earlier in this chapter. Light therapy gained modern popularity with the advent of the laser and **light-emitting diodes (LEDs)**. The history of the laser begins in 1916 when Albert Einstein introduced the concept of **stimulated emission** and proposed that it should be possible to make a powerful light amplifier. He improved on a fundamental statistical theory of heat that predicted that as light passed through a substance it could stimulate the emission of more light. This effect is at the heart of the modern laser. Einstein moved on to other things, and it was not until 1954 that the first stimulated emission device was made.

In 1954, Arthur Schawlow and Charles Townes at Columbia University in New York, and Nicolay Basov and Aleksandr Prochorov at the Lebedev Institute in Moscow, all winners of the Nobel prize in physics, simultaneously made the first stimulated emission device, a **maser**. This device used ammonia gas as its medium to produce stimulated emission of radiation in the microwave frequency range.

Shortly thereafter, in 1960, Theodore Maiman made the first laser using ruby as the lasing medium. This laser output red light with a wavelength of 694 nm. Later in the same year, Ali Javan invented the first gas laser, the helium-neon (He-Ne) laser. This also output red light but with a wavelength of 632.8 nm. Laser technology evolved rapidly in the following few years, using different lasing media to produce laser light of different colors and wavelengths and of different **powers**.

High-power lasers were quickly adopted for a range of medical applications. Lasers were first used in medicine by ophthalmologists to "weld" detached retinas back in place, and are now used by ophthalmologists for many other applications as well as by surgeons where finely controlled cutting and coagulation is required, and by dermatologists for treating vascular lesions. The high-intensity "hot" lasers used for surgery heat and can destroy tissue. Because the laser has a narrow beam, and because laser light is absorbed selectively by **chromophores**, it generates heat in and destroys only the tissue directly in the beam while avoiding damage to surrounding tissues.[8] **Hot lasers** have a number of advantages over traditional surgical implements: the beam is sterile, it allows fine control, it cauterizes as it cuts, and, it produces less scarring. Because hot lasers destroy tissue, they are not used for rehabilitation.

In the late 1960s and early 1970s, Endre Mester began to explore potential clinical applications of the nonthermal effects of laser light on tissue. He found that low-level irradiation with the He-Ne laser appeared to stimulate tissue healing.[9-12] Based on Mester's early work, others started to study the effects of low-level laser irradiation, primarily with the He-Ne laser, and the He-Ne laser was promoted throughout Eastern Europe and much of Asia as the treatment of choice for a wide range of conditions.

The He-Ne gas tube lasers enjoyed limited popularity in the West because of their cost, bulk, fragility, and the limited evidence regarding effectiveness. However, in the late 1980s, with the advent of relatively inexpensive semiconductor-technology-based photodiodes and mounting research evidence, low-intensity laser therapy and later, other forms of light therapy, including treatment with light from LEDs and then **supraluminous diodes** (SLDs), started to gain popularity in the West and were widely studied.[13]

Because of conflicting and limited research data, until 2002 the FDA limited the clinical use of low-intensity lasers in the US to investigational use only. In June 2002, the use of one laser device was cleared for the treatment of carpal tunnel syndrome. Since then, laser devices have received FDA clearance for the treatment of head and neck pain, knee pain, and postmastectomy lymphedema, and many other light therapy devices that include infrared output have been introduced to the US market and cleared by the FDA as heating devices based on the known effects of IR lamps.

The laser light therapy market in the US is evolving rapidly at this time, with a constantly changing array of devices and features becoming available. In general, these devices include one or more probes (applicators), each of which contains one or more diodes. The diodes may be LEDs, SLDs, or **laser diodes**, each producing light in the visible or IR range of the electromagnetic spectrum. Applicators with more than one diode, generally called **cluster probes**, usually contain various diodes of different types, wavelengths, and power.

PHYSICAL PROPERTIES OF LASERS AND LIGHT

Light is electromagnetic energy in or close to the visible range of the spectrum. Light from all sources except lasers comprises a range of wavelengths. Light that appears white is made up of a combination of light wave frequencies across the entire visible range of the spectrum. Sunlight includes visible light, as well as shorter wavelengths of light in the UV part of the spectrum and longer wavelengths of light in the IR part of the spectrum. Light that appears to the human eye to be one color but that is not from a laser includes light waves with a narrow range of wavelengths, with most of the light energy around a given wavelength. Lasers produce coherent light of a single wavelength only. Light sources used for therapy generally produce light in narrow ranges of the visible or near visible part of the spectrum.

Light Sources

Light can be produced by emission from a gas-filled glass tube or a photodiode, with tubes being the older type of device. Spontaneously emitted mixed wavelength light, such as light from a household light bulb, is generated by applying energy in the form of electricity to molecules of a contained gas. The electricity moves electrons in these molecules to a higher energy level, and as the electrons spontaneously fall back down to their original level, they emit photons of light of various frequencies, depending on how far they fall (Fig. 12-7). The original clinical laser devices used vacuum tube technology similar to a tube fluorescent light bulb to produce monochromatic coherent laser light. With this type of laser, energy in the form of electricity is also applied to molecules of a contained gas. However, in this case, only certain gases can be used and the gas is contained in a tube with mirrored ends. One end of the tube is fully mirrored and the other end is semimirrored. When electricity is applied to the gas, it causes electrons to jump up to a higher energy level. When these electrons fall, they produce photons that are reflected by the mirrored ends of the tube. As the photons travel back and forth from one mirrored end of the tube to the other, each excited atom they encounter releases two identical photons. These two photons can then travel back and forth and encounter two more excited atoms, causing the release of a total of four identical photons. Eventually, many identical photons are traveling back and forth between the mirrored ends of the tube, stimulating the emission of yet more identical photons. When the number of identical photons is sufficient, this strong light, which is coherent and of a single frequency, escapes through the semimirrored end of the tube as monochromatic coherent directional laser light (Fig. 12-8).

Today, therapeutic light sources generally use photodiodes instead of glass tubes (Fig. 12-9). Photodiodes are made up of two layers of semiconductor, one layer with P-type material, with more positive charges, and the other layer with N-type material, with more negative charges (Fig. 12-10). When electrons fall from the N type to the

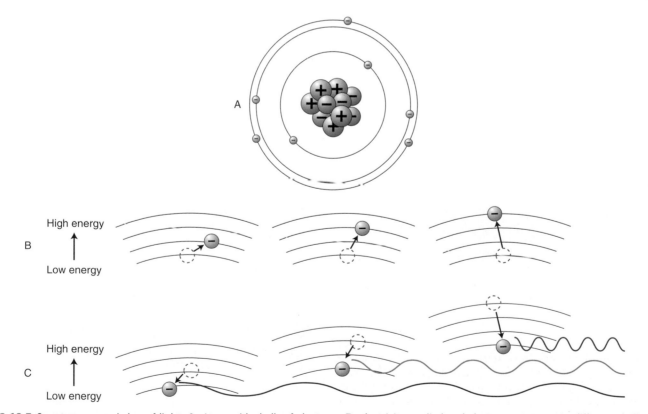

FIG 12-7 Spontaneous emission of light. **A,** Atom with shells of electrons; **B,** electricity applied and electrons move up to different shells; **C,** electrons fall down and photons of various wavelengths are emitted.

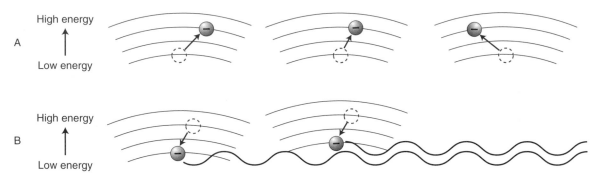

FIG 12-8 Stimulated emission of light. **A,** Electricity applied and electrons all move up to the same level; **B,** electrons fall down and photons all with the same wavelength are emitted.

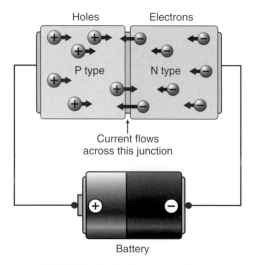

FIG 12-9 Photodiodes. *Courtesy LaserMate Group, Pomona, CA.*

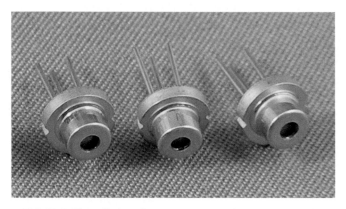

FIG 12-10 Light diode technology.

P type, photons of various frequencies are emitted. If the diode has mirrored ends, it can also be engineered to produce monochromatic laser light. Photodiodes offer the advantages of being small, hardy, and relatively inexpensive. Photodiodes may be laser diodes, LEDs, or SLDs.

> ◎ **Clinical Pearl**
>
> Photodiodes can be laser diodes, LEDs, or SLDs. All of these diodes are small, hardy, and relatively inexpensive.

Laser diodes produce light that is monochromatic, coherent, and directional, providing high-intensity light in one area. LEDs produce low-intensity light that may appear to be one color but that is not coherent or monochromatic. LED light is also not directional and spreads widely. LED therapeutic light applicators are generally arrays that include many (>30) LEDs, with each LED having a low-output power. The low power of LEDs increases the application time required when using these for treatment, but the large number of diodes and their divergence allows the light energy to be delivered to a wide area. SLDs produce high-intensity, almost monochromatic light that is not coherent and that spreads a little but less than the light produced by an LED (Fig. 12-11). Thus SLDs require shorter application times than LEDs and deliver energy to a wider area than do laser diodes. Many applicators include a few laser diodes, SLDs, and LEDs together in a cluster. Clusters usually include 10 to 20 diodes.

Wavelength

The wavelength of light most affects the depth to which the light penetrates and impacts the nature of the cellular effects of light.[4] Light with wavelengths between 600 and 1300 nm, which is red or IR, has the optimal depth of penetration in human tissue and is therefore most commonly used for patient treatment.[14,15] Light with a wavelength at the longer end and a frequency at the lower end of this range penetrates deeper, whereas light with a shorter wavelength and higher frequency penetrates less deeply.[16,17]

> ◎ **Clinical Pearl**
>
> Light with a longer wavelength penetrates more deeply than light with a shorter wavelength.

IR light penetrates 2 to 4 cm into soft tissue, whereas red light penetrates only a few millimeters, just through and below the skin. Light may also produce physiological

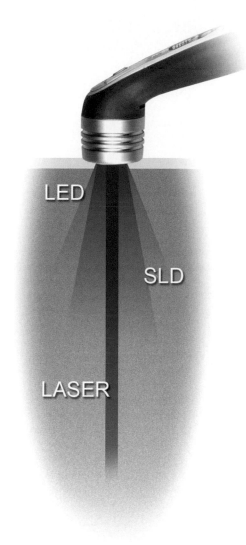

FIG 12-11 Comparison of the spread of laser, SLD, and LED light. *Courtesy Chattanooga Group, Hixson, TN.*

TABLE 12-1		Laser Classifications
Class	Power	Effects
1	<0.5 mW	No hazard.
1M		No hazard because the beam has a large diameter or is divergent.
2	<1 mW	Safe for momentary viewing; will provoke a blink reflex.
3A	<5 mW	Commonly used for laser pointers. Poses an eye hazard with prolonged exposure.
3B	<500 mW	Used for therapy. Can cause permanent eye injury with brief exposure. Direct viewing of the beam should be avoided. Viewing of the diffuse beam reflected from the skin is safe. Can cause minor skin burns with prolonged exposure.
4	>500 mW	Surgical and industrial cutting lasers. Can cause permanent eye injury before you can react. Can cause serious skin burns. Can burn clothing. Use with extreme caution.

ⓒ Clinical Pearl

Most laser diodes used for therapy have a power between 5 and 500 mW.

effects beyond its depth of penetration because the energy may promote chemical reactions that mediate processes distant from the site of application.

Power and Power Density

Light intensity can be expressed in terms of power, measured in watts or milliwatts, or **power density**, measured in milliwatts per centimeter squared (mW/cm^2). Power is the rate of energy flow, and power density is the amount of power per unit area. Laser and other light therapy applicators generally have a fixed power, although in some cases this can be reduced by pulsing the output.

Because high-intensity lasers have the potential to cause harm, lasers have been divided into four classes, according to their power ranges (Table 12-1). The power of most laser diodes used for therapy is between 5 and 500 mW and are thus classified as class 3B.

When a laser or light therapy applicator includes a number of diodes, the power of the applicator is equal to the sum of the power of all its diodes and the power density is equal to the total power divided by the total area.

High power-density light applicators have the advantage of taking less time to deliver a given amount of energy. It is not known if the clinical effects are the same with longer applications of low power light as with delivery of the same amount of energy in a shorter period of time using a high power light source. There is more research on the use of lower power lasers than the newer higher power lasers or SLDs because these were available first. However, some studies have found that the effects of the laser are more pronounced with short-duration, high-power doses than with long-duration, low-power doses delivering the same total amount of energy.[18]

Energy and Energy Density

Energy is the power multiplied by the time of application and is measured in Joules:

$$\text{Energy (J)} = \text{Power (W)} \times \text{Time (s)}$$

Energy density, also known as fluence, is the amount of power per unit area. Energy density is measured in Joules per centimeter squared (J/cm^2). Energy density is the treatment dose measure preferred by most authors and researchers in this field. This measure takes into account the power, the treatment duration and the area of application.

$$\text{Energy density } (J/cm^2) = \frac{\text{Energy (J)}}{\text{Area of irradiation } (cm^2)}$$

Most laser and light therapy devices allow for selection of energy or energy density. Because energy (Joules) includes time (watts × seconds), when using a laser light therapy device, the clinician generally does not need to select the treatment time (duration).

> ◎ **Clinical Pearl**
>
> Energy density is the measure of laser and light treatment dose used most often, and most therapy devices allow for selection of energy or energy density.

EFFECTS OF LASERS AND LIGHT

Low-intensity lasers and other forms of light have been studied and recommended for use in rehabilitation because there is evidence that this form of electromagnetic energy may be biomodulating and facilitate healing.[19,20] The clinical effects of light are thought to be related to the direct effect of light energy, photons, on intracellular chromophores in many different types of cells.[4,21,22] A chromophore is the light-absorbing part of a molecule that gives it color and that can be stimulated by light energy to undergo chemical reactions. To produce an effect, the photons of light must be absorbed by a target cell to promote a cascade of biochemical events that affects tissue function. There is evidence that light has a wide range of effects at cellular and subcellular levels, including stimulating ATP[23] and RNA production, altering the synthesis of cytokines involved in inflammation, and initiating reactions at the cell membrane by affecting calcium channels[24] and intercellular communication.[25,26]

> ◎ **Clinical Pearl**
>
> Light can stimulate ATP and RNA production within cells.

PROMOTE ADENOSINE TRIPHOSPHATE PRODUCTION

The primary function of mitochondria, the power house of the cell, is to generate ATP, which can then be used as the energy source for all other cellular reactions. ATP generation is a multistep process that occurs on the inner mitochondrial membrane. Red laser (632.8 nm)[27] and LED (670 nm)[28] light have been shown to improve mitochondrial function and increase their production of ATP by up to 70%. It appears that light promotes this increase in ATP production by increasing cytochrome oxidase production and enhancing electron transfer by cytochrome-C oxidase (Fig. 12-12).[27,29-31] This effect may also be partly mediated by cellular or mitochondrial calcium uptake.[24,32] The

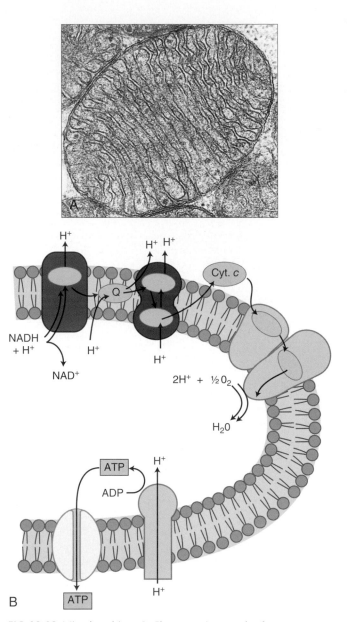

FIG 12-12 Mitochondrion. **A,** Electron micrograph of structure; **B,** electron transport chain and ATP production within a mitochondrion. *From Stevens & Lowe: Human Histology, ed 3. London, Mosby, 2005.*

increased ATP production promoted by laser and other forms of light is thought to be the primary contributor to many of the clinical benefits of laser and light therapy, particularly enhancement of tissue healing.[23] In addition, this effect may explain the reduction in fatigue from electrically stimulated muscle contraction produced by laser irradiation.[33]

PROMOTE COLLAGEN PRODUCTION

Laser and light therapy is also thought to enhance tissue healing by promoting collagen production, likely by stimulating production of mRNA that codes for procollagen. Red laser light has been shown to promote an increase in collagen synthesis[34-36] and mRNA production[37] and to induce a more than threefold increase in procollagen production.[36]

MODULATE INFLAMMATION

Laser irradiation can modulate inflammation and is associated with increased levels of prostaglandin-$F_{2\alpha}$ ($PGF_{2\alpha}$),[38,39] interleukin-1α (IL-1α), and interleukin-8 (IL-8)[40] and decreased levels of PGE_2[38,39] and tumor necrosis factor-alpha (TNF-α).[41] The changes in prostaglandin balance likely result in increased blood flow. The stimulation of IL-1α and IL-8 release has been shown to induce keratinocyte migration and proliferation.[40] There is also evidence that red (He-Ne) laser irradiation activates T and B lymphocytes,[42] enhancing their ability to bind bacteria,[43] and that laser light promotes degranulation of mast cells[44,45] and synthesis and release of chemical mediators of fibroblast proliferation by macrophages.[46,47] Laser and LED light in the red to IR wavelength range can also stimulate proliferation of various cells involved in tissue healing, including fibroblasts,[48-50] keratinocytes,[51] and endothelial cells.[52]

INHIBIT BACTERIAL GROWTH

Laser light can also inhibit bacterial growth. A study published in 1999 reported that red (632.8 or 670 nm) laser light had a dose-dependent bactericidal effect on photosensitized *Staphylococcus aureus* (*S. aureus*) and *Pseudomonas aeruginosa* (*P. aeruginosa*).[53] A more recent study examining the effects of different wavelengths of laser light on bacterial growth found that 630 nm laser irradiation at 1 to 20 J/cm^2 was more effective than 660, 810, or 905 nm laser light at inhibiting the growth of *P. aeruginosa*, *S. aureus*, and *Escherichia coli*.[54] In addition, two more recent studies found that shorter wavelength blue (405 nm or 405 nm combined with 470 nm) light also had a dose-dependent bactericidal effect on *S. aureus* and *P. aeruginosa* when doses of 10 to 20 J/cm^2 were used, reducing bacterial colonies by approximately 62% to 95%.[55,56] However, one study found that certain doses and pulse frequencies of IR (810 nm) wavelength laser irradiation can enhance bacterial growth.[57]

Based on the overall results of the research on the effects of laser light on bacterial growth, it appears that light generally inhibits bacterial growth and that wavelengths of 670 to 405 nm (visible red to blue) are the most effective. It appears that only wavelengths that are longer but not shorter than this range have been studied for this effect.

PROMOTE VASODILATION

Some authors also report that laser light can induce vasodilation, particularly of the microcirculation.[20,58] This effect may be mediated by the release of preformed nitric oxide, which has been found to be enhanced by irradiation with red light.[59] Such vasodilation could accelerate tissue healing by increasing the availability of oxygen and other nutrients and by speeding the removal of waste products from the irradiated area.

ALTER NERVE CONDUCTION VELOCITY AND REGENERATION

Some studies have shown increased peripheral nerve conduction velocities, increased frequency of action potentials, decreased distal sensory latencies, accelerated nerve regeneration, and reduced nerve scarring in response to laser stimulation, all of which indicate increased activation of the nervous tissue by laser light.[37,60-67] This effect has appeared to be more pronounced with red laser light than with blue or IR.[37] These positive effects occur in response to laser irradiation over the site of nerve compression and are enhanced by irradiation of the corresponding spinal cord segments.[68,69] In addition, laser irradiation has been found to induce axonal sprouting and outgrowth in cultured nerves[70] and in in vitro brain cortex.[71]

As with other areas of laser and light research, there are conflicting findings in the literature. Some studies have found that laser light irradiation results in decreased nerve conduction velocities and increased distal conduction latencies,[72-74] indicating decreased activation of the nervous tissue, and other studies report no change in nerve conduction in response to laser light irradiation.[75-79] Given the currently available data, further research is necessary to clarify the effects of lasers and light on nerve conduction and to determine the specific parameters required to achieve these effects.

CLINICAL INDICATIONS FOR THE USE OF LASERS AND LIGHT

TISSUE HEALING: SOFT TISSUE AND BONE

A number of studies,[9-12,24,80-91] review articles,[92-95] and meta-analyses[96-99] have been published concerning the use of low-level laser and light therapy to promote the healing of chronic and acute wounds in humans and animals. This area of research was based on Mester's early findings that low-level laser irradiation appeared to accelerate wound healing.[10] Although many studies supported the effectiveness of this intervention,[9-12,24,81-88] a number of studies failed to show improved wound healing with laser light therapy.[80,82,89-91] Therefore various groups of authors have attempted to analyze the overall data through metaanalysis. Initial metaanalyses, published in 1999 and 2000, of the studies on the effects of **low-level laser therapy** (LLLT) on venous leg ulcer healing, reported no evidence of any benefit associated with this specific application of laser therapy, although they reported that one small study suggested that a combination of IR light and red He-Ne laser may have some benefit.[99,96] However, two more recent metaanalyses,[97,98] both published in 2004, including 34 and 24 studies, respectively, reported strong (Cohen's d = +1.81[97] and +2.22[98]) positive effects of laser therapy on tissue repair. Laser therapy was associated with increased collagen synthesis, rate of healing and wound closure, tensile strength, tensile stress, number of degranulated mast cells, and reduced wound healing time.

Based on these extensive and thorough reviews, it appears that laser therapy can promote tissue repair. However, most of the published studies are of poor quality, lack adequate controls, and vary in or poorly report treatment parameters. The limited data available from clinical trials in humans continue to limit the strength with which laser and light therapy is recommended and limits the ability to develop clear guidelines for the clinical application of lasers and light for the treatment of wounds in patients.

Although most of the publications on tissue healing have focused on the effects of laser and light therapy on general soft tissue healing, as occurs with pressure ulcers or surgical incisions, some studies have examined the effects of laser or light therapy on the healing of specific types of tissue such as tendon,[100-102] ligament,[103] or bone.[104-109] The few studies on tendon and ligament healing have consistently shown positive outcomes. However, the studies on fracture healing have produced conflicting results with some showing acceleration of fracture healing or physiologic processes associated with fracture healing,[104-106] whereas others have found no effect or even signs of delayed ossification after laser irradiation.[107,108] The one study comparing the effects of laser therapy with those of low-level ultrasound in promoting fracture healing found both to be equally effective and for the combination of both to be no more effective than either intervention alone.[109] It is thought that low-level laser accelerates bone healing by increasing the rate of hematoma absorption, bone remodeling, blood vessel formation, and calcium deposition, as well as by stimulating macrophage, fibroblast, and chondrocyte activity[89] and increasing osteoblast number and osteoid volume[109] and the amount of intracellular calcium in osteoblastic cells.[110]

Although the ideal treatment parameters for promoting tissue healing are uncertain, the evidence at this time indicates that red or IR light with an energy density between 5 and 24 J/cm^2 is most effective.[98,111] There is some evidence that a dose too high or too low may be ineffective and a dose above 16-20 J/cm^2 may even inhibit wound healing.[112-114] Therefore current recommendations are to use 4-16 J/cm^2 for most wound healing applications, starting at the lower end of this range and progressing up as tolerated. The addition of shorter wavelength light, in the blue to red range, may provide additional benefit in open areas infected or colonized by aerobic bacteria.

ARTHRITIS

A number of studies regarding the application of laser and light therapy for the management of pain and dysfunction associated with arthritis have been published. Some of these studies have found that laser therapy can benefit patients with arthritis, resulting in increased hand grip strength and flexibility and decreased pain and swelling in patients with rheumatoid arthritis, decreased pain and increased grip strength in patients with osteoarthritis (OA) affecting the hands, and decreased pain and improved function in patients with cervical OA.[92,115-119] However, some blinded, controlled studies using lasers for the treatment for osteoarthritis reported that this intervention did not relieve pain in the subjects studied.[120,121]

Metaanalyses and reviews of the studies concerning the effects of laser therapy on pain, strength, stiffness and function in patients with rheumatoid arthritis (RA) and OA concluded that there is sufficient evidence to recommend consideration of LLLT for short-term (up to 4 weeks) relief of pain and morning stiffness in RA, but that for OA the results are conflicting, with only 5 out of 8 included studies finding benefit.[122-125] Different outcomes may be a result of different laser doses, different methods of application, or differences in the pathology of RA and OA. Improvements in arthritic conditions may be the result of reduced inflammation caused by changes in the activity of inflammatory mediators[41,126] or reduced pain caused by changes in nerve conduction or activation. Given the variability in treatment parameters used in different studies, ideal treatment parameters are not clear. In general, shorter wavelengths, application to the nerve as well as the joint, and longer durations of application may be more effective.

LYMPHEDEMA

Two recent studies have examined the effects of LLLT on postmastectomy lymphedema.[127,128] Based on the findings of the first of these studies,[127] the FDA authorized the use of one laser device (the LTU-904, RianCorp, Richmond, South Australia) for use as part of a therapy regimen to treat postmastectomy lymphedema. This device has a 904 nm wavelength (i.e., in the IR range), a peak pulse power of 5 W, and a fixed average power of 5 mW. In this study, laser treatment was applied at 1.5 J/cm^2 (300 mJ per 0.2 cm^2 spot, to 17 spots for a total of 5.1 J) to the area of the axilla 3 times per week for 1 or 2 cycles of 3 weeks each. Although there was no significant improvement immediately after any of the treatments, the mean affected limb volume was significantly reduced 1 and 3 months after completion of 2 (although not 1) treatment cycles. Approximately one third of the 37 actively treated subjects had a clinically significant (>200 ml) reduction in limb volume 2 to 3 months after treatment with the laser.

The latter study[128] was much smaller, with a total of 8 subjects who completed the 22 week intervention. After applying an 890 nm IR laser at 1.5 J/cm^2 to the arm and axilla for 22 weeks, actively treated patients had a greater reduction in limb circumference and generally less pain than placebo-treated patients.

Although these studies provide only limited data, they suggest that IR laser therapy may help to reduce postmastectomy lymphedema. It is interesting to note that the effects of laser treatment were delayed by 1 to 3 months after completion of the treatment sessions, suggesting that laser affects the development of lymphatic drainage pathways rather than directly facilitating lymphatic circulation at the time of application. Based on these studies, it is recommended that laser treatment for lymphedema be at an energy density of around 1.5 J/cm^2 to a total area of 3 cm^2 3 times per week for a total of 3 weeks for 1 to 2 cycles.

NEUROLOGICAL CONDITIONS

Several studies have attempted to determine the impact of laser light irradiation on nerve conduction, regeneration, and function. The first FDA clearance for laser therapy was based on a 1995 study of IR laser (830 nm) therapy for approximately 100 General Motors' employees with carpal tunnel syndrome.[65] This randomized double-blind controlled study compared the effect of physical therapy combined with laser to physical therapy alone for the treatment of carpal tunnel syndrome. Grip and pinch strength, radial deviation range of motion (ROM), median nerve motor conduction velocity across the wrist, and incidence of return to work were all significantly higher in the laser-treated group than in the control group. The treatment protocol was to apply 3 J (90 mW for 33 seconds) during therapy for 5 weeks. A recent review of seven studies of laser or light therapy for the treatment of carpal tunnel syndrome found that two controlled studies and three open-protocol studies found laser to be more effective than placebo, whereas two studies did not find such a benefit. The studies finding benefit applied higher-dose laser (≥ 9 J) than those not finding benefit (≤ 6 J/cm²). Laser light treatment was applied to the area of the carpal tunnel or proximally up to the area of the nerve cell body at the neck.

Laser therapy has also been investigated for the treatment of a number of other neurological conditions. A number of studies have investigated the effect of laser and light therapy on diabetic peripheral neuropathy, and these trials are ongoing.[129,130] Overall, these trials have found that IR light may help reduce the pain associated with this condition. IR[131] and red[132] laser irradiation have also been found to be more effective than placebo at reducing the pain associated with postherpetic neuralgia, and preliminary studies have found improved functional outcome after stroke with application of IR laser therapy to the head within 24 hours of stroke onset.[133] Studies in all of these areas are ongoing.

PAIN MANAGEMENT

Many studies have found that laser and light therapy may reduce the pain and disability associated with a wide variety of neuromusculoskeletal conditions other than arthritis and neuropathy,[134] including lateral epicondylitis,[135-137] chronic low-back and neck pain,[138-140] trigger points,[141,142] and delayed-onset muscle soreness.[143]

Laser light's effects on pain may be mediated by its effects on inflammation,[126] tissue healing, nerve conduction, or endorphin release or metabolism.[144] Analgesic effects are generally most pronounced when laser or light is applied to the skin overlying the involved nerves or nerves innervating the area of the involved dermatome.[136] Although some studies have not found a significant difference in subjective or objective treatment outcomes when comparing treatment with low-level laser to alternative sham treatments,[145-147] a recent metaanalysis of studies on the effects of laser therapy on pain found an overall positive treatment effect ($d = +1.11$) of laser light therapy on pain in humans.[97]

CONTRAINDICATIONS AND PRECAUTIONS FOR LASERS AND LIGHT

Various authors and manufacturers list different contraindications and precautions for the application of laser and light therapy. The following general recommendations are a summary. However, the clinician should adhere to the recommendations provided with the specific unit(s) being used.

CONTRAINDICATIONS FOR THE USE OF LASERS AND LIGHT

CONTRAINDICATIONS
for the Use of Lasers and Light

- Direct irradiation of the eyes
- Malignancy
- Within 4 to 6 months after radiotherapy
- Over hemorrhaging regions
- Over the thyroid or other endocrine glands

Direct Irradiation of the Eyes

Because lasers can damage the eyes, all patients treated with lasers should wear goggles opaque to the wavelength of the light emitted from the laser being used throughout treatment.[16] The clinician applying the laser should also wear goggles that reduce the intensity of light of the wavelength produced by the specific device to a nonhazardous level. Goggles should be marked with the wavelength range they attenuate and their optical density within that **band**.

Clinical Pearl

Both the clinician and patient should wear goggles during laser treatment, and the goggles should be marked with the range of wavelengths they block.

Clinicians should remember that the higher the optical density, the greater the attenuation of the light. Also, safety goggles suitable for one wavelength should not be assumed to be safe at any other wavelength. Particular care should be taken with IR lasers because the radiation they produce is not visible but it can easily damage the retina. The laser beam should never be directed at the eyes, and one should never look directly along the axis of the laser light beam.

This contraindication does not apply to nonlaser light sources, including SLDs and LEDs. Lasers can damage the eye, particularly the retina, because the light is directional and thus very concentrated in one area. In contrast, other light sources are **divergent** and thus diffuse the light energy so that concentrated light energy would not reach the eye.

Malignancy

Laser and light therapy have been shown to have a range of physiological and cellular effects, including increasing blood flow and cellular energy production. These effects may increase the growth rate or rate of metastasis of malignant tissue.

Because a patient may not know that he or she has cancer or may be uncomfortable discussing this diagnosis directly, the therapist should first check the chart for a diagnosis of cancer.

Ask the Patient

- Are you under the care of a physician for any major medical problem? If so, what is the problem?
- Have you experienced any recent unexplained weight loss or weight gain?
- Do you have constant pain that does not change?
- If the patient has experienced recent unexplained changes in body weight or has constant pain that does not change, laser or light therapy should be deferred until a physician has performed a follow-up evaluation to rule out malignancy. If the patient is known to have cancer, the following questions should be asked.

Ask the Patient

- Do you know if you have a tumor in this area?

Laser or light therapy should not be applied in the area of a known or possible malignancy.

Within 4 to 6 Months After Radiotherapy

It is recommended that lasers and light not be applied to areas that have recently been exposed to radiotherapy because radiotherapy increases tissue susceptibility to malignancy and burns.

Ask the Patient

- Have you recently had radiation applied in this area (the area being considered for treatment application)?

If the patient has recently had radiation therapy applied to the area, laser or light therapy should not be applied in that area.

Over Hemorrhaging Regions

Laser and light therapy are contraindicated in hemorrhaging regions because this intervention may cause vasodilation and thus increase bleeding.

Assess

- Check for signs of bleeding, including blood in a wound or worsening or recent bruising.

Laser or light therapy should not be applied in the area of bleeding.

Over the Thyroid or Other Endocrine Glands

Studies have found that the application of LLLT to the area of the thyroid gland can alter thyroid hormone levels in animals.[148] Therefore irradiation of the area near the thyroid gland (the midanterior neck) should be avoided. LLLT may also result in changes in serum concentrations of luteinizing hormone (LH), follicle-stimulating hormone (FSH), adrenocorticotropic hormone (ACTH), prolactin, testosterone, cortisol, and aldosterone.

PRECAUTIONS FOR THE USE OF LASERS AND LIGHT

PRECAUTIONS

for the Use of Lasers and Light[149,150]

- Low back or abdomen during pregnancy
- Epiphyseal plates in children
- Impaired sensation
- Impaired mentation
- Photophobia, or abnormally high sensitivity to light
- Pretreatment with one or more photosensitizers

Low Back or Abdomen During Pregnancy

Because the effects of LLLT on fetal development and fertility are not known, it is recommended that this type of treatment not be applied to the abdomen or low back during pregnancy.

Ask the Patient

- Are you pregnant?
- Do you think you may be pregnant?
- Are you trying to get pregnant?

If the patient is or may be pregnant, laser light therapy should not be applied to the abdomen or low back.

Epiphyseal Plates in Children

The effect of laser light therapy on epiphyseal plate growth or closure is not known. However, because laser light therapy can affect cell growth, application over the epiphyseal plates before their closure is not recommended.

Impaired Sensation or Mentation

Caution is recommended when treating patients with impaired sensation or mentation because these patients may not be able to report discomfort during the treatment. Although discomfort is rare during the application of laser light therapy, the area of the applicator in contact with the patient's skin can become warm and may burn the skin if applied for prolonged periods or if malfunctioning.

Ask the Patient

- Do you have normal feeling in this area?

Assess

- Check sensation in the application area. Use test tubes containing hot and cold water or metal spoons put in hot and cold water to test thermal sensation.
- Check alertness and orientation.

Laser light therapy should not be applied to any area where thermal sensation is impaired. Laser light therapy should not be applied if the patient is unresponsive or confused.

Photophobia or Pretreatment with Photosensitizers

Certain authors recommend that laser and light therapy should not be applied to any patient who has abnormally high sensitivity to light, either intrinsically or as the result of treatment with a photosensitizing medication. However, because increased skin sensitivity to light is generally limited to the UV range of the electromagnetic spectrum, only UV irradiation must be avoided in such patients. When wavelengths of light outside the UV range are being used in patients with photosensitivity, the clinician should check closely for any adverse effects and stop treatment if they occur.

Ask the Patient
• Are you taking any medication that increases your sensitivity to light or your risk of sunburn?
• Do you sunburn easily?

Assess
• Observe the skin for any signs of burning including erythema or blistering.

Treatment with laser or light therapy should be stopped if the patient show any signs of burning.

ADVERSE EFFECTS OF LASERS AND LIGHT

Although most reports concerning the use of low-level laser or other light devices note no adverse effects in the treatment area from the application of this physical agent,[123,151] there have been reports of transient tingling, mild erythema, skin rash, or a burning sensation, and increased pain or numbness in response to the application of low-level lasers and light therapy.[105,118,152-156]

The primary hazards of laser irradiation are the adverse effects that can occur with irradiation of the eyes. Laser devices are classified on a scale from 1 to 4 according to their power and associated risk of adverse effects to unprotected skin and eyes (see Table 12-1). The low-level lasers used in clinical applications are generally class 3B, which means that although they are harmless to unprotected skin, they do pose a potential hazard to the eyes if viewed along the beam. Exposure of the eyes to laser light of this class can cause retinal damage as a result of the concentrated intensity of the light and the limited attenuation of the beam intensity by the outer structures of the eye. As noted previously, this hazard does not apply to nonlaser light sources (LED and SLD) where the light is divergent and therefore not concentrated in one particular area.

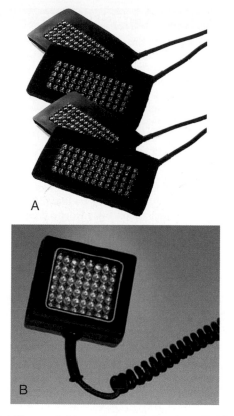

FIG 12-13 LED-array light applicators. **A,** Anodyne; **B,** MedX in Canada. *Courtesy Anodyne Therapy, Tampa, FL.*

The other potential hazard of laser or light therapy is burns. Although the mechanism of therapeutic action of laser and light therapy is not thermal, the diodes used to apply laser or other light therapy will get warm if they are on for a prolonged period. This is more likely to occur with lower-power LEDs that take a long time to deliver a therapeutic dose of energy and where many diodes may be used together in an array (Fig. 12-13). For this reason, particular caution should be taken when applying laser or any other form of light therapy to patients with impaired sensation or mentation and to areas of fragile tissue such as open wounds.

APPLICATION TECHNIQUE FOR LASERS AND LIGHT

APPLICATION TECHNIQUE 12-1 LASERS AND LIGHT

Procedure

1. Evaluate the patient's clinical findings and set the goals of treatment.
2. Determine if laser or light therapy is the most appropriate treatment.
3. Determine that laser or light therapy is not contraindicated for the patient or the condition. Check with the patient and check the patient's chart for contraindications regarding the application of laser or light therapy.

4. Select an applicator with the appropriate diode(s) including type(s) (LED, SLD, or laser diode), wavelength(s), and power. See discussion of parameters in next section.
5. Select the appropriate energy density (fluence) (J/cm²). Recommendations for different clinical applications are summarized in Table 12-2 and the parameter discussion in the next section.
6. Before treating any area with a risk of cross-infection, swab the face of the applicator with 0.5% alcoholic chlorhexidine or the antimicrobial approved for this use in the facility.

Continued

APPLICATION TECHNIQUE 12-1   **LASERS OR LIGHT**—*cont'd*

7. If using an applicator that includes laser diodes, the patient and the therapist should wear protective goggles (Fig. 12-14). These goggles should shield the eyes from light of the wavelength of the laser. DO NOT substitute sunglasses for the goggles provided with or intended for your laser device. Sunglasses do not adequately filter IR light. Never look into the beam or the laser aperture. Remember, a laser beam can damage the eyes even if the beam cannot be seen.

8. Expose the area to be treated. Remove overlying clothing, opaque dressings, and any shiny jewelry from the area. Nonopaque dressings, such as thin films, do not need to be removed because it has been shown that most of the laser light can penetrate through these wound dressings.[157]

9. Apply the applicator to the skin with firm pressure, keeping the light beam(s) perpendicular to the skin (see Fig. 12-14). If the treatment area does not have intact skin, is painful to touch, or does not tolerate contact for any other reason, treatment may be applied with the applicator slightly above the tissue, without touching the skin but with the light beam(s) still kept perpendicular to the tissue surface (Fig. 12-15).

10. Start the light output and keep the applicator in place throughout the application of each dose. If the treatment area is larger than the applicator, repeat the dose to areas approximately 1 inch apart throughout the treatment area. The device will automatically stop after delivery of the set dose (J/cm^2).

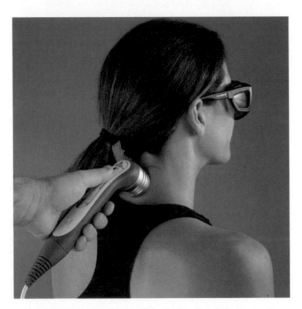

FIG 12-14 Patient wearing goggles during laser therapy. *Courtesy Chattanooga Group, Hixson, TN.*

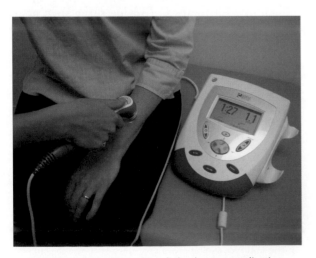

FIG 12-15 Noncontact laser light therapy application.

PARAMETERS FOR THE USE OF LASERS AND LIGHT

Note that because laser and light therapy is an active area of research in which new information about the effects of different treatment parameters becomes available almost every day, recommendations for ideal parameters are evolving and change over time. The recommendations given here are based on this author's interpretation of the current literature, which is likely to change as new discoveries are made about the effects of specific parameters of laser and light therapy.

Type of Diode

There is much controversy in the literature and among experts concerning the importance of selecting a specific type of diode for clinical application. Although it is clear that the different diodes produce light of different degrees of wavelength range, coherence, and collimation, it is not clear if these differences have a clinical impact, and there are very few studies directly comparing the effects of coherent (laser) and noncoherent (LED and SLD) light.[154,155] There are more studies on the effects of laser light than on the effects of light emitted by LEDs and SLDs, largely because laser applicators were available many years earlier, but there are studies showing beneficial effects of all three. What remains uncertain and controversial is whether the effects of coherent laser light can be assumed to also occur in response to noncoherent LED and SLD light, and whether one type of light is superior to another.[48,158-160]

LEDs provide the most diffuse light with the widest frequency range and are low power individually. Because they output diffuse light, LEDs are most suitable for treating larger more superficial areas. Applicators that use LEDs as the treatment light source generally contain many LEDs in an array (see Fig. 12-13) or cluster (Fig. 12-16) to provide more power for the entire applicator and to treat a larger area. The power of the applicator equals the sum of the power of all of its diodes. Some cluster applicators may include a small number of low-power LEDs in the visible wavelength range to serve as indicators for when the device is emitting, particularly when the other higher-

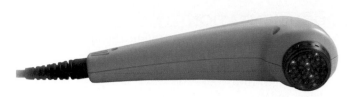

FIG 12-16 A cluster light applicator that includes LEDs that emit low-power red light and SLDs that emit higher power infrared light. *Courtesy Dynatronics, Salt Lake City, UT.*

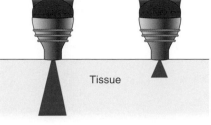

Wavelength Absorption
Laser probe 100 mW   Laser probe 100 mW

Tissue

900 nm   630 nm

FIG 12-18 Depth of penetration according to wavelength.

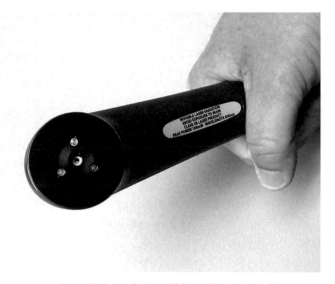

FIG 12-17 A laser diode applicator. This applicator includes one infrared laser diode and three blue LEDs that serve as indicators to show when the applicator is on. *Courtesy Mettler Electronics, Anaheim, CA.*

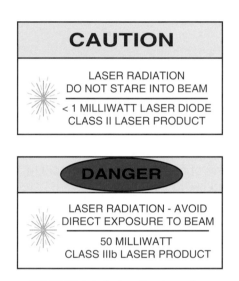

CAUTION

LASER RADIATION
DO NOT STARE INTO BEAM

< 1 MILLIWATT LASER DIODE
CLASS II LASER PRODUCT

DANGER

LASER RADIATION - AVOID
DIRECT EXPOSURE TO BEAM

50 MILLIWATT
CLASS IIIb LASER PRODUCT

FIG 12-19 Labels denoting laser class.

power SLDs or laser diodes emit only in the invisible IR range (Fig. 12-17).

SLDs provide light that is less diffuse and of a narrower wavelength range than LEDs and they are also higher power than LEDs (see Fig. 12-11). SLDs are suitable for treating superficial or moderately deep areas, depending on their wavelength.

Laser diodes provide light of a single wavelength that is very concentrated. Laser diodes are suitable for treating small areas and, for the same wavelength and power, will deliver the most light deepest to a focused area of tissue. Protective goggles should be worn by both the patient and the clinician when using any applicator that includes one or more laser diodes because this concentrated light can damage the eyes.

Wavelength
Laser light applicators output light in the visible or near-visible wavelength range of the electromagnetic spectrum, between 500 and 1,100 nm. Most applicators include near IR (≈700 to 1,100 nm) or red (≈600 to 700 nm) light. IR, with its longer wavelength, penetrates deeper than red light (Fig. 12-18) and is therefore most suitable for treating deeper tissues up to 30 to 40 mm deep. Red light is most suitable for treating more superficial tissues, at a depth of

5 to 10 mm, such as the skin and subcutaneous tissue. Applicators that output blue light have recently also become available. These are most suitable for treating surface tissue such as skin or exposed soft tissue.

Power
Laser light applicator power is measured in milliwatts (1 mW = 1/1000th of a watt). Lasers are classified by international agreement as class 1 to class 4, according to their power and resulting effects (see Table 12-1). All lasers carry a label denoting their class (Fig. 12-19).

Lasers used for therapy are generally power class 3B, with the power of any individual diode being more than 5 mW and less than 500 mW. A number of laser diodes may be combined in a single applicator to provide a total power of more than 500 mW.

The laser classification system does not apply to LEDs and SLDs because these diodes do not produce light that is concentrated in a small area and that can therefore be damaging to the eye. The power of a single LED is generally in the range of 1 to 5 mW but can be as high as 30 to 40 mW. A number of LEDs, often around 20 to 60, but up to 200 or more, are generally placed in a pad or array applicator to provide an applicator with more total power. The power of SLDs is generally in the range of 5 to 35 mW

TABLE 12-2	Energy Density Suggestions Based on Condition
Type of Condition	**Suggested Treatment Dose Range (J/cm^2)**
Soft tissue healing	5-16
Fracture healing	5-16
Arthritis: acute	2-4
Arthritis: chronic	4-8
Lymphedema	1.5
Neuropathy	10-12
Acute soft tissue inflammation	2-8
Chronic soft tissue inflammation	10-20

each, but may be as high as 90 mW or more each. A number of SLDs, generally about 3 to 10, are usually placed together in a cluster applicator to provide more total power.

As discussed earlier in this chapter, lower-power light applicators require longer application times to deliver the same amount of energy as higher-power light applicators. Thus the applicator power should be selected to optimize the practicality of the treatment time.

Energy Density

In general, low energy densities are thought to be stimulatory, whereas too high an energy density can be suppressive or damaging. Most recommend using lower doses for acute and superficial conditions and higher doses for chronic and deeper conditions and that treatment be initiated at the lower end of the recommended range and increased in subsequent treatments if the prior treatment was well tolerated (Table 12-2).

DOCUMENTATION

When using laser, LED, or SLD light therapy, document the following:
- Type of diode (laser, LED, SLD)
- Wavelength (nm)
- Power (mW)
- Area of body treated
- Energy density (J/cm^2)

Note that duration of treatment is not listed because this is included in the energy density parameter, and the unit will stop automatically when the total dose (energy density) has been delivered.

EXAMPLES

When applying laser to a pressure ulcer over the left greater trochanter in a patient with T10 level paraplegia, in the second week of treatment document the following:

S: *Pt reports his wound over the left thigh was stable for the 2 months before initiating laser therapy but is now closing up.*

O: *Stage IV pressure ulcer over left greater trochanter, 3 cm × 4 cm, 2 cm deep.*

Treatment: *IR laser 904 nm, 200 mW, to area of wound, 9 J/cm^2 to 4 areas over the wound.*

A: *Wound size decreased from 4 cm × 5 cm × 2.5 cm deep at initiation of laser therapy.*

P: *Continue current laser therapy and pressure management.*

When applying light therapy to a patient with lateral epicondylitis, document the following:

S: *Pt reports 5/10 pain over the right lateral elbow and increased pain with gripping.*

O: *Tender to deep palpation over extensor carpi radialis brevis tendon.*

Treatment: *Red SLD, 630 nm, 500 mW cluster, 3 J/cm^2.*

Posttreatment: *Minimal tenderness, pain decreased to 2/10.*

A: *Reduced pain and tenderness after light therapy.*

P: *Continue light therapy. Modify work activities to reduce strain on wrist extensors.*

CLINICAL CASE STUDIES

The following case studies summarize the concepts of laser and light therapy discussed in this chapter. Based on the scenarios presented, an evaluation of the clinical findings and goals of treatment are proposed. These are followed by a discussion of the factors to be considered in the selection of laser or light therapy as an indicated intervention and in the selection of the ideal laser or light therapy parameters to promote progress toward the set goals.

CASE STUDY 12-1

Open Wound
Examination
History

JM is a 78-year-old man with an open wound on his right foot. JM states that the wound has been present for

6 months and has not improved with compression bandaging and regular dressing changes. His doctor has diagnosed chronic venous insufficiency and diabetes, and JM has had similar ulcers in the past that have healed slowly. JM relies on his wife to help him with daily dressing changes, and his wife notes that there is yellow-colored drainage on the dressings when they are changed. Although the wound does not cause much pain, JM has been walking less to avoid aggravating the wound. As a result, he has not been as active in many of his usual activities, including gardening and Sunday night bingo.

Tests and Measures

The patient is an alert man with mild bilateral lower extremity edema. He has an ulcerated area approximately 4 × 5 cm on the plantar aspect of his right foot with purulent drainage and no evidence of granulation tissue or bleeding. His left foot and lower extremity are free of

CLINICAL CASE STUDIES—*cont'd*

wounds. Sensation in both feet and around the wound is moderately impaired.

Why might the clinician need to use caution when applying laser or light to this patient? Should the patient continue compression? How will you know if this patient is or is not improving?

Evaluation, Diagnosis, Prognosis, and Goals
Evaluation and Goals

ICF Level	Current Status	Goals
Body structure and function	Chronic right foot ulcer Decreased bilateral lower extremity sensation	Closed right foot ulcer
Activity	Decreased ambulation	Increase ambulation to pre-wound distances
Participation	Decreased participation in hobbies such as gardening and bingo	Return to gardening and bingo

Diagnosis
Preferred Practice Pattern 7D: Impaired integumentary integrity associated with full-thickness skin involvement and scar formation.

Prognosis/Plan of Care
This patient presents with a chronic ulcer of the foot that is likely a result of his diabetes and chronic venous insufficiency. Compression bandages and daily dressing changes over several months have not resulted in wound healing. At this point, it is appropriate to add a new modality. Laser or light, electrical stimulation, and ultrasound might be options for this patient, but laser or light has the advantage of short treatment time and the ability to be applied without touching the wound, thus minimizing cross-infection risk. With this intervention and ongoing management of his impaired venous return, the wound can be expected to close completely over a period of weeks.

Intervention
Laser and light therapy was selected as an adjunctive treatment modality to promote tissue healing. Laser and light therapy have been shown in a number of studies and a recent metaanalysis to accelerate wound healing. This effect is likely in part a result of increased ATP and collagen production.

A cluster probe that included laser diodes and SLDs was selected because this provides both focal and broad coverage with light.

Red light with around 600 nm wavelength was selected because it has shallow penetration, consistent with the depth of tissue involved with this wound. In addition, some studies have found that light in this wavelength range can reduce bacterial viability.

A cluster probe with a total power of 500 mW was selected so that treatment time could be fairly short.

The dose for the first treatment was 4 J/cm², which was increased by 2 J/cm² at each subsequent treatment up to 16 J/cm².

Treatment was provided twice a week for 8 weeks.

Documentation
S: Pt reports a right foot ulcer present for 6 months.

O: Pretreatment: 4 × 5 cm ulcer on plantar surface of right foot.

Intervention: Laser SLD cluster, 630-650 nm, 500 mW, 4 J/cm², applied to right foot ulcer without contact.

A: Pt tolerated intervention with no signs of discomfort.

P: Continue laser and light treatment 2 × /week, increasing by 2 J/cm² at each subsequent treatment up to 16 J/cm², until wound has healed. Educate pt to keep his lower extremities elevated and in the proper use of compression bandages or stockings.

CASE STUDY 12-2

Rheumatoid Arthritis
Examination
History
RM is a 42-year-old electrical engineer with RA. She has been referred to therapy for stiffness and pain, particularly in the joints of her hands. In the past when RM received therapy, she was taught ROM exercises that she now performs three times weekly. The patient's work involves using her hands on the computer and when troubleshooting projects involving fine wires. She finds she has become slower at these fine motor tasks and is unable to do some of the finest work. She is worried that this will affect her ability to continue her current job or to maintain other types of employment.

RM's medications include methotrexate and ibuprofen, which provide some relief of hand pain and stiffness.

Tests and Measures
The patient appears to be generally healthy, although she walks somewhat stiffly. She reports hand pain that varies from 4/10 at rest to 7/10 with motion. She reports that her hands are particularly stiff for the first 1 to 1½ hours each morning. ROM appears to be generally decreased in all joints of both hands, and there is mild ulnar drift at the metacarpophalangeal joints. Passive ROM was measured in a number of joints and was as follows:

Joint	Right	Left
Thumb interphalangeal (IP) flexion	80°	80°
Thumb IP extension	−20°	−20°
Index finger proximal IP (PIP) joint flexion	90°	90°
Index finger PIP joint extension	−20°	−25°
Middle finger PIP flexion	100°	90°
Middle finger PIP extension	−20°	−30°

Continued

CLINICAL CASE STUDIES—*cont'd*

Grip strength is 4/5 bilaterally and is limited by pain and stiffness.

What would be reasonable goals for therapy with laser or light therapy? What other interventions would you consider in addition to laser or light therapy? What are advantages and disadvantages for this patient of laser or light therapy compared with other interventions?

Evaluation, Diagnosis, Prognosis, and Goals
Evaluation and Goals

ICF Level	Current Status	Goals
Body structure and function	Bilateral hand joint pain, stiffness, and decreased ROM	Decrease pain by 50%, shorten duration of morning stiffness to 30 minutes, and increase ROM by ≥5 degrees in measured joints in both hands
Activity	Decreased fine motor skill and speed	Improve fine motor skill and speed Be aware of adaptive tools and other methods to perform certain fine motor skills
Participation	Slowed and limited work performance	Continue working at current job at an acceptable level

Diagnosis

Preferred Practice Pattern 4E: Impaired joint mobility, motor function, muscle performance, and ROM associated with localized inflammation.

Prognosis/Plan of Care

This patient presents with reduced functional abilities and participation as a result of reduced ROM, pain, and stiffness in her fingers from RA. Laser light therapy has been found in individual studies and in a metaanalysis of current studies to reduce pain and morning stiffness in patients with RA. This form of therapy would be a good choice for RM because laser light could be delivered quickly and easily to many of her joints with the appropriate applicator. Given the chronic progressive nature of RA, treatment should be provided in conjunction with body mechanics and adaptive equipment evaluation and intervention to optimize function and participation over the long term.

Intervention

Laser light therapy was selected as an adjunctive treatment modality to modify inflammation.

A cluster probe that included laser diodes and SLDs was selected because this provides both focal and broad coverage with light and could be used to treat a number of involved joints at once. Alternatively, a single diode could be used and applied to individual joints separately or an array of LEDs could be applied to most or all of each hand, although this would likely require a longer application time because these arrays output light with a low energy density.

IR light with around 800-900 nm wavelength was selected because it has deep penetration and may penetrate to the involved joint structures.

A cluster probe with a total power of 200-500 mW was selected so that treatment time could be fairly short.

The dose for the first treatment was 2 J/cm². This low dose was used at first as higher doses have been found by some clinicians to exacerbate inflammation. If this dose is well tolerated, the dose may be increased to 4 or possibly 8 J/cm².

Treatment was provided twice per week for 4 weeks.

Documentation

S: Pt reports stiffness of her hands that is worst for the first 60-90 minutes each morning and that interferes with fine motor tasks at work.

O: Pretreatment PROM:

Joint	Right	Left
Thumb IP flexion	80°	80°
Thumb IP extension	−20°	−20°
Index finger PIP joint flexion	90°	90°
Index finger PIP joint extension	−20°	−25°
Middle finger PIP flexion	100°	90°
Middle finger PIP extension	−20°	−30°

Intervention: Laser SLD cluster, 800-900 nm, 500 mW, 2 J/cm² applied to both hands, 2 different areas to focus on IP joints.

A: Pt tolerated laser with no signs of discomfort.

P: Continue laser treatment 2 × week. Recheck ROM in 1 week and if improved and pt tolerating treatment well, increase dose to 4-8 J/cm². Educate patient in joint protection techniques.

CHAPTER REVIEW

1. Electromagnetic radiation is composed of electric and magnetic fields that vary over time and are oriented perpendicular to each other.
2. Different frequencies of electromagnetic radiation have different names, different properties and different applications. Shortwave, microwave, infrared, visible light, and UV radiation all have clinical therapeutic applications.
3. Laser light has the unique features of being monochromatic (one frequency), coherent and directional while light produced by LEDs and SLDs has a range of frequencies, is noncoherent and spreads. Low-intensity laser or noncoherent light may be used as physical agents in rehabilitation.

4. Lasers and light affect cells via their interaction with intracellular chromophores. This interaction leads to a range of cellular effects, including increased ATP and RNA synthesis. These effects can promote tissue healing, reduce pain and improve function in patients with a range of conditions, including arthritis, neuropathy, and lymphedema.

5. Contraindications to the use of lasers include direct irradiation of the eyes, malignancy, within 4 to 6 months after radiotherapy, hemorrhaging regions, and application to the endocrine glands. Precautions include application to the low back or abdomen during pregnancy, epiphyseal plates in children, impaired sensation and mentation, photophobia or abnormally high sensitivity to light, and pretreatment with one or more photosensitizers. Clinicians should always read and follow the contraindications and precautions listed for a particular unit.

6. When selecting a device, the clinician should first consider whether light therapy will be effective for the patient's condition. After deciding on the type of diode (laser, LED, or SLD), the clinician should set the appropriate parameters, including wavelength, power, and energy density.

7. The reader is referred to the Evolve web site for further exercises and links to resources and references.

ADDITIONAL RESOURCES *evolve*

Web Sites

Laser World (Swedish Laser Medical Society): www.laser.nu
    Excellent bibliography of laser papers with abstracts produced by the Société Francophone des Lasers Médicaux: www.sflm.org/s3/dl/applisusr/angio/BiblioBiostimulation.pdf

Books

Baxter DG: *Therapeutic lasers: theory and practice,* London, 1994, Churchill Livingstone.
    Tuner J, Hode L: *Laser therapy clinical practice and scientific background,* Grangesburg, Sweden, 2002, Prima Books.
    Tuner J, Hode L: *The laser therapy handbook,* Grangesburg, Sweden, 2004, Prima Books.

Manufacturers

Chattanooga Group: www.chattgroup.com
Dynatronics: www.dynatronics.com
Mettler Electronics: www.mettlerelectronics.com
MedX: www.medxonline.com
Thor: www.thorlaser.com
Microlight Corporation: www.microlightcorp.com
Photothera: www.photothera.com

GLOSSARY *evolve*

Band (frequency band): A range within the electromagnetic spectrum defined by wavelength (e.g., the band for UVA radiation is 320-400 nm).

Chromophores: Light-absorbing parts of a molecule that give it its color.

Cluster probe: Light therapy applicator with multiple diodes that may be any combination of laser diodes, LEDs, or SLDs. The use of multiple diodes allows coverage of a larger treatment area, takes advantage of the properties of the different types of diodes, and may reduce treatment time.

Coherent: Light in which all the waves are in phase with each other; lasers produce coherent light.

Diathermy: The application of shortwave or microwave electromagnetic energy to produce heat within tissues, particularly deep tissues.

Directional (collimated): Light with parallel waves.

Divergent: Light that spreads; the opposite of collimated.

Electromagnetic radiation: Radiation composed of electric and magnetic fields that vary over time and are oriented perpendicular to each other. This type of radiation does not need a medium to propagate.

Energy: The total amount of electromagnetic energy delivered over the entire treatment time. Energy is usually measured in Joules (J). Energy is equal to power multiplied by time.

$$1 \text{ J} = 1 \text{ W} \times 1 \text{ sec}$$

Energy density: The total amount of electromagnetic energy delivered per unit area over the entire treatment time. Energy density isgenerally measured in Joules per centimeter squared (J/cm^2). Most authors agree that this should be the standard dosage measure for laser light therapy.

Frequency: Number of waves per unit time, generally measured in hertz (Hz), which is waves per second.

Hot laser: Heats and destroys tissue directly in beam and is used for surgery. Also called high-intensity laser.

Ionizing radiation: Electromagnetic radiation that can penetrate cells and displace electrons from atoms or molecules to create ions. Ionizing radiation includes x-rays and gamma rays. Ionizing radiation can damage the internal structures of living cells.

Laser: Acronym for light amplification by stimulated emission of radiation. Laser light has the unique properties of being monochromatic, coherent, and directional.

Laser diodes: Light source that uses semiconductor diode technology and optics to produce laser light.

Light-emitting diode (LED): Semiconductor diode light source that produces relatively low-power light in a range of frequencies. LED light may appear to be one color (e.g., red) but will always have a range of wavelengths and not be coherent or directional.

Low-level laser therapy (LLLT): Application of laser light for therapeutic purposes. LLLT is also known as cold laser, low-intensity, low-power, or soft laser. LLLT generally uses laser light diodes that have less than 500 mW power per diode. LLLT cluster probes may contain a number of diodes with a total combined power above 500 mW.

Maser: Acronym for microwave amplification by stimulated emission of radiation.

Monochromatic: Light of single frequency, wavelength, and color. Laser light is monochromatic. Other light sources produce light with a range of wavelengths.

Photobiomodulation: Stimulatory or inhibitory effects on the body caused by light phototherapy; the therapeutic use of light.

Power: Rate of energy production, generally measured in milliwatts (mW) for laser light.

Power density (irradiance): The concentration of power per unit area, measured in watts per centimeter squared (W/cm^2).

Speckling: Variability of light intensity that occurs when a coherent light illuminates a rough object.

Stimulated emission: Occurs when a photon hits an atom that is already excited (i.e., electrons are at a higher energy level than usual). The atom being hit releases a new photon that is identical to the incoming photon—the same color, going in the same direction.

Supraluminous diode (SLD): Light source that uses semiconductor diode technology to produce high-power light in a narrow frequency range.

Ultraviolet (UV) radiation: Electromagnetic radiation with wavelength from < 290 nm to 400 nm, which lies between x-ray and visible light.

Wavelength: The length of a wave of light from peak to peak determines frequency and color. Longer wavelengths are associated with deeper penetration.

REFERENCES *evolve*

1. Sears FW, Zemansky MW, Young HD: *College physics*, Reading, MA, 1987, Addison-Wesley.
2. Hitchcock RT, Patterson RM: *Radio-frequency and ELF electromagnetic energies: a handbook for health professionals*, New York, 1995, Van Nostrand Reinhold.
3. Thomas CL: *Taber's cyclopedic medical dictionary*, Philadelphia, 1993, FA Davis.
4. Hawkins D, Houreld N, Abrahamse H. Low level laser therapy (LLLT) as an effective therapeutic modality for delayed wound healing, *Ann NY Acad Sci* 1056:486-493, 2005.
5. Holick MF: The cutaneous photosynthesis of previtamin D: a unique photoendocrine system, *J Invest Dermatol* 76:51-58, 1981.
6. Adley WR: Physiological signalling across cell membranes and cooperative influences of extremely low frequency electromagnetic fields. In Frohlich H, ed: *Biological coherence and response to external stimuli*, Heidelberg, 1988, Springer-Verlag.
7. Tsong TY: Deciphering the language of cells, *TIBS* 14:89-92, 1989.
8. Alster TS, Kauvar AN, Geronemus RG: Histology of high-energy pulsed CO_2 laser resurfacing, *Semin Cutan Med Surg* 15(3):189-193, 1996.
9. Mester E, Spiry T, Szende B, et al: Effects of laser rays on wound healing, *Am J Surg* 122:532-535, 1971.
10. Mester E, Ludany G, Sellyei M, et al: The stimulating effects of low power laser rays on biological systems, *Laser Rev* 1:3, 1968.
11. Mester AF, Mester A: Wound healing, *Laser Ther* 1:7-15, 1989.
12. Mester AF, Mester A: Clinical data of laser biostimulation in wound healing, *Lasers Surg Med* 7:78, 1987.
13. Beckerman H, de Bie RA, Bouter LM, et al: The efficacy of laser therapy for musculoskeletal and skin disorders: a criteria-based meta-analysis of randomized clinical trials, *Phys Ther* 72(7):483-491, 1992.
14. Kolari PJ: Penetration of unfocused laser light into the skin, *Arch Dermatol Res* 277:342-344, 1985.
15. King PR: Low level laser therapy—a review, *Lasers Med Sci* 4:141-150, 1989.
16. Goldman L, Michaelson SM, Rockwell RJ, et al: Optical radiation with particular reference to lasers. In Suess M, Benwell-Morrison D, eds: *Nonionizing radiation protection*, ed 2, European Series No. 25, Geneva, 1989, WHO.
17. Goldman L, Rockwell JR: *Lasers in medicine*, New York, 1971, Gordon & Breach.
18. Trelles MA, Mayayo E, Miro L: The action of low reactive laser therapy on mast cells, *Laser Ther* 1:1, 27-30, 1989.
19. Oshiro T, Calderhead RG: *Low level laser therapy: a practical introduction*, Chichester, UK, 1988, Wiley.
20. Basford JR: Low energy laser therapy: controversies and new research findings, *Lasers Surg Med* 9:1-5, 1989.
21. Belkin M, Schwartz M: New biological phenomena associated with laser radiation, *Health Phys* 56:687-690, 1989.
22. Karu T: Photobiology of low-power laser effects, *Health Phys* 56:691-704, 1989.
23. Karu TI: Molecular mechanisms of the therapeutic effects of low intensity laser radiation, *Lasers Life Sci* 2:53-74, 1988.
24. Smith KC: The photobiological basis of low level laser radiation therapy, *Laser Ther* 3:19-24, 1991
25. Baxter D: Low intensity laser therapy. In Kitchen S, Bazin S, eds: *Clayton's electrotherapy*, ed 10, London, 1996, WB Saunders.
26. Kitchen SS, Partridge CJ: A review of low level laser therapy, *Physiotherapy* 77:161-168, 1991.
27. Passarella S, Casamassima E, Molinari S, et al: Increase of proton electrochemical potential and ATP synthesis in rat liver mitochondria irradiated in vitro by Helium-Neon laser, *FEBS Lett* 175:95-99, 1984.
28. Eells JT, Henry MM, Summerfelt MTT, et al: Therapeutic photobiomodulation for methanol-induced retinal toxicity, *PNAS* 100(6):3439-3444, 2003.
29. Eells JT, Wong-Riley MT, VerHoeve J, et al: Mitochondrial signal transduction in accelerated wound and retinal healing by near-infrared light therapy, *Mitochondrion* 4(5-6):559-567, 2004.
30. Winterle JS, Einarsdottir O: Photoreactions of cytochrome C oxidase, *J Photochem Photobiol* 82(3):711-719, 2006.
31. Silveira PC, Streck EL, Pinho RA: Evaluation of mitochondrial respiratory chain activity in wound healing by low-level laser therapy, *J Photochem Photobiol* 86(3):279-282, 2006.
32. Greco M, Vacca R, Moro L, et al: Helium-neon laser irradiation of hepatocytes can trigger increase of the mitochondrial membrane potential and can stimulate c-fos expression in a Ca [2+]-dependent manner, *Lasers Surg Med* 29(5):433-441, 2001.
33. Lopes-Martins RA, Marcos RL, Leonardo PS, et al: Effect of low-level laser (Ga-Al-As 655 nm) on skeletal muscle fatigue induced by electrical stimulation in rats, *J Appl Physiol* 101(1):283-288, 2006.
34. Carney SA, Lawrence JC, Ricketts CR: The effect of light from a ruby laser on the metabolism of skin tissue culture, *Biochem Biophys Acta* 148:525-530, 1967.
35. Abergel RP, Meeker CA, Lam TS, et al: Control of connective tissue metabolism by lasers: recent developments and future prospects, *J Am Acad Dermatol* 11:1142-1150, 1984.
36. Lam TS, Abergel RP, Castel JC, et al: Laser stimulation of collagen synthesis in human skin fibroblast cultures, *Laser Life Sci* 1:61-77, 1986.
37. Anders JJ, Geuna S, Rochkind S: Phototherapy promotes regeneration and functional recovery of injured peripheral nerve, *Neuro Res* 26:234-240, 2004.
38. Mester E, Mester AF, Mester A: The biomedical effects of laser application, *Lasers Surg Med* 5:31-39, 1985.
39. Bjordal JM, Lopes-Martins RA, Iversen VV: A randomised, placebo controlled trial of low level laser therapy for activated Achilles tendinitis with microdialysis measurement of peritendinous prostaglandin E2 concentrations, *Br J Sports Med* 40(1):76-80; discussion 76-80, 2006.
40. Yu HS, Chang KL, Yu CL, et al: Low-energy helium-neon laser irradiation stimulates interleukin-1 alpha and interleukin-8 release from cultured human keratinocytes, *J Invest Dermatol* 107(4):593-6, 1996.
41. Aimbire F, Albertini R, Pacheco MT, et al: Low-level laser therapy induces dose-dependent reduction of TNFalpha levels in acute inflammation, *Photomed Laser Surg* 24(1):33-37, 2006.
42. Kupin IV, Bykov VS, Ivanov AV, et al: Potentiating effects of laser radiation on some immunologic traits, *Neoplasma* 29:403-406, 1982.
43. Passarella S, Casamassima E, Quagliariello E, et al: Quantitative analysis of lymphocyte-Salmonella interaction and the effects of lymphocyte irradiation by He-Ne laser, *Biochem Biophys Res Commun* 130:546-552, 1985.
44. El Sayed SO, Dyson M. Effect of laser pulse repetition rate and pulse duration on mast cell number and degranulation, *Lasers Surg Med* 19:433-437, 1996.

45. El Sayed SO, Dyson M: Comparison of the effect of multi-wavelength light produced by a cluster of semiconductor diodes and of each individual diode on mast cell number and degranulation in intact and injured skin, *Lasers Surg Med* 10:559-568, 1990.
46. Young S, Bolton P, Dyson M, et al: Macrophage responsiveness to light therapy, *Lasers Surg Med* 9:497-505, 1989.
47. Rajaratnam S, Bolton P, Dyson M: Macrophage responsiveness to laser therapy with varying pulsing frequencies, *Laser Ther* 6:107-111, 1994.
48. Vinck EM, Cagnie BJ, Cornelissen MJ, et al: Increased fibroblast proliferation induced by light emitting diode and low power laser irradiation, *Laser Med Sci* 18:95-99, 2003.
49. Pereira AN, Eduardo Cde P, Matson E, et al: Effect of low-power laser irradiation on cell growth and procollagen synthesis of cultured fibroblasts, *Lasers Surg Med* 31(4):263-267, 2002.
50. Webb C, Dyson M, Lewis WHP: Stimulatory effect of 660 nm low level laser energy on hypertrophic scar-derived fibroblasts: possible mechanisms for increase in cell counts, *Lasers Surg Med* 22:294-301, 1998.
51. Grossman N, Schneid N, Reuveni H, et al: 780 nm low power diode laser irradiation stimulates proliferation of keratinocyte cultures: involvement of reactive oxygen species, *Lasers Surg Med* 29(2):105-106, 2001.
52. Schindl A, Merwald H, Schindl L, et al: Direct stimulatory effect of low-intensity 670 nm laser irradiation on human endothelial cell proliferation, *Br J Dermatol* 148(2):334-336, 2003.
53. de Simone NA, Christiansen C, Dore D: Bactericidal effect of 0.95mW helium-neon and 5-mW indium-gallium-aluminum-phosphate laser irradiation at exposure times of 30, 60 and 120 seconds on photosensitized *Staphylococcus aureus* and *Pseudomonas aeruginosa* in vitro, *Phys Ther* 79(9):839-846, 1999.
54. Nussbaum EL, Lilge L, Mazzuli T: Effects of 630-, 660-, 810- and 905-nm laser irradiation delivering radiant exposure of 1-50 J/cm² on three species of bacteria in vitro, *J Clin Laser Med Surg* 20:325-333, 2002.
55. Guffey SJ, Wilborn J: Effect of combined 405-nm and 880-nm light on *Staphylococcus aureus* and *Pseudomonas aeruginosa* in vitro, *Photomed Laser Surg* 24(6):680-683, 2006.
56. Guffey JS, Wilborn J: In vitro bactericidal effects of 405 nm and 470 nm blue light, *Photomed Laser Surg* 24(6):684-688, 2006.
57. Nussbaum EL, Lilge L, Mazzulli T: Effects of 810 nm laser irradiation on in vitro growth of bacteria: comparison of continuous wave and frequency modulated light, *Lasers Surg Med* 31(5):343-351, 2002.
58. Schindl A, Heinze G, Schindl M, et al: Systemic effects of low-intensity laser irradiation on skin microcirculation in patients with diabetic microangiopathy, *Microvasc Res* 64(2):240-246, 2002.
59. Lingard A, Hulten LM, Svensson L, et al: Irradiation at 634 nm releases nitric oxide from human monocytes, *Laser Med Sci* 22:30-36, 2007.
60. Nissan M, Rochkind S, Razon N, et al: Ne-He laser irradiation delivered transcutaneously: its effects on the sciatic nerve of the rat, *Lasers Surg Med* 6:435-438, 1986.
61. Schwartz M, Doron A, Erlich M, et al: Effects of low energy He-Ne laser irradiation on posttraumatic degeneration of adult rabbit optic nerve, *Lasers Surg Med* 7(1):51-55, 1987.
62. Rochkind S, Nissan M, Lubar R, et al: The in-vivo nerve response to direct low energy laser irradiation, *Acta Neurochir* 94:74-77, 1988.
63. Walker JB, Akhanjee LK: Laser induced somatosensory evoked potentials: evidence of photosensitivity in peripheral nerves, *Brain Res* 344(2):281-285, 1985.
64. Hamilton GF, Robinson TK, Ray RH: The effects of helium-neon laser upon regeneration of the crushed peroneal nerve, *J Orth Sports Phys Ther* 15(5):209-214, 1992.
65. Anderson TE, Good WT, Kerr HH, et al: Low level laser therapy in the treatment of carpal tunnel syndrome, Unpublished data, Microlight corporation. Available at http://www.laserhealthproducts.com/gmstudy.pdf, 1995.
66. Naeser MA: Photobiomodulation of pain in carpal tunnel syndrome: Review of seven laser therapy studies, *Photomed Laser Surg* 24(2):101-110, 2006.
67. Rochkind S, Nissan M, Barr-Nea L, et al: Response of peripheral nerve to He-Ne laser: experimental studies, *Lasers Surg Med* 7:441-443, 1987.
68. Shamir MH, Rochkind S, Sandbank J, et al: Double-blind randomized study evaluating regeneration of the rat transected sciatic nerve after suturing and postoperative low-power laser treatment, *J Reconstr Microsurg* 17:133-137, 2001.
69. Rochkind S, Nissan M, Alon M, et al: Effects of laser irradiation on the spinal cord for the regeneration of crushed peripheral nerve in rats, *Lasers Surg Med* 28:216-219, 2001.
70. Wollman Y, Rochkind S, Simantov R: Low power laser irradiation enhances migration and neurite sprouting of cultured rat embryonal brain cells, *Neurol Res* 18:467-470, 1996.
71. Wollman Y, Rochkind S: In vitro cellular processes sprouting in cortex microexplants of adult rat brains induced by low power laser irradiation, *Neurol Res* 20:470-472, 1998.
72. Snyder-Mackler L, Cork C: Effect of helium neon laser irradiation on peripheral sensory nerve latency, *Phys Ther* 68:223-225, 1988.
73. Baxter D, Bell AJ, Allen JM, et al: Laser mediated increase in median nerve conduction velocities, *Ir J Med Sci* 160:145-146, 1991.
74. Vinck E, Coorevits P, Cagnie B, et al: Evidence of changes in sural nerve conduction mediated by light emitting diode irradiation, *Lasers Med Sci* 20:35-40, 2005.
75. Basford JR, Daube JR, Hallman HO, et al: Does low intensity helium neon laser irradiation alter sensory nerve action potentials or distal latencies? *Lasers Surg Med* 10:35-39, 1990.
76. Lundeberg T, Haker E, Thomas M: Effects of laser versus placebo in tennis elbow, *Scand J Rehabil Med* 19:135-138, 1987.
77. Wu WH, Ponnudurai R, Katz J, et al: Failure to confirm report of light-evoked response of peripheral nerve to low power helium neon laser light stimulus, *Brain Res* 401(2):407-408, 1987.
78. Jarvis D, MacIver MB, Tanelian DL: Electrophysiologic recording and thermodynamic modeling demonstrate that helium-neon laser irradiation does not affect peripheral A-delta or C-fiber nociceptors, *Pain* 43(2):235-242, 1990.
79. Walsh D, Baxter G, Allen J: Lack of effect of pulsed low-intensity infrared (820 nm) laser irradiation on nerve conduction in the human superficial radial nerve, *Laser Surg Med* 26(5):485-490, 2000.
80. Nussbaum EL, Biemann I, Mustard B: Comparison of ultrasound/ultraviolet-C and laser for treatment of pressure ulcers in patients with spinal cord injury, *Phys Ther* 74:812-823, 1994.
81. Lyons RF, Abergel RP, White RA, et al: Biostimulation of wound healing in vivo by a helium-neon laser, *Ann Plast Surg* 18(1):47-50, 1987.
82. Surchinak JS, Alago ML, Bellamy RF, et al: Effects of low level energy lasers on the healing of full thickness skin defects, *Laser Surg Med* 2:267-274, 1983.
83. Ma SY, Hou H: Effect of He-Ne laser irradiation on healing skin wounds in mice, *Laser* 7:146, 1981.
84. Dyson M, Young S: Effect of laser therapy on wound contraction and cellularity in mice, *Lasers Med Sci* 1:125-130, 1986.
85. Gogia PP, Hurt BS, Zirn TT: Wound management with whirlpool and infrared cold laser treatment: a clinical report, *Phys Ther* 68(8):1239-1242, 1988.
86. Kahn J: Case reports: open wound management with the HeNe cold laser, *J Orthop Sport Phys* 6(3):203-204, 1984.
87. Reddy GK, Stehno-Bittel D, Enwemeka CS: Laser photostimulation accelerates wound healing in diabetic rats, *Wound Repair Regen* 9(3):248-255, 2001.
88. Schindl A, Schindl M, Schon H, et al: Low-intensity laser irradiation improves skin circulation in patients with diabetic microangiopathy, *Diabetes Care* 21:580-584, 1998.
89. Cambier DC, Vanderstraeten GG, Mussen MJ, et al: Low power laser and healing of burns: a preliminary assay, *Plast Reconstr Surg* 97(3):555-558, 1996.
90. McCaughan JS Jr, Bethel BH, Johnson T, et al: Effect of low dose argon irradiation on rate of wound closure, *Lasers Surg Med* 5(6):607-614, 1985.
91. Basford JR, Hallman HO, Sheffield SG, et al: Comparisons of cold-quartz ultraviolet, low-energy laser, and occlusion in wound

healing in a swine model, *Arch Phys Med Rehabil* 106(6):358-363, 1986.

92. Walker JB, Akhanjee LK, Cooney MM, et al: Laser therapy for pain of rheumatoid arthritis, *Clin J Pain* 3:54-59, 1987.

93. Matic M, Lazetic B, Poljacki, C, et al: Low level laser irradiation and its effect on repair processes in the ski, *Med Pregl* (in Croatian) 56:137-141, 2003.

94. Enwemeka CS, Laser biostimulation of healing wounds: specific effects and mechanisms of action, *J Orthop Sports Phys Ther* 9:333-338, 1988.

95. Lucas C, Criens-Poublon LJ, Cockrell CT, et al: Wound healing in cell studies and animal model experiments by low level laser therapy: were clinical studies justified? A systematic review, *Lasers Med Sci* 17:110-134, 2002.

96. Flemming K, Cullum N: Laser therapy for venous leg ulcers, *Cochrane Database Syst Rev* 2:CD001182, 2000.

97. Enwemeka CS, Parker JC, Dowdy DS, et al: The efficacy of low-power lasers in tissue repair and pain control: a meta-analysis study, *Photomed Laser Surg* 22(4):323-329, 2004.

98. Woodruff LD, Bounkeo JM, Brannon WM, et al: The efficacy of laser therapy in wound repair: a meta-analysis of the literature, *Photomed Laser Surg* 22(3):241-247, 2004.

99. Flemming KA, Cullum NA, Nelson EA: A systematic review of laser therapy for venous leg ulcers, *J Wound Care* 8(3):111-114, 1999.

100. Reddy GK, Stehno-Bittel D, Enwemeka CS: Laser photostimulation of collagen production in healing rabbit Achilles tendons, *Laser Surg Med* 22:281-287, 1998.

101. Carrinho PM, Renno AC, Koeke P, et al: Comparative study using 685-nm and 830-nm lasers in the tissue repair of tenotomized tendons in the mouse, *Photomed Laser Surg* 24(6):754-758, 2006.

102. Enwemeka CS, Cohen E, Duswalt EP, et al: The biomechanical effects of Ga-As laser photostimulation on tendon healing, *Laser Ther* 6:181-188, 1995.

103. Bayat M, Delbari A, Elmaseyeh MA, et al: Low-level laser therapy improves early healing of medial collateral ligament injuries in rats, *Photomed Laser Surg* 23(6):556-560, 2005.

104. Trelles MA, Mayayo E: Bone fracture consolidates faster with low-power laser, *Lasers Surg Med* 7:36-45, 1987.

105. Chen JW, Zhou YC: Effect of low level carbon dioxide laser irradiation on biochemical metabolism of rabbit mandibular bone callus, *Laser Ther* 1:83-87, 1989.

106. Tang XM, Chai BP: Effect of CO_2 laser irradiation on experimental fracture healing: a transmission electron microscopy study, *Lasers Surg Med* 6:346-352, 1986.

107. Niccoli-Filho W, Okamoto T: The effect of exposure to continuous Nd: YAG laser radiation on the wound healing process after removal of the teeth (a histological study on rats), *Stomatologiia* 74(5):26-29, 1995.

108. Kucerova H, Dostalova T, Himmlova L, et al: Low-Level laser therapy after molar extraction, *J Clin Laser Med Surg* 18(6):309-315, 2000.

109. Lirani-Galvao AP, Jorgetti V, daSilva OL: Comparative study of how low-level laser therapy and low intensity pulsed ultrasound affect bone repair in rats, *Photomed Laser Surg* 24(6):735-740, 2006.

110. Coombe AR, Ho CT, Darendeliler MA, et al: The effects of low level laser irradiation on osteoblastic cells, *Clin Orthod Res* 4(1):3-14, 2001.

111. Hawkins DH, Abrahamse H: The role of laser fluence in cell viability, proliferation, and membrane integrity of wounded human skin fibroblasts following helium-neon laser irradiation, *Lasers Surg Med* 38(1):74-83, 2006.

112. Hawkins D, Abrahamse H: Effect of multiple exposures of low-level laser therapy on the cellular responses of wounded human skin fibroblasts, *Photomed Laser Surg* 24(6):705-714, 2006.

113. Houreld NN, Abrahamse H: Laser light influences cellular viability and proliferation in diabetic-wounded fibroblast cells in a dose- and wavelength dependent manner, *Lasers Med Sci* March 15, 2007 (Epub ahead of print).

114. Mendez TM, Pinheiro AL, Pacheco MT, et al: Dose and wavelength of laser light have influence on the repair of cutaneous wounds, *J Clin Laser Med Surg* 22(1):19-25, 2004.

115. Goldman JA, Chiarpella J, Casey H, et al: Laser therapy of rheumatoid arthritis, *Lasers Surg Med* 1:93-101, 1980.

116. Palmgren N, Jensen GF, Kaae K, et al: Low power laser therapy in rheumatoid arthritis, *Lasers Med Sci* 4:193-195, 1989.

117. Asada K, Yutani Y, Shimazu A: Diode laser therapy for rheumatoid arthritis: a clinical evaluation of 102 joints treated with low level laser therapy, *Laser Ther* 1:147-151, 1989.

118. Lonauer G: Controlled double blind study on the efficacy of He-Ne laser beams v He-Ne + infrared laser beams in therapy of activated OA of the finger joint, *Lasers Surg Med* 6:172, 1986.

119. Ozdemis F, Birtane M, Kokino S: The clinical efficacy of low-power laser therapy on pain and function in cervical osteoarthritis, *Clin Rheumatol* 20(3):181-184, 2001.

120. Basford JR, Sheffield CG, Mair SD, et al: Low energy helium neon laser treatment of thumb osteoarthritis, *Arch Phys Med Rehabil* 68(11):794-797, 1987.

121. McAuley R, Ysala R: Soft laser: a treatment for osteoarthritis of the knee? *Arch Phys Med Rehabil* 66:553-554, 1985.

122. Brosseau L, Welch V, Wells G, et al: Low level laser therapy for osteoarthritis and rheumatoid arthritis: a metaanalysis, *J Rheumatol* 27(8):1961-1969, 2000.

123. Brosseau L, Welch V, Wells G, et al: Low level laser therapy (classes I, II and III) in the treatment of rheumatoid arthritis, *Cochrane Database Syst Rev* 2:CD002049, 2005.

124. Brosseau L, Welch V, Wells G, et al: Low level laser therapy (class III) for the treatment of osteoarthritis, *Cochrane Database Syst Rev* 3:CD002046, 2006.

125. Marks R, de Palma F: Clinical efficacy of low power laser therapy in osteoarthritis, *Physiother Res Int* 4(2):141-157, 1999.

126. Ferreira DM, Zangaro RA, Villaverde AB, et al: Analgesic effect of He-Ne (632.8 nm) low-level laser therapy on acute inflammatory pain, *Photomed Laser Surg* 23(2):177-181, 2005.

127. Carati CJ, Anderson, SN, Gannon BJ, et al: Treatment of postmastectomy lymphedema with low-level laser therapy: a double blind, placebo controlled trial, *Cancer* 98:1114-1122, 2003.

128. Kaviani A, Fateh M, Nooraie RY, et al: Low-level laser therapy in management of postmastectomy lymphedema, *Lasers Med Sci* 21(2), 2006.

129. Leonard DR, Farooqi MH, Myers S: Restoration of sensation, reduced pain, and improved balance in subjects with diabetic peripheral neuropathy: a double-blind, randomized, placebo-controlled study with monochromatic near-infrared treatment, *Diabetes Care* 27(1):168-172, 2004.

130. Zinman LH, Ngo M, Ng ET, et al: Low-intensity laser therapy for painful symptom diabetic sensorimotor polyneuropathy: a controlled trial, *Diabetes Care* 27:921-924, 2004.

131. Kemmotsu O, Sato K, Furumido H, et al: Efficacy of low reactive-level laser therapy for pain attenuation of postherpetic neuralgia, *Laser Ther* 3(2):71-75, 1991.

132. Iijima K, Shimoyama M, Shimoyama N, et al: Effect of repeated irradiation of low-power He-Ne laser in pain relief from postherpetic neuralgia, *Clin J Pain* 5(3):271-274, 1989.

133. Lampl Y, Zivin J, Fisher M, et al: Infrared laser therapy for ischemic stroke: A new treatment strategy, *Stroke* 38:1843, 2007.

134. Walker J: Relief from chronic pain by low power laser irradiation, *Neurosci Lett* 43:339-344, 1983.

135. Haker E, Lundeberg T: Is low-energy laser treatment effective in lateral epicondylalgia? *J Pain Symptom Manage* 6(4):241-246, 1991.

136. Vasseljen O, Hoeg N, Kjelstad B, et al: Low level laser versus placebo in the treatment of tennis elbow, *Scand J Rehabil Med* 24(1):37-42, 1992.

137. Lam LK, Ceing GL: Effects of 904-nm low-level laser therapy in the management of lateral epicondylitis: a randomized controlled trial, *Photomed Laser Surg* 25(2):65-71, 2007.

138. Gur A, Sarac AJ, Cevik R, et al: Efficacy of 904 nm gallium arsenide low level laser therapy in the management of chronic myofascial pain in the neck: a double-blind and randomize-controlled trial, *Lasers Surg Med* 35(3):229-235, 2004.

139. Chow RT: The effect of 300 mW, 830 nm laser on chronic neck pain: a double-blind, randomized, placebo-controlled study, *Pain* 124(1-2):201-210, 2006.

140. Basford JR, Sheffield CG, Harmsen WS: Laser therapy: a randomized, controlled trial of the effects of low-intensity Nd:YAG laser irradiation on musculoskeletal back pain, *Arch Phys Med Rehabil* 80(6):647-652, 1999.
141. Snyder-Mackler L, Barry AJ, Perkins AI, et al: Effects of helium-neon laser irradiation on skin resistance and pain in patients with trigger points in the neck or back, *Phys Ther* 69(5):336-341, 1989.
142. Snyder-Mackler L, Bork C, Bourbon B, et al: Effect of helium-neon laser on musculoskeletal trigger points, *Phys Ther* 66(7):1087-1090, 1986.
143. Vinck E, Cagnie B, Coorevits P, et al: Pain reduction by infrared light-emitting diode irradiation: a pilot study on experimentally induced delayed-onset muscle soreness in humans, *Lasers Med Sci* 21:11-18, 2006.
144. Laakso EL, Cabot PJ: Nociceptive scores and endorphin-containing cells reduced by low-level laser therapy (LLLT) in inflamed paws of Wistar rat, *Photomed Laser Surg* 23(1):32-35, 2005.
145. Moore KC, Hira N, Kumar PS, et al: A double blind crossover trial of low level laser therapy in the treatment of post-herpetic neuralgia, *Laser Ther* Pilot Issue:7-9, 1989.
146. Siebert W, Seichert N, Siebert B, et al: What is the efficacy of soft and mid lasers in therapy of tendinopathies? *Arch Orthop Trauma Surg* 106:358-363, 1987.
147. Haker EH, Lundeberg TC: Lateral epicondylalgia: report of noneffective midlaser treatment, *Arch Phys Med Rehabil* 72(12):984-988, 1991.
148. Azevedo LH, Correaaranha AC, Stolf SF, et al: Evaluation of low intensity laser effects on the thyroid gland of male mice, *Photomed Laser Surg* 23(6): 567-570, 2005.
149. Moolenar H: *Endolaser 476 therapy protocol,* Delft, Netherlands, 1990, Enraf-Nonius Delft.
150. Waylonis GW, Wilke S, O'Toole DO, et al: Chronic myofascial pain: management by low output helium-neon laser therapy, *Arch Phys Med Rehabil* 69:1017-1020, 1988.
151. Zinman LH, Ngo M, Ng ET, et al: Low-intensity laser therapy for painful symptoms of diabetic sensorimotor polyneuropathy. A controlled trial, *Diabetes Care* 27:921-924, 2004.
152. Chartered Society of Physiotherapy, Safety of Electrotherapy Equipment Working Group: *Guidelines for the safe use of lasers in physiotherapy,* London, 1991, Chartered Society of Physiotherapy.
153. Moholkar R, Zukowski S, Turbill H, et al: The safety and efficacy of low level laser therapy in soft tissue injuries: a double-blind randomized study, *Phys Ther* 81(5):A49, 2001.
154. Klebanov GI, Shuraeva NI, Chichuk TV, et al: A comparative study of the effects of laser and light-emitting diode irradiation on the wound healing and functional activity of wound exudate leukocytes, *Biofizika* 50(6):1137-1144, 2005.
155. Osipov AN, Rudenko TG, Shekhter AB, et al: A comparison of the effects of laser and light-emitting diodes on superoxide dismutase activity and nitric oxide production in rat wound fluid, *Biofizika* 51(1):116-122, 2006.
156. Blidall H, Hellesen C, Ditlevesen P, et al: Soft laser therapy of rheumatoid arthritis, *Scand J Rheumatol* 16:225-228, 1987.
157. Lilge L, Tierney K, Nussbaum E: Low-level laser therapy for wound healing: feasibility of wound dressing transillumination, *J Clin Laser Med Surg* 18(5):235-240, 2000.
158. Pontinen PJ, Aaltokallio T, Kolari PJ: Comparative effects of exposure to different lights sources (He-Ne laser, InGaAl diode laser, a specific type of noncoherent LED) on skin blood flow for the head, *Acupunct Electrother Res* 21:105-118, 1996.
159. Whelan HT, Buchmann EV, Dhokalia A, et al: Effect of NASA light-emitting diode irradiation on molecular changes for wound healing in diabetic mice, *J Clin Laser Med Surg* 21:67-74, 2003.
160. Vladimirov YA, Osipov AN, Klebanov GI: Photobiological principles of therapeutic applications of laser radiation, *Biochemistry* 69(1):81-90, 2004.

Ultraviolet Radiation

PHYSICAL PROPERTIES OF ULTRAVIOLET RADIATION

Ultraviolet (UV) radiation is electromagnetic radiation with a frequency range of 7.5×10^{14} to over 10^{15} Hz and wavelengths from 400 nm to below 290 nm. The frequency of UV radiation lies between that of x-rays and visible light (see Fig 12-6). UV radiation is divided into three bands—UVA, UVB, and UVC—with wavelengths of 320 to 400, 290 to 320, and less than 290 nm, respectively (Fig. 13-1). UVA, also known as long-wave UV, produces fluorescence in many substances, whereas UVB, or middle-wave UV, produces the most skin **erythema**. UVC, or

short-wave UV, is germicidal. Because UV does not produce heat, it is thought to produce physiological effects by nonthermal mechanisms. The most significant source of UV radiation is the sun, which emits a broad spectrum of UV, including UVA, UVB, and UVC. Both UVA and the UVB reach the earth from the sun; however, UVC is filtered out by the ozone layer. Patients can be treated with UV of specific wavelength ranges using a UV lamp.

The physiological effects of UV radiation are influenced not only by the wavelength of the radiation but also by the intensity of radiation reaching the skin and its depth of penetration. The depth of UV penetration is affected by the intensity of radiation reaching the skin, the wavelength and power of the radiation source, the size of the area being treated, the thickness and pigmentation of the skin, and the duration of treatment. When treating a patient with a UV lamp, the intensity of UV radiation reaching the patient's skin is proportional to the power output of the lamp, the inverse square of the distance of the lamp from the patient, and the cosine of the angle of incidence of the radiation beam with the tissue (Fig. 13-2). Thus the intensity reaching the skin is greatest when a high-power lamp is used, when the lamp is close to the patient, and when the radiation beam is perpendicular to the surface of the skin.

> **◎ Clinical Pearl**
>
> The intensity of UV radiation reaching the skin is highest with a high-power lamp positioned close to the patient with the radiation beam perpendicular to the skin's surface.

Penetration is deepest for UV radiation with the highest intensity, longest wavelength, and lowest frequency. Thus UVA penetrates farthest and reaches through several millimeters of skin, whereas UVB and UVC penetrate less deeply and are almost entirely absorbed in the superficial epidermal layers. The penetration of UV radiation is also less deep if the skin is thicker or darker.[1,2]

EFFECTS OF ULTRAVIOLET RADIATION

UV radiation exposure produces skin erythema, tanning, **epidermal hyperplasia**, and vitamin D synthesis. It is

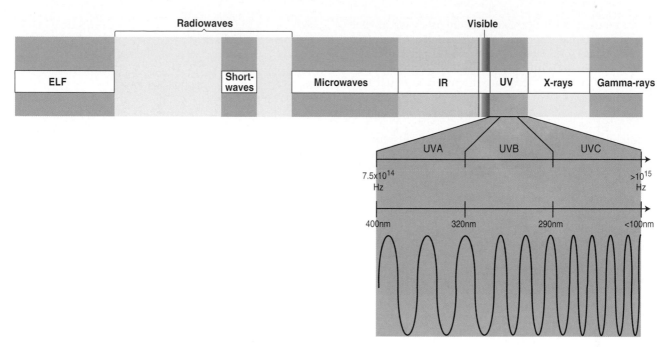

FIG 13-1 Bands of ultraviolet (UV) radiation. *ELF,* Extremely low frequency; *IR,* infrared.

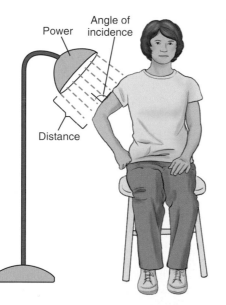

FIG 13-2 Factors affecting the intensity of ultraviolet radiation reaching the patient's skin: inverse square of the distance of the lamp from the patient, power output of the lamp, and cosine of the angle of incidence of the beam with the tissue.

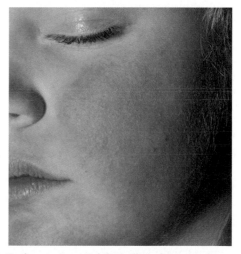

FIG 13-3 Erythema. *From Habif TP:* Clinical Dermatology, *ed 4, Edinburgh, 2004, Mosby.*

thought that these effects are the result of absorption of electromagnetic energy by the cells of exposed skin, causing chemical excitation and facilitation of photobiological processes. UVC radiation is also bactericidal.

ERYTHEMA PRODUCTION

Erythema (Fig. 13-3), or redness of the skin as a result of dilation of the superficial blood vessels caused by the release of histamines, is one of the most common and obvious effects of exposure to UV radiation.[3] Erythema is produced primarily in response to UVB exposure, or in response to UVA exposure after drug sensitization. Without drug sensitization, UVA is 100 to 1000 times less potent in inducing erythema than UVB. With sensitization, the erythemal efficacy of UVA is similar to that of UVB alone, with less risk of overexposure or burning. The precise mechanism of UV-induced erythema is unknown; however, it is known that this effect is mediated by prostaglandin release from the epidermis and that it may be related to the DNA-damaging effects of UV radiation. The severity of erythema, which can produce blistering, tissue burning, and pain, and the risk of cell damage are the primary factors limiting the intensity and duration of UV exposure that can be used clinically. Because patients vary in their degree of erythemal response to UV, a **minimal erythemal dose** (MED) is determined for each patient before initiating treatment with UV radiation. Determination of the MED and treatment dose are discussed in detail later in this chapter.

TANNING

Tanning, a delayed pigmentation of the skin, also occurs in response to UV radiation exposure. This effect is the result of increased production and upward migration of melanin granules and oxidation of premelanin in the skin.[4,5] Because the darkening of skin pigmentation that occurs with tanning reduces the penetration of UV to deeper tissue layers, it is thought that tanning is a protective response of the body.

EPIDERMAL HYPERPLASIA

Epidermal hyperplasia, a thickening of the superficial layer of the skin, occurs approximately 72 hours after exposure to UV radiation and increases with repeated exposure, eventually resulting in thickening of the epidermis and the stratum corneum that persists for several weeks. This effect is thought to be caused by the release of prostaglandin precursors leading to increased DNA synthesis by epidermal cells, resulting in increased epithelial cell turnover and cellular hyperplasia.[6] Epidermal hyperplasia is most pronounced in response to UVB exposure. It is also thought to be a protective response to UV exposure.

Because tanning and epidermal hyperplasia impair UV penetration, progressively higher doses of UV radiation are generally required during a course of clinical treatment with UV.

> ### Clinical Pearl
>
> Progressively higher doses of UV radiation are generally needed during a course of UV treatment.

VITAMIN D SYNTHESIS

UV irradiation of the skin is necessary for the conversion of ingested provitamin D to active vitamin D (Fig. 13-4).[7,8] Because vitamin D controls calcium absorption and exchange, it is an essential vitamin for bone formation. Vitamin D also influences brain, kidney, intestine, endocrine, immune, and cellular function.[9,10] Vitamin D deficiency can result in poor intestinal absorption of calcium and, when severe, can cause rickets, a disease characterized by failure of bone mineralization. Rickets results from inadequate exposure to UV radiation, inadequate intake of provitamins, or poor kidney function. Although for most individuals the exposure to UV in sunlight is sufficient to maintain adequate levels of vitamin D production, UV exposure may be inadequate in certain populations. Risk factors for inadequate vitamin D include exclusively breast-fed infants, dark skin, aging and institutionalization, covering all exposed skin or using sunscreen whenever outdoors, fat malabsorption syndromes, inflammatory bowel disease, and obesity.[10] Recently, there

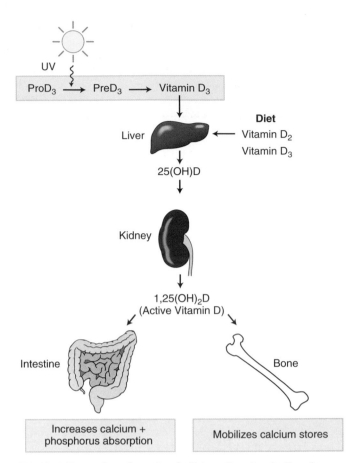

FIG 13-4 Conversion of provitamin D to active vitamin D and some of the physiologic roles of Vitamin D.

has been a growing interest in the effects of prolonged, slightly low levels of vitamin D in the body (subclinical vitamin D deficiency), as well as in the effects of vitamin D supplementation in people who do not meet criteria for vitamin D deficiency. Studies have found that increased intake of vitamin D can decrease blood pressure in hypertensive patients, improve blood glucose levels in people with diabetes, and improve symptoms of rheumatoid arthritis and multiple sclerosis.[11,12] Vitamin D deficiency is also associated with an increased risk of cancer, and supplementation may help reduce cancer risk.[13]

BACTERICIDAL EFFECTS

In the laboratory setting UVC in adequate doses can be bactericidal.[14-16] UVC radiation is used to kill bacteria in food and, in one small study, UVC was found to be as effective as standard hospital cleaners in removing pathogens from hospital surfaces.[17] One clinical study also found that UVC radiation may help reduce bacterial load in open wounds and improve wound healing.[18]

OTHER EFFECTS OF ULTRAVIOLET RADIATION

UVB radiation has been shown to affect the immune system, reducing contact sensitivity, changing the distribution of circulating lymphocytes, and suppressing mast cell–mediated whealing.[19-21] It is proposed that these effects are dose dependent: with low doses the immune response is suppressed and with higher doses the immune response is activated. UVA has also been shown to inhibit cyclooxygenase 2 expression and prostaglandin E_2 production.[22] This mechanism is thought to underlie the beneficial effects of **psoralen with UVA (PUVA)** in the treatment of scleroderma.[22] In patients with **vitiligo**, PUVA is thought to act by creating a favorable milieu for the growth of melanocytes, whereas UVB directly stimulates the proliferation and migration of melanocytes.[23,24]

CLINICAL INDICATIONS FOR ULTRAVIOLET RADIATION

The earliest modern clinical use of UV radiation, for which Neils Finsen was awarded the Nobel Prize in 1903, was for the treatment of cutaneous tuberculosis. In the 1920s and 1930s, the use of UV radiation for the treatment of skin disorders, including **psoriasis**, acne, and alopecia, became very popular; however, with the advent of antibiotics and other medications, the role of UV radiation in dermatological medicine has since decreased. At this time, UV radiation is used primarily in the treatment of psoriasis, and there are also recent reports of UV therapy being used for the treatment of other dermatological conditions, including scleroderma, eczema, atopic dermatitis, cutaneous T-cell lymphoma (mycosis fungoides), vitiligo, and palmoplantar pustulosis.[22,25,26] These treatments may be applied in conjunction with the use of photosensitizing drugs. UV is also used occasionally as a component of the treatment of chronic open wounds.[25,27-29] Although the clinical application of UV radiation for the treatment of skin disorders is within the scope of physical therapy, such treatments are generally provided by dermatologists or their assistants. Treatment of chronic wounds with UV radiation, however, generally is performed by a physical therapist.

UVB alone or PUVA may be used for the treatment of psoriasis and other skin disorders, including eczema, acne, pityriasis lichenoides, vitiligo (Fig. 13-5), pruritus, and polymorphic light eruption.[30-32,24] PUVA or UVA radiation alone is also used for the treatment of eczema, urticaria, lichen planus, graft-versus-host disease, cutaneous T-cell lymphoma, urticaria pigmentosa, and a variety of photosensitive disorders.[33,34] Clinical recommendations for the treatment of psoriasis are given in the next section, and recommendations for the treatment of other skin disorders are available in the literature.[35-37,24] Clinical protocols for the treatment of other disorders should be developed and agreed on in conjunction with the referring physician.

PSORIASIS

Psoriasis is a common benign, acute, or chronic inflammatory skin disease that appears to be based on genetic predisposition. It is characterized by bright red plaques

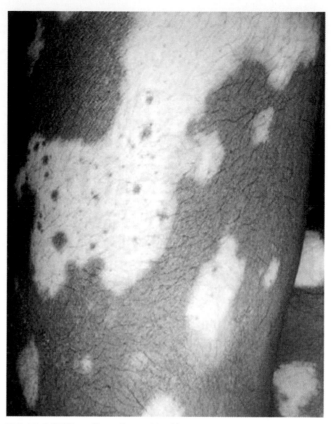

FIG 13-5 Vitiligo. *From Kumar V, Abbas AK, Fausto N:* Robbins and Cotran Pathologic Basis of Disease, *ed 7, Philadelphia, 2005, Saunders.*

with silvery scales, usually on the knees, elbows, and scalp, and is associated with mild itching (Fig. 13-6). These dermatological manifestations may also be associated with joint changes known as **psoriatic arthritis**.

There are numerous reports of successful treatment of psoriasis with UV radiation alone or in conjunction with sensitizing drugs.[32,38-42] **Phototherapy** of psoriasis with UV has a history of more than 75 years; in 1925, Goeckerman introduced a combination of topical crude coal tar and subsequent UV irradiation. This treatment became a standard therapy for psoriasis for half a century. The therapeutic efficacy of UV radiation in the treatment of this condition is thought to be a result of its ability to inactivate the cell division and inhibit the DNA synthesis and mitosis of hyperproliferating epidermal cells that are characteristic of psoriasis.[32] Other proposed mechanisms include altered leukocyte behavior and immune activity, altered prostaglandin and cytokine release, release of platelet-activating factor to cause cell death, as well as effects on cellular metabolism.[43,44] However, much is still not understood about the precise cellular targets and effector mechanisms of UV radiation in psoriasis.

Psoriasis is most responsive to UVA administered in conjunction with oral or topical **psoralen** sensitization (PUVA) and is almost as responsive to narrowband UVB alone, at a wavelength of 311 to 313 nm.[30,45-47] Psoriasis is

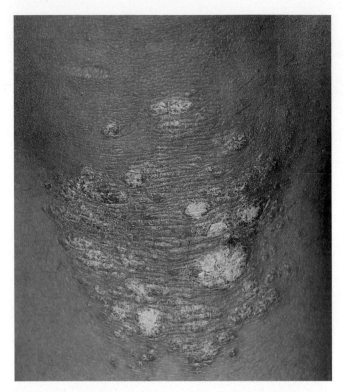

FIG 13-6 Psoriatic plaques. *From Habif TP:* Clinical dermatology, *ed 4, Edinburgh, 2004, Mosby.*

not responsive to UVC and is minimally responsive to UVA without drug sensitization. Use of UVA alone is also not recommended because the dose that does effectively clear psoriatic plaques also causes severe erythema, pigmentation, and an increased risk of melanoma.[48]

The use of UV sensitizers in conjunction with UV radiation for the treatment of psoriasis has been studied extensively. The most commonly used sensitizers were tar-based topicals and psoralen-derived drugs. However, studies on the use of tar-based derivatives in conjunction with UV radiation in the management of psoriasis yielded mixed results, with some reporting that these products are valuable adjuncts to treatment and others reporting that tar-based products are no more effective than simple oil-based ointments. As a result, the use of tar-based products has lapsed and psoralen-derived drugs are now the product of choice for this application.[49,50] The fact that tar-based products are messy and expensive also limits their popularity.

Treatment with psoralen-based topical and systemic drugs in conjunction with UVA (PUVA) is used today for some patients with psoriasis. This treatment combination was first described by Tronnier and Schule in 1972 and has since been shown to be effective by a number of other researchers.[51] It is thought that psoralen reduces the appearance of psoriatic plaques because it causes crosslinks to form between adjacent strands of DNA when activated by UVA, thus interfering with cell replication and preventing the excessive cell proliferation characteristic of psoriasis.

PUVA treatment has a number of side effects, including epidermal pigmentation and hyperplasia, immune suppression, and the release of free radicals. Free radicals can damage cell membranes and cytoplasmic structures. Psoralens alone have also been found to be carcinogenic. Therefore work is in process to search for safer alternative sensitizers. Although acitretin, corticosteroids, and fish oil have been evaluated for this application, there is insufficient evidence at this time to support the use of these UV sensitizers in the treatment of psoriasis.[52-54]

Because of the short- and long-term adverse effects associated with PUVA treatment and the advent of narrowband UVB lamps, UVB therapy without sensitizing agents has become a more popular option for the treatment of moderate to severe psoriasis.[55] Narrowband UVB lamps first became readily available in the United States (US) in 1998, although they were available in Europe a number of years earlier. Narrowband UVB (311 to 313 nm wavelength) has been found to be more effective at clearing psoriasis plaques than broadband UVB therapy.[56,57] Narrowband UVB has fewer short-term side effects than PUVA and is easier to apply. However, because this treatment is relatively new, its long-term side effects are not yet known. When compared to PUVA, narrowband UVB therapy is almost as effective at clearing psoriatic plaques, but plaque remission does not last as long.[58] Depending on the patient, UVB may be used instead of PUVA in the treatment of psoriasis. The most recent development in phototherapy for psoriasis is the use of excimer UVB laser. This type of laser delivers UV radiation with 308 nm wavelength.[59] Lasers have the advantage and disadvantage of providing very targeted therapy to a local area that can be ideal when a small area of skin is involved but less useful when psoriasis is widespread (see Chapter 12 for more information on lasers).

WOUND HEALING

UV is occasionally used as a component of the treatment of chronic wounds despite limited research on the effectiveness of this intervention.[60] When UV is used for wound treatment, UVC is the **frequency band** most commonly chosen[27,28] because it may contribute to wound healing while causing little erythema or tanning. UVC also has a low carcinogenic effect and is absorbed almost equally by all skin colors.[61] UV radiation is thought to facilitate wound healing by increasing epithelial cell turnover,[18] causing epidermal cell hyperplasia,[27] accelerating granulation tissue formation, increasing blood flow,[62] killing bacteria,[18] increasing vitamin D production by the skin, and promoting sloughing of necrotic tissue.[63] Although the data on the efficacy of UVC for this application are limited and mixed, with some studies reporting faster or more complete healing with the addition of UVC to their treatment protocol for wounds and others reporting no significant benefit, this physical agent has proved beneficial in some cases; thus it may be appropriate to consider adding UVC to the treatment of wounds that have not responded to or are inappropriate for other types of treatment.[64]

CONTRAINDICATIONS AND PRECAUTIONS FOR THE USE OF ULTRAVIOLET RADIATION

CONTRAINDICATIONS FOR THE USE OF ULTRAVIOLET RADIATION

CONTRAINDICATIONS

for the Use of Ultraviolet Radiation

- Irradiation of the eyes
- Skin cancer
- Pulmonary tuberculosis
- Cardiac, kidney, or liver disease
- Systemic lupus erythematosus
- Fever

Irradiation of the Eyes

UV irradiation of the eyes should be avoided because UV can damage the cornea, the eyelids, or the lens. Exposure of the eyes can be avoided by having the patient wear UV-opaque goggles throughout treatment and by having the therapist wear UV-opaque goggles when at risk of irradiation, such as when turning the UV lamp on or off. Patients taking UV-sensitizing drugs, such as psoralens, should continue to wear UV-opaque eye protection for 12 hours after taking these drugs.

Certain Systemic Conditions

UV radiation should not be applied to areas in which skin cancer is present because UV is known to be carcinogenic.[65] Details of the carcinogenic effects of UV radiation can be found in the section on adverse effects. It is generally recommended that UV radiation not be used in patients with pulmonary tuberculosis; cardiac, kidney, or liver disease; systemic lupus erythematosus; or fever because these conditions may be exacerbated by exposure to UV radiation.

PRECAUTIONS FOR THE USE OF ULTRAVIOLET RADIATION

PRECAUTIONS

for the Use of Ultraviolet Radiation

- Photosensitizing medications and dietary supplements.
- Photosensitivity.
- Recent x-ray therapy.
- No dose of UV radiation should be repeated until the effects of the previous dose have disappeared.

Photosensitizing Medications and Dietary Supplements

Care should be taken when applying UV radiation to patients who are taking photosensitizing medications or supplements. Photosensitizing medications include sulfonamide, tetracycline, and quinolone antibiotics; gold-based medications used for the treatment of rheumatoid arthritis; amiodarone hydrochloride and quinidines used for the treatment of cardiac arrhythmias; phenothiazines used for the treatment of anxiety and psychosis; and psoralens used for the treatment of psoriasis. Certain dietary supplements, including St John's wort, are also known to be photosensitizing.[66] While patients are taking these medications or supplements, they have increased sensitivity to UV radiation, resulting in a decrease in the minimal erythemal dose and an increased risk of burning if too high a dose is used. A patient's minimal erythemal dose must be remeasured if the patient starts to take a photosensitizing medication or supplement during a course of UV treatment.

Photosensitivity

Some individuals, particularly those with fair skin and hair coloring and those with red hair, have greater sensitivity to UV exposure. Because these individuals have an accelerated and exaggerated skin response to UV radiation, low levels of UV radiation should be used both when determining the minimal erythemal dose and for treatment.

Recent X-Ray Therapy

It is recommended that UV radiation be applied with caution to areas that have had recent x-ray radiation exposure because the skin in these areas may be more susceptible to the development of malignancies.

Erythema from Prior Ultraviolet Dose

To minimize the risk of burns or an excessive erythemal response, UV irradiation should not be repeated until the erythemal effects of the previous dose have resolved.

ADVERSE EFFECTS OF ULTRAVIOLET RADIATION[32,67]

BURNING

Burning by UV radiation will occur if too high a dose is used. Burning can usually be avoided by careful assessment of the minimal erythemal dose before initiating treatment and by avoiding further exposure when signs of erythema from a prior dose are still present.

PREMATURE AGING OF SKIN

Chronic exposure to UV radiation, including sunlight, is associated with premature aging of the skin. This effect, known as **actinic damage**, causes the skin to have a dry, coarse, leathery appearance with wrinkling and pigment abnormalities (Fig. 13-7). It is thought that these changes are primarily the result of the collagen degeneration that accompanies long-term exposure to UV radiation.

CARCINOGENESIS

Most of the information regarding the carcinogenic effect of UV radiation concerns the effect of prolonged or intense sunlight exposure. Prolonged exposure to UV radiation, as occurs with excessive exposure to sunlight, is considered to be a major risk factor for the development of basal cell

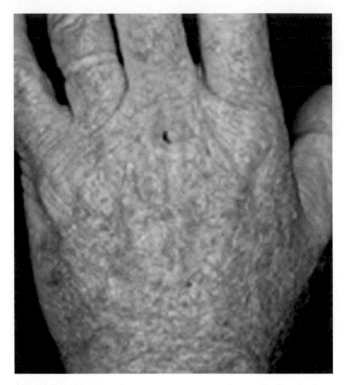

FIG 13-7 Actinic skin damage. *From Habif TP: Clinical dermatology, ed 4, Edinburgh, 2004, Mosby.*

and squamous cell carcinoma and malignant melanoma. A review of the literature on the carcinogenicity of UV phototherapy, with and without psoralens, concluded that the therapeutic use of UVB has a low risk of producing cutaneous cancers, except possibly on the skin of the male genitals; however, there is a definite cutaneous carcinogenic risk from PUVA treatment when oral systemic psoralens medications are used.[68,69] The increased cancer risk with PUVA may be a result of the carcinogenicity of the psoralens or may be a response specific to the wavelength of UV radiation used for this treatment application. PUVA treatments may also exacerbate the effects of previous exposure to carcinogens.[65]

Because of the potential cumulative adverse effects of repeated low-level exposure to UV radiation, it is recommended that clinicians avoid frequent or excessive exposure during patient treatment. This can be achieved by wearing UV-opaque goggles and UV-opaque clothing.

EYE DAMAGE

UV irradiation of the eyes can cause a number of eye problems, including **photokeratitis**, **conjunctivitis**, and possibly some forms of **cataracts**.[70] Photokeratitis and conjunctivitis can occur acutely after exposure to UVB or UVC. The symptoms of photokeratitis, an inflammation of the cornea that can be extremely painful, generally appear 6 to 12 hours after UV exposure and resolve fully within 2 days, without permanent or long-term damage. Conjunctivitis, an inflammation of the insides of the eyelids and the membrane that covers the cornea, results in a sensation of gritty eyes and varying degrees of photophobia, tearing, and blepharospasm. Chronic UVA and

UVB exposure have been associated with the development of cataracts, characterized by a loss of transparency of the lens or lens capsule of the eye. This association is even stronger for PUVA because psoralens are deposited in the lens of the eye.

Because of the risks of eye irritation or damage, UV-opaque eye protection should always be worn by the patient and the clinician during UV treatment. Patients should also wear UV-opaque eye protection for 12 hours after psoralen administration to protect their eyes from sunlight exposure.

ADVERSE EFFECTS OF PSORALEN WITH ULTRAVIOLET A

PUVA is associated with all the adverse effects of UV radiation, as described previously. In addition, oral psoralens are also associated with nausea and vomiting that lasts for 1 to 4 hours after ingestion. Prolonged high-dose PUVA therapy can also result in skin damage, including small hyperpigmented nonmalignant lesions, keratotic lesions that may have premalignant histological characteristics, and squamous cell carcinomas.[71]

APPLICATION TECHNIQUES

When applying UV radiation for therapeutic purposes, one must first determine the individual patient's sensitivity to UV radiation.[72] This varies widely among individuals and can be affected by skin pigmentation, age, prior exposure to UV radiation, and use of sensitizing medications. For example, even for Caucasians, there can be a fourfold to sixfold variation in minimal erythemal dose.[2] Sensitivity to UV radiation is assessed using the dosimetry procedure described in the next section.

Because the response to UV radiation can vary significantly with even slightly different frequencies of radiation, the same lamp must be used for assessing an individual's sensitivity and for all subsequent treatments. For example, the skin is 100 times more sensitive to UV with a wavelength of 300 nm than to UV with a wavelength of 320 nm. If the lamp must be changed, the individual's response to the new lamp must be assessed before it is used for treatment. Reassessment is also necessary if there is a long gap between treatments because lamp output intensity decreases with prolonged use and skin tanning and hyperplasia decreases over prolonged periods. Once the individual's responsiveness to a particular UV lamp has been determined, the treatment dose can be selected to produce the desired erythemal response.

Clinical Pearl

The same lamp that will be used for treatment should be used to assess a person's UV sensitivity.

DOSE-RESPONSE ASSESSMENT

The UV dose is graded according to the individual's erythemal response and is categorized as follows[73]:

- **Suberythemal dose** (SED): No change in skin redness occurs in the 24 hours after UV exposure.

- **Minimal erythemal dose** (MED): The smallest dose producing erythema within 8 hours after exposure that disappears within 24 hours after exposure.
- **First-degree erythema** (E₁): Definite redness with some mild desquamation appears within 6 hours after exposure and lasts for 1 to 3 days. This dose is generally about 2½ times the MED.
- **Second-degree erythema** (E₂): Intense erythema with edema, peeling, and pigmentation appears within 2 hours or less after treatment and is like a severe sunburn. This dose is generally about 5 times the MED.
- **Third-degree erythema** (E₃): Erythema with severe blistering, peeling, and exudation. This dose is generally about 10 times the MED.

For patients receiving PUVA therapy, the MED should be determined after they have taken psoralen. When using an oral psoralen, the MED should be determined 2 hours after ingestion. When using a topical psoralen, the MED should be determined immediately after bathing in the psoralen. In addition, for PUVA the erythemal response may be delayed, typically first appearing 24 to 48 hours after exposure and resolving at about 72 hours after exposure.

> **◎ Clinical Pearl**
>
> The MED for patients receiving PUVA therapy should be determined after the patient has taken psoralen orally or bathed in psoralen.

Once an individual's MED for a particular lamp has been determined, the treatment dose is set according to the disease being treated and the protocol being used. Guidelines for treatment of psoriasis with UVB or with PUVA are given in the next section. Guidelines for using UV to treat other problems can be obtained from UV lamp manufacturers or from texts focusing on the treatment of the particular problem or disease.

APPLICATION TECHNIQUE 13-1

DETERMINING MINIMAL ERYTHEMAL DOSE OF ULTRAVIOLET FOR AN INDIVIDUAL

1. Place UV-opaque goggles on the patient and the clinician.
2. Remove all clothing and jewelry from and wash an area of the body least exposed to natural sunlight. The areas usually used are the volar forearm, the abdomen, or the buttocks.
3. Take a piece of cardboard approximately 4 × 20 cm and cut four square holes 2 × 2 cm in it.
4. Place the cardboard on the test area and drape the area around the cardboard so that the surrounding skin will not be exposed to the UV radiation.
5. Place the lamp 60 to 80 cm away from, and perpendicular to, the area to be exposed. Measure and record the exact distance of the lamp from the area to be exposed.
6. Cover all but one of the holes in the cardboard.
7. Turn on the lamp. If using an arc lamp, allow the lamp to warm up for 5 to 10 minutes to reach full power before turning it toward the patient. A fluorescent lamp will reach full power and can be used within 1 minute of being turned on.
8. Once the lamp has reached full power, direct the beam directly toward the area to be exposed and start the timer.
9. After 120 seconds, uncover the second hole.
10. After another 60 seconds, uncover the third hole.
11. After another 30 seconds, uncover the fourth hole.
12. After another 30 seconds, turn off the lamp.

According to this protocol, the first window will have been exposed for 240 seconds, the second for 120 seconds, the third for 60 seconds, and the fourth for 30 seconds (Fig. 13-8). This protocol can be adjusted according to the individual's self-reported tanning and burning response to sunlight. For individuals who tan and never or rarely burn, longer exposures can be used, whereas for those who burn easily but do not tan or those taking photosensitizing drugs, shorter exposures are recommended. More holes with shorter time differences between exposures can also be used to increase the accuracy of the dose sensitivity assessment. For example, there could be eight holes in the cardboard, and one hole could be exposed every 10 seconds.

13. The patient should observe the area for the 24 hours after exposure. The area that shows mild reddening of the skin within 8 hours that disappears within 24 hours was treated with the MED.

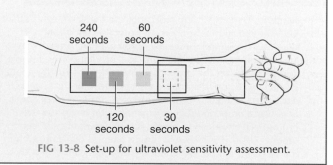

FIG 13-8 Set-up for ultraviolet sensitivity assessment.

ULTRAVIOLET THERAPY APPLICATION

DOSIMETRY FOR THE TREATMENT OF PSORIASIS WITH ULTRAVIOLET RADIATION

In general, treatment time is selected as a proportion of the MED. The MED for an individual is determined in the manner described in the next section. Because repeated exposure to UV radiation generally decreases sensitivity to UV, prior exposure should also be taken into account when determining UV treatment dosage parameters.

Because people build up a tolerance to UV radiation with repeated exposure as a result of darkening of the skin with tanning and thickening of the skin by epidermal hyperplasia, their MED will also increase. Thus, to maintain effective treatment with a consistent proportion of the MED, either the exposure time should be increased or the distance of the lamp from the skin should be decreased with repeated treatments. Exposure time should be increased between 10% and 50% at each treatment, with a maximum of 5 minutes total exposure if possible. If exposure for more than 5 minutes is needed to produce a MED, because the intensity of the radiation reaching the patient increases as the lamp gets closer to the patient according to the inverse square law shown in Fig. 13-2, the effective dose can be increased by moving the lamp closer to the patient rather than by increasing the treatment time. For example, the distance of the lamp from the patient can be halved to increase the intensity of radiation reaching the patient by a factor of four. If the patient is receiving whole body exposure in a cabinet, where the distance between the lamps and the patient cannot be changed, then the treatment time must be adjusted to produce the desired erythemal response.

Using Ultraviolet B

Initial dose recommendations of UVB for the treatment of psoriasis vary from 50% of the MED to an E1 dose (about $2\frac{1}{2}$ times the MED), with increases of 10% to 40% at each treatment, depending on the skin response.[32,74] Treatment is given three to five times weekly, once the erythema from the prior dose resolves, and is terminated when the plaques clear. It usually takes about 15 to 20 treatments to achieve 50% clearance of psoriatic plaques,[55] and total plaque clearance may take several weeks. Treatment may be continued for a few sessions after complete clearance of the plaques to increase the period of remission, and some clinicians continue with less frequent maintenance therapy with the goal of keeping the patient symptom-free.[75] If severe, painful erythema with blistering develops at any time, the treatment should be stopped until these signs clear and a lower UV dose should be used when treatment is resumed.

Using Psoralen with Ultraviolet A

When providing PUVA treatments using oral psoralens for the treatment of psoriasis the UV irradiation is usually applied 2 hours after ingestion of the drug. When the psoralen is delivered topically, the UV exposure is provided immediately after the patient has soaked in a bath of weak psoralen solution for 15 minutes. Topical delivery of psoralens is less common than oral administration, although this route of drug delivery is associated with fewer acute side effects and may result in a longer period of remission after therapy.[76] Erythema in response to PUVA has a delayed onset compared with UVB-induced erythema and at first usually appears 24 to 48 hours after the exposure and peaks 72 hours after the exposure. PUVA-induced erythema also differs from erythema induced by UV alone in that even 2 to 3 times the MED causes only a slightly greater effect. PUVA treatments are usually given 2 or 3 times per week to allow time for the erythema of one treatment to resolve before the next treatment is applied. The treatment dose is determined by assessing the MED after the patient has taken the psoralen. Treatment is generally applied to the whole body and is usually started at 40% to 70% of the MED and increased by 10% to 40% each week to maintain the response. Complete clearance usually takes about 6 weeks, although there is much variation among individuals.

| **APPLICATION TECHNIQUE 13-2** | **ULTRAVIOLET THERAPY** |

The setups for UVB and PUVA application are the same, except that for PUVA the radiation is applied after psoralen sensitization.

1. Warm up the lamp if necessary. If using an arc lamp, it can take several minutes for the lamp to reach full power. If there is a glass filter on the lamp, the lamp should be run for about 20 minutes before being used for treatment for the filter to reach thermal equilibrium. A fluorescent lamp requires only a brief warm-up period (about 1 minute after being switched on) but will also need to be run for 20 minutes before being used for treatment if there is a glass filter on the lamp. During the warm-up period, either cover the lamp beam with a UV-opaque card or direct the lamp away from the patient or other people or toward a wall or the floor.
2. Place UV-opaque goggles on the patient and the clinician.
3. Remove clothing and jewelry from the area to be treated.
4. Wash and dry the area to be treated.
5. Cover all areas not needing treatment that may otherwise be exposed to the radiation with a UV-opaque material such as a cloth or paper towel.
6. Position the area to be exposed comfortably. When treating psoriatic plaques with UVB, a non–UVB absorbing lubricant,

such as mineral oil, may be applied to the plaques to decrease reflectance by the scale on the plaques. Do not apply agents containing salicylic acid, which absorbs UVB light.

7. Adjust the position of the lamp or the patient so that the distance between the lamp and the area to be exposed is the same as it was when the MED was determined. Also, place the lamp so that the UV beam will be as perpendicular to the treatment area as possible. Measure and record the distance of the lamp from the patient.
8. Stay close to the patient, or give the patient a call bell and a means to turn off the lamp. Also, provide the patient with a means to open the cabinet if a whole body treatment is being given.
9. Direct the beam at the treatment area and start the timer. Select the treatment time according to the recommendations for dosimetry following.
10. When the treatment is complete, observe the treated area, and document the treatment given and any observable response to the treatment.

DOCUMENTATION

The following should be documented:
- If and how psoralen was given
- Area of the body treated
- Type of UV radiation used
- Serial number of the lamp
- Distance of the lamp from the patient
- Treatment duration
- Response to treatment

EXAMPLE

S: Patient reports itching of the psoriatic plaque on R dorsal elbow.

O: Pretreatment: Well-demarcated scaling plaque approximately 3 × 4 cm on R dorsal elbow area.

Intervention: UVB to R dorsal elbow, lamp No. 6555, 60 cm from pt, 4 minutes.

Posttreatment: Mild erythema 6 hours after exposure lasted for 24 hours. Psoriatic plaque 50% resolved since initial treatment 3 weeks ago.

A: Pt tolerated treatment well, with appropriate erythema response and excellent plaque clearance.

P: Continue treatment every other day until plaque resolves. Increase dose by 10% of MED for next treatment.

ULTRAVIOLET LAMPS

SELECTING A LAMP

A number of different lamps that output UV radiation at different ranges in the UV spectrum and that use different technology to produce the radiation are currently available in the US (Fig. 13-9). The output ranges include broad-spectrum UVA with wavelengths of 320 to 400 nm, wide band (250 to 320 nm) and narrowband (311 to 312 nm) UVB, and UVC with wavelengths of 200 to 290 nm with a peak at 250 nm. The lamps can be of the arc or fluorescent type. Arc lamps are generally small and emit radiation of a consistent intensity, whereas fluorescent lamps are long and emit higher-intensity radiation in the middle than at the ends.[77] Single arc lamps are recommended for treating small areas such as the hand, and units incorporating an array of arc lamps are recommended for treatment of larger body areas. Fluorescent tubes are generally not recommended because of the variability of intensity along their length. Ideally, a lamp that produces a narrow band of radiation and provides uniform treatment of the area within a reasonable amount of time should be selected.

LAMP MAINTENANCE

Lamp surfaces should be cleaned regularly to remove dust which will attenuate the radiation. Lamps should be replaced when their intensity decreases to the point where treatment times become unacceptably long. The useful lifetime of most UV lamps is between 500 and 1,000 hours. Beyond this time the lamp output falls by about 20% compared with the initial output.

> ◎ **Clinical Pearl**
> Most UV lamps last 500 to 1,000 hours.

CLINICAL CASE STUDY

The following case study summarizes some of the concepts of the clinical use of UV therapy discussed in this chapter. Based on the scenario presented, an evaluation of the clinical findings and goals of treatment are proposed. These are followed by a discussion of the factors to be considered in treatment selection.

CASE STUDY 13-1

Psoriasis
Examination
History

FR is a 25-year-old woman with psoriasis. She has had this disease for about 8 years and has been successfully treated with PUVA in the past. Prior courses of treatment have generally taken about 6 weeks and have resulted in clearance of plaques for 6 months, with a gradual recurrence thereafter. Her last course of PUVA treatments was completed 1 year ago, and she now has plaques on the dorsal aspects of both elbows and on the anterior aspects of both knees. She complains that these areas itch and are unsightly and that she therefore always wears clothing that covers her elbows and knees when in public. She has not been participating in her local soccer league because she is embarrassed to have other people see her arms and legs.

Tests and Measures

The patient has plaques approximately 4 × 8 cm on both dorsal elbows and approximately 5 × 7 cm on both anterior knees.

What types of UV therapy would you consider for this patient? What history do you need to obtain from this patient? How do you determine the appropriate dose?

Continued

CLINICAL CASE STUDY—*cont'd*

Evaluation, Diagnosis, Prognosis, and Goals
Evaluation and Goals

ICF Level	Current Status	Goals
Body structure and function	Itchiness Impaired skin integrity	Complete clearing of psoriatic plaques in 6 weeks
Activity	Avoids wearing clothes that expose unsightly psoriatic plaques	Return to feeling of comfort when wearing clothes that expose the elbows or knees
Participation	Stopped playing soccer	Return to playing in local soccer league

Diagnosis

Preferred Practice Pattern 7B: Impaired integumentary integrity associated with superficial skin involvement.

Prognosis/Plan of Care

UVA in conjunction with psoralen sensitization or UVB are indicated treatments for psoriasis and have been shown to result in the temporary clearance of psoriatic plaques. PUVA is recommended for this patient because this treatment has produced good results for her in the past and because the risk of burning with PUVA treatment is less than that with UVB. However, UVB may be considered because of the carcinogenic nature of psoralens and treatment with PUVA.

Intervention

To provide treatment with PUVA, FR's skin sensitivity to UV radiation should first be assessed. Sensitivity testing should be carried out approximately 2 hours after the patient has taken oral psoralen and should be conducted using the same lamp that will be used for treatment. Because FR has a number of areas with plaques, treatment should be provided in a UV cabinet and the areas without plaques should be covered. Alternatively, a single lamp could be used to treat each of the four involved areas sequentially. Once FR's sensitivity to UV radiation while taking psoralen has been determined, treatment with 40% to 70% of her MED, increasing by 10% to 40% each week, applied 2 or 3 times per week, is recommended. This treatment regimen should be continued until complete clearance has been achieved and possibly for a few more sessions to increase the period of remission. After treatment with PUVA has been completed, the patient should be encouraged to wear clothes that expose her elbows and knees when outside because the UV radiation in sunlight may help to control her psoriasis; however, she should try to avoid exposing her skin to sunlight during the period of PUVA treatment because this would increase her UV exposure and thus increase her risk of burning.

Documentation

S: Pt reports itchy, scaly psoriatic plaques on both knees and elbows that have been successfully treated with PUVA in the past.

O: Pretreatment: Well-demarcated, scaling plaques approx 4 × 8 cm bilateral dorsal elbows and 5 × 7 cm bilateral anterior knees.

Intervention: Pt's MED determined before treatment: 2 hrs after psoralen ingestion pt placed in UV cabinet, lamp No. 9624, PUVA to bilateral knees and elbows for 4 minutes.

Posttreatment: No change in appearance of plaques. No erythema.

A: Pt tolerated PUVA well, with no adverse effects.

P: Continue PUVA 3 times per week, increasing dose by 10%-40% (of MED) each week depending on pt's response. Pt should minimize sun exposure while receiving PUVA.

CHAPTER REVIEW

1. UV radiation is electromagnetic radiation with wavelength between below 290 nm and up to 400 nm, lying between x-ray and visible light. UV is emitted by the sun and by UV lamps. UV radiation is divided into three categories defined by wavelength. UVA has the longest wavelength (320 to 400 nm), UVB is in the middle (290 to 320 nm), and UVC has the shortest wavelength (less than 290 nm). UVA has the greatest depth of skin penetration, whereas UVC affects the most superficial skin layers.

2. Effects of UV radiation include erythema, tanning, epidermal hyperplasia, and vitamin D synthesis. UVC may be bactericidal, whereas UVA and UVB can affect immune activity and inflammation, depending on the dose applied.

3. UV is used primarily for the treatment of psoriasis and other skin disorders. For this application, either narrowband (≈312 nm) UVB or UVA in combination with psoralen (PUVA) are preferred. UVB is gaining popularity for this application because it has fewer side effects than PUVA, is easier to apply, and is almost as effective as PUVA. UVC is sometimes used to augment standard wound care interventions in patients with chronic wounds.

4. Contraindications to the use of UV radiation include irradiation of the eyes; skin cancer; pulmonary tuberculosis; cardiac, kidney, or liver disease; systemic lupus erythematosus; and fever. Precautions include photosensitizing medication use, photosensitivity, and recent x-ray therapy. No dose of UV radiation should be repeated until the effects of the previous dose have disappeared.

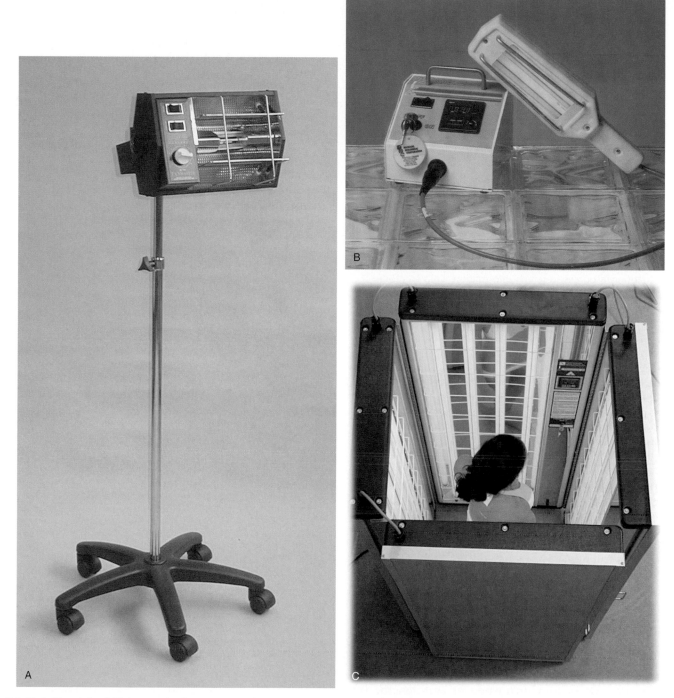

FIG 13-9 Ultraviolet (UV) lamps. **A,** Fluorescent; **B,** handheld UVA/UVB wand; **C,** UVB cabinet for whole body therapy. **A,** *Courtesy Brandt Industries, Inc, Bronx, NY;* **B** *and* **C,** *Courtesy National Biological Corporation, Twinsburg, OH.*

5. The MED (minimal erythemal dose) is the smallest dose of UV radiation needed to produce erythema that appears within 8 hours of exposure and that disappears within 24 hours after exposure. Dosing of UV radiation is determined by the MED. If a patient is undergoing PUVA therapy, the MED should be determined after the patient has taken psoralen. For skin conditions, a series of treatments over the course of weeks is typically needed. Doses usually increase as treatment proceeds, and the patient should be closely monitored for erythema and therapeutic response.

6. The reader is referred to the Evolve web site for further exercises and links to resources and references.

ADDITIONAL RESOURCES *evolve*

Web Sites

National Psoriasis Foundation: Website covers the treatment of psoriasis with PUVA and UVB, along with general psoriasis information, resources, research information, links to other sites, patient advocacy, and healthcare provider information. www.psoriasis.org

GLOSSARY *evolve*

Actinic damage: Skin damage caused by chronic exposure to UV radiation. The skin becomes dry, coarse, and leathery with wrinkling and pigment abnormalities.

Arc lamp: A lamp that produces light when electric current flows across the gap between two electrodes.

Cataracts: A loss of transparency of the lens of the eye that causes blurry, hazy or distorted vision and that is caused by aging and by chronic UV exposure.

Conjunctivitis: Inflammation of the insides of the eyelids and the membrane covering the cornea that causes light sensitivity, tearing, eyelid twitching, and a sensation of gritty eyes.

Epidermal hyperplasia: Thickening of the superficial layer of the skin.

Erythema: Redness of the skin.

First-degree erythema (E_1): Definite redness with some mild desquamation that appears within 6 hours after exposure to UV and lasts for 1 to 3 days.

Fluorescent lamp: A lamp that uses electricity to excite mercury vapor in argon or neon gas and that can produce ultraviolet light.

Frequency band: A range within the electromagnetic spectrum defined by frequency or wavelength. For example, the band for UVA radiation is 320 to 400 nm wavelength. Also called band.

Minimal erythemal dose (MED): The smallest dose of UV to produce erythema that appears within 8 hours of exposure and that disappears within 24 hours after exposure.

Photokeratitis: A temporary inflammation of the cornea that occurs after UV exposure and that causes discomfort, blurred vision, and light sensitivity.

Phototherapy: The therapeutic use of light.

Psoralen: A photosensitizing chemical administered orally or topically to increase the skin's reaction to light for a therapeutic effect.

Psoriasis: A chronic skin disorder marked by itchy, scaly red patches.

Psoriatic arthritis: Arthritis that may accompany the skin manifestations of psoriasis.

Psoralen with UVA (PUVA): A combination of psoralen and UVA radiation. PUVA is used to treat some skin conditions.

Second-degree erythema (E_2): Intense erythema with edema, peeling, and pigmentation appearing within 2 hours or less after exposure to UV.

Suberythemal dose (SED): A dose of UV that produces no change in skin redness in the 24 hours after exposure.

Third-degree erythema (E_3): Erythema with severe blistering, peeling, and exudation.

Ultraviolet (UV) radiation: Electromagnetic radiation with a frequency range of 7.5×10^{14} to over 10^{15} Hz and wavelengths from 400 nm to below 290 nm, which lies between x-ray and visible light.

Vitiligo: A chronic skin condition that causes loss of pigmentation, resulting in patches of pale skin. Also known as leukoderma.

REFERENCES *evolve*

1. Anderson RR, Parrish JA: The optics of human skin, *J Invest Dermatol* 77:13-19, 1981.
2. Kaidbey K, Agin P, Sayre R, et al: Photoprotection by melanin: a comparison of black and Caucasian skin, *Am Acad Dermatol* 1:249-260, 1979.
3. Farr P, Diffey B: The erythemal response of human skin to ultraviolet radiation, *Br J Dermatol* 113:65-76, 1985.
4. Faber M: Ultraviolet radiation. In Suess M, Benwell-Morrison D, eds: *Non-ionising radiation protection*, ed 2, Geneva, 1989, World Health Organization.
5. Murphy T: Nucleic acids: interaction with solar UV radiation, *Curr Top Radiat Res Q* 10:199, 1975.
6. Eaglestein W, Weinstein G: Prostaglandin and DNA synthesis in human skin: possible relationship to ultraviolet light effects, *J Invest Dermatol* 64:386-396, 1975.
7. Ganong WF: *Review of medical physiology*, ed 13, East Norwalk, CT, 1987, Appleton & Lange.
8. Holick MF: The cutaneous photosynthesis of previtamin D: a unique photoendocrine system, *J Invest Dermatol* 76:51-58, 1981.
9. Holick MF: Evolution and function of vitamin D, *Rec Res Cancer Res* 164:3-28, 2003.
10. Higdon, J: Vitamin D. Linus Pauling Institute, Micronutrient research for optimum health, Oregon State University, http://lpi.oregonstate.edu/infocenter/vitamins/vitaminD/. Last updated March 3, 2004. Accessed February 12, 2007.
11. Zittermann A: Vitamin D in preventive medicine: are we ignoring the evidence? *Br J Nut* 89(5):552-572, 2003.
12. Holick MF: High prevalence of vitamin D inadequacy and implications for health, *Mayo Clin Proc* 81(3):353-373, 2006.
13. Garland CF, Garland FC, Gorham ED, et al: The role of vitamin D in cancer prevention. *Am J Pub Health* 96(2):252-261, 2006.
14. High AS, High JP: Treatment of infected skin wounds using ultraviolet radiation: an in-vitro study, *Physiotherapy* 69(10):359-360, 1983.
15. Yaun BR, Sumner SS, Eifert JD, et al: Response of Salmonella and Escherichia coli O157:H7 to UV energy, *J Food Prot* 66(6):1071-1073, 2003.
16. Sullivan PK, Conner-Kerr TA: A comparative study of the effects of UVC irradiation on select procaryotic and eucaryotic wound pathogens, *Ostomy Wound Manage* 46(10):28-34, 2000.
17. Anderson BM, Banrud H, Boe E, et al: Comparison of UV C light and chemicals for disinfection of surfaces in hospital isolation units, *Infect Control Hosp Epidemiol* 27(7):729-734, 2006.

18. Thai TP, Keast DH, Campbell KE, et al: Effect of ultraviolet light C on bacterial colonization in chronic wounds, *Ostomy Wound Manage* 51(10):32-45, 2005.

19. Rasanen L, Reunala T, Lehto M, et al: Immediate decrease in antigen-presenting function and delayed enhancement of interleukin-I production in human epidermal cells after in vivo UV-B irradiation, *Br J Dermatol* 120:589-596, 1989.

20. Horkay I, Bodolay E, Koda A: Immunologic aspects of prophylactic UV-B and PUVA therapy in polymorphic light eruption, *Photodermatology* 3:47-49, 1986.

21. Gollhausen R, Kaidbey K, Schechter N: UV suppression of mast cell mediated whealing in human skin, *Photodermatology* 2:58-67, 1985.

22. Kanekura T, Higashi Y, Kanzaki T: Cyclooxygenase-2 expression and prostaglandin E2 biosynthesis are enhanced in scleroderma fibroblasts and inhibited by UVA irradiation, *J Rheumatol* 28(7):1568-1572, 2001.

23. Wu CS, Lan CC, Wang LF, et al: Effects of psoralen plus ultraviolet A irradiation on cultured epidermal cells in vitro and patients with vitiligo in vivo, *Br J Dermatol* 156(1):122-129, 2007.

24. Grimes PE: New insights and new therapies in vitiligo, *JAMA* 293(6):730-735, 2005.

25. Reynolds NJ, Franklin V, Gray JC, et al: Narrow-band ultraviolet B and broad-band ultraviolet A phototherapy in adult atopic eczema: a randomised controlled trial, *Lancet* 357(9273):2012-2016, 2001.

26. Marsland AM, Chalmers RJ, Hollis S, et al: Interventions for chronic palmoplantar pustulosis, *Cochrane Database Syst Rev* (1):CD001433, 2006.

27. Freytes H, Fernandez B, Fleming W: Ultraviolet light in the treatment of indolent ulcers, *South Med J* 223-226, 1965.

28. Nussbaum EL, Biemann I, Mustard B: Comparison of ultrasound/ultraviolet-C and laser for treatment of pressure ulcers in patients with spinal cord injury, *Phys Ther* 74:812-823, 1994.

29. Scott BO: Ultraviolet application. In Stillwell K, ed: *Therapeutic electricity and ultraviolet radiation*, ed 3, Baltimore, 1983, Williams & Wilkins.

30. Sjovall P, Moller H: The influence of locally administered ultraviolet light (UV-B) on allergic contact dermatitis in the mouse, *Acta Dermatol Venereol* 65:465-471, 1985.

31. Sjovall P, Christensen O: Local and systemic effect of UV-B irradiation in patients with chronic hand eczema, *Acta Dermatol Venereol* 67:538-541, 1987.

32. Epstein JH: Phototherapy and photochemotherapy, *N Engl J Med* 322:1149-1151, 1990.

33. Wolska H, Kleniewaska D, Kowalski J: Successful desensitization in a case of solar urticaria with sensitivity to UV-A and positive passive transfer test, *Dermatosensitivity* 30:84-86, 1982.

34. Norris PG, Hawk JLM, Baker C, et al: British photodermatology group guidelines for PUVA, *Br J Dermatol* 130:246-255, 1994.

35. Honig B, Morison WL, Karp D: Photochemotherapy beyond psoriasis, *J Am Acad Dermatol* 31:775-790, 1994.

36. Berneburg M, Rocken M, Benedix F: Phototherapy with narrowband vs broadband UVB, *Acta Dermato-Venereologica* 85(2):98-108, 2005.

37. Griffiths CE, Clark CM, Chalmers RJ: A systematic review of treatments for severe psoriasis, *Health Technology Assessment* (Winchester, England) 4(40):1-125, 2000.

38. Fusco RJ, Jordon PA, Kelly A, et al: PUVA treatment for psoriasis, *Physiotherapy* 66:40, 1980.

39. Klaber MR: Ultra-violet light for psoriasis, *Physiotherapy* 66:36-38, 1980.

40. Shurr DG, Zuehlke RL: Photochemotherapy treatment for psoriasis, *Phys Ther* 62:33-36, 1981.

41. Fotaides J, Lim HW, Jiang SB, et al: Efficacy of ultraviolet B phototherapy for psoriasis in patients infected with human immunodeficiency virus, *Photodermatol Photoimmunol Photomed* 11(3):107-111, 1995.

42. Honigsmann H: Phototherapy for psoriasis, *Clin Exp Dermatol* 26(4):343-350, 2001.

43. Wolf P, Nghiem DX, Walterscheid JP, et al: Platelet-activating factor is crucial in psoralen and ultraviolet A-induced immune suppression, inflammation, and apoptosis, *Am J Pathol* 169(3):795-805, 2006.

44. Marathe GK, Johnson C, Billings SD, et al: Ultraviolet B radiation generates platelet-activating factor-like phospholipids underlying cutaneous damage, *J Biol Chem* 280(42):35448-35457, 2005.

45. Ortel B, Perl S, Kinciyan T, et al: Comparison of narrow-band (331 nm) UVB and broad band UVA after oral or bath-water 8-methoxypsoralen in the treatment of psoriasis, *J Am Acad Dermatol* 29(5 pt 1):736-740, 1993.

46. Tanew A, Radakovic-Fijan S, Schemper M, et al: Paired comparison study on narrow-band (TL-01) UVB phototherapy versus photochemotherapy (PUVA) in the treatment of chronic plaque type psoriasis, *Arch Dermatol* 135:519-524, 1999.

47. Yones SS, Palmer RA, Garibaldinos TT, et al: Randomized double-blind trial of the treatment of chronic plaque psoriasis: efficacy of psoralen-UV-A therapy vs narrowband UV-B therapy, *Arch Dermatol* 142(7):836-842, 2006.

48. Fisher T, Alsisns J, Berne B: Ultraviolet action spectrum and evaluation of ultraviolet lamps for psoriasis healing, *Int J Dermatol* 23:633-637, 1984.

49. Lowe NJ, Wortzman MS, Breeding J, et al: Coal tar phototherapy for psoriasis reevaluated: erythemogenic versus suberythemogenic ultraviolet with a tar extract in oil and crude coal tar, *J Am Acad Dermatol* 8:781-789, 1983.

50. Stern RS, Gange RW, Parrish JA, et al: Contribution of topical tar oil to ultraviolet B phototherapy for psoriasis, *J Am Acad Dermatol* 14(5):742-747, 1986.

51. Tronnier H, Schule D: First results of therapy with long wave UV-A after photosensitization of the skin, Abstracts of the Sixth International Congress of Photobiology, Germany, 1972.

52. Iest J, Boer J: Combined treatment of psoriasis with acitretin and UV-B phototherapy compared with acitretin alone and UV-B alone, *Br J Dermatol* 120:665-670, 1989.

53. Dover JS, McEvoy MT, Rosen CF, et al: Are topical corticosteroids useful in phototherapy for psoriasis? *J Am Acad Dermatol* 21(3):592-593, 1989.

54. Gupta AK, Ellis CN, Tellner DC, et al: Double blind placebo controlled study to evaluate the efficacy of fish oil and low dose UV-B in the treatment of psoriasis, *Br J Dermatol* 120:801-807, 1989.

55. Zanolli M: Phototherapy treatment of psoriasis today, *J Am Acad Dermatol* 49(suppl):S78-S86, 2003.

56. Walters IB, Burack LH, Coven TR, et al: Suberythemogenic narrow-band UVB is markedly more effective than conventional UVB in treatment of psoriasis vulgaris, *J Am Acad Dermatol* 40:893-900, 1999.

57. Coven TR, Burack LH, Gilleaudeau R, et al: Narrowband UV-B produces superior clinical and histopathological resolution of moderate-to-severe psoriasis in patients compared with broad-band UV-B, *Arch Dermatol* 133:1514-1522, 1997.

58. Tanew A, Radakovic-Fijan S, Schemper M, et al: Narrowband UVB phototherapy vs photochemotherapy in the treatment of chronic plaque type psoriasis, *Arch Dermatol* 135:519-524, 1999.

59. Gerber W, Arheilger B, Ha TA, et al: Ultraviolet B 308-nm excimer laser treatment of psoriasis: a new phototherapeutic approach, *Br J Dermatol* 149(6):1250-8, 2003.

60. Houghton PE, Campbell KE: Choosing an adjunctive therapy for the treatment of chronic wounds, *Ostomy Wound Manage* 15(8):43-52, 1999.

61. Parrish J, Zaynoun S, Anderson R: Cumulative effect of repeated subthreshold doses of ultraviolet radiation, *J Invest Dermatol* 76:356-358, 1981.

62. Ramsay C, Challoner A: Vascular changes in human skin after ultraviolet irradiation, *Br J Dermatol* 94:487-493, 1976.

63. Kloth LC: Physical modalities in wound management: UVC, therapeutic heating and electrical stimulation, *Ostomy Wound Manage* 41(5):18-20, 22-24, 26-27, 1995.

64. Wills EE, Anderson TW, Beatie LB, et al: A randomised placebo controlled trial of ultraviolet in the treatment of superficial pressure sores, *J Am Geriatr Soc* 31:131-133, 1983.

65. Burns F: Cancer risks associated with therapeutic irradiation of the skin, *Arch Dermatol* 125:979-981, 1989.

66. Beattie PE, Dawe RS, Traynor NJ, et al: Can St John's wort (hypericin) ingestion enhance the erythemal response during high-dose ultraviolet A1 therapy? *Br J Dermatol* 153(6):1187-1191, 2005.

67. Swanbeck G: To UV-B or not to UV-B? *Photodermatology* 1:2-4, 1984.

68. Studniberg HM, Weller P: PUVA, UVB, psoriasis, and nonmelanoma skin cancer, *J Am Acad Dermatol* 29(6):1013-1022, 1993.

69. Stern RS, Laird N: The carcinogenic risk of treatments for severe psoriasis, *Cancer* 73:2759-2764, 1994.

70. Taylor HR: The biological effects of ultraviolet-B on the eye, *Photochem Photobiol* 50(4):489-492, 1989.

71. Stern RS, Liebman EJ, Vakeva L: Oral psoralen and ultraviolet-A light (PUVA) treatment of psoriasis and persistent risk of nonmelanoma skin cancer: PUVA follow-up study, *J Natl Cancer Inst* 90:1278-1284, 1998.

72. Tromovitch TA, Thompson LR, Jacobs PH: Testing for photosensitivity, *J Am Phys Ther Assoc* 143:348-349, 1963.

73. Low J: Quantifying the erythema due to UVR, *Physiotherapy* 72:60-64, 1986.

74. Levine M, Parrish JA: Out-patient phototherapy of psoriasis, *Arch Dermatol* 116:552-554, 1980.

75. Stern RS, Armstrong RB, Anderson TF, et al: Effect of continued ultraviolet B phototherapy on the duration of remission of psoriasis: a randomised study, *J Am Acad Dermatol* 15(3):546-556, 1986.

76. Karrer S, Eholzer C, Ackermann G: Phototherapy of psoriasis: comparative experience of different phototherapeutic approaches, *Dermatology* 202(2):108-115, 2001.

77. Chue B, Borok M, Lowe NJ: Phototherapy units: comparison of fluorescent ultraviolet B and ultraviolet A units with high-pressure mercury system, *J Am Acad Dermatol* 18:641-645, 1998.

Diathermy

Diathermy, from the Greek meaning "through heating," is the application of shortwave (about 1.8 to 30 MHz frequency and 3 to 200 m wavelength) or microwave (300 MHz to 300 GHz frequency and 1 mm to 1 m wavelength) electromagnetic energy to produce heat and other physiological changes within tissues. **Shortwave radiation** is within the radiofrequency range (3 kHz to 300 MHz frequency and 1 m to 100 km wavelength), and radiofrequency is between extremely **low frequency** (ELF) and **microwave radiation** (Fig. 14-1). Microwave radiation

has a frequency between that of radiofrequency and infrared (IR) radiation. Both shortwave and microwave radiation are nonionizing.

The use of diathermy dates back to 1892, when d'Arsonval used radiofrequency electromagnetic fields with 10 kHz frequency to produce a sensation of warmth without the muscular contractions that occur at lower frequencies. The clinical use of shortwave diathermy (SWD) became popular in the early 20th century, and this intervention was frequently used to treat infections in the United States (US) in the 1930s. However, despite a number of reports indicating that SWD can be effective for a range of problems, by the 1950s, with the advent of antibiotics and with growing concerns about potential hazards to the patient and the operator if the equipment was applied inappropriately, its use declined. Diathermy also lost popularity because, by its nature, the electromagnetic field cannot be readily contained to eliminate interference with other electronic equipment and because most diathermy devices were large, expensive, and cumbersome to use. Nonetheless, in recent years, there has been some resurgence of interest in this technology, with the development of smaller better-shielded devices. Some clinicians in skilled nursing facilities and other practice settings are now using diathermy to produce gentle heat in large areas, and in response to the publication of a number of studies regarding the nonthermal effects of pulsed diathermy, clinicians in specialized wound care practices are applying diathermy to facilitate tissue healing by nonthermal mechanisms. Currently, SWD devices are manufactured and available in the US, whereas microwave diathermy (MWD) devices are not manufactured in the US but can be obtained from abroad.

The radiation used for diathermy falls within the radiofrequency range and could therefore interfere with radiofrequency signals used for communications. To avoid such interference the Federal Communications Commission (FCC) has assigned certain frequencies of shortwave and microwave radiation to medical applications. SWD devices have been allocated the three frequency bands centered on 13.56, 27.12, and 40.68 MHz, with ranges of ±6.78, 160, and 20 kHz, respectively.[1] The 27.12 MHz band is most commonly used for SWD devices because it has the widest bandwidth and is therefore the easiest and least expensive to generate. MWD devices for medical application have been allocated the frequency of 2,450 MHz.

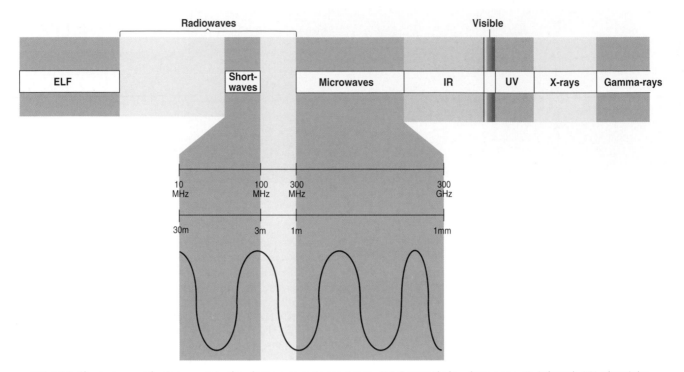

FIG 14-1 Shortwaves and microwaves in the electromagnetic spectrum. *ELF,* Extremely low frequency; *IR,* infrared; *UV,* ultraviolet.

Both SWD and MWD can be delivered in a **continuous** or pulsed mode and when delivered at a sufficient average intensity, can generate heat in the body.[2-4] When delivered in a pulsed mode at low average intensities, heat is dissipated before it can accumulate; however, pulsed low-intensity electromagnetic energy in the shortwave or microwave frequency range may produce physiological effects by nonthermal mechanisms. Pulsed SWD, when applied at nonthermal levels, is generally referred to as **pulsed shortwave diathermy** (PSWD); however, the terms pulsed electromagnetic field (PEMF), pulsed radio-frequency (PRF), or pulsed electromagnetic energy (PEME) have also been used to describe this type of radiation. The term PSWD is used in this text.

PHYSICAL PROPERTIES OF DIATHERMY

The key factor that determines whether a diathermy device will increase tissue temperature is the amount of energy absorbed by the tissue. This is determined by the intensity of the electromagnetic field produced by the device and the type of tissue to which the field is applied.

◎ **Clinical Pearl**

Electromagnetic field intensity and tissue type determine how much energy will be absorbed by the tissue and how warm it will become.

A pulsed signal can allow heat to dissipate during the off cycle of the pulse. Previously published literature categorized devices with an average power driving the appli-

cator below 38 W as nonthermal.[5] In clinical practice, however, the strength of the magnetic field reaching the tissue, the type of tissue, and tissue perfusion, rather than the power driving the applicator, determine whether the tissue will be heated. Therefore the clinician should use the patient's report and information provided by the device's manufacturer to ascertain whether a particular diathermy application increases tissue temperature.

When applied at sufficient power to increase tissue temperature, diathermy has a number of advantages over other thermal agents. It can heat deeper tissues than superficial thermal agents such as hot packs, and it can heat larger areas than ultrasound.

◎ **Clinical Pearl**

Diathermy heats deeper than hot packs and heats a larger area than ultrasound.

SWD is not reflected by bones and therefore does not concentrate at the periosteum or pose a risk of periosteal burning, as does ultrasound; however, MWD is reflected at tissue interfaces, including those between air and skin, between skin and subcutaneous fat, and between soft tissue and superficial bones, and therefore does produce more heat in the areas close to these interfaces. The reflection of microwaves can also lead to the formation of standing waves, resulting in hot spots in other areas. Both SWD and MWD treatments generally need little time for application and do not require the clinician to be in direct contact with the patient throughout the treatment period.

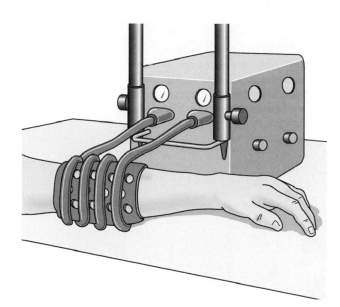

FIG 14-2 An inductive coil shortwave diathermy applicator set-up with cables around the patient's limb. This type of applicator produces a uniform, incident electromagnetic field that induces an electric field and current within the target tissue.

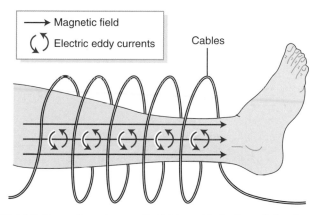

FIG 14-3 Generation of magnetic fields and induction of electric fields by an inductive coil.

TYPES OF DIATHERMY APPLICATORS

There are three different types of diathermy applicators: inductive coils, capacitive plates, and a **magnetron**.[5] Inductive coils or capacitive plates can be used to apply SWD, whereas a magnetron is used to apply MWD. PSWD devices use **inductive coil applicator**s in a drum form or capacitive plates.

INDUCTIVE COIL

An inductive diathermy applicator is made up of a coil through which an alternating electric current flows (Fig. 14-2). The alternating current in the coil produces a magnetic field perpendicular to the coil, which in turn induces electric eddy currents in the tissues (Fig. 14-3). These induced electric currents cause charged particles in the tissue to oscillate. The friction produced by this oscillation produces an elevation in tissue temperature.

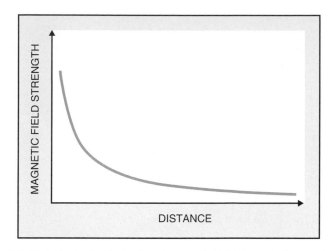

FIG 14-4 The typical behavior of magnetic field strength delivered by a shortwave diathermy device as the distance from the applicator increases. Note that this is an inverse square relationship.

TABLE 14-1	Conductivity of Muscle at Different Frequencies
Frequency (MHz)	**Conductivity (siemens/meter)**
13.56	0.62
27.12	0.60
40.68	0.68
200	1.00
2,450	2.17

From Durney CH, Massoudi H, Iskander MF: *Radiofrequency radiation dosimetry handbook.* USAFSAM-TR-85-73, Salt Lake City, 1985, University of Utah Electrical Engineering Department.

TABLE 14-2	Conductivity of Different Tissues at 25 MHz
Tissue	**Conductivity (siemens/meter)**
Muscle	0.7-0.9
Kidney	0.83
Liver	0.48-0.54
Brain	0.46
Fat	0.04-0.06
Bone	0.01

From Durney CH, Massoudi H, Iskander MF: *Radiofrequency radiation dosimetry handbook.* USAFSAM-TR-85-73, Salt Lake City, 1985, University of Utah Electrical Engineering Department.

Heating with an inductive coil diathermy applicator is known as heating by the magnetic field method because the electric current that generates the heat is induced in the tissues by a magnetic field. The amount of heat generated in an area of tissue is affected by the strength of the magnetic field that reaches the tissue and by the strength and density of the induced eddy currents. The strength of the magnetic field is determined by the distance of the tissue from the applicator and decreases in proportion to the square of the distance of the tissue from the applicator, according to the inverse square law, but does not vary with

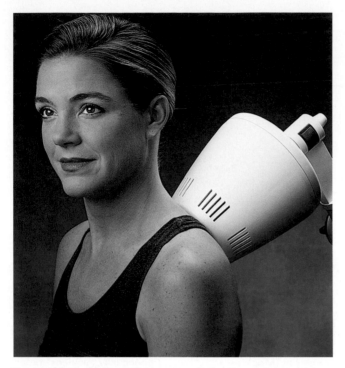

FIG 14-5 An inductive coil shortwave diathermy applicator in drum form. *Courtesy Mettler Electronics Corporation, Anaheim, CA.*

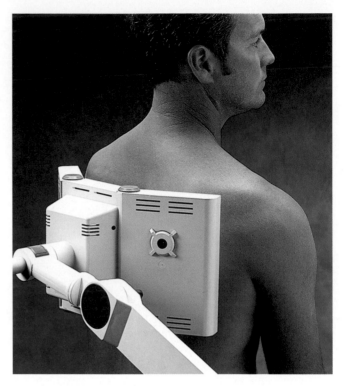

FIG 14-6 Application of SWD using an inductive coil applicator that can conform to the body. *Courtesy Mettler Electronics Corporation, Anaheim, CA.*

tissue type (Fig. 14-4). The strength of the induced eddy currents is determined by the strength of the magnetic field in the area and by the electrical conductivity of the tissue in the area. The electrical conductivity of tissue depends primarily on the tissue type and the frequency of the signal being applied. Metals and tissues with a high water and electrolyte content, such as muscle or synovial fluid, have high electrical conductivity, whereas tissues with a low water content, such as fat, bone, and collagen, have low electrical conductivity (Tables 14-1 and 14-2). Thus inductive coils can heat both deep and superficial tissues, but they produce the most heat in tissues closest to the applicator and in tissues with the highest electrical conductivity.

◎ Clinical Pearl

Inductive coil diathermy applicators produce the most heat in tissues that have high electrical conductivity and that are closest to the applicator.

Inductive coil applicators have been produced in two basic forms, cables and drums. The cables are bundles of plastic-coated wires that are applied by wrapping them around the patient's limb. When an alternating electric current flows through these wires, eddy currents are induced inside the limb. Cable diathermy applicators are not available at this time. A drum applicator is made of a flat spiral coil contained within a plastic housing (Fig. 14-5). Diathermy devices with drum applicators may have one or two drums or a single drum that can be bent to conform to the area being treated (Fig. 14-6). The drum is placed directly over the area being treated, and the

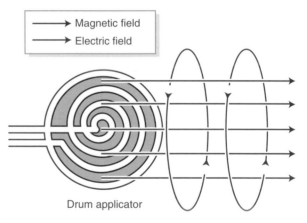

FIG 14-7 Magnetic field generated by an inductive drum shortwave diathermy applicator and the resultant induced electric field.

flow of alternating electric current in the coil produces a magnetic field, which in turn induces eddy currents within the tissues directly in front of it (Fig. 14-7).

CAPACITIVE PLATES

Capacitive plate diathermy applicators are made of metal encased in a plastic housing or transmissive carbon rubber electrodes that are placed between felt pads. A high-frequency alternating electric current flows from one plate to the other through the patient, producing an electric field and a flow of current in the body tissue that is between the plates (Figs. 14-8 and 14-9). Thus the patient becomes a part of the electrical circuit connecting the two plates. As current flows through the tissue, it causes oscillation of charged particles and thus an increase in tissue temperature.

Heating with capacitive plate diathermy applicators is known as heating by the electric field method because the electric current that generates the heat is produced directly

by an electric field. As with the inductive coils, the amount of heat generated in an area of tissue depends on the strength and density of the current, with most heating occurring in tissues with the highest conductivity. Because current will always take the path of least resistance, when a capacitive plate type of applicator is used, the current will generally concentrate in the superficial tissues and will not penetrate as effectively to deeper tissues if there are poorly conductive tissues, such as fat, superficial to them. Thus capacitive plates generally produce most heat in skin and less heat in deeper structures, in contrast to inductive applicators, which heat the deeper structures more effectively because the incident magnetic field can achieve greater penetration to induce the electric field and current within the targeted tissue[6-9] (Fig. 14-10).

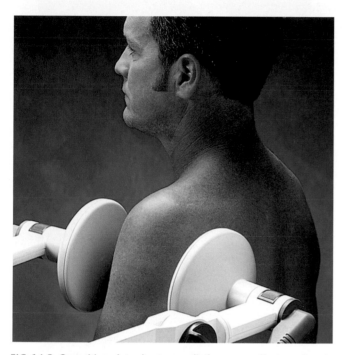

FIG 14-8 Capacitive plate shortwave diathermy applicators placed around the target to produce an electric field directly. *Courtesy Mettler Electronics Corporation, Anaheim, CA.*

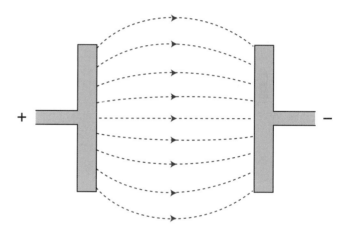

FIG 14-9 Electric field distribution between capacitive shortwave diathermy plates.

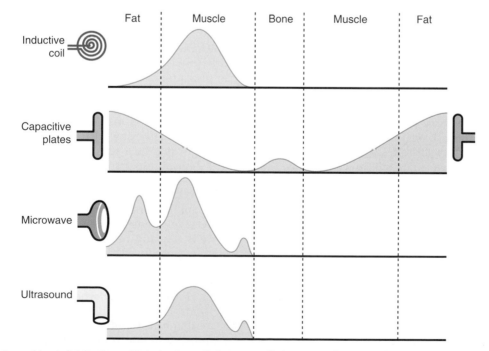

FIG 14-10 Comparison of heat distribution with inductive coil shortwave diathermy applicator, capacitive plate shortwave diathermy applicator, microwave diathermy, and ultrasound.

MAGNETRON (CONDENSER)

A magnetron, which produces a high-frequency alternating current in an antenna, is used to deliver MWD. The alternating current in the antenna produces an electromagnetic field that is directed toward the tissue by a curved reflecting director surrounding the antenna (Fig. 14-11). The presence of a director and the short wavelength of microwave radiation allow this type of diathermy to be focused and applied to small, defined areas. Therefore these devices can be useful during rehabilitation when only small areas of tissue are involved; they are also popular for the medical treatment of malignant tumors by hyperthermia. The magnetrons used clinically are similar to those used in microwave ovens intended for cooking food.

The microwaves produced by a magnetron generate the most heat in tissues with high electrical conductivity; however, this high-frequency, short-wavelength radiation penetrates less deeply than SWD. Microwaves usually generate the most heat in the superficial skin, although some authors have also reported significant temperature increases in muscles and joint cavities in response to microwave application.[3,10,11] These differences in reported depth of heating appear to be related to variations in the microwave frequency used, from 915 to 2,450 MHz, and to variability in tissue composition among different areas of the body and among different species.[12] The shallow depth of microwave penetration, the reflection at tissue interfaces, and the potential for standing waves all contribute to an increased risk of uneven heating and burning of the superficial skin or fat with this type of diathermy device.

EFFECTS OF DIATHERMY

THERMAL EFFECTS

If applied at sufficient average intensity, SWD and MWD will produce a sensation of heat and increase tissue temperature.[13-15] The physiological effects of increasing tissue temperature are described in detail in Chapter 6 and include vasodilation, increased rate of nerve conduction, elevation of pain threshold, alteration of muscle strength, acceleration of enzymatic activity, and increased soft tissue extensibility. All of these effects have been observed in response to the application of diathermy.[16-20] The mechanisms underlying these physiological effects of increasing tissue temperature are also described in detail in Chapter 6.

The difference between the effects of superficial heating agents and diathermy is that superficial heating agents only increase the temperature of the superficial first few millimeters of tissue, whereas diathermy heats deeper tissues. Therefore the physiological effects of superficial heating agents occur primarily in the superficial tissues, whereas diathermy also produces thermal effects in deeper

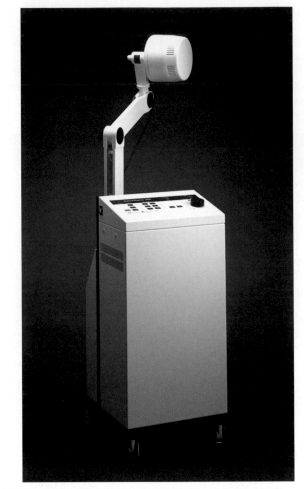

FIG 14-11 Microwave diathermy applicator. *Courtesy Mettler Electronics, Anaheim, CA.*

tissues. For example, superficial heating agents primarily increase cutaneous circulation, whereas SWD and MWD significantly increase circulation in muscles.[16,21,22] Although diathermy is primarily used for its deep heating effects, it can also produce some heat in the skin and superficial tissues, particularly when higher frequencies (450 MHz versus 220 or 100 MHz) are used.[23] Even when skin temperature does not increase the body responds to deep heating by diathermy with sweating and vasodilation. It is thought that heat sensors deep in the body signal these physiological responses to heat.[24]

NONTHERMAL EFFECTS

When applied in a pulsed mode with a low **duty cycle,** the average intensity of energy delivered by a diathermy device is low and no maintained increase in tissue temperature is produced. Any transient heating of tissues that may occur during a brief pulse is quickly dissipated by the blood perfusing the area during the off time between pulses. However, PSWD, when applied at such nonthermal levels, may have certain physiological effects.[25] Although the mechanisms by which PSWD achieves these effects are unknown, it has been proposed that these effects are produced by modification of ion binding and cellular function by the incident electromagnetic fields and the resulting electric currents.[26,27]

Increased Microvascular Perfusion

The application of PSWD for 40 to 45 minutes at settings which the device manufacturer states does not increase tissue temperature has been found to increase local microvascular perfusion in healthy subjects and around the ulcer site in patients with diabetic ulcers.[28,29] Increasing microvascular perfusion, and thus local circulation, can increase local tissue oxygenation, nutrient availability, and phagocytosis. It has been proposed that the clinical benefits of PSWD are in part the result of increased microvascular perfusion.

Altered Cell Membrane Function and Cellular Activity

It has been reported that electromagnetic fields can affect ion binding to the cell membrane, and that this can trigger a cascade of biological processes, including growth factor activation in fibroblasts, chondrocytes, and nerve cells; macrophage activation; and changes in myosin phosphorylation.[30-36] PSWD is also thought to affect the regulation of the cell cycle by altering calcium ion binding, and it has been shown that exposure to electric fields can accelerate cell growth and division when it is too slow and inhibit it when it is too fast.[37,38] It has been proposed that alteration of cellular activity and stimulation of adenosine triphosphate (ATP) and protein synthesis may also underlie the observed clinical benefits of PSWD.[39]

CLINICAL INDICATIONS FOR THE USE OF DIATHERMY

THERMAL-LEVEL DIATHERMY

The clinical benefits of applying diathermy at a sufficient intensity to increase tissue temperature are the same as those of applying other thermal agents (see Chapter 6). These benefits include pain control, accelerated tissue healing, decreased joint stiffness, and if applied in conjunction with stretching, increased joint range of motion (ROM).[40,41] Because diathermy can increase the temperature of large areas of deep tissue, its use is indicated when trying to achieve the clinical benefits of heat in deep structures such as the hip joint or diffuse areas of the spine.

The thermal effects of diathermy may be produced by continuous diathermy or pulsed diathermy at sufficient average intensity. Five studies, all performed by the same research group, found that PSWD, with appropriate treatment parameters, produced increases in soft tissue extensibility, as measured by ankle dorsiflexion or hamstring flexibility. The PSWD used in these studies had an average output of 48 W and was found to increase tissue temperature by up to 3.5° C in 20 minutes.[42] Therefore the clinical outcome was likely a result of thermal rather than nonthermal effects of diathermy. Three of the studies found that PSWD applied in this manner in conjunction with stretching resulted in increased muscle length or ROM, with two of the studies showing greater effect with diathermy than without.[43-45] However, the impact of this intervention beyond 3 weeks was not evaluated,[46] and one of the studies found no long-term difference in the effectiveness of diathermy followed by stretching as compared to stretching alone.[47]

NONTHERMAL PULSED SHORTWAVE DIATHERMY

The first documented clinical application of diathermy at a nonthermal level in the US was in the 1930s, when Ginsberg used a pulsed form of SWD to fight infection without producing a significant temperature rise in tissue.[48] He reported successfully treating a variety of acute and chronic infections with this type of electromagnetic radiation and stated that this was the most effective treatment he had ever used. However, this was before antibiotics were commonly available or used. In 1965, A.S. Milinowski patented a device designed to deliver electrotherapy without heat generation. He stated that this device produced good clinical results in a range of conditions while eliminating the factors of patient heat tolerance and contraindications when treating with heat.[49] Such nonthermal levels of PSWD have been evaluated and are now used clinically, primarily to control pain and edema and to promote wound, nerve, and fracture healing.

Control of Pain and Edema

A number of studies concerning the effects of PSWD on recovery from soft tissue injury have shown improved edema resolution and reduction of pain in response to the application of this type of electromagnetic energy.[50-53] Two double-blind studies on the effects of nonthermal PSWD on acute ankle sprains found a significant decrease in edema, pain, or disability in the treated group compared with a placebo-treated group, and a double-blind study assessing the effects of PSWD treatment found that it decreased pain, erythema, and edema after foot surgery.[50-53] Maximum power and pulse frequency available on the device were used in all of these studies. It should be noted, however, that not all studies on the use of PSWD have shown such improvements. Both Barker et al and McGill found no significant differences in pain, swelling, or gait between patients treated with PSWD and those treated with a placebo after acute ankle injuries.[54,55]

Pain Control

A number of studies have evaluated the effect of PSWD on pain associated with a variety of conditions. Double-blind studies on the effects of using a home PSWD device placed in a soft cervical collar on patients with persistent neck pain or acute cervical injuries found significantly greater decreases in pain and increases in ROM in patients using this device for 3 weeks than in patients treated with a sham device.[56,57] The authors of these studies suggested that these effects could be a result of modification of cell membrane function by the electromagnetic field. Studies without double-blind controls have also reported that PSWD can decrease low back and postoperative pain,[58,59] and a recent double-blind, placebo-controlled study found that pain and disability decreased significantly more in subjects with chronic low back pain who received pulsed electromagnetic therapy than in control participants.[60] However, another randomized controlled trial with 350 participants found that PSWD provided no additional benefit for patients with neck pain when added to advice and exercise.[61]

Soft Tissue Healing

Nonthermal PSWD has been shown to increase the rate of soft tissue healing in both animal and human subjects.[62-65] This effect has been found with incisional wounds,[62] pressure ulcers,[63,65] burn-related injuries,[64] and tendon injuries.[66] Surgical wound sites in animals demonstrated increased collagen formation, white blood cell infiltration, and phagocytosis after treatment with PSWD and transected tendons showed significantly (69%) increased tensile strength after treatment with PSWD. Researchers proposed that these effects were the result of increased circulation and improved tissue oxygenation. In vitro studies have also shown increased fibroblast and chondrocyte proliferation in response to PSWD application.[66] These effects are likely a result of direct effects of PSWD on cell or cell membrane function.

Nerve Healing

Acceleration of peripheral nerve regeneration in rats and cats, and of spinal cord regeneration in cats, in response to the application of PSWD have been reported[67-71]; however, the authors of this book are not aware of any published clinical studies regarding the effect of PSWD on the recovery or regeneration of human nerves at this time.

Bone Healing

Animal studies have shown acceleration of bone healing after application of PSWD. A study in 1971 reported acceleration of osteogenesis by PSWD after tooth extraction wounds in dogs,[72] and a recent study found that PSWD accelerated the healing of the rabbit fibula after osteotomy.[73] The authors of this book are not aware of any published clinical studies regarding the effect of PSWD on human bone healing at this time.

Osteoarthritis Symptoms

Several studies have evaluated the effectiveness of PSWD for improving symptoms of osteoarthritis.[74-78] These studies have examined the effects of this intervention on inflammation, ROM, pain, stiffness, functional ability, mobility, and synovial thickness. Two studies did not find any benefits to applying PSWD to patients with osteoarthritis of the knee.[74,75] Another study found that PSWD was only effective at reducing stiffness in patients with osteoarthritis of the knee who were less than 65 years old.[78] However, one study did find that pain was decreased after the application of PSWD to patients with knee or cervical spine osteoarthritis,[76] and another study found that, in patients with knee synovitis and osteoarthritis, synovial thickness and knee pain decreased after the application of PSWD.[77] Overall, it appears that PSWD may provide some benefit to patients with osteoarthritis of the knee.

Other Applications

It has been suggested that nonthermal PSWD may also have therapeutic benefits when applied in the treatment of various forms of neuropathy, ischemic skin flaps, cerebral diseases, and myocardial diseases.[26] There is also one report on the use of PSWD in the management of head injuries.[79]

CONTRAINDICATIONS AND PRECAUTIONS FOR THE USE OF DIATHERMY

Although diathermy is a safe treatment modality when applied appropriately, to avoid adverse effects, it should not be used when contraindicated, and appropriate precautions should be taken when necessary.[80,81] When applying any form of diathermy at an intensity that may increase tissue temperature, all the contraindications and precautions that apply to the use of thermotherapy apply (see Chapter 6). In addition, there are a number of other contraindications and precautions that apply uniquely to this type of physical agent and some unique reasons for these restrictions. These are described in detail in the related boxes that follow.

CONTRAINDICATIONS FOR THE USE OF ALL FORMS OF DIATHERMY

CONTRAINDICATIONS

for the Use of Diathermy

- Implanted or transcutaneous neural stimulators, including cardiac pacemakers
- Pregnancy

Diathermy of any sort should NEVER be used in patients with implanted or transcutaneous stimulators because the electromagnetic energy of the diathermy may interfere with the functioning of the device. Two cases of coma and death have been reported when diathermy has been applied to patients with implanted deep brain stimulators. Also, burns can occur if diathermy is applied to patients with implanted or external electrical stimulation wires or metal containing electrodes.

Diathermy should not be used on patients with pacemakers because these devices have metal components that can become overheated in response to the application of diathermy and because the electromagnetic fields produced by diathermy devices may interfere directly with the performance of pacemakers, particularly those of the demand type. Although the risk of adverse effects is greatest if the thorax is being treated, it is generally recommended that diathermy not be used to treat any area of the body if a patient has a pacemaker, although some authors state that the extremities may be treated in patients with pacemakers.[82]

Pregnancy

The application of diathermy during pregnancy is contraindicated because of concerns regarding the effects of deep heat and electromagnetic fields on fetal development. Maternal hyperthermia has been shown to increase the risk of abnormal fetal development, and SWD has been shown to be linked to increased rates of spontaneous abortion and abnormal fetal development in animals.[84-87] Diathermy exposure, particularly of the lower abdominal and pelvic regions, should be avoided during pregnancy, and because the distribution of an electromagnetic field is not predictably constrained in the body, it is recommended that diathermy exposure of any other part of the body also be avoided. A discussion of the risks and precautions for pregnant therapists applying diathermy to patients follows the section on precautions for applying diathermy to patients.

CONTRAINDICATIONS FOR THE USE OF THERMAL-LEVEL DIATHERMY

> **CONTRAINDICATIONS**
>
> **for the Use of Thermal-Level Diathermy**
>
> - Metal implants
> - Malignancy
> - Eyes
> - Testes
> - Growing epiphyses

Metal Implants

Metal is highly conductive electrically and therefore can become very hot with the application of diathermy, leading to potentially hazardous temperature increases in adjacent tissues. The risk of extreme temperature increases is greatest when there is metal in the superficial tissues, as can occur with pieces of shrapnel; however, it is recommended that diathermy not be used in any areas containing or close to metal. This contraindication applies to metal both inside and outside the patient. Therefore all jewelry should be removed before diathermy is applied, and care should be taken that there is no metal in the furniture or other objects close to the patient being treated.

Malignancy

The use of diathermy in an area of malignancy is contraindicated unless the treatment is for the tumor itself. Diathermy is occasionally used by physicians to treat tumors by hyperthermia; however, such treatment requires fine control of tissue temperature and is outside the realm of the rehabilitation professional. Fine temperature control is required because certain cancer cells have been shown to die at temperatures of 42° to 43° C but to proliferate at temperatures of 40° to 41° C.[83]

Over the Eyes

The eyes should not be treated with diathermy because increasing the temperature of intraocular fluid may damage the internal structures of the eyes.

Over the Testes

It is recommended that diathermy not be applied over the testes because of the risk of adversely affecting fertility by increasing local tissue temperature.

Over Growing Epiphyses

The effects of diathermy on growing epiphyses is unknown; however, its use is not recommended in these areas because of the concern that diathermy may alter the rate of epiphyseal closure.

CONTRAINDICATIONS FOR THE USE OF NONTHERMAL PULSED SHORTWAVE DIATHERMY

> **CONTRAINDICATIONS**
>
> **for the Use of Nonthermal Pulsed Shortwave Diathermy**
>
> - Deep tissues such as internal organs
> - Substitute for conventional therapy for edema and pain
> - Pacemakers, electronic devices, or metal implants (warning)

Deep Tissues Such as Internal Organs

Although contraindicated for the treatment of internal organs, nonthermal PSWD can be used to treat soft tissue overlying an organ.

Assess
- Check the patient's chart for any record of organ disease.
- Check with the patient's physician before applying PSWD in an area with organ disease present.

Substitute for Conventional Therapy for Edema and Pain

PSWD should not be used as a substitute for conventional therapy for edema and pain. It is intended to be used as an adjunctive modality in conjunction with conventional methods, including compression, immobilization, and medications.

Pacemakers, Electronic Devices, or Metal Implants

The electromagnetic radiation of PSWD may interfere with the functioning of a cardiac pacemaker and thus may adversely affect patients with cardiac pacemakers. The electromagnetic field emitted by nonthermal PSWD devices can also interfere with other electromedical and electronic devices. Therefore PSWD should not be used over or near medical electronic devices, including pacemakers, and should be used with caution with and around patients with other external or implanted medical electronic devices.

Nonthermal PSWD devices can be used to treat soft tissue adjacent to most metal implants without significantly heating the metal; however, when the metal forms closed loops, as occurs with the wires used for fixating rods and plates in surgical fracture repairs, heating may occur because current can flow in the wire loops. Therefore if a patient has a metal implant, the clinician should determine the type of implant before applying PSWD.

Ask the Patient
- Do you have a pacemaker or any other metal in your body?

Assess
• Check the patient's chart for any information regarding a pacemaker or other metal implants.

If the patient has a pacemaker or is using other medical electronic devices, PSWD should not be used except in extreme circumstances, such as when trying to save a limb from amputation. When considering the use of PSWD in such circumstances, the patient's physician should be consulted, and the clinician should try to shield all medical electronic devices from the electromagnetic field. In the presence of metal implants, an x-ray should be requested and treatment with PSWD should not be done if the metal forms loops. If the patient has nonlooping metal implants, PSWD may be applied with caution.

PRECAUTIONS FOR THE USE OF ALL FORMS OF DIATHERMY

PRECAUTIONS

for the Use of All Forms of Diathermy
• Near electronic or magnetic equipment
• Obesity
• Copper-bearing intrauterine contraceptive devices

Near Electronic or Magnetic Equipment

A number of studies and reports have demonstrated the presence of unwanted electrical and magnetic radiation around diathermy applicators.[88-91] Because the treatment field may interfere with any electronic or magnetic equipment, such as computers or computer-controlled medical devices, it is recommended that the leads and applicators of diathermy devices be at least 3 m and preferably 5 m from other electrical equipment. Precise guidelines are not available because interference depends on the exact arrangement and the shielding of both the diathermy device and the other equipment being used. If interference occurs, then the two types of equipment should be used at different times.

Obesity

Diathermy should be used with caution in obese patients because it may heat fat excessively. Capacitive plate applicators, which generally result in greater increases in the temperature of fat than other types of applicators, should not be used with obese patients.[5,92]

Copper-Bearing Intrauterine Contraceptive Devices

Although copper-bearing intrauterine contraceptive devices do contain a small amount of metal, calculations and in vivo measurements have shown that these devices and the surrounding tissue increase only slightly in temperature when exposed to therapeutic levels of diathermy.[93,94] Therefore diathermy may be used by therapists and by patients with such devices.

PRECAUTIONS FOR THE USE OF NONTHERMAL PULSED SHORTWAVE DIATHERMY

PRECAUTIONS

for the Use of Nonthermal Pulsed Shortwave Diathermy
• Pregnancy
• Skeletal immaturity

The use of thermal-level diathermy is contraindicated during pregnancy. In addition, because the effects of electromagnetic energy on fetal or child development are not known, nonthermal PSWD should also be used with caution during pregnancy and in skeletally immature patients.

PRECAUTIONS FOR THE USE OF THE THERAPIST APPLYING DIATHERMY

There is concern regarding potential hazards to therapists applying diathermy because of their greater exposure as a result of treating multiple patients throughout the day. These devices produce diffuse radiation and can thus irradiate the therapist if she or he is standing close to the machine.[90,91] It is therefore recommended that therapists stay at least 1 to 2 m away from all continuous diathermy applicators, at least 30 to 50 cm away from all PSWD applicators, and out of the direct beam of any MWD device during patient treatment.[95-97]

Some reports have noted above-average rates of spontaneous abortion and abnormal fetal development in therapists after the use of SWD equipment; however, other studies have failed to demonstrate a statistically significant correlation between SWD exposure and either congenital malformation or spontaneous abortion.[98,99] One comparison of SWD and MWD exposure of therapists found that only MWD increased the risk of miscarriage.[100] However, a recent study found that shortwaves have potentially harmful effects on pregnancy outcome and are specifically associated with low birth weight. This effect increased in a dose-related manner.[101] On balance, given the current research findings, it is recommended that therapists avoid SWD and MWD exposure during pregnancy.[102]

Malignancy and Electromagnetic Fields

Substantial controversy exists regarding the effects of electromagnetic fields on malignancy. The literature on this topic is primarily concerned with the risks associated with living near and working with power lines. Although some reports suggest that the electromagnetic fields generated from power lines may be linked to childhood cancers and leukemia, others have failed to show such an association.[103,104] In 1995, the Council of the American Physical Society (APS) determined that "The scientific literature and the reports of reviews by other panels show no consistent, significant link between cancer and power line fields. . . . No plausible biophysical mechanisms for the systematic initiation or promotion of cancer by these power line fields have been identified." In 2005, they reviewed and again supported this opinion, stating that "Since that time, there have been several large in vivo studies of animal populations subjected for their life span to high magnetic fields and epidemiological studies, done with larger populations and with direct, rather than surrogate, measurements of the magnetic field exposure. These studies have produced no results that change the earlier assessment by APS. In addition, no biophysical mechanisms for the initiation or promotion of cancer by electric or magnetic fields from power lines have been identified."[105]

The electromagnetic fields associated with power lines are of much lower frequency (50 to 60 Hz) than those used in pulsed or continuous SWD devices (27.12 MHz); thus the application of the data from the studies on power lines to the effects of SWD are limited. At this time, there are no recommendations against using nonthermal levels of PSWD in the area of a malignancy, and there are no indications that PSWD is carcinogenic.

ADVERSE EFFECTS OF DIATHERMY

BURNS
Diathermy can cause soft tissue burns when used at normal or excessive doses, and because the distribution of this type of energy varies significantly with the type of tissue, it can burn some layers of tissue while sparing others.[106]

Fat layers are at the greatest risk of burning, particularly when capacitive plate applicators are used, because they are more effectively heated by this type of device and because fat is less well-vascularized than muscle or skin and therefore is not cooled as effectively by vasodilation. Because water is preferentially heated by all forms of diathermy, the patient's skin should be kept dry by wrapping with towels to avoid scalding from hot perspiration.

◎ Clinical Pearl
To avoid burns during the application of diathermy the patient's skin must be kept dry by wrapping with towels.

APPLICATION TECHNIQUES
Thermal-level diathermy is the most effective modality for increasing the temperature of large areas of deep tissue. Therefore treatment with this physical agent is most appropriate when the goal(s) of treatment can be achieved by increasing the temperature of large areas of deep tissue.

Nonthermal PSWD can reduce pain and edema and may accelerate tissue healing. It can be used at the acute, subacute, and chronic stages of an injury; however, the literature and anecdotal reports suggest that better results are achieved when acute conditions are treated. Although not documented in the literature, favorable results have also been reported anecdotally for patients with lymphedema, cerebrovascular accidents, and reflex sympathetic dystrophy (RSD).

APPLICATION TECHNIQUE 14-1	DIATHERMY

Procedure

1. Evaluate the patient's problem and determine the goals of treatment.
2. Determine that diathermy is the most appropriate intervention.

    Because diathermy induces an electrical current in the tissues without touching the patient's body, the use of this physical agent may be particularly appropriate in cases where direct contact with the patient is not possible or desirable—for example, if infection control is an issue, if the patient cannot tolerate direct contact with the skin, or if the area is in a cast. Because heat accumulates with the application of nonthermal PSWD and because little or no sensation is associated with its use, nonthermal PSWD can be used where heat is contraindicated or potentially hazardous and can be applied to insensate patients or to those who cannot tolerate the sensations associated with other physical agents such as cryotherapy or electrical stimulation.

3. Determine that diathermy is not contraindicated.
4. Select the most appropriate diathermy device.

    Choose between a thermal and a nonthermal device according to the desired effects of the treatment and the different types of applicators (inductive coil, capacitive plate, or magnetron) according to the desired depth of penetration and the tissue to be treated.

See later section for more information on selecting a diathermy device.

5. Explain the procedure and the reason for applying diathermy to the patient and the sensations the patient can expect to feel.

    During the application of thermal-level diathermy, the patient should feel a comfortable sensation of mild warmth without any increase in pain or discomfort.

    The application of nonthermal PSWD is not generally associated with any change in patient sensation, although some patients report feeling slight tingling or mild warmth. This sensation may be the result of increased local circulation in response to the treatment.

6. Remove all metal jewelry and clothing from the area to be treated.

    All clothing with metal fastenings or components, such as buttons, zippers, or clips, must be removed from the treatment area. Nonmetal clothing, bandages, or casts do not need to be removed before treatment with diathermy because magnetic fields penetrate these materials unaltered; however, when thermal-level diathermy is used, it is recommended that clothing be removed from the area so that towels can be applied to absorb local sweating.

Continued

7. Clean and dry the skin and inspect it if necessary.
8. Position the patient comfortably on a chair or plinth with no metal components. Position the patient so that the area to be treated is readily accessible.
9. If applying thermal-level diathermy, wrap the area to be treated with toweling to absorb local perspiration. If applying nonthermal PSWD, it is not necessary to place towels between the applicator and the body, but a disposable cloth or plastic covering can be used over the applicator when treating conditions in which there is a risk of cross-contamination or infection.
10. Position the device and the applicator(s) for effective and safe treatment application. See later section for more information on positioning.
11. Tune the device.

SWD devices allow tuning of the applicator to each particular load. Tuning adjusts the precise frequency of the device, within the accepted range, to optimize coupling between the device and the load. Most modern diathermy devices tune automatically. To tune a device that requires manual tuning, first turn it on and allow it to warm up according to the manufacturer's directions; then turn up the intensity to a low level and adjust the tuning dial until a maximal reading on the power/intensity indicator is obtained.

12. Select the appropriate treatment parameters.

When applying thermal-level diathermy, the intensity should be adjusted to produce a sensation of mild warmth in the patient. The gauge of heating used in clinical practice is the patient's reported sensation because calculations of energy delivery and temperature increases are not reliable.[107] The pattern of energy and heat distribution by both SWD and MWD is difficult to predict because it is influenced by the amount of reflection, the electrical properties of different types of tissue in the field, the tissue size and composition, the frequency of the field, and the type, size, geometry, and orientation of the applicator. This issue is further complicated by evidence that the thermal sensation threshold may be affected by the frequency of radiation applied.[107] Thermal-level diathermy is generally applied for about 20 minutes.

> **◎ Clinical Pearl**
>
> Thermal-level diathermy is usually applied for 20 minutes.

When applying nonthermal PSWD, most clinicians select the intensity, pulse frequency, and total treatment time based on the manufacturer's recommendations and on their individual experience because the clinical research using these devices does not indicate clearly which parameters are most effective. Most manufacturers and studies recommend using the maximum strength and frequency available on the device for all conditions and if the patient reports any discomfort, reducing the pulse rate until the discomfort resolves. Most nonthermal PSWD treatments are administered for 30 to 60 minutes once or twice a day, 5 to 7 times a week.

> **◎ Clinical Pearl**
>
> PSWD is usually applied for 30 to 60 minutes, once or twice daily.

Two similar nonthermal PSWD devices manufactured in the US have 6 intensity settings, to provide various field strengths, and 6 pulse frequency settings, to provide between 80 and 600 65 μsecond long pulses.[108,109] Another SWD device (Mettler Electronics, Anaheim, CA) can be used for application of PSWD and allows adjustment of pulse duration, frequency and field strength (as defined by the maximum power during a pulse).

13. Provide the patient with a bell or other means to call for assistance during treatment and a means to turn off the diathermy device. Instruct the patient to turn off the device and call immediately if he or she experiences excessive heating or an increase in pain or discomfort.
14. After 5 minutes, check to be certain that the patient is not too hot or is experiencing any increase in symptoms.
15. When the treatment is complete, turn off the device, remove the applicator and towels, and inspect the treatment area. It is normal for the area to appear slightly red, and it may also feel warm to the touch.
16. Assess the outcome of the intervention.

Reassess the patient, checking particularly for any signs of burning and for progress toward the goals of treatment. Remeasure quantifiable subjective complaints and objective impairments and disabilities.

17. Document the treatment.

POSITIONING

Inductive Applicator

When positioning an inductive applicator with a cable, the cable should be wrapped around the towel-covered limb to be treated, with the turns of the cable spaced at least 3 cm apart. Rubber or wooden spacers should be used to ensure that adjacent turns of the cable do not come into contact with each other.

Alternatively, the cable can be coiled into a flat spiral approximately the size of the area to be treated. Spacers can be used to separate adjacent pieces of cable to ensure that adjacent turns of the cable do not come into contact with each other. The coil should be placed over the area to be treated and separated by six to eight layers of towels (Fig. 14-12).

With a drum applicator, the drum should be placed directly over and close to the skin or tissues to be treated, with a slight air gap to allow for heat dissipation. Contact should be avoided when infection control is an issue. The center of the applicator should be placed over the area to be treated. The treatment surface of the applicator should be placed facing and as parallel to the tissues being treated as possible.

The patient should be advised to move as little as possible during the treatment because the strength of the field will change if the distance between the applicator and the treatment area changes, decreasing in proportion to the square of the distance between the treatment surface of the applicator and the tissues being treated (see Fig. 14-4). For example, if the distance doubles, the strength of the magnetic field will decrease by a factor of four. Thus

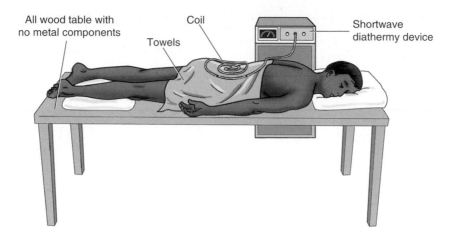

FIG 14-12 Inductive coil applicator for shortwave diathermy. Set-up with "pancake" coil on the patient's back. Note the layer of towels.

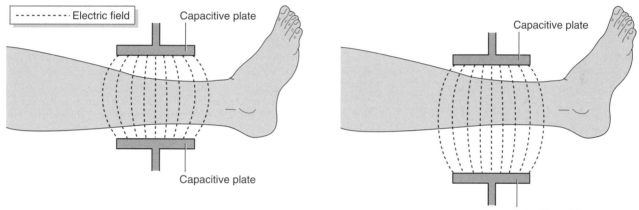

FIG 14-13 Electric field distribution in tissue with evenly and unevenly placed capacitive shortwave diathermy plates.

	Thermal			**Nonthermal**
TABLE 14-3	**Comparison of Different Types of Diathermy Devices**			
Type	**Shortwave**		**Microwave**	**Pulsed shortwave**
Frequency	27.12 MHz*		2450 MHz	27.12 MHz
Applicator	Inductive coil	Capacitive plate	Magnetron	Inductive coil drum
Incident field	Electromagnetic	Electric	Electromagnetic	Electromagnetic
Tissues most affected	Deep and superficial	Superficial	Small areas	Deep and superficial

*Shortwave diathermy can also have a frequency of 13.56 or 40.68 MHz; however, the most commonly used frequency is 27.12 MHz.

maintaining the applicator at a constant distance from the patient is important for consistent treatment.

Capacitive Applicator

The two plates of a capacitive applicator should be placed at an equal distance on either side of the area to be treated, approximately 2 to 10 cm (1 to 3 inches) from the skin surface (see Fig. 14-8). Equal placement at a slight distance from the body is recommended for even field distribution in the treatment area because the field is most concentrated near the plates. Unequal placement will result in uneven heating, with the areas closest to the plate becoming hotter than those farther from the plate (Fig. 14-13).

Magnetron Microwave Applicator

The magnetron microwave applicator should be placed a few inches from the area to be treated and directed toward the area, with the beam perpendicular to the patient's skin.

DOCUMENTATION

The following should be documented:
- Area of the body treated
- Frequency range
- Average power or power setting
- Pulse rate
- Time of irradiation

- Type of applicator
- Treatment duration
- Patient positioning
- Distance of the applicator from the patient
- Patient's response to the treatment

Documentation is typically written in the SOAP note (Subjective, Objective, Assessment, Plan) format. The following examples summarize only the modality component of treatment and are not intended to represent a comprehensive plan of care.

EXAMPLES

When applying SWD to the low back, document the following:

S: Pt reports low back pain at level 7/10.

O: Pretreatment: Limited lumbar ROM in all planes, limited by pain.

Intervention: 27.12 MHz continuous SWD, power level 3, to low back, drum applicator 3 in from patient, patient prone, 20 min.

Posttreatment: Report of mild warmth, pain decreased to 4/10.

A: Pt tolerated SWD well, with dec low back pain.

P: Continue SWD as above before ther ex program.

When applying microwave diathermy to the posterior left (L) knee, document the following:

S: Pt reports stiffness and pain with L knee extension.

O: Pretreatment: L knee extension ROM −40 degrees.

Intervention: 2450 MHz continuous MWD to posterior knee, 3 in from skin surface, power level 4, 15 min. Patient prone with 3 lb cuff weight at ankle.

Posttreatment: Extension ROM increased to −30 degrees.

A: Pt tolerated MWD well, with increased ROM.

P: Continue MWD as above, followed by active ROM exercises into extension.

When applying pulsed SWD to ulcer on the lateral aspect of the right (R) distal leg, document the following:

S: Pt reports he is scheduled to have a cardiac pacemaker implanted in 2 weeks.

O: Pretreatment: R distal LE lateral ulcer 9 × 5 cm.

Intervention: PSWD intensity 6, pulse rate 600 pps, to R distal leg in area of venous insufficiency ulcer, applicator 3 in from lateral leg, 45 min.

Posttreatment: Ulcer dimensions decreased to 7 × 4 cm over last week.

A: Pt tolerated PSWD well, with decreased ulcer size.

P: Continue PSWD as above 1× per day. Discontinue PSWD component of care after pacemaker is implanted.

SELECTING A DIATHERMY DEVICE

When considering purchasing a diathermy device, the first consideration should be whether it outputs a thermal or nonthermal level of energy, or both (Table 14-3). The Food and Drug Administration (FDA) differentiates between diathermy devices according to their thermal or nonthermal mechanism of action. Specifically, the FDA separates diathermy devices into "diathermy for use in applying therapeutic deep heat for selected medical conditions" and "diathermy intended for the treatment of medical conditions by means other than the generation of deep heat."[109]

When purchasing a device intended for thermal treatments, one should consider the type of applicator (plates, coils, or drum), the frequency band of the energy (shortwave or microwave), and whether the device is self-tuning. In general, drums are the easiest to apply, although coils may provide deeper penetration when applied to the limbs. SWD is generally preferred over MWD because it has a more predictable distribution pattern and self-tuning devices provide greater ease of use.

The nonthermal PSWD devices currently manufactured in the US are similar. They have peak powers between 150 and 400 W, allow adjustment of pulse frequency between 10 and 800 pps and adjustment of pulse duration between 65 μs and 2 ms. Depending on the combination of peak power, pulse frequency, and pulse duration selected, these devices may deliver thermal or nonthermal treatment. If the average power (peak power × pulse duration × pulse frequency) is set to be less than 38 W, then the treatment will be nonthermal.

CLINICAL CASE STUDIES

The following case studies summarize the concepts of diathermy discussed in this chapter. Based on the scenario presented, an evaluation of the clinical findings and goals of treatment are proposed. These are followed by a discussion of the factors to be considered in the selection of diathermy as the indicated intervention, the ideal diathermy device, and the parameters to promote progress toward the goals.

CASE STUDY 14-1

Adhesive Capsulitis
Examination
History

SJ is a 45-year-old physical therapist. She has been diagnosed with adhesive capsulitis of the right shoulder and has been referred to physical therapy. She reports shoulder stiffness, with a tight sensation at the end of range. Although she is able to perform most of her work functions, she has difficulty reaching overhead, which interferes with placing objects on high shelves and with serving when playing tennis, and she has difficulty reaching behind her to fasten clothing.

Tests and Measures

The objective examination reveals restricted right shoulder active ROM (AROM) and passive ROM (PROM) and restricted passive glenohumeral joint inferior and posterior gliding. All other tests, including cervical and elbow ROM and upper extremity strength and sensation, are within normal limits.

CLINICAL CASE STUDIES—*cont'd*

Shoulder ROM		
	R	**L**
AROM		
Flexion	120°	170°
Abduction	100°	170°
Hand behind back	R 5 inches below L	—
PROM		
Flexion	130°	175°
Abduction	110°	175°
Internal rotation	50°	80°
External rotation	10°	80°

What are some reasonable goals of treatment for this patient? What type of diathermy would be most appropriate? How would you position the patient during treatment? What should be done in addition to diathermy?

Evaluation, Diagnosis, Prognosis, and Goals
Evaluation and Goals

ICF Level	Current Status	Goals
Body structure and function	Restricted right shoulder ROM Restricted right glenohumeral passive intraarticular gliding	Increase right shoulder passive and active ROM
Activity	Difficulty reaching and lifting over her head and behind her back	Improve patient's ability to place objects on overhead shelves, get dressed without assistance
Participation	Decreased tennis playing Difficulty dressing	Return patient to playing tennis Dresses with ease

Diagnosis
Preferred Practice Pattern 4D: Impaired joint mobility, motor function, muscle performance, and ROM associated with connective tissue dysfunction.

Prognosis/Plan of Care
The goals of treatment at this time are to regain full AROM and PROM of the right shoulder and to return to full sports participation and daily living activities. The loss of active and passive joint motion associated with adhesive capsulitis is thought to be a result of adhesion and loss of length of the anterior inferior joint capsule. Effective treatment should attempt to increase the length of the joint capsule. Increasing tissue temperature before stretching will increase the extensibility of soft tissue, allowing the greatest increase in soft tissue length with the least force while minimizing the risk of tissue damage. Diathermy is the optimal modality for heating the shoulder capsule because this thermal agent can reach large areas of deep tissue. A superficial heating agent, such as a hot pack, would not be as effective because it does not increase the temperature of tissue at the depth of the joint capsule, and ultrasound would not generally be as effective because its heating is limited by the effective radiating area of the sound head.

Intervention
A continuous diathermy device must be used to increase tissue temperature. An SWD device with an inductive coil applicator in a drum form is recommended because this mode of application provides deep, even heat distribution and is easy to apply. The device should be applied to the right shoulder, ideally with the shoulder positioned at end of range flexion and abduction to apply a gentle stretch to the anterior inferior capsule. The diathermy device should be set to produce a sensation of mild, comfortable warmth, and the treatment should be applied for approximately 20 minutes. This diathermy treatment should be followed immediately by a low-load, prolonged stretch to maximize ROM gains.

Documentation
S: *Patient reports R shoulder stiffness and a diagnosis of adhesive capsulitis.*

O: Pretreatment: *R shoulder decreased AROM and PROM when compared with L for flexion, abduction, internal rotation, external rotation (see above for measurements).*

Intervention: *27.12 MHz continuous SWD, power level 3, to R shoulder, drum applicator 3 in from patient, patient sitting with R shoulder at end of range flexion and abduction × 20 min followed by 10 min low-load prolonged stretch.*

Posttreatment: *R shoulder flexion PROM increased from 120 to 140 degrees, abduction increased from 100 to 120 degrees.*

A: *Pt tolerated SWD well, noting a sensation of warmth, increased PROM after treatment.*

P: *Continue SWD 3 times weekly as above until patient regains full PROM and returns to prior level of function.*

CASE STUDY 14-2

Acute Ankle Inversion Sprain
Examination
History
MB is a 24-year-old woman recreational soccer player who sustained a grade II left ankle inversion sprain approximately 48 hours ago. She has been applying ice and a compression bandage to the ankle, resting and elevating the ankle as much as possible, and using a cane to reduce weight bearing when walking. She has been referred to physical therapy to attain a pain-free return to sports as rapidly as possible. She reports moderate pain at the lateral ankle that is aggravated by weight bearing and ankle swelling that is aggravated when her ankle is in a dependent position.

Continued

Tests and Measures

The objective examination reveals a mild increase in superficial skin temperature at the left lateral ankle and edema of the left ankle, with a girth of 25.5 cm (10 inches) on the left compared with 21.5 cm (8.5 inches) on the right. Left ankle ROM is restricted in all planes, with 0 degrees dorsiflexion on the left and 10 degrees on the right, 20 degrees plantar flexion on the left and 45 degrees on the right, 10 degrees inversion on the left, with pain at the lateral ankle at the end of range, and 30 degrees on the right, and 20 degrees eversion on the left and 30 degrees on the right. Isometric testing of muscle strength against manual resistance at midrange revealed no abnormalities.

What are the goals of treatment at this time? What type of diathermy is appropriate? What type of diathermy is contraindicated for this patient? How would you position this patient during treatment? What else should this patient do?

Evaluation, Diagnosis, Prognosis, and Goals
Evaluation and Goals

ICF Level	Current Status	Goals
Body structure and function	Left ankle pain, swelling, increased temperature, decreased ROM	Decrease symptoms and regain normal ROM
Activity	Decreased weight-bearing tolerance, limited ambulation	Return to normal ambulation and weight-bearing
Participation	Unable to play soccer	Return to playing soccer in 4 weeks

Diagnosis

Preferred Practice Pattern 4D: Impaired joint mobility, motor function, muscle performance, and ROM associated with connective tissue dysfunction.

Prognosis/Plan of Care

The goals of treatment at this time are to control pain, resolve edema, and restore normal ROM for the patient to return to full sports participation. The diagnosis of a grade II ankle sprain indicates that there has been some damage to the ankle ligaments; therefore the goals of treatment should also include healing of these soft tissues.

Nonthermal PSWD is an indicated adjunctive treatment for pain and edema and has also been shown to accelerate soft tissue healing. Because this patient is already applying rest, ice, compression, and elevation (RICE) to her ankle at home and desires a rapid return to full sports participation, the addition of PSWD treatment may help maximize her rate of recovery. Thermal-level diathermy should not be applied to this patient because the use of all thermal agents is contraindicated in the presence of acute injury or inflammation.

Intervention

It is proposed that treatment with nonthermal PSWD be started immediately after the evaluation to reduce pain and swelling. The patient's limb should be placed in a comfortable elevated position to optimize the reduction of swelling. The PSWD applicator should be positioned over the lateral aspect of the ankle, as close to the skin as possible, with the center of the applicator over the area of the ankle presenting with the most marked swelling and as parallel as possible to the damaged tissues.

Daily application of PSWD for 30 minutes, with power and pulse rate settings of 6, is generally used for treatment of this type of acute injury. If the patient complains of any increase in discomfort, the pulse rate should be decreased until the discomfort resolves. The PSWD treatment can be followed by the application of ice, after which the ankle should be wrapped in a compression bandage. The patient should continue with RICE and should be instructed in appropriate ambulation, weight bearing, and ROM exercises. She may also need to wear a splint if the ankle is unstable.

Documentation

S: *Patient sustained a grade II L ankle inversion sprain 48 hours ago, has been applying RICE, and reports L ankle pain, swelling, and decreased weight-bearing tolerance.*

O: Pretreatment: *L ankle girth 25.5 cm, R ankle girth 21.5 cm. L ankle ROM restricted in all planes, with 0 degrees dorsiflexion, 20 degrees plantar flexion, 10 degrees inversion with pain at the lateral ankle at the end of range, and 20 degrees eversion.*

Intervention: *PSWD to L lateral ankle, 3 in from skin, power and pulse settings of 6, for 30 min. Ice and compression applied after PSWD.*

Posttreatment: *Mildly improved L ankle ROM, ankle circumference unchanged.*

A: *Pt experienced no discomfort with treatment.*

P: *Continue daily PSWD and RICE protocol at all other times. Patient will be instructed in ambulation, weight bearing, and ROM exercises.*

CASE STUDY 14-3

Sacral Pressure Ulcer
Examination
History

FG is an 85-year-old man with a stage IV sacral pressure ulcer. He is bedridden, minimally responsive, and dependent for all bed mobility and feeding activities. He is able to swallow but eats poorly. Treatment until this time has consisted of sharp débridement and hydrocolloid dressings. Although this treatment has resulted in a reduction of the yellow slough, there has been little change in wound area over the last month.

Tests and Measures

The pressure ulcer is 15 × 8 cm and 3 cm deep in the deepest area. There is no tunneling or undermining. Approximately 70% of the wound bed is red and granulating, and 30% is covered with yellow slough.

What are reasonable goals of treatment for this patient? What type of diathermy should be used and why? How often should diathermy be applied? What other aspects of wound care are important for this patient?

Evaluation, Diagnosis, Prognosis, and Goals
Evaluation and Goals

ICF Level	Current Status	Goals
Body structure and function	Sacral ulcer (impaired tissue integrity), reduced strength	Achieve a completely red wound base (short-term), decrease ulcer size (long-term), wound closure (long-term)
Activity	Bedridden, poor appetite, at risk for infection	Prevent infection
Participation	Dependent for bed mobility and eating	Decrease patient's medical care requirements

Diagnosis

Preferred Practice Pattern 7E: Impaired integumentary integrity associated with skin involvement extending into fascia, muscle, or bone and scar formation.

Prognosis/Plan of Care

Nonthermal PSWD has been shown to accelerate the healing of chronic open wounds, including pressure ulcers. One advantage of this treatment modality over other adjunctive treatments is that it can be applied without removing the dressing, thus limiting the mechanical and temperature disturbance to the wound and reducing the time required to set up the treatment. Also, because nonthermal PSWD produces little sensation, it can be applied even if the patient is insensate or cognitively incapable of giving sensory feedback about the treatment. Limiting the mechanical disruption of the wound is particularly important in this case because 70% of the wound bed is covered with red granulation tissue that is fragile but does have the potential to heal.

Intervention

A comprehensive wound care program that addresses pressure relief, dressings, the nutritional status of the patient, and débridement, when necessary, is required to optimize the healing of this patient's wound. Nonthermal PSWD may be used as an adjunct to these interventions to facilitate wound healing and closure. The patient should be positioned with the treatment surface of the applicator as close and as parallel to the tissues to be treated as possible, with the center of the applicator over the deepest part of the wound. The wound dressing may be left in place. If tunneling were present, the center of the applicator should be positioned over the deepest portion of the tunnel to promote closure of the tunnel before the more superficial wound site closes. The treatment surface of the applicator head can be covered with a plastic bag or surgical covering if infection control is an issue. It is recommended that this wound be treated either twice a day for 30 minutes or once a day for 45 to 60 minutes. If the patient appears to have any discomfort, the pulse rate should be lowered. The pulse rate setting should also be reduced if the surface of the wound appears to be closing before the depth of the wound has completely filled.

Documentation

S: *Bedridden, poorly responsive pt with stage IV sacral pressure ulcer.*

O: **Pretreatment:** *Sacral ulcer 15 × 8 cm and 3 cm deep in the deepest area. No tunneling or underminimg. 70% of the wound bed is red and granulating, and 30% is covered with yellow slough.*

Intervention: *PSWD twice daily for 30 min to sacral ulcer, power 6 and pulse rate 600 pps, pt prone, applicator covered with sheath and 3 in from wound.*

Posttreatment: *Wound appears unchanged after 2 treatments.*

A: *PSWD applied with no noticeable adverse effects.*

P: *Continue PSWD twice daily for 1 more week. Continue if wound improves, discontinue if no benefit appreciated.*

CHAPTER REVIEW

1. Diathermy is the application of shortwave or microwave electromagnetic energy to a person's body.
2. The effects of diathermy may be thermal or nonthermal. Continuous diathermy produces thermal effects and is used for heating large areas of deep tissue. PSWD is generally used to produce nonthermal effects and may provide pain control, edema reduction, decreased symptoms of osteoarthritis, and accelerated wound, nerve, and bone healing.
3. Contraindications for the use of diathermy depend on whether the application is thermal or nonthermal. Diathermy is contraindicated for both thermal and nonthermal applications if a patient has implanted or transcutaneous neural stimulators (including cardiac pacemakers) or is pregnant. Contraindications for thermal-level diathermy include metal implants, malignancy, and application over the eyes, testes, and growing epiphyses. Contraindications for nonthermal diathermy include application to deep tissue such as

organs, as a substitute for conventional therapy for edema and pain, and the presence of electronic devices, or metal implants.

4. Precautions for all forms of diathermy include electronic or magnetic equipment in the vicinity, obesity, and copper-bearing intrauterine contraceptive devices. Precautions for the use of PSWD include pregnancy and skeletal immaturity.

5. The reader is referred to the Evolve web site for further exercises and links to resources and references.

ADDITIONAL RESOURCES *evolve*

Web Sites

Accelerated Care Plus: Manufacturer of a thermal and nonthermal SWD unit. The web site has information on that unit and has useful links to professional organizations and medical databases. www.acplus.com

Mettler Electronics: This company produces thermal and nonthermal SWD units, and their website includes information and specifications on their products. www.mettlerelectronics.com

GLOSSARY *evolve*

Continuous shortwave diathermy (SWD): The clinical application of continuous shortwave electromagnetic radiation to increase tissue temperature.

Diathermy: The application of shortwave or microwave electromagnetic energy to increase tissue temperature, particularly in deep tissues.

Duty cycle: The proportion of time energy is being delivered.

$$\text{Duty cycle} = \text{on time}/[\text{on time} + \text{off time}]$$

Inductive coil applicator: A coil through which an alternating electric current flows producing a magnetic field perpendicular to the coil and, in turn, inducing electric eddy currents in the tissue within or in front of the coil. This type of applicator can be used to apply shortwave diathermy.

Low-frequency electromagnetic radiation: Electromagnetic radiation that is nonionizing and that cannot break molecular bonds or produce ions. This includes extremely low frequency waves, shortwaves, microwaves, infrared, visible light, and ultraviolet.

Magnetron: An applicator that produces a high-frequency alternating current in an antenna. This type of applicator is used to apply microwave diathermy.

Microwave radiation: Nonionizing electromagnetic radiation with a frequency range 300 MHz to 300 GHz, which lies between the ranges of radiofrequency and IR radiation.

Pulsed shortwave diathermy (PSWD): The clinical application of pulsed shortwave electromagnetic radiation in which heating is not the therapeutic mechanism of action.

Shortwave radiation: Nonionizing electromagnetic radiation with a frequency range of approximately 3 to 30 MHz. Shortwave is a band within the radiofrequency range. The radiofrequency range lies between ELF and microwave radiation.

REFERENCES *evolve*

1. Hitchcock RT, Patterson RM: *Radio-frequency and ELF electromagnetic energies: a handbook for health professionals*, New York, 1995, Van Nostrand Reinhold.

2. Silverman DR, Pendleton LA: A comparison of the effects of continuous and pulsed shortwave diathermy on peripheral circulation, *Arch Phys Med Rehabil* 49:429-436, 1968.

3. Conradi E, Pages IH: Effects of continuous and pulsed microwave irradiation on distribution of heat in the gluteal region of minipigs, *Scand J Rehabil Med* 21:59-62, 1989.

4. Draper DO, Knight K, Fujiwara T, et al: Temperature change in human muscle during and after pulsed short-wave diathermy, *J Orthop Sports Phys Ther* 29(1):13-18; discussion 19-22, 1999.

5. Kloth LC, Zisken MC: Diathermy and pulsed radio frequency radiation. In Michlovitz SL, ed: *Thermal agents in rehabilitation*, Philadelphia, 1996, FA Davis.

6. Verrier M, Falconer K, Crawford SJ: A comparison of tissue temperature following two shortwave diathermy techniques, *Physiotherapy Canada* 29(1):21-25, 1977.

7. Guy AW, Lehmann JF, Stonebridge JB: Therapeutic applications of electromagnetic power, *Proc IEEE* 62:55-75, 1974.

8. Van der Esch M, Hoogland R: *Pulsed shortwave diathermy with the Curapuls 419*, Delft, Netherlands, 1990, Delft Instruments Physical Medicine BV.

9. Hand JW: Biophysics and technology of electromagnetic hyperthermia. In Guthrie M, ed: *Methods of external hyperthermic heating*, Berlin, 1990, Springer-Verlag.

10. McMeeken JM, Bell C: Effects of selective blood and tissue heating on blood flow in the dog hind limb, *Exp Physiol* 75:359-366, 1990.

11. Fadilah R, Pinkas J, Weinberger A, et al: Heating rabbit joint by microwave applicator, *Arch Phys Med Rehabil* 68(10):710-712, 1987.

12. Scott RS, Chou CK, McCumber M, et al: Complications resulting from spurious fields produced by a microwave applicator used for hyperthermia, *Int J Radiat Oncol Biol Phys* 12(10):1883-1886, 1986.

13. Murray CC, Kitchen S: Effect of pulse repetition rate on the perception of thermal sensation with pulsed shortwave diathermy, *Physiother Res Int* 5(2):73-84, 2000.

14. Garrett CL, Draper DO, Knight KL: Heat distribution in the lower leg from pulsed short-wave diathermy and ultrasound treatments, *J Athl Train* 35(1):50-55, 2000.

15. Draper DO, Knight K, Fujiwara T, et al: Temperature change in human muscle during and after pulsed short-wave diathermy, *J Orthop Sports Phys Ther* 29(1):13-18; discussion 19-22, 1999.

16. McNiven DR, Wyper DJ: Microwave therapy and muscle blood flow in man, *J Microwave Power* 11:168, 1976.

17. McMeeken JM, Bell C: Microwave irradiation of the human forearm and hand, *Physiother Theory Practice* 75:359-366, 1990.

18. Wyper DJ, McNiven DR: Effects of some physiotherapeutic agents on skeletal muscle blood flow, *Physiotherapy* 60(10):309-310, 1976.

19. Benson TB, Copp EP: The effect of therapeutic forms of heat and ice on the pain threshold of the normal shoulder, *Rheumatol Rehabil* 13:101-104, 1974.

20. Abramson DL, Chu LSW, Tuck S, et al: Effect of tissue temperature and blood flow on motor nerve conduction velocity, *J Am Med Soc* 198:1082-1088, 1966.

21. Chastain PB: The effect of deep heat on isometric strength, *Phys Ther* 58(5):543-546, 1978.

22. McMeeken JM, Bell C: Effects of microwave irradiation on blood flow in the dog hind limb, *Exp Physiol* 75:367-374, 1990.

23. Adair ER, Blick DW, Allen SJ, et al: Thermophysiological responses of human volunteers to whole body RF exposure at 220 MHz, *Bioelectromagnetics* 26(6):448-461, 2005.

24. Adair ER, Mylacraine KS, Allen SJ: Thermophysiological consequences of whole body resonant RF exposure (100 MHz) in human volunteers, *Bioelectromagnetics* 24(7):489-501, 2003.

25. Hayne CR: Pulsed high frequency energy: its place in physiotherapy, *Physiotherapy* 70(12):459-466, 1984.
26. Markov MS: Electric current electromagnetic field effects on soft tissue: implications for wound healing, *Wounds* 7(3):94-110, 1995.
27. Pilla AA, Markov MS: Bioeffects of weak electromagnetic fields, *Rev Environ Health* 10(3-4):155-169, 1994.
28. Mayrovitz HN, Larsen PB: A preliminary study to evaluate the effect of pulsed radio frequency field treatment on lower extremity peri-ulcer skin microcirculation of diabetic patients, *Wounds* 7(3):90-93, 1995.
29. Mayrovitz HN, Larsen PB: Effects of pulsed electromagnetic fields on skin microvascular blood perfusion, *Wounds* 4(5):197-202, 1992.
30. Rozengurt E, Mendoza S: Monovalent ion fluxes and the control of cell proliferation in cultured fibroblasts, *Ann NY Acad Sci* 339:175-190, 1980.
31. Boonstra J, Skper SD, Varons SJ: Regulation of Na+, K+ pump activity by nerve growth factor in chick embryo dorsal root ganglia cells, *J Cell Physiol* 113:452-455, 1982.
32. Gemsa D, Seitz M, Kramer W, et al: Ionophore A 23187 rasis cyclic AMP levels in macrophages by stimulation of prostaglandin E formation, *Exp Cell Res* 118:55-62, 1979.
33. Pilla A: Electrochemical information and energy transfer in vivo, Proceedings of the seventh IECEC, Washington, DC, 1972, American Chemical Society.
34. Markov MS, Muechsam DJ, Pilla AA: Modulation of cell-free myosin phosphorylation with pulsed radio frequency electromagnetic fields. In Allen MJ, Cleary SF, Sowers AE, eds: *Charge and field effects in biosystems*, ed 4, Singapore, 1995, World Scientific Publishing Co.
35. Markov MS, Pilla AA: Modulation of cell-free myosin light chain phosphorylation with weak low frequency and static magnetic fields, In Frey AH, ed: *On the nature of electromagnetic field interactions with biological systems*, Austin/New York, 1995, RG Landes/Springer.
36. Hill J, Lewis M, Mills P, et al: Pulsed short-wave diathermy effects on human fibroblast proliferation, *Arch Phys Med Rehabil* 83(6):832-836, 2002.
37. Whitfield JF, Boynton AL, McManus JP, et al: The roles of calcium and cyclic AMP in cell proliferation, *Ann NY Acad Sci* 339:216-240, 1981.
38. Canaday DJ, Lee RC: Scientific basis for clinical application of electric fields in soft tissue repair. In Brighton CT, Pollack SR, eds: *Electromagnetics in biology medicine*, San Francisco, 1991, San Francisco Press.
39. Markov MS, Pilla AA: Electromagnetic field stimulation of soft tissues: pulsed radio frequency treatment of post-operative pain and edema, *Wounds* 7(4):143-151, 1995.
40. Vance AR, Hayes SH, Spielholz NI: Microwave diathermy treatment for primary dysmenorrhea, *Phys Ther* 76(9):1003-1008, 1996.
41. Goats GC: Continuous short-wave (radio-frequency) diathermy, *Br J Sports Med* 23:123-127, 1989.
42. Draper DO, Knight K, Fujiwara T, et al: Temperature change in human muscle during and after pulsed short-wave diathermy, *J Orthop Sports Phys Ther* 29(1):13-22, 1999.
43. Sieger C, Draper DO: Use of pulsed shortwave diathermy and joint mobilization to increase ankle range of motion in the presence of surgical implanted metal: a case series, *J Orthop Sports Phys Ther* 36(9):669-677, 2006.
44. Draper DO, Castro JL, Feland B, et al: Shortwave diathermy and prolonged stretching increase hamstring flexibility more than prolonged stretching alone, *J Orthop Sports Phys Ther* 34(1):13-20, 2004.
45. Peres SE, Draper DO, Knight KL, et al: Pulsed shortwave diathermy and prolonged long-duration stretching increase dorsiflexion range of motion more than identical stretching without diathermy, *J Athl Train* 37(1):43-50, 2002.
46. Brucker JB, Knight KL, Rubley MD, et al: An 18-day stretching regimen, with or without pulsed, shortwave diathermy, and ankle dorsiflexion after 3 weeks, *J Athl Train* 40(4):276-280, 2005.
47. Draper DO, Miner L, Knight KL, et al: The carry-over effects of diathermy and stretching in developing hamstring flexibility, *J Athl Train* 37(1):37-42, 2002.
48. Ginsberg AJ: Ultrasound radiowaves as a therapeutic agent, *Med Rec* 19:1-8, 1934.
49. Milinowski AS: Athermapeutic device, United States Patent no. 3181535, 1965.
50. Pilla AA, Martin DE, Schuett AM, et al: Effect of PRF therapy on edema from grades I and II ankle sprains: a placebo controlled randomized, multi-site, double-blind clinical study, *J Athl Train* 31:S53, 1996.
51. Wilson DH: Treatment of soft tissue injuries by pulsed electrical energy, *Br Med J* 2:269-270, 1972.
52. Pennington GM, Danley DL, Sumko MH: Pulsed, non-thermal, high frequency electromagnetic field (Diapulse) in the treatment of Grade I and Grade II ankle sprains, *Milit Med* 153:101-104, 1993.
53. Kaplan EG, Weinstock RE: Clinical evaluation of Diapulse as adjunctive therapy following foot surgery, *J Am Podiatr Assoc* 58(5):218-221, 1968.
54. Barker AT, Barlow PS, Porter J, et al: A double blind clinical trial of low power pulsed shortwave therapy in the treatment of soft tissue injury, *Physiotherapy* 71(12):500-504, 1985.
55. McGill SN: The effects of pulsed shortwave therapy on lateral ankle sprains, *N Z J Physiother* 51:21-24, 1988.
56. Foley-Nolan D, Barry C, Coughlan RJ, et al: Pulsed high frequency (27 MHz) electromagnetic therapy for persistent neck pain: a double blind placebo-controlled study of 20 patients, *Orthopedics* 13:445-451, 1990.
57. Foley-Nolan D, Moore K, Codd M, et al: Low energy, high frequency, pulsed electromagnetic therapy for acute whiplash injuries, *Scand J Rehabil Med* 24:51-59, 1992.
58. Wagstaff P, Wagstaff S, Downey M: A pilot study to compare the efficacy of continuous and pulsed magnetic energy (shortwave diathermy) on the relief of low back pain, *Physiother* 72(1):563-566, 1986.
59. Santiesteban AJ, Grant C: Post-surgical effect of pulsed shortwave therapy, *J Am Podiatr Assoc* 75(6):306-309, 1985.
60. Lee PB, Kim YC, Lim YJ, et al: Efficacy of pulsed electromagnetic therapy for chronic lower back pain: a randomized, double-blind, placebo-controlled study, *J Int Med Res* 34(2):160-167, 2006.
61. Dziedzic K, Hill J, Lewis M, et al: Effectiveness of manual therapy or pulsed shortwave diathermy in addition to advice and exercise for neck disorders: a pragmatic randomized controlled trial in physical therapy clinics, *Arthritis Rheum* 53(2):214-222, 2005.
62. Cameron BM: Experimental acceleration of wound healing, *Am J Orthop* 3(12):336-343, 1961.
63. Itoh M, Montemayor JS, Matsumoto E, et al: Accelerated wound healing of pressure ulcers by pulsed high peak power electromagnetic energy (Diapulse), *Decubitus* 2:24-28, 1991.
64. Ionescu A, Ionescu D, Milinescu S, et al: Study of efficiency of Diapulse therapy on the dynamics of enzymes in burned wound, *Proc Inter Cong Burns* 6:25-26, 1982.
65. Salzberg CA, Cooper-Vastola SA, Perez FJ, et al: The effect of non-thermal pulsed electromagnetic energy (Diapulse) on wound healing of pressure ulcers in spinal cord injured patients: a randomized, double-blind study, *Wounds* 7(1):11-16, 1995.
66. Strauch B, Patel MK, Rosen DJ, et al: Pulsed magnetic field therapy increases tensile strength in a rat Achilles tendon repair model, *J Hand Surg Am* 31(7):1131-1135, 2006.
67. Raji ARM, Bowden REM: Effects of high peak pulsed electromagnetic fields on the degeneration and regeneration of the common peroneal nerve in rats, *J Bone Joint Surg* 65:478-492, 1983.
68. Wilson DH, Jagadeesh P, Newman PP, et al: The effects of pulsed electromagnetic energy on peripheral nerve regeneration, *Ann NY Acad Sci* 238:575-580, 1974.
69. Wilson DH, Jagadeesh P: Experimental regeneration in peripheral nerves and the spinal cord in laboratory animals exposed to a pulsed electromagnetic field, *Paraplegia* 14:12-20, 1976.
70. Byers JM, Clark KF, Thompson GC: Effect of pulsed electromagnetic stimulation on facial nerve regeneration, *Arch Otolaryngol Head Neck Surg* 124(4):383-389, 1998.
71. Crowe MJ, Sun ZP, Battocletti JH, et al: Exposure to pulsed magnetic fields enhances motor recovery in cats after spinal cord injury, *Spine* 28(24):2660-2666, 2003.

72. Cook HH, Narendan NS, Montogomery JC: The effects of pulsed, high-frequency waves on the rate of osteogenesis in the healing of extraction wounds in dogs, *Oral Surg* 32(6):1008-1016, 1971.

73. Pilla AA: 27.12 MHz pulsed radiofrequency electromagnetic fields accelerate bone repair in a rabbit fibula osteotomy model. Presented at the Bioelectromagnetics Society meeting, Boston, 1995.

74. Thamsborg G, Florescu A, Oturai P, et al: Treatment of knee osteoarthritis with pulsed electromagnetic fields: a randomized, double-blind, placebo-controlled study, *Osteoarthritis Cart* 13(7):575-581, 2005.

75. Trock DH, Bollet AJ, Markoll R: The effect of pulsed electromagnetic fields in the treatment of osteoarthritis of the knee and cervical spine. Report of randomized, double blind, placebo controlled trials, *J Rheumatol* 21(10):1903-1911, 1994.

76. Jan MH, Chai HM, Wang CL, et al: Effects of repetitive shortwave diathermy for reducing synovitis in patients with knee osteoarthritis: an ultrasonographic study, *Phys Ther* 86(2):236-244, 2006.

77. Callaghan MJ, Whittaker PE, Grimes S, et al: An evaluation of pulsed shortwave on knee osteoarthritis using radioleucoscintigraphy: a randomised, double blind, controlled trial, *Joint Bone Spine* 72(2):150-155, 2005.

78. Laufer Y, Zilberman R, Porat R, et al: Effect of pulsed short-wave diathermy on pain and function of subjects with osteoarthritis of the knee: a placebo-controlled double-blind clinical trial, *Clin Rehabil* 19(3):255-263, 2005.

79. Sambasivan M: Pulsed electromagnetic field in management of head injuries, *Neurol India* 41(suppl):56, 1993.

80. Hayward L, Statham A: Microwave, *Physiotherapy* (South Africa) 37(1):7-9, 1981.

81. Low J, Reed A: *Electrotherapy explained: principles and practice*, London, 1990, Butterworth-Heinemann.

82. Health Notice (Hazard) 80(10): Implantable cardiac pacemakers: interference generated by diathermy equipment, Washington, DC, 1980, DHHS.

83. Burr B: *Heat as a therapeutic modality against cancer: Report 16*, Bethesda, MD, 1974, National Cancer Institute.

84. Mcmurray RG, Katz VL: Thermoregulation in pregnancy: implications for exercise, *Sports Med* 10(3):146-158, 1990.

85. Edwards MJ: Congenital defects in guinea pigs following induced hyperthermia during gestation, *Arch Pathol Lab Med* 84:42-48, 1967.

86. Edwards MJ: Congenital defects due to hyperthermia, *Adv Vet Sci Comp Med* 22:29-52, 1978.

87. Brown-Woodman PD, Hadley JA, Waterhouse J, et al: Teratogenic effects of exposure to radiofrequency radiation (27.12 MHz) from a short wave diathermy unit, *Ind Health* 26(1):1-10, 1988.

88. Tofani S, Agnesod G: The assessment of unwanted radiation around diathermy RF capacitive applicators, *Health Phys* 47(2):235-241, 1984.

89. Lau RW, Dunscombe PB: Some observations on stray magnetic fields and power outputs from shortwave diathermy equipment, *Health Phys* 46(4):939-943, 1984.

90. Lerman Y, Caner A, Jacubovich R, et al: Electromagnetic fields from shortwave diathermy equipment in physiotherapy departments, *Physiotherapy* 82(8):456-458, 1996.

91. Martin JC, McCallum HM, Strelley S, et al: Electromagnetic fields from therapeutic diathermy equipment: a review of hazards and precautions, *Physiotherapy* 77(1):3-7, 1991.

92. Christensen DA, Durney CH: Hyperthermia production for cancer therapy: a review of fundamentals and methods, *J Microwave Power* 16:89-105, 1981.

93. Nielson NC, Hansen R, Larsen T: Heat induction in copper bearing IUDs during short wave diathermy, *Acta Obstet Gynecol Scand* 58(5):495, 1979.

94. Heick A, Espesen T, Pedersen HL, et al: Is diathermy safe in women with copper-bearing IUDs? *Acta Obstet Gynecol Scand* 70(2):153-155, 1991.

95. Alster TS, Kauvar AN, Geronemus RG: Histology of high-energy pulsed CO2 laser resurfacing, *Semin Cutan Med Surg* 15(3):189-193, 1996.

96. Delpizzo V, Joyner KH: On the safe use of microwave and shortwave diathermy units, *Aust J Physiother* 33:152-161, 1987.

97. Chartered Society of Physiotherapy: Guidelines for safe use of microwave therapy equipment, London, 1994, Chartered Society of Physiotherapy.

98. Kallen B, Malmquist G, Moritz U: Delivery outcome among physiotherapists in Sweden: is non-ionising radiation a fetal hazard? *Arch Environ Health* 37:81-84, 1982. Reprinted in *Physiotherapy* 78(1):15-18, 1992.

99. Larsen A, Olsen J, Svane O: Gender specific reproductive outcome and exposure to high frequency electromagnetic radiation among physiotherapists, *Scand J Work Environ Health* 17:318-323, 1991.

100. Ouellet-Hellstrom R, Stewart WF: Miscarriages among female physical therapists who report using radio and microwave frequency electromagnetic radiation, *Am J Epidemiol* 10:775-785, 1993.

101. Lerman Y, Jacubovich R, Green MS: Pregnancy outcome following exposure to shortwaves among female physiotherapists in Israel, *Am J Ind Med* 39(5):499-504, 2001.

102. Takininen H, Kyyronene P, Hemminki K: The effects of ultrasound, shortwaves and physical exertion on pregnancy outcomes in physiotherapists, *J Epidemiol Commun Health* 44:196-201, 1990.

103. Werheimer N, Leeper E: Electrical wiring configurations and childhood cancer, *Am J Epidemiol* 109:273-284, 1979.

104. Milham S Jr: Mortality from leukemia in workers exposed to electrical and magnetic fields (letter), *N Engl J Med* 307:249, 1982.

105. American Physical Society. National Policy Statement 05.3 Electric and magnetic fields and public health, adopted 2005 April. http://www.aps.org/policy/statements/05_3.cfm Accessed March 1, 2007.

106. Surrell JA, Alexander RC, Cohle SD: Effects of microwave radiation on living tissues, *J Trauma* 27:935-939, 1987.

107. Justesen D, Adair ER, Stevens J, et al: Human sensory thresholds of microwave and infra-red radiation, *Bioelectromagnetics* 3:117, 1982.

108. sofPulse: Electropharmacology, Inc, Pompano Beach, FL.

109. Diapulse: Diapulse Corporation of America, Great Neck, NY.

Introduction

This quick-reference manual is based on information presented in Physical Agents in Rehabilitation: From Research to Practice, 3e by Michelle H. Cameron.

The information in this handbook is intended for use by qualified clinicians with prior training in the use of physical agents in rehabilitation and for students practicing under qualified supervision.

The outline format of the handbook is meant to make the information easily accessible to rehabilitation professionals during clinical practice. For more detailed information and complete references please refer to Physical Agents in Rehabilitation: From Research to Practice, 3e.

How to use this handbook
For ultrasound treatment

1. Read Chapter 7 on ultrasound in Physical Agents in Rehabilitation: From Research to Practice, 3e to review how this modality works and what the adjustable treatment parameters are.
2. Select appropriate treatment parameters for increasing tissue temperature or promoting tissue healing from the ultrasound parameters section in this handbook.
3. Determine ultrasound treatment location by referring to the ultrasound section in this handbook concerning your patient's problem.
4. *These are treatment suggestions only. Adjust parameters based on clinical judgment.*

1

Michelle H. Cameron
Jennifer A. Rohl

Electrical Stimulation, Ultrasound & Laser Light Handbook

SAUNDERS
ELSEVIER

Note to readers: This handbook is available on Evolve to create and print custom study or clinical quick reference.

For electrical stimulation treatment

1. Read Chapter 8 on electrical stimulation in *Physical Agents in Rehabilitation: From Research to Practice, 3e* to review how this modality works and what the adjustable treatment parameters are.

2. Select appropriate stimulation parameters for pain management, muscle contraction, edema control or promoting tissue healing from the appropriate electrical stimulation parameters section in this handbook.

3. Determine electrode placement by referring to the electrode placement section in this handbook concerning your patient's problem.

4. *These are treatment suggestions only. Adjust parameters based on clinical judgment.*

For laser light treatment

1. Read Chapter 12 on laser light in *Physical Agents in Rehabilitation: From Research to Practice, 3e* to review how this modality works and what the adjustable treatment parameters are.

2. Select appropriate parameters for pain management or promoting tissue healing from the appropriate laser light parameters section in this handbook.

3. Determine laser light treatment location by referring to the laser light section in this handbook concerning your patient's problem.

4. *These are treatment suggestions only. Adjust parameters based on clinical judgment.*

Ultrasound

What is ultrasound?

Ultrasound is a type of sound. It is similar to audible sound, except that it has a higher frequency. Ultrasound has a frequency of greater than 20 kHz (20,000 cycles/second). The human ear can hear sounds with a frequency of up to 20 kHz. Therapeutic ultrasound generally has a frequency of between 1 and 3 MHz (millions of cycles/second) in order to achieve a depth of penetration through soft tissue of between 1 and 5 cm (with 1 MHz penetrating deeper than 3 MHz).

How therapeutic ultrasound works

When ultrasound passes through tissue some of it is absorbed by the tissue producing molecular motion. This motion causes friction between particles and thus, with sufficient ultrasound intensity, an increase in tissue temperature. The tissue heating produced by ultrasound can increase local blood flow and collagen extensibility, reduce pain and muscle spasm, increase local circulation and enzyme activity and produce a mild inflammatory response.

It has also been found that ultrasound has a range of effects that are not related to its ability to increase tissue temperature. These effects are known as non–thermal or mechanical effects and include stable cavitation, microstreaming and acoustic streaming. Research indicates that these non–thermal effects may promote soft and bony tissue repair and increase cell and tissue membrane permeability.

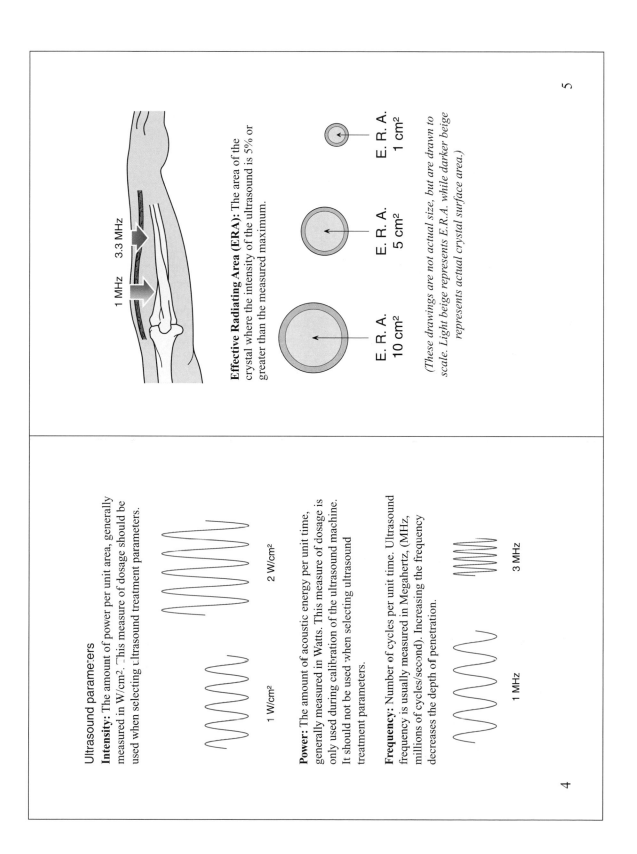

Ultrasound parameters

Intensity: The amount of power per unit area, generally measured in W/cm². This measure of dosage should be used when selecting ultrasound treatment parameters.

1 W/cm² 2 W/cm²

Power: The amount of acoustic energy per unit time, generally measured in Watts. This measure of dosage is only used during calibration of the ultrasound machine. It should not be used when selecting ultrasound treatment parameters.

Frequency: Number of cycles per unit time. Ultrasound frequency is usually measured in Megahertz, (MHz, millions of cycles/second). Increasing the frequency decreases the depth of penetration.

1 MHz 3 MHz

1 MHz 3.3 MHz

Effective Radiating Area (ERA): The area of the crystal where the intensity of the ultrasound is 5% or greater than the measured maximum.

E. R. A.
10 cm²

E. R. A.
5 cm²

E. R. A.
1 cm²

(These drawings are not actual size, but are drawn to scale. Light beige represents E.R.A. while darker beige represents actual crystal surface area.)

4

5

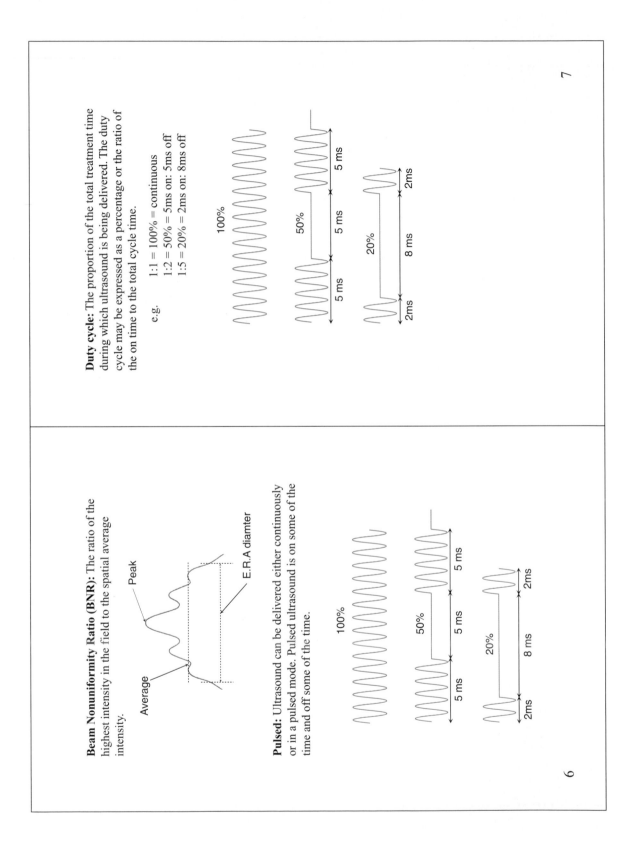

Duty cycle: The proportion of the total treatment time during which ultrasound is being delivered. The duty cycle may be expressed as a percentage or the ratio of the on time to the total cycle time.

e.g.   1:1 = 100% = continuous
1:2 = 50% = 5ms on: 5ms off
1:5 = 20% = 2ms on: 8ms off

100%

50%   5 ms   5 ms

5 ms

20%   8 ms

2ms   2ms

7

Beam Nonuniformity Ratio (BNR): The ratio of the highest intensity in the field to the spatial average intensity.

Peak

Average

E.R.A diamter

Pulsed: Ultrasound can be delivered either continuously or in a pulsed mode. Pulsed ultrasound is on some of the time and off some of the time.

100%

50%   5 ms   5 ms

5 ms

20%   8 ms

2ms   2ms

6

Contact

Complete contact should be maintained between the entire transducer surface and the patient's skin throughout treatment.

Area of treatment

Ultrasound should generally be used to treat areas equal to twice the ERA of the transducer. Treatment recommendations are based on treating areas of this size. If treatment of a larger area is required the treatment time should be increased proportionately.

Motion of transducer

The transducer should be moved throughout the treatment. It may be moved in a circular or stroking manner.

The speed of transducer movement should be sufficient to maintain constant motion while avoiding increasing the treatment area or losing consistent and constant contact with the skin.

Clinical application of ultrasound

Transmission medium

When applying therapeutic ultrasound to a patient, a transmission medium must be placed between the patient's skin and the ultrasound transducer. This transmission medium ensures effective ultrasound transmission to the patient. Good ultrasound transmission media include manufactured ultrasound gel, ultrasound lotion and water. Other topical preparations, such as creams or ointments, not intended for ultrasound transmission should not be used since many of these transmit ultrasound poorly.

Since air is a poor transmitter of ultrasound the amount of transmission medium applied must be sufficient to eliminate any air between the transducer and the patient's skin

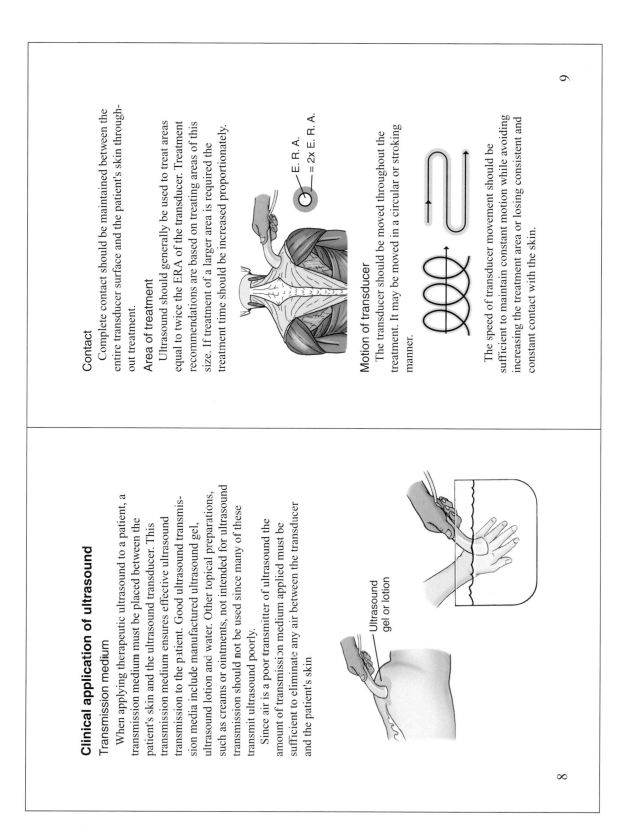

Ultrasound gel or lotion

E. R. A.

= 2x E. R. A.

9

8

Recommended ultrasound treatment parameters

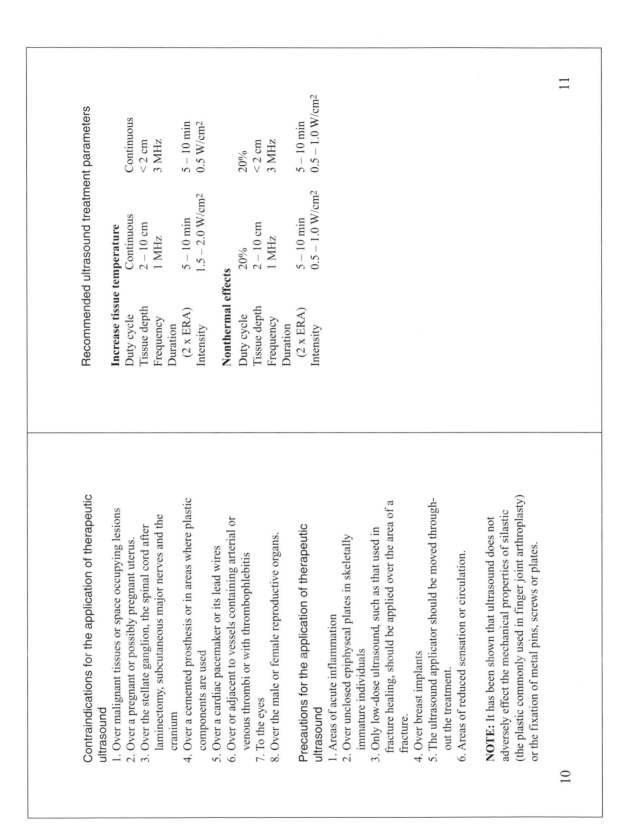

Increase tissue temperature

Duty cycle	Continuous	Continuous
Tissue depth	2 – 10 cm	<2 cm
Frequency	1 MHz	3 MHz
Duration (2 x ERA)	5 – 10 min	5 – 10 min
Intensity	1.5 – 2.0 W/cm²	0.5 W/cm²

Nonthermal effects

Duty cycle	20%	20%
Tissue depth	2 – 10 cm	<2 cm
Frequency	1 MHz	3 MHz
Duration (2 x ERA)	5 – 10 min	5 – 10 min
Intensity	0.5 – 1.0 W/cm²	0.5 – 1.0 W/cm²

11

Contraindications for the application of therapeutic ultrasound

1. Over malignant tissues or space occupying lesions
2. Over a pregnant or possibly pregnant uterus.
3. Over the stellate ganglion, the spinal cord after laminectomy, subcutaneous major nerves and the cranium
4. Over a cemented prosthesis or in areas where plastic components are used
5. Over a cardiac pacemaker or its lead wires
6. Over or adjacent to vessels containing arterial or venous thrombi or with thrombophlebitis
7. To the eyes
8. Over the male or female reproductive organs.

Precautions for the application of therapeutic ultrasound

1. Areas of acute inflammation
2. Over unclosed epiphyseal plates in skeletally immature individuals
3. Only low-dose ultrasound, such as that used in fracture healing, should be applied over the area of a fracture.
4. Over breast implants
5. The ultrasound applicator should be moved throughout the treatment.
6. Areas of reduced sensation or circulation.

NOTE: It has been shown that ultrasound does not adversely effect the mechanical properties of silastic (the plastic commonly used in finger joint arthroplasty) or the fixation of metal pins, screws or plates.

10

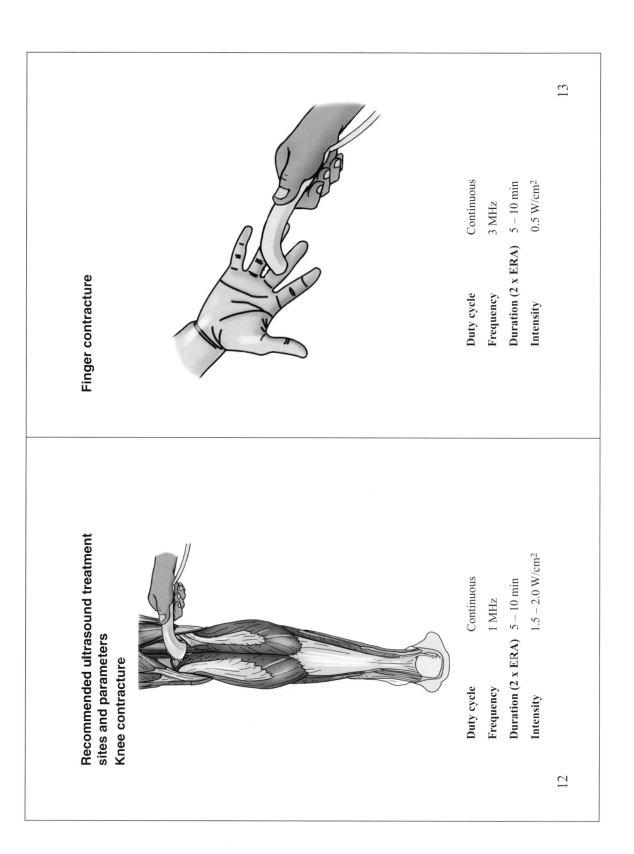

Finger contracture

Duty cycle	Continuous
Frequency	3 MHz
Duration (2 x ERA)	5 – 10 min
Intensity	0.5 W/cm²

13

Recommended ultrasound treatment sites and parameters

Knee contracture

Duty cycle	Continuous
Frequency	1 MHz
Duration (2 x ERA)	5 – 10 min
Intensity	1.5 – 2.0 W/cm²

12

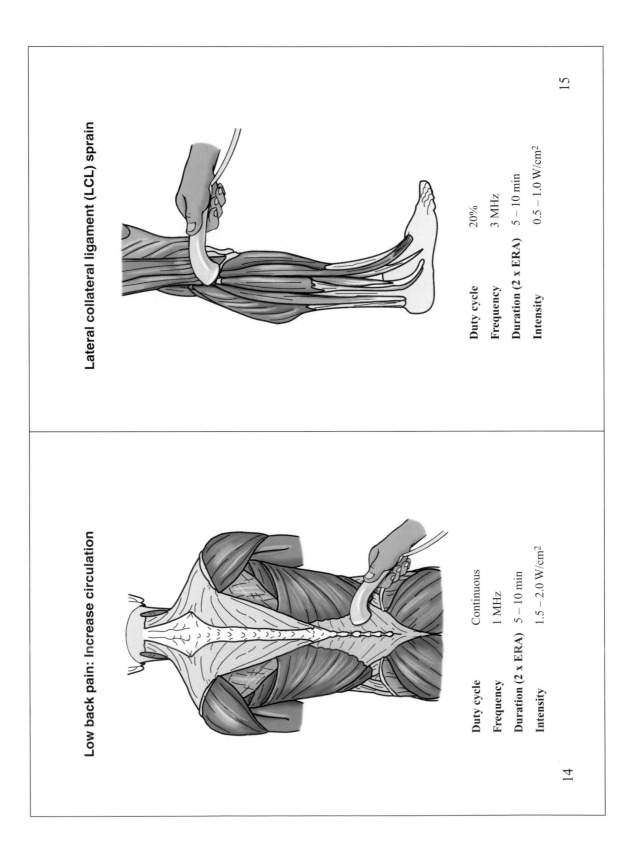

Lateral collateral ligament (LCL) sprain

Duty cycle	20%
Frequency	3 MHz
Duration (2 x ERA)	5 – 10 min
Intensity	0.5 – 1.0 W/cm²

15

Low back pain: Increase circulation

Duty cycle	Continuous
Frequency	1 MHz
Duration (2 x ERA)	5 – 10 min
Intensity	1.5 – 2.0 W/cm²

14

Electrical stimulation

What is electrical stimulation?

Electrical stimulation is the application of an electrical current to the body via transcutaneous electrodes for therapeutic benefit.

How electrical stimulation works

Electrical stimulation works primarily by stimulating peripheral nerves to produce action potentials which are transmitted along these nerves. Sensory nerves transmit action potentials from the periphery towards the central nervous system to produce a sensation frequently described as tingling. Motor nerves transmit action potentials towards the periphery to cause contraction of the muscles they innervate. When nociceptive (pain transmitting) nerves transmit action potentials towards the central nervous system the individual feels pain.

The different types of nerves, sensory, motor and nociceptive, have different minimum thresholds for responding to electrical stimulation. These thresholds depend on the duration and amplitude of the applied pulse of electrical current. Sensory nerves respond to shorter and lower amplitude pulses than motor nerves and motor nerves respond to shorter and lower amplitude pulses than pain transmitting nerves. The minimum threshold for stimulation of these types of nerves is most readily demonstrated by the amplitude duration curves on the following page.

17

Sacral pressure ulcer

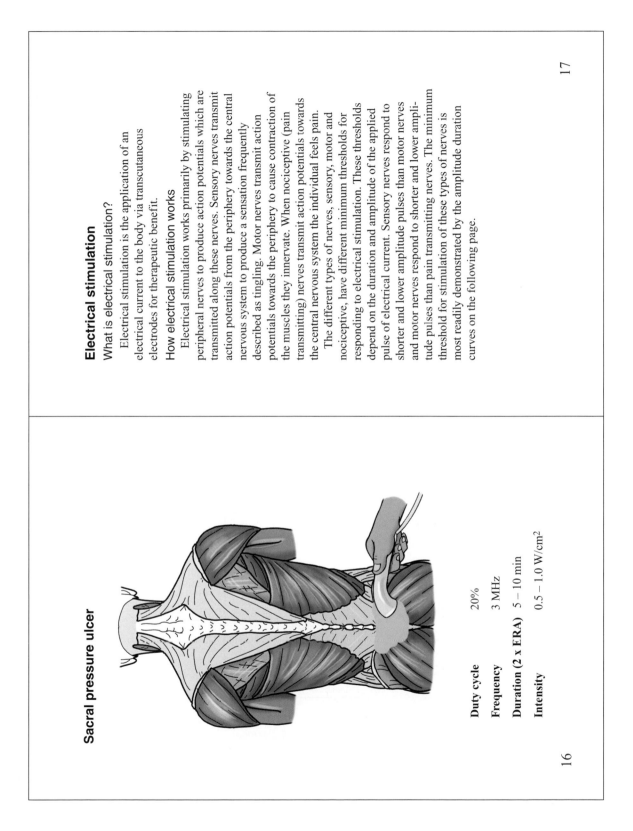

Duty cycle	20%
Frequency	3 MHz
Duration (2 x ERA)	5 – 10 min
Intensity	0.5 – 1.0 W/cm^2

16

Electrical stimulation parameters

Waveform

The waveform may be one of three general types—direct current, alternating current or pulsed current.

Direct current (DC) : A continuous unidirectional flow of charged particles. DC is used for iontophoresis, for stimulating contraction of denervated muscle, and also occasionally to facilitate wound healing.

Alternating current (AC) : A continuous bidirectional flow of charged particles. AC is generally used for interferential, premodulated, and Russion protocol stimulation.

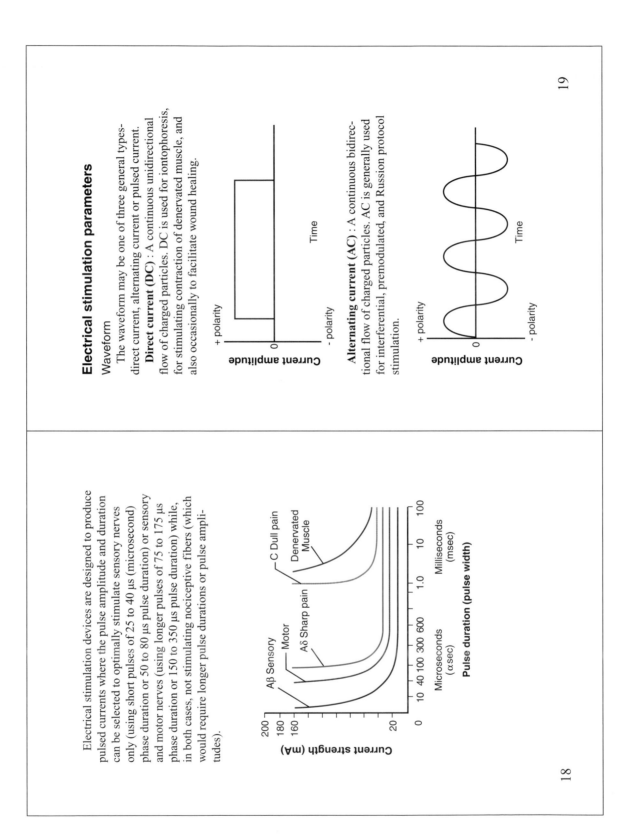

Electrical stimulation devices are designed to produce pulsed currents where the pulse amplitude and duration can be selected to optimally stimulate sensory nerves only (using short pulses of 25 to 40 μs (microsecond) phase duration or 50 to 80 μs pulse duration) or sensory and motor nerves (using longer pulses of 75 to 175 μs phase duration or 150 to 350 μs pulse duration) while, in both cases, not stimulating nociceptive fibers (which would require longer pulse durations or pulse amplitudes).

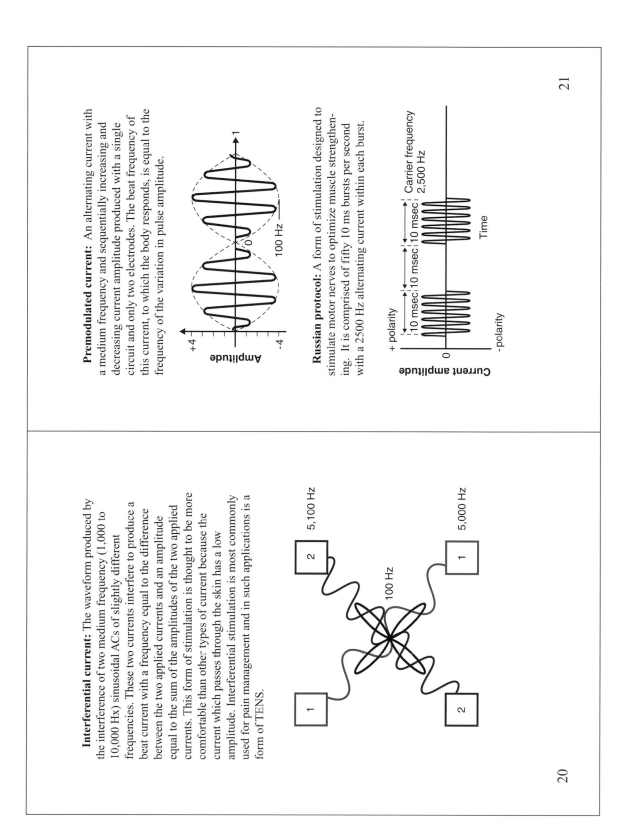

Premodulated current: An alternating current with a medium frequency and sequentially increasing and decreasing current amplitude produced with a single circuit and only two electrodes. The beat frequency of this current, to which the body responds, is equal to the frequency of the variation in pulse amplitude.

100 Hz

Amplitude +4 / −4

Russian protocol: A form of stimulation designed to stimulate motor nerves to optimize muscle strengthening. It is comprised of fifty 10 ms bursts per second with a 2500 Hz alternating current within each burst.

+ polarity
10 msec 10 msec 10 msec
Carrier frequency 2,500 Hz
Time
Current amplitude
− polarity

21

Interferential current: The waveform produced by the interference of two medium frequency (1,000 to 10,000 Hx) sinusoidal ACs of slightly different frequencies. These two currents interfere to produce a beat current with a frequency equal to the difference between the two applied currents and an amplitude equal to the sum of the amplitudes of the two applied currents. This form of stimulation is thought to be more comfortable than other types of current because the current which passes through the skin has a low amplitude. Interferential stimulation is most commonly used for pain management and in such applications is a form of TENS.

2   5,100 Hz
100 Hz
1   5,000 Hz
1
2

20

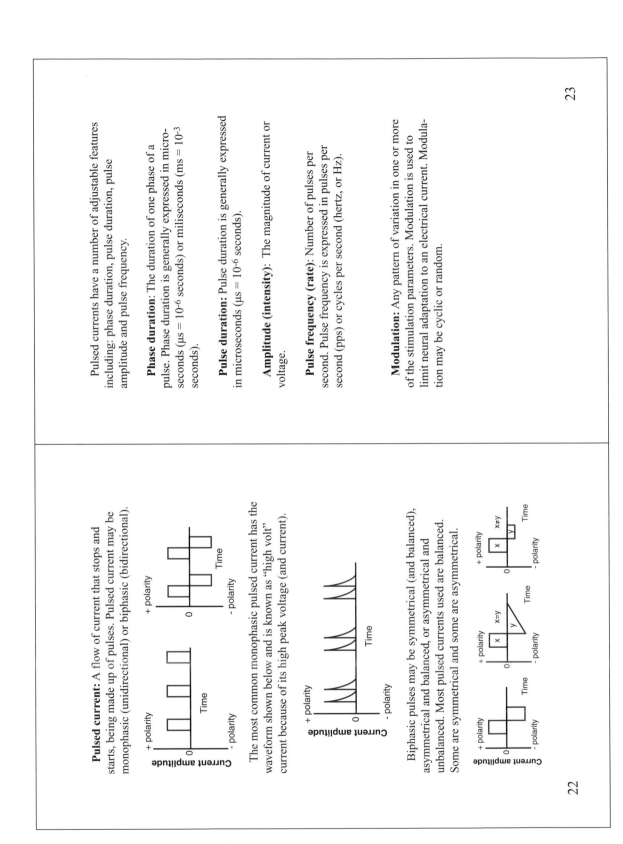

Pulsed current: A flow of current that stops and starts, being made up of pulses. Pulsed current may be monophasic (unidirectional) or biphasic (bidirectional).

The most common monophasic pulsed current has the waveform shown below and is known as "high volt" current because of its high peak voltage (and current).

Biphasic pulses may be symmetrical (and balanced), asymmetrical and balanced, or asymmetrical and unbalanced. Most pulsed currents used are balanced. Some are symmetrical and some are asymmetrical.

22

Pulsed currents have a number of adjustable features including: phase duration, pulse duration, pulse amplitude and pulse frequency.

Phase duration: The duration of one phase of a pulse. Phase duration is generally expressed in microseconds ($\mu s = 10^{-6}$ seconds) or miliseconds (ms = 10^{-3} seconds).

Pulse duration: Pulse duration is generally expressed in microseconds ($\mu s = 10^{-6}$ seconds).

Amplitude (intensity): The magnitude of current or voltage.

Pulse frequency (rate): Number of pulses per second. Pulse frequency is expressed in pulses per second (pps) or cycles per second (hertz, or Hz).

Modulation: Any pattern of variation in one or more of the stimulation parameters. Modulation is used to limit neural adaptation to an electrical current. Modulation may be cyclic or random.

23

When using interferential current, modulating the current amplitude moves the area of maximal stimulation within the treatment area. On most devices this is called vector or scan.

24

Electrode selection

Most electrodes used clinically at this time are self-adhesive.

Self-adhesive electrodes can be applied directly to the patient's skin. This type of electrode can be reused as long as it maintains its adhesive property. The length of time this type of electrode maintains its adhesive property varies with manufacture. Keep these electrodes in a sealed plastic bag between uses and slightly moisten the adhesive surface prior to use in order to maximize longevity.

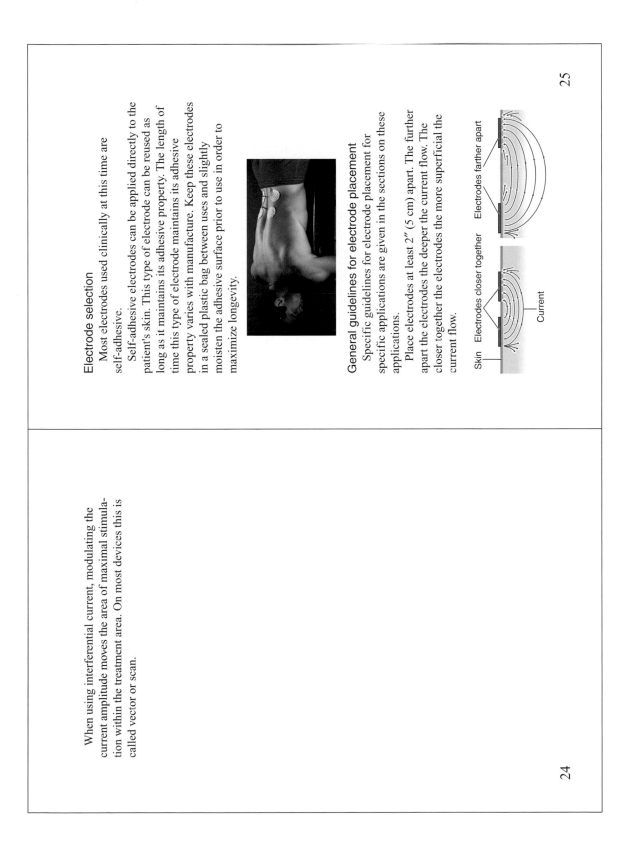

General guidelines for electrode placement

Specific guidelines for electrode placement for specific applications are given in the sections on these applications.

Place electrodes at least 2″ (5 cm) apart. The further apart the electrodes the deeper the current flow. The closer together the electrodes the more superficial the current flow.

Skin   Electrodes closer together   Electrodes farther apart

Current

25

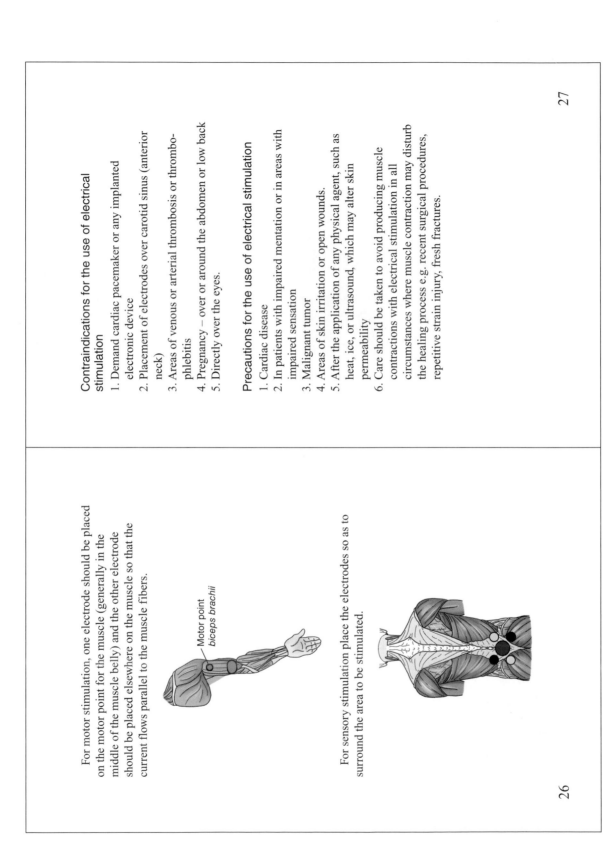

For motor stimulation, one electrode should be placed on the motor point for the muscle (generally in the middle of the muscle belly) and the other electrode should be placed elsewhere on the muscle so that the current flows parallel to the muscle fibers.

Motor point
biceps brachii

For sensory stimulation place the electrodes so as to surround the area to be stimulated.

26

Contraindications for the use of electrical stimulation

1. Demand cardiac pacemaker or any implanted electronic device
2. Placement of electrodes over carotid sinus (anterior neck)
3. Areas of venous or arterial thrombosis or thrombophlebitis
4. Pregnancy – over or around the abdomen or low back
5. Directly over the eyes.

Precautions for the use of electrical stimulation

1. Cardiac disease
2. In patients with impaired mentation or in areas with impaired sensation
3. Malignant tumor
4. Areas of skin irritation or open wounds.
5. After the application of any physical agent, such as heat, ice, or ultrasound, which may alter skin permeability
6. Care should be taken to avoid producing muscle contractions with electrical stimulation in all circumstances where muscle contraction may disturb the healing process e.g. recent surgical procedures, repetitive strain injury, fresh fractures.

27

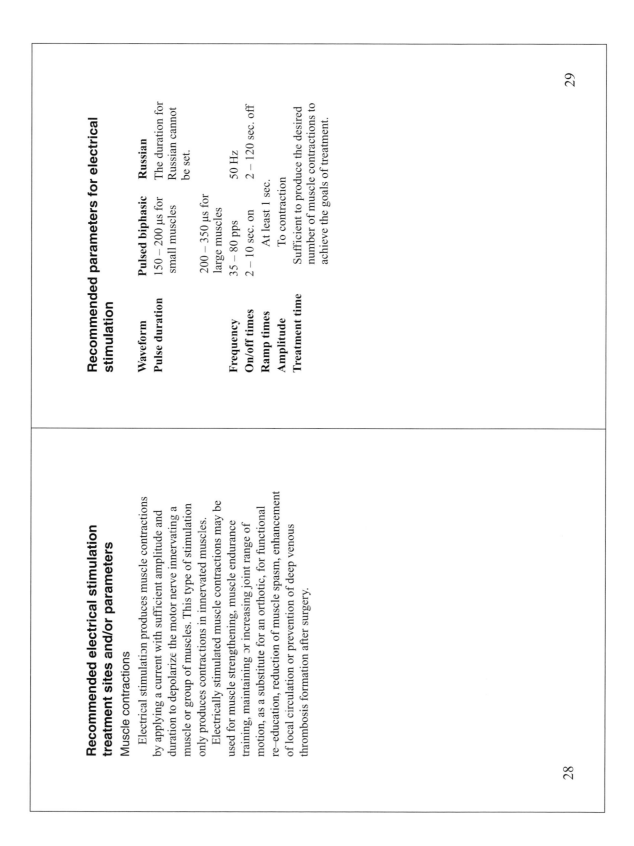

Recommended parameters for electrical stimulation

Muscle contractions

Waveform	Pulsed biphasic	Russian
Pulse duration	150 – 200 µs for small muscles	The duration for Russian cannot be set.
	200 – 350 µs for large muscles	
Frequency	35 – 80 pps	50 Hz
On/off times	2 – 10 sec. on	2 – 120 sec. off
Ramp times	At least 1 sec.	
Amplitude	To contraction	
Treatment time	Sufficient to produce the desired number of muscle contractions to achieve the goals of treatment.	

29

Recommended electrical stimulation treatment sites and/or parameters

Muscle contractions

Electrical stimulation produces muscle contractions by applying a current with sufficient amplitude and duration to depolarize the motor nerve innervating a muscle or group of muscles. This type of stimulation only produces contractions in innervated muscles.

Electrically stimulated muscle contractions may be used for muscle strengthening, muscle endurance training, maintaining or increasing joint range of motion, as a substitute for an orthotic, for functional re–education, reduction of muscle spasm, enhancement of local circulation or prevention of deep venous thrombosis formation after surgery.

28

Muscle strengthening: Quadriceps

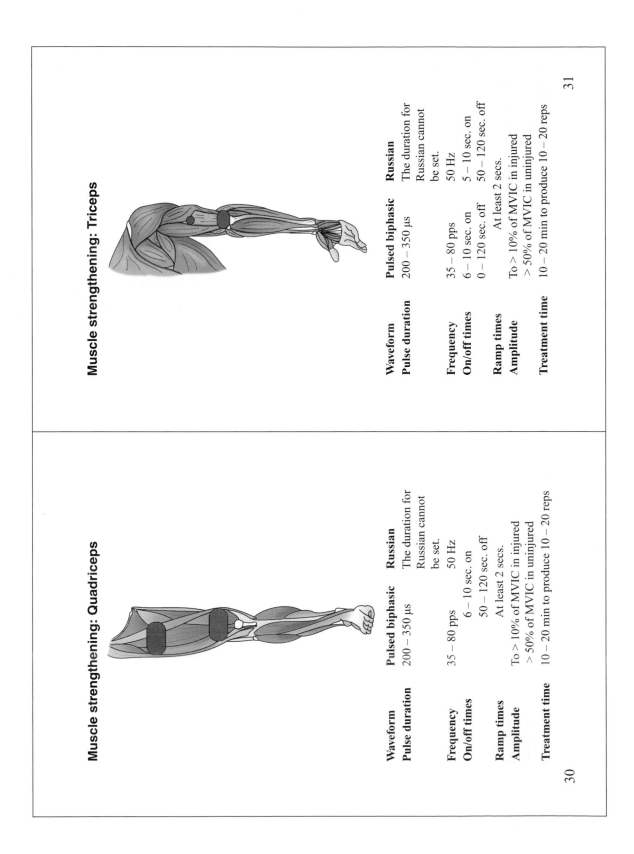

	Pulsed biphasic	Russian
Waveform		
Pulse duration	200 – 350 μs	The duration for Russian cannot be set.
Frequency	35 – 80 pps	50 Hz
On/off times	6 – 10 sec. on	
	50 – 120 sec. off	
Ramp times	At least 2 secs.	
Amplitude	To > 10% of MVIC in injured	
	> 50% of MVIC in uninjured	
Treatment time	10 – 20 min to produce 10 – 20 reps	

30

Muscle strengthening: Triceps

	Pulsed biphasic	Russian
Waveform		
Pulse duration	200 – 350 μs	The duration for Russian cannot be set.
Frequency	35 – 80 pps	50 Hz
On/off times	6 – 10 sec. on	5 – 10 sec. on
	0 – 120 sec. off	50 – 120 sec. off
Ramp times		At least 2 secs.
Amplitude	To > 10% of MVIC in injured	
	> 50% of MVIC in uninjured	
Treatment time	10 – 20 min to produce 10 – 20 reps	

31

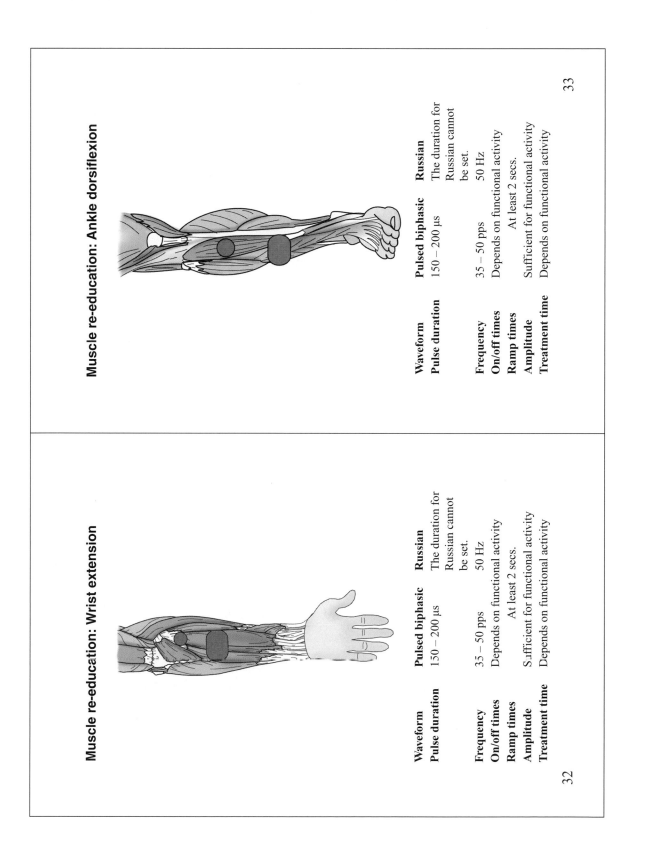

Muscle re-education: Wrist extension

Waveform	Pulsed biphasic	Russian
Pulse duration	150 – 200 μs	The duration for Russian cannot be set.
Frequency	35 – 50 pps	50 Hz
On/off times	Depends on functional activity	
Ramp times	At least 2 secs.	
Amplitude	Sufficient for functional activity	
Treatment time	Depends on functional activity	

32

Muscle re-education: Ankle dorsiflexion

Waveform	Pulsed biphasic	Russian
Pulse duration	150 – 200 μs	The duration for Russian cannot be set.
Frequency	35 – 50 pps	50 Hz
On/off times	Depends on functional activity	
Ramp times	At least 2 secs.	
Amplitude	Sufficient for functional activity	
Treatment time	Depends on functional activity	

33

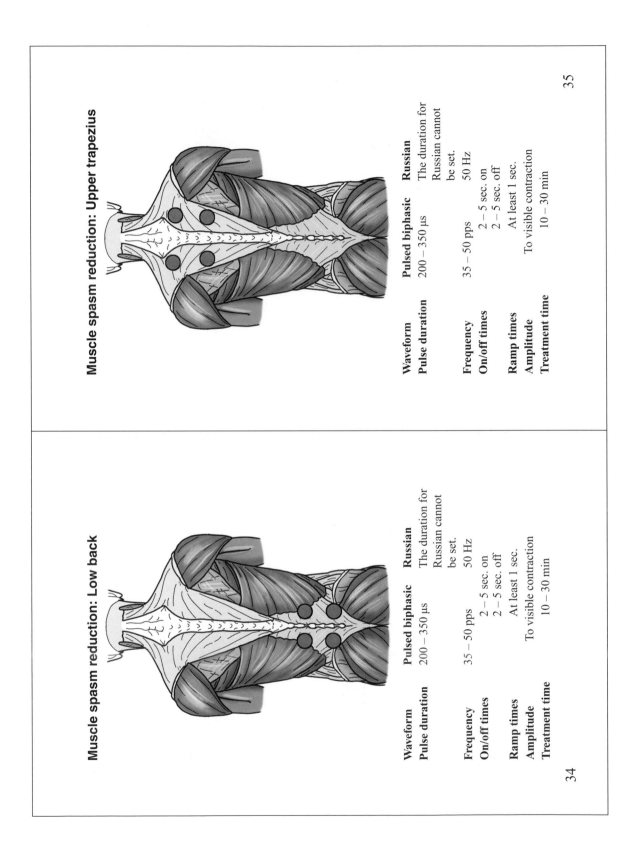

Muscle spasm reduction: Low back

Waveform	Pulsed biphasic	Russian
Pulse duration	200 – 350 μs	The duration for Russian cannot be set.
Frequency	35 – 50 pps	50 Hz
On/off times		2 – 5 sec. on 2 – 5 sec. off
Ramp times		At least 1 sec.
Amplitude		To visible contraction
Treatment time		10 – 30 min

34

Muscle spasm reduction: Upper trapezius

Waveform	Pulsed biphasic	Russian
Pulse duration	200 – 350 μs	The duration for Russian cannot be set.
Frequency	35 – 50 pps	50 Hz
On/off times		2 – 5 sec. on 2 – 5 sec. off
Ramp times		At least 1 sec.
Amplitude		To visible contraction
Treatment time		10 – 30 min

35

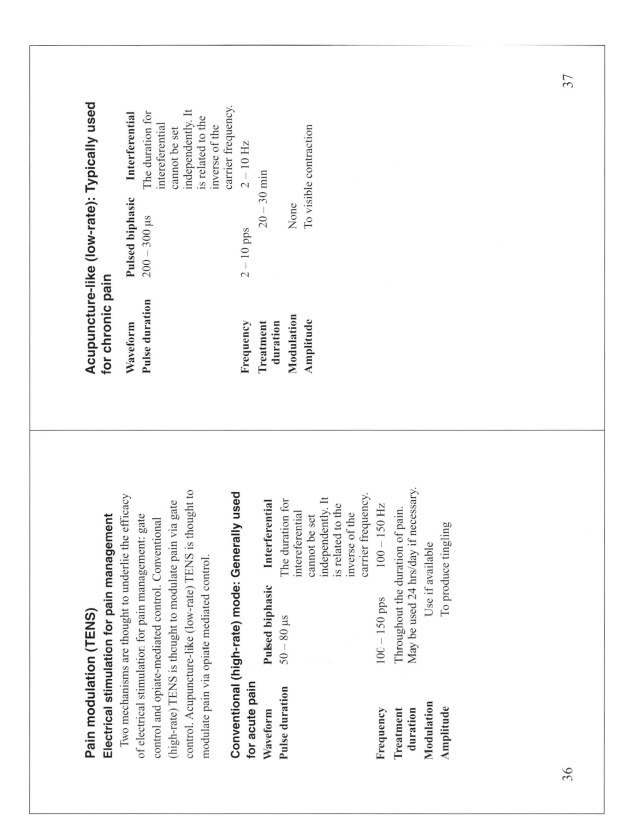

37

Acupuncture-like (low-rate): Typically used for chronic pain

	Pulsed biphasic	Interferential
Waveform		
Pulse duration	200 – 300 µs	The duration for interferential cannot be set independently. It is related to the inverse of the carrier frequency.
Frequency	2 – 10 pps	2 – 10 Hz
Treatment duration	20 – 30 min	
Modulation	None	
Amplitude	To visible contraction	

36

Pain modulation (TENS)
Electrical stimulation for pain management

Two mechanisms are thought to underlie the efficacy of electrical stimulation for pain management: gate control and opiate-mediated control. Conventional (high-rate) TENS is thought to modulate pain via gate control. Acupuncture-like (low-rate) TENS is thought to modulate pain via opiate mediated control.

Conventional (high-rate) mode: Generally used for acute pain

	Pulsed biphasic	Interferential
Waveform		
Pulse duration	50 – 80 µs	The duration for interferential cannot be set independently. It is related to the inverse of the carrier frequency.
Frequency	100 – 150 pps	100 – 150 Hz
Treatment duration	Throughout the duration of pain. May be used 24 hrs/day if necessary.	
Modulation	Use if available	
Amplitude	To produce tingling	

Low back pain: Acute

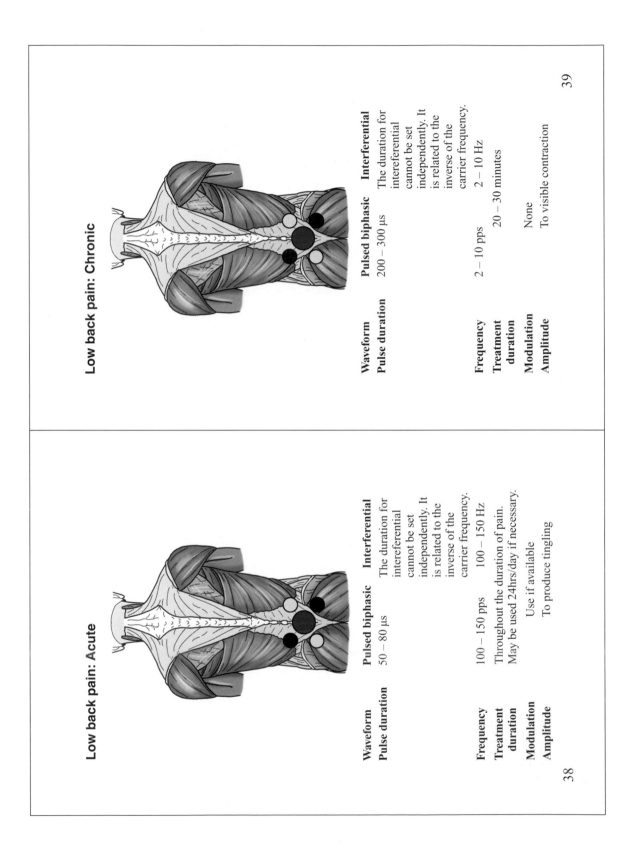

	Pulsed biphasic	Interferential
Waveform		
Pulse duration	50 – 80 µs	The duration for intereferential cannot be set independently. It is related to the inverse of the carrier frequency.
Frequency	100 – 150 pps	100 – 150 Hz
Treatment duration	Throughout the duration of pain. May be used 24hrs/day if necessary.	
Modulation	Use if available	
Amplitude	To produce tingling	

38

Low back pain: Chronic

	Pulsed biphasic	Interferential
Waveform		
Pulse duration	200 – 300 µs	The duration for intereferential cannot be set independently. It is related to the inverse of the carrier frequency.
Frequency	2 – 10 pps	2 – 10 Hz
Treatment duration	20 – 30 minutes	
Modulation	None	
Amplitude	To visible contraction	

39

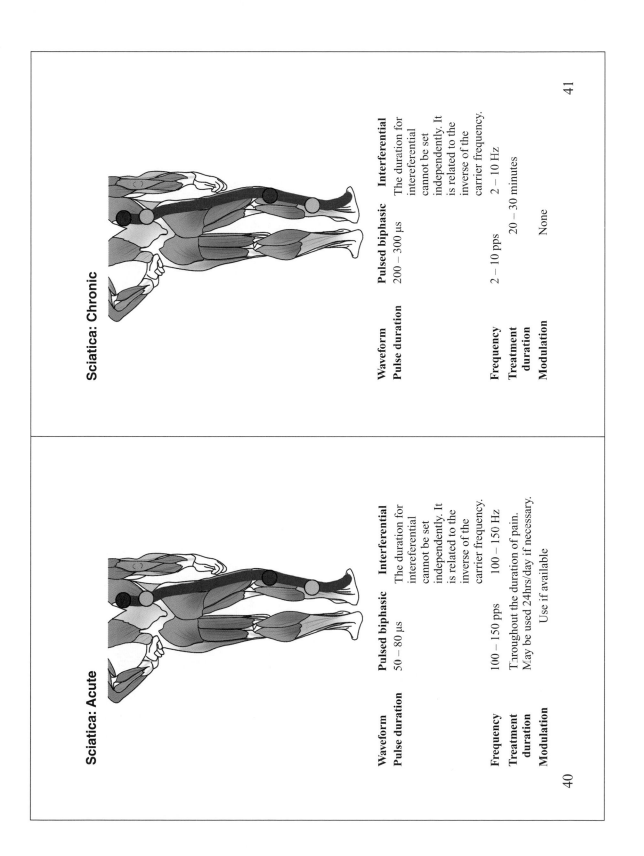

Sciatica: Chronic

	Pulsed biphasic	Interferential
Waveform		
Pulse duration	200 – 300 µs	The duration for interferential cannot be set independently. It is related to the inverse of the carrier frequency.
Frequency	2 – 10 pps	2 – 10 Hz
Treatment duration		20 – 30 minutes
Modulation	None	

41

Sciatica: Acute

	Pulsed biphasic	Interferential
Waveform		
Pulse duration	50 – 80 µs	The duration for interferential cannot be set independently. It is related to the inverse of the carrier frequency.
Frequency	100 – 150 pps	100 – 150 Hz
Treatment duration	Throughout the duration of pain. May be used 24hrs/day if necessary.	
Modulation	Use if available	

40

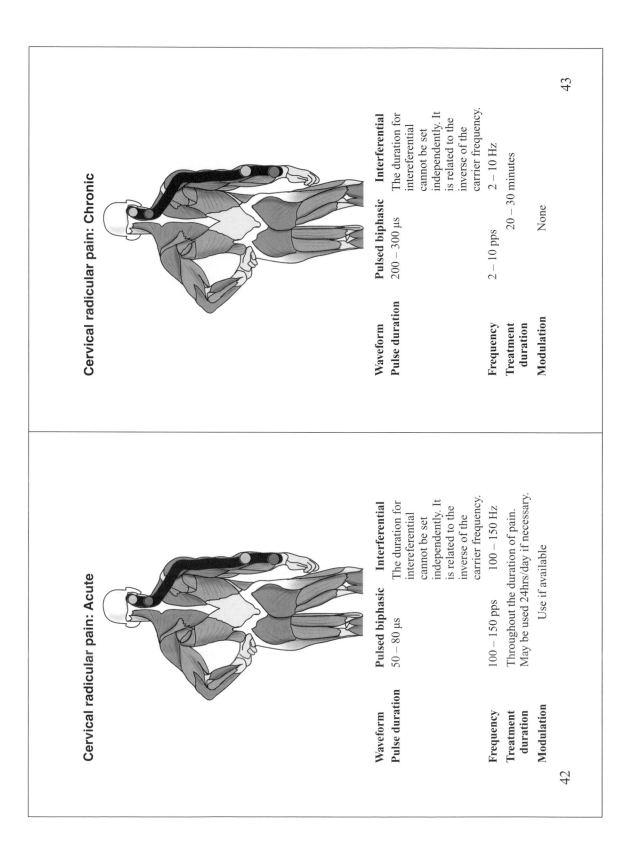

Cervical radicular pain: Acute

	Pulsed biphasic	Interferential
Waveform		
Pulse duration	50 – 80 μs	The duration for interferential cannot be set independently. It is related to the inverse of the carrier frequency.
Frequency	100 – 150 pps	100 – 150 Hz
Treatment duration	Throughout the duration of pain. May be used 24hrs/day if necessary.	
Modulation	Use if available	

42

Cervical radicular pain: Chronic

	Pulsed biphasic	Interferential
Waveform		
Pulse duration	200 – 300 μs	The duration for interferential cannot be set independently. It is related to the inverse of the carrier frequency.
Frequency	2 – 10 pps	2 – 10 Hz
Treatment duration	20 – 30 minutes	
Modulation	None	

43

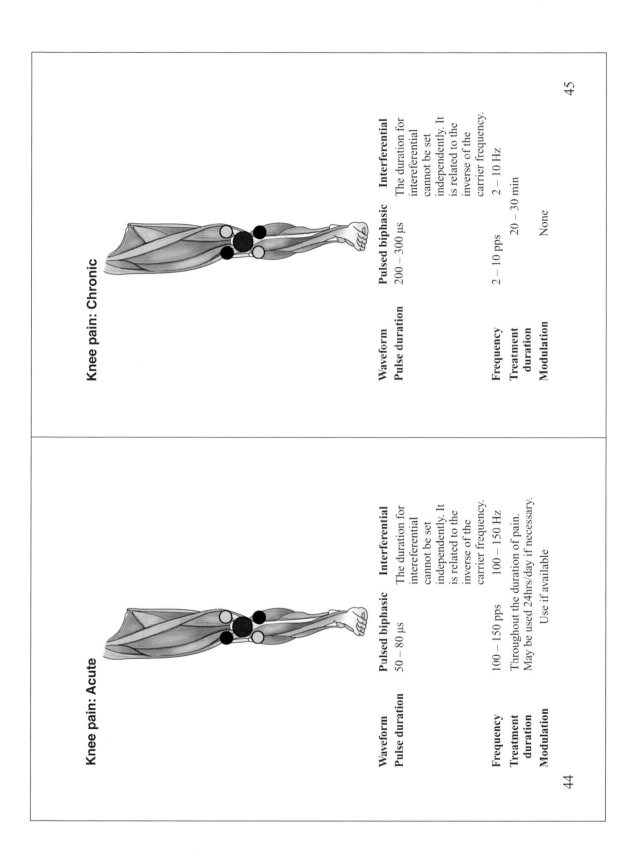

Knee pain: Chronic

Waveform	**Pulsed biphasic**	**Interferential**
Pulse duration	200 – 300 μs	The duration for interferential cannot be set independently. It is related to the inverse of the carrier frequency.
Frequency	2 – 10 pps	2 – 10 Hz
Treatment duration	20 – 30 min	
Modulation	None	

45

Knee pain: Acute

Waveform	**Pulsed biphasic**	**Interferential**
Pulse duration	50 – 80 μs	The duration for interferential cannot be set independently. It is related to the inverse of the carrier frequency.
Frequency	100 – 150 pps	100 – 150 Hz
Treatment duration	Throughout the duration of pain. May be used 24hrs/day if necessary.	
Modulation	Use if available	

44

Sacral pressure ulcer: Inflammatory phase

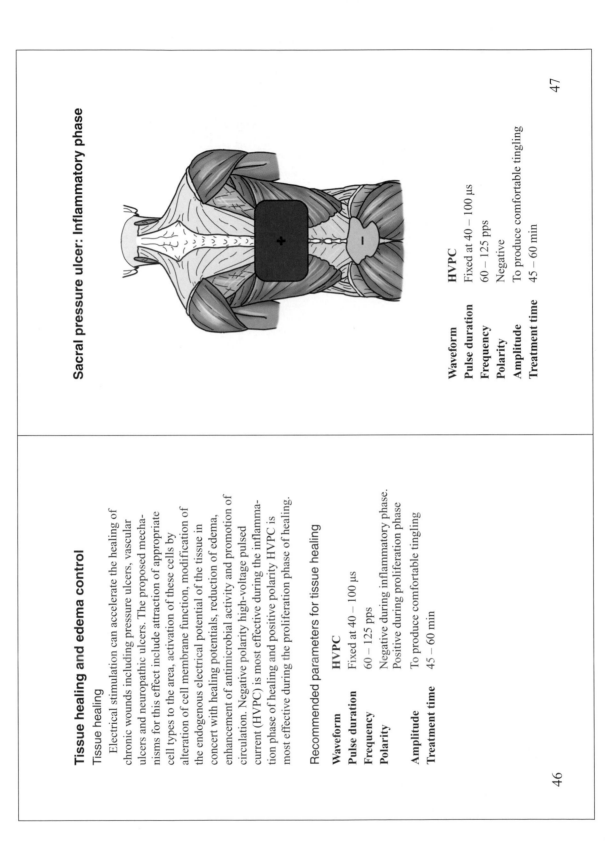

Waveform	**HVPC**
Pulse duration	Fixed at 40 – 100 µs
Frequency	60 – 125 pps
Polarity	Negative
Amplitude	To produce comfortable tingling
Treatment time	45 – 60 min

47

Tissue healing and edema control

Tissue healing

Electrical stimulation can accelerate the healing of chronic wounds including pressure ulcers, vascular ulcers and neuropathic ulcers. The proposed mechanisms for this effect include attraction of appropriate cell types to the area, activation of these cells by alteration of cell membrane function, modification of the endogenous electrical potential of the tissue in concert with healing potentials, reduction of edema, enhancement of antimicrobial activity and promotion of circulation. Negative polarity high-voltage pulsed current (HVPC) is most effective during the inflammation phase of healing and positive polarity HVPC is most effective during the proliferation phase of healing.

Recommended parameters for tissue healing

Waveform	**HVPC**
Pulse duration	Fixed at 40 – 100 µs
Frequency	60 – 125 pps
Polarity	Negative during inflammatory phase. Positive during proliferation phase
Amplitude	To produce comfortable tingling
Treatment time	45 – 60 min

46

Acute edema due to inflammation

When there is acute edema due to inflammation, indicated by swelling, warm and red skin, and local pain, treatment is directed at repelling negatively charged blood cells and plasma proteins. This, in turn, results in flow of fluid away from the swollen and inflamed area. Electrical stimulation can produce this effect by use of a high voltage pulsed current (HVPC), with sufficient pulse duration and amplitude to produce sensation but not a muscle contraction, with the negative polarity electrode placed over the swollen and inflamed area.

Recommended parameters for controlling acute edema due to inflammation

Waveform	HVPC
Pulse duration	Fixed at 40 – 100 μs
Frequency	100 – 120 pps
Polarity	Negative
Amplitude	To produce comfortable tingling
Treatment time	20 – 30 min

49

Sacral pressure ulcer: Proliferation phase

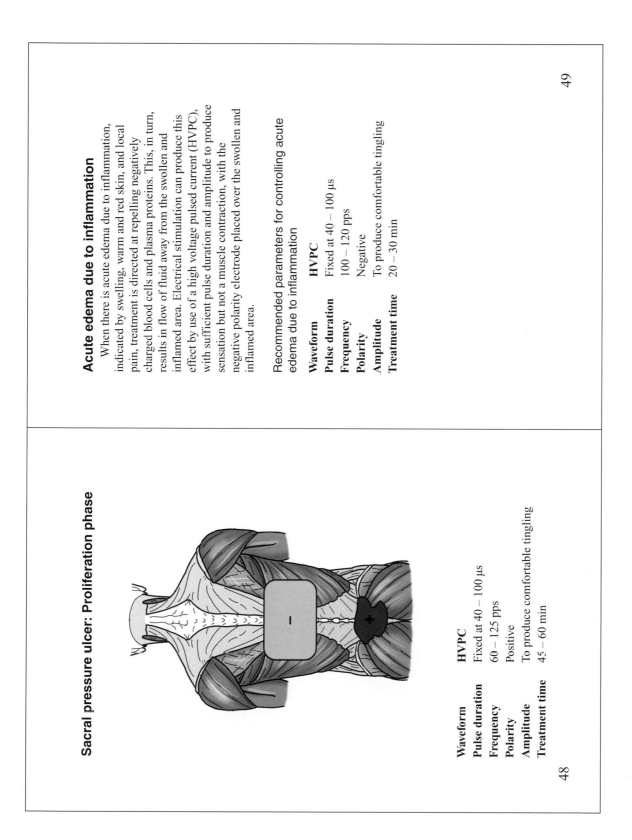

Waveform	HVPC
Pulse duration	Fixed at 40 – 100 μs
Frequency	60 – 125 pps
Polarity	Positive
Amplitude	To produce comfortable tingling
Treatment time	45 – 60 min

48

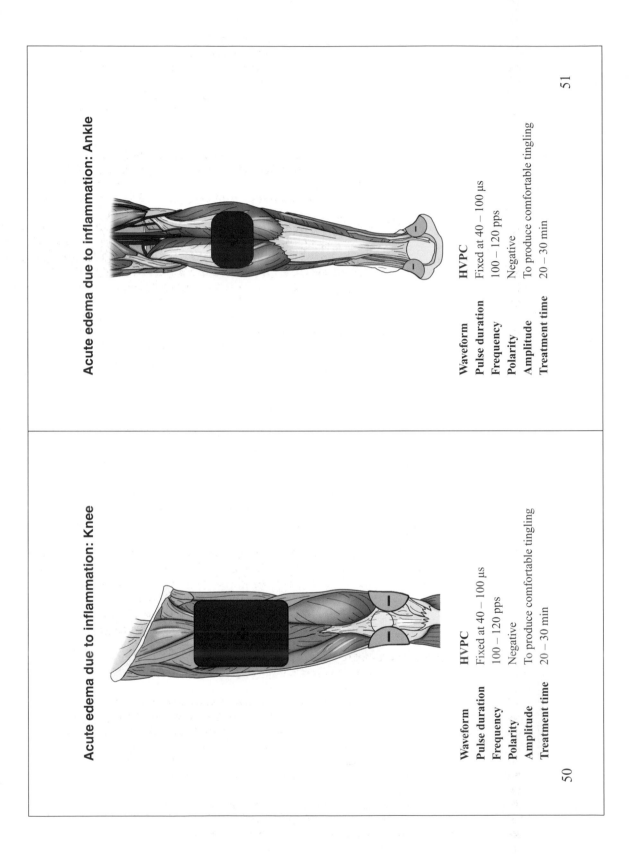

Acute edema due to inflammation: Ankle

Waveform	HVPC
Pulse duration	Fixed at 40 – 100 μs
Frequency	100 – 120 pps
Polarity	Negative
Amplitude	To produce comfortable tingling
Treatment time	20 – 30 min

51

Acute edema due to inflammation: Knee

Waveform	HVPC
Pulse duration	Fixed at 40 – 100 μs
Frequency	100 – 120 pps
Polarity	Negative
Amplitude	To produce comfortable tingling
Treatment time	20 – 30 min

50

Chronic edema due to lack of motion

Electrical stimulation is generally used to increase local circulation when edema is present. When there is chronic edema due to lack of motion present, indicated by swelling and cool and pale skin, treatment is directed at increasing the activity of the muscles around the venous system. Intermittent contraction of these muscles can help pump fluid through the veins from the periphery to reduce peripheral swelling. Intermittent electrical stimulation of the motor nerves can be used to produce such intermittent muscle contractions.

Recommended parameters for controlling chronic edema due to lack of motion

Waveform	Pulsed biphasic	Russian
Pulse duration	150 – 350 µs	The duration for Russian cannot be set.
Frequency	35 – 50 pps	50 Hz
On/off times	2 – 5 sec. on	
	2 – 5 sec. off	
Ramp times	At least 1 sec.	
Amplitude	To visible contraction	
Treatment time	10 – 30 min	

52

Chronic edema due to lack of motion:
Foot and ankle

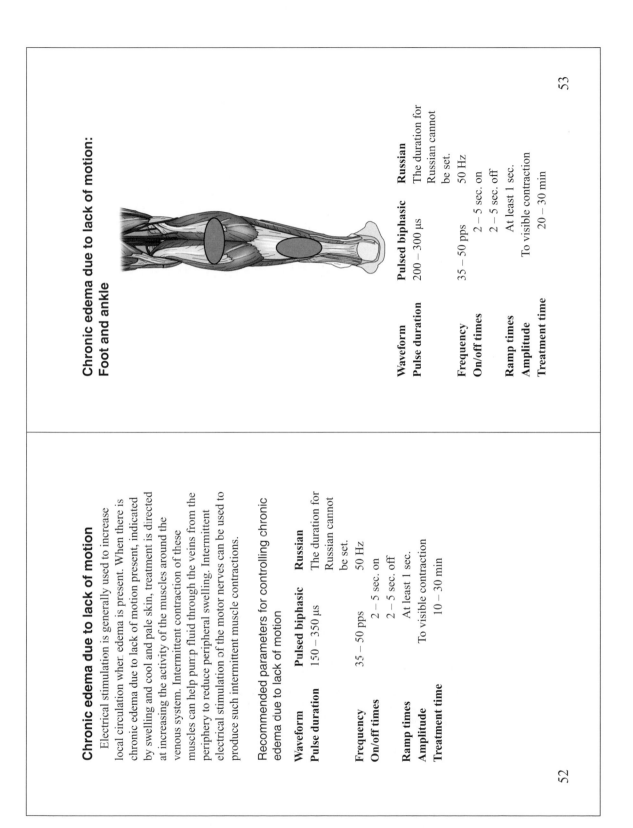

Waveform	Pulsed biphasic	Russian
Pulse duration	200 – 300 µs	The duration for Russian cannot be set.
Frequency	35 – 50 pps	50 Hz
On/off times	2 – 5 sec. on	
	2 – 5 sec. off	
Ramp times	At least 1 sec.	
Amplitude	To visible contraction	
Treatment time	20 – 30 min	

53

Laser and Light

Introduction to laser light therapy

What is laser light therapy?

Light is electromagnetic energy in the visible or near visible part of the electromagnetic spectrum.

Electromagnetic spectrum

Light of a specific or narrow range of frequencies can be produced by a laser, a supraluminous diode (SLD) or a light-emitting diode (LED).

Supraluminous diode/light-emitting diode/laser

Lasers produce light that is of one frequency only (monochromatic), coherent (all the waves are in sync) and, directional (non-divergent). SLDs and LEDs produce light with a narrow range of frequencies that is not coherent and that is slightly divergent.

Coherent and directional light

Laser light therapy is the application of light from a laser, an SLD or an LED to the body for therapeutic benefit.

Laser

Regular light source

55

Chronic edema due to lack of motion: Hand and wrist

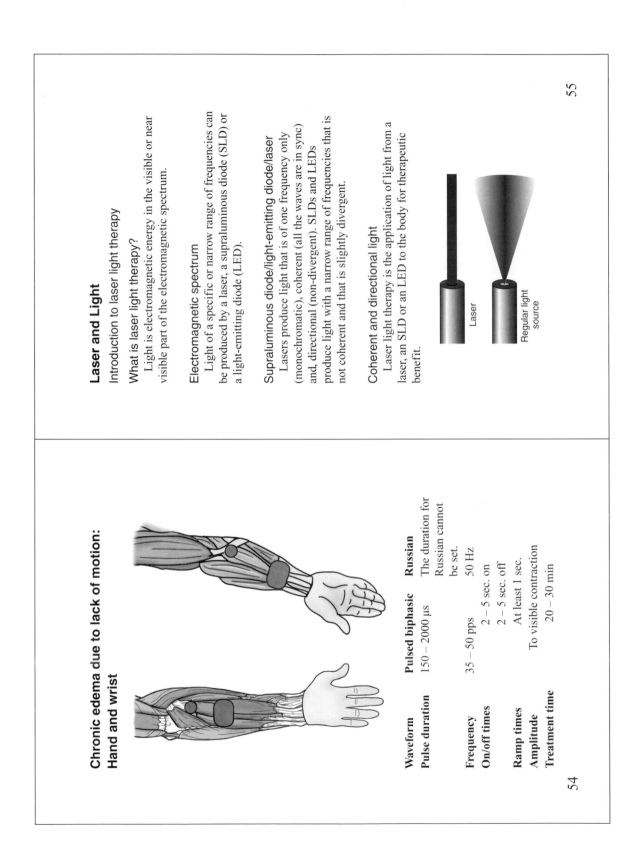

	Pulsed biphasic	Russian
Waveform		
Pulse duration	150 – 2000 µs	The duration for Russian cannot be set.
Frequency	35 – 50 pps	50 Hz
On/off times	2 – 5 sec. on	
	2 – 5 sec. off	
Ramp times	At least 1 sec.	
Amplitude	To visible contraction	
Treatment time	20 – 30 min	

54

Laser light parameters explained

Wavelength: The length of each cycle of the electro-magnetic wave. The wavelength of the light affects its color and depth of penetration, the longer the wavelength the greater the depth of penetration. Wavelength is generally measured in nanometers (nm, 10^{-9}) and, for most therapeutic lasers, ranges from around 600 nm to around 1,000 nm to produce red or infra-red light.

57

How laser light works

Laser light therapy works by photobiomodulation. The light is absorbed by chromophores in cells. This can increase the production of adenosine triphosphate (ATP) by mitochondria, increase the production of ribonucleic acid (RNA) specific for collagen synthesis, alter prostaglandin synthesis, alter serotonin and endorphin metabolism and reduce nociceptor activity. Together, these effects help to control pain and inflammation and promote tissue healing.

Coherent vs. non-coherent light

Coherent   Non-coherent

56

Contraindications for the application of laser light therapy

1. Irradiation of the eyes: the patient and the clinician should always wear protective eyewear when treating with a laser device.
2. Cancer
3. Within 4 to 6 months after radiotherapy
4. Areas of hemorrhage
5. Irradiation of endocrine glands

Precautions for the application of laser light therapy

1. Low back or abdomen during pregnancy
2. Epiphyseal plates in children
3. Impaired sensation
4. Impaired mentation
5. Photophobia or abnormally high sensitivity to light
6. Pretreatment with one or more photosensitizer

59

Power: The amount of electromagnetic energy per unit time, usually measured in mW (milliWatts). The power of a laser light device is preset on each applicator and generally ranges from 5 to 500 mW. Some applicators produce a higher total power by containing a cluster of multiple lower powered diodes. Some devices can produce a lower total power from an applicator by pulsing the output.

Energy: The total amount of electromagnetic energy delivered over the entire treatment time. Energy is generally measured in J (Joules). Energy is power multiplied by time.

$$1 \text{ J} = 1 \text{ W} \times 1 \text{ sec}$$

Therefore, the higher the power of the applicator the shorter the treatment time to deliver the same amount of energy.

Energy density: The total amount of electromagnetic energy delivered to an area over the entire treatment time. Energy density is generally measured in J/cm^2 (Joules per centimeter squared). Most authors agree that this should be the standard measure of treatment dose. Most treatments use $2 - 30 \, J/cm^2$.

58

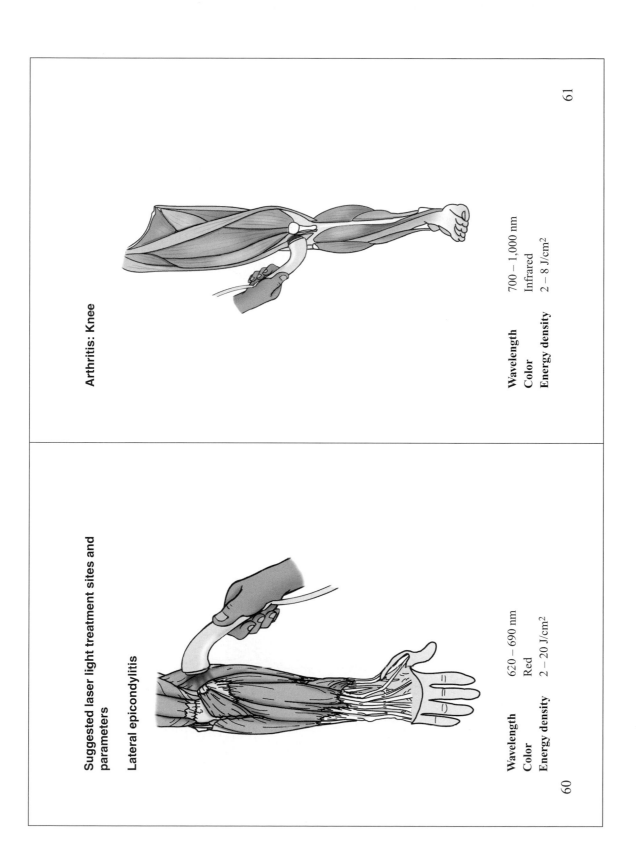

Arthritis: Knee

Wavelength	700 – 1,000 nm
Color	Infrared
Energy density	2 – 8 J/cm²

61

Suggested laser light treatment sites and parameters

Lateral epicondylitis

Wavelength	620 – 690 nm
Color	Red
Energy density	2 – 20 J/cm²

60

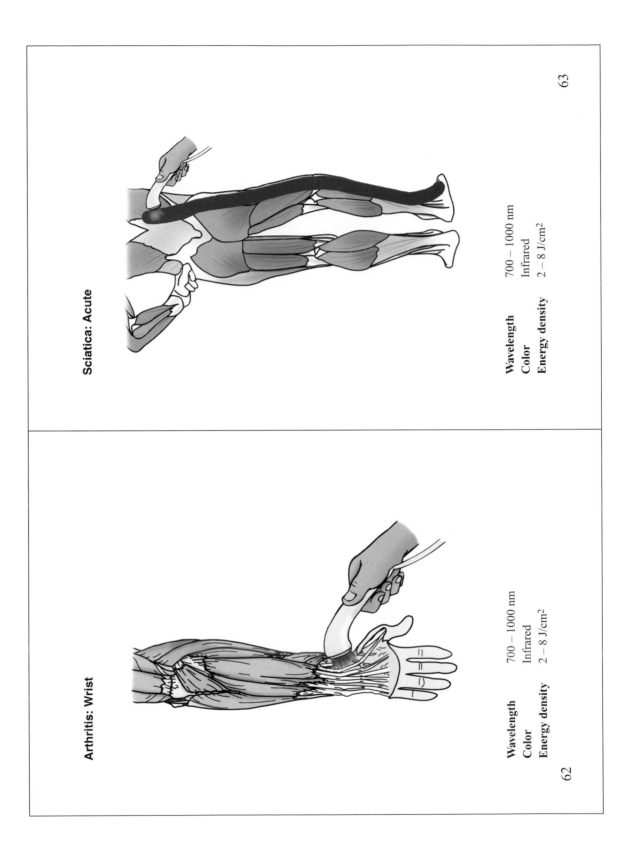

Sciatica: Acute

Wavelength	700 – 1000 nm
Color	Infrared
Energy density	2 – 8 J/cm²

63

Arthritis: Wrist

Wavelength	700 – 1000 nm
Color	Infrared
Energy density	2 – 8 J/cm²

62

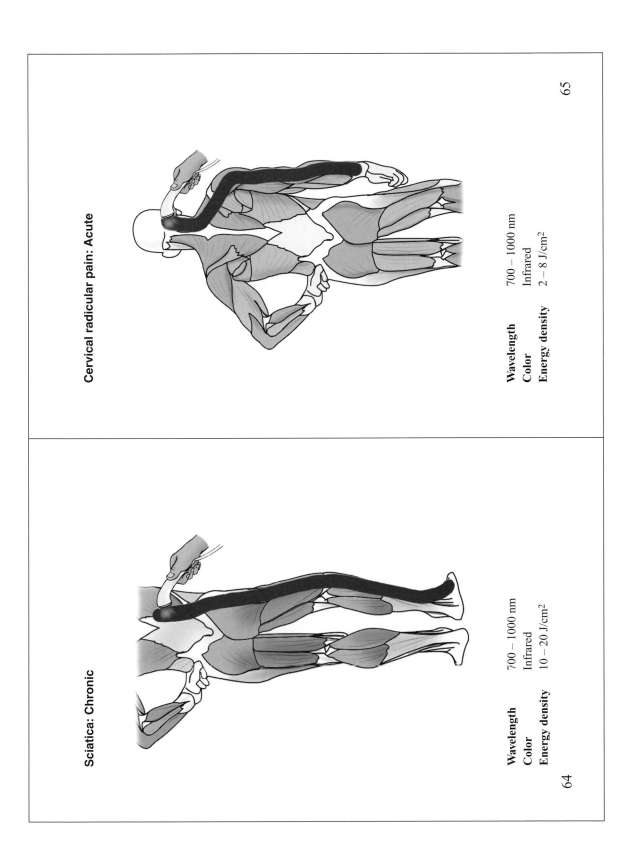

Cervical radicular pain: Acute

Wavelength	700 – 1000 nm
Color	Infrared
Energy density	2 – 8 J/cm²

65

Sciatica: Chronic

Wavelength	700 – 1000 nm
Color	Infrared
Energy density	10 – 20 J/cm²

64

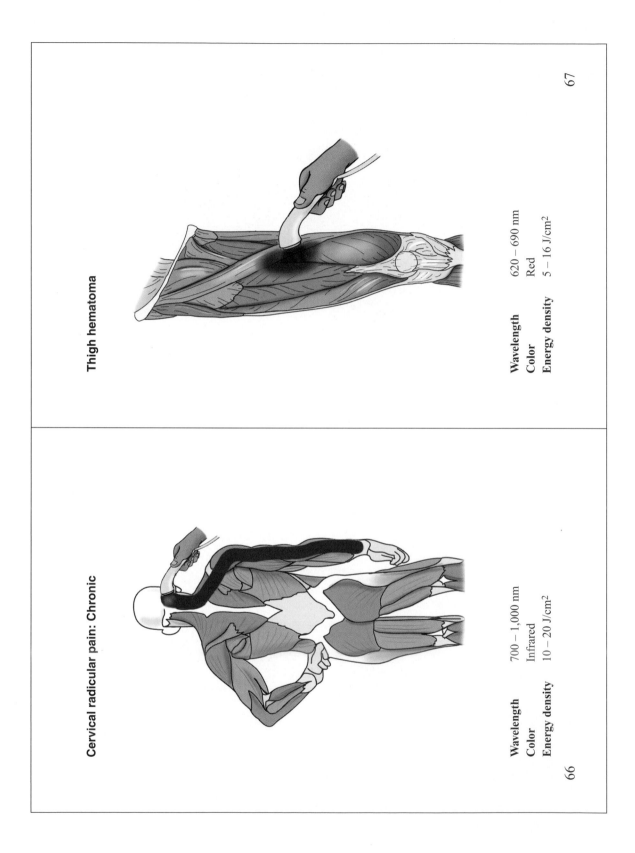

Thigh hematoma

67

Wavelength	620 – 690 nm
Color	Red
Energy density	5 – 16 J/cm^2

Cervical radicular pain: Chronic

Wavelength	700 – 1,000 nm
Color	Infrared
Energy density	10 – 20 J/cm^2

66

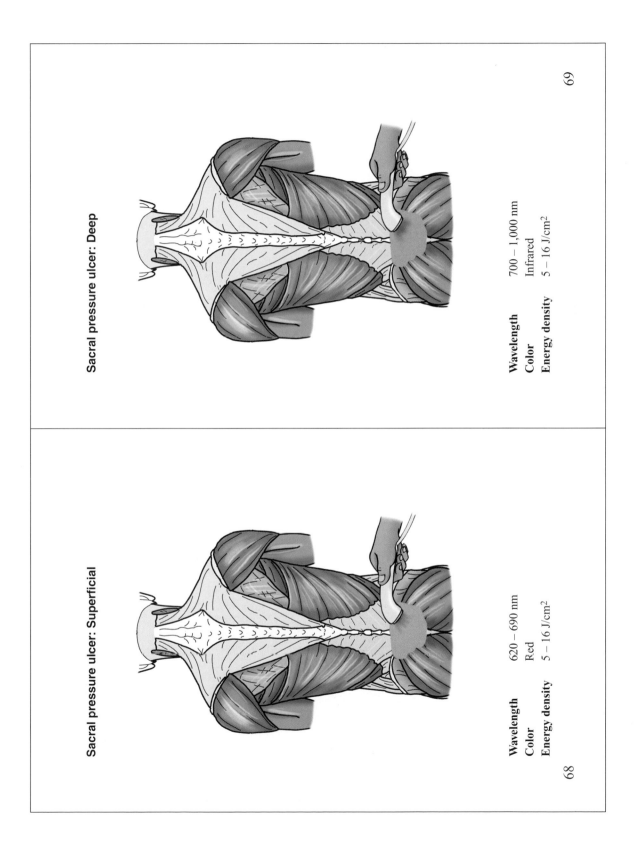

Sacral pressure ulcer: Deep

Wavelength	700 – 1,000 nm
Color	Infrared
Energy density	5 – 16 J/cm²

69

Sacral pressure ulcer: Superficial

Wavelength	620 – 690 nm
Color	Red
Energy density	5 – 16 J/cm²

68

Index

Page number followed by t indicates
table; f indicates figure; b indicates box.

441